Controversies in Otolaryngology

Controversies in Otolaryngology

Myles L. Pensak, M.D., F.A.C.S.

Professor, Department of Otolaryngology–Head and Neck Surgery
Director, Division of Otology, Neurotology, and Skull Base Surgery
University of Cincinnati
College of Medicine
Cincinnati, OH

2001
Thieme
New York • Stuttgart

Thieme New York
333 Seventh Avenue
New York, NY 10001

Editor: Esther Gumpert
Editorial Assistant: Michelle Schmitt
Director, Production & Manufacturing: Anne Vinnicombe
Production Editor: Felicity Edge
Marketing Director: Phyllis Gold
Sales Manager: Ross Lumpkin
Chief Financial Officer: Peter van Woerden
President: Brian D. Scanlan
Cover Designer: Kevin Kall
Designer: Marsha Cohen
Compositor: Emilcomp Prepare, Inc.
Printer: Maple-Vail

The front cover shows Janus, the god of gates and doorways from Roman mythology. With two faces looking in opposite directions, Janus represents awareness of different ideas. Janus was chosen for the cover because being aware of disparate opinions is important in otolaryngology, broadening the individual's viewpoint and improving the ability to deal with arising controversies.

Library of Congress Cataloging-in-Publication Data

Controversies in otolaryngology / [edited by] Myles L. Pensak.
p. ; cm.
Includes bibliographical references and index.
ISBN 0-86577-853-1 (hard cover : alk. paper)
1. Otolaryngology. 2. Otolaryngology--Miscellanea. I. Pensak, Myles L.
[DNLM: 1. Otorhinolaryngologic Diseases. WV 140 C764 2001]
RF46.5 .C65 2001
617.5'1--dc21

2001027038

Important note: Medical knowledge is ever-changing. As new research and clinical experience broaden our knowledge, changes in treatment and drug therapy may be required. The authors and editors of the material herein have consulted sources believed to be reliable in their efforts to provide information that is complete and in accord with the standards accepted at the time of publication. However, in view of the possibility of human error by the authors, editors, or publisher of the work herein, or changes in medical knowledge, neither the authors, editors, publisher, nor any other party who has been involved in the preparation of this work, warrants that the information contained herein is in every respect accurate or complete, and they are not responsible for any errors or omissions or for the results obtained from use of such information. Readers are encouraged to confirm the information contained herein with other sources. For example, readers are advised to check the product information sheet included in the package of each drug they plan to administer to be certain that the information contained in this publication is accurate and that changes have not been made in the recommended dose or in the contraindications for administration. This recommendation is of particular importance in connection with new or infrequently used drugs.

Printed in the United States of America

5 4 3 2 1

TNY ISBN 0-86577-853-1
GTV ISBN 3-13-126011-4

CONTENTS

CONTRIBUTORS

Khaled M. Abdel Aziz, M.D., Ph.D.
Fellow of Skull Base Surgery
Department of Neurosurgery
University of Cincinnati
Cincinnati, OH

Amit Agrawal, M.D.
Assistant Professor
Department of Otolaryngology
Ohio State University
Arthur G. James Cancer Hospital and Richard J. Solove Research Institute
Columbus, OH

James C. Alex, M.D.
Director, Facial Plastic and Reconstructive Surgery
Assistant Professor
Otolaryngology–Head and Neck Surgery
Yale University School of Medicine
New Haven, CT

Joseph P. Allegretti, M.D.
Assistant Professor
Otolaryngology–Head and Neck Surgery
Rush Medical College of Rush University
Rush Presbyterian–St. Luke's Medical Center
Chicago, IL

Sebastian Arena, M.D.
Chief Surgeon
Otolaryngology–Head and Neck Surgery
Department of Surgery
Mercy Hospital
Pittsburgh, PA

David J. Arnold, M.D.
Assistant Professor
Otolaryngology–Head and Neck Surgery
University of Miami
Miami, FL

Moisés A. Arriaga, M.D., F.A.C.S.
Clinical Associate Professor
Department of Otolaryngology
University of Pittsburgh School of Medicine, *and*
Adjunct Associate Professor
MCP/Hahnemann
Department of Otolaryngology
Alleghery General Hospital
Pittsburgh, PA

Shelly Ash, M.S., C.C.C.
Audiologist
Audiology Department
All Children's Hospital
St. Petersburg, FL

Byron J. Bailey, M.D.
Wiess Professor and Chairman
Department of Otolaryngology
University of Texas Medical Branch
Galveston, TX

Thomas J. Balkany, M.D., F.A.C.S., F.A.A.P.
Hotchkiss Distinguished Professor and Chairman
Department of Otolaryngology
University of Miami
Miami, FL

Steven S. Ball, M.D.
Resident
Otolaryngology–Head and Neck Surgery
Department of Surgery
University of North Carolina
Chapel Hill, NC

William H. Beeson, M.D.
Clinical Assistant Professor
Otolaryngology–Head and Neck Surgery
Clinical Assistant Professor of Dermatology
Indiana School of Medicine
Indianapolis, IN

Philomena Mufalli Behar, M.D.
Memphis, TN

F. Owen Black, M.D.
Director, Neurotology Research
Legacy Clinical Research and Technology Center
Portland, OR

Brian W. Blakley, M.D., Ph.D., F.R.C.S.C.
Professor and Chairman
Department of Otolaryngology
Health Sciences Center
University of Manitoba
Winnipeg, MB, Canada

Eve Bluestein, M.D., D.D.S.
Bluestein Oral and Facial Surgery, P.C.
Louisville, CO

Charles D. Bluestone, M.D.
Eberly Professor of Pediatric Otolaryngology
Department of Otolaryngology
University of Pittsburgh School of Medicine
Pittsburgh, PA

Derald E. Brackmann, M.D., F.A.C.S.
Clinical Professor of Otolaryngology–Head and Neck Surgery
Clinical Professor of Neurosurgery
University of Southern California School of Medicine, *and*
President, House Ear Clinic
Board of Directors, House Ear Institute
Los Angeles, CA

Stacy L. Butts, B.A., M.A.
Instructor
Department of Otolaryngology
University of Miami
Miami, FL

Phillip Chang, F.R.A.C.S.
Clinical Neurotology Fellow
Department of Ear, Nose, and Throat
Universitätsspital Zürich
Zürich, Switzerland

Douglas A. Chen, M.D., F.A.C.S.
Clinical Associate Professor
Department of Otolaryngology
University of Pittsburgh Medical Center, *and*
Adjunct Associate Professor
MCP/Hahnemann
Department of Otolaryngology
Alleghery General Hospital
Pittsburgh, PA

Mack L. Cheney, M.D.
Associate Professor
Department of Otology and Laryngology
Harvard Medical School
Massachusetts Eye and Ear Infirmary
Boston, MA

Michael R. Chicoine, M.D.
Assistant Professor of Neurological Surgery
Department of Neurosurgery
Washington University
St. Louis, MO

Daniel Choo, M.D.
Assistant Professor
Department of Pediatric Otolaryngology
Children's Hospital Medical Center
Cincinnati, OH

Sharon L. Collins, M.S., M.D.
Otolaryngology–Head and Neck Surgery
Decatur, IL

Robin T. Cotton, M.D.
Professor
Pediatric Otolaryngology–Head and Neck Surgery
Children's Hospital Medical Center
University of Cincinnati
Cincinnati, OH

Aongus J. Curran, M.D., F.R.C.S.I
Head and Neck Fellow
Department of Otolarynoglogy
University of Toronto Health Network
Toronto, ON, Canada

Angelo Cuzalina, M.D., D.D.S.
Cosmetic Surgeon
Tulsa Surgical Arts
Tulsa, OK

Robert L. Daniels, M.D.
Clinical Assistant Professor
Department of Surgery
Michigan State University
Grand Rapids, MI

Douglas D. Dedo, M.D.
Clinical Assistant Professor
Otolaryngology–Head and Neck Surgery
University of Miami Medical School
Miami, FL

Antonio De la Cruz, M.D.
Clinical Professor
Otolaryngology–Head and Neck Surgery
University of Southern California
Los Angeles, CA

J. Oliver Donegan, M.D.
Professor of Surgery
Otolaryngology–Head and Neck Surgery
Dartmouth Hitchcock Medical Center
Lebanon, NH

Laurie S. Eisenberg, Ph.D.
Scientist II
Children's Auditory Research and Evaluation Center
House Ear Institute
Los Angeles, CA

Jose N. Fayad, M.D.
Assistant Professor
Otolaryngology–Head and Neck Surgery
Columbia University College of Physicians and Surgeons
New York, NY

Ugo Fisch, M.D.
Professor
Department of Ear, Nose, and Throat
Universitätsspital Zürich
Zürich, Switzerland

John C. Flickinger, M.D.
Professor of Radiation Oncology and Neurological Surgery
Department of Radiation Oncology
University of Pittsburgh
Pittsburgh, PA

L. Arick Forrest, M.D.
Clinical Associate Professor
Department of Otolaryngology
Ohio State University Medical Center
Columbus, OH

Andrew S. Frankel, M.D., F.A.C.S.
Assistant Clinical Professor
Division of Head and Neck Surgery
University of California
Los Angeles, CA

Richard R. Gacek, M.D.
Professor of Surgery
Otolaryngology–Head and Neck Surgery
University of South Alabama
Mobile, AL

Richard M. Gallagher, M.D., M.B.B.S., F.R.A.C.S.
Otolaryngology–Head and Neck Surgery
St. Vincent's Hospital
Sydney, NSW, Australia

Eric M. Genden, M.D.
Assistant Professor
Otolaryngology–Head and Neck Surgery
Mount Sinai School of Medicine
New York, NY

Stuart G. Gherini, M.D.
Private Practice
Sacramento, CA

Richard E. Gliklich, M.D.
Associate Professor
Department of Otology and Laryngology
Harvard Medical School
Boston, MA

Jack L. Gluckman, M.D., F.C.S.(S.A.), F.A.C.S.(Ed.)(Hon.)
Professor and Chairman
Otolaryngology–Head and Neck Surgery
University of Cincinnati
Cincinnati, OH

Gary S. Gordon, M.D.
Fellow, Department of Medicine
Section of Hematology/Oncology
University of Chicago
Chicago, IL

Charles W. Gross, M.D., F.A.C.S.
Professor
Departments of Otolaryngology–Head and Neck Surgery *and* Pediatrics
University of Virginia School of Medicine
Charlottesville, VA

Patrick J. Gullane, M.D., F.R.C.S.C., F.A.C.S.
Professor of Otolaryngology and Surgery
Department of Otolaryngology
University of Toronto Health Network
Toronto, ON, Canada

Tessa A. Hadlock, M.D.
Fellow in Facial Plastic Surgery
Department of Otology and Laryngology
Harvard Medical School
Massachusetts Eye and Ear Infirmary
Boston, MA

Ehab Y. Hanna, M.D.
Associate Professor
Otolaryngology–Head and Neck Surgery
University of Arkansas for Medical Sciences
Little Rock, AR

Stephen G. Harner, M.D.
Professor
Department of Otolaryngology
Mayo Medical School
Rochester, MN

Scott E. Harrison, M.D., M.B.A.
Jackson Ear, Nose, and Throat Clinic
Jackson, MS

Christopher J. Hartnick, M.D.
Fellow
Department of Pediatric Otolaryngology
Children's Hospital Medical Center
Cincinnati, OH

Annelle V. Hodges, Ph.D., C.C.C.-A.
Associate Professor of Otolaryngology
Director, Division of Audiology
University of Miami
Miami, FL

Henry T. Hoffman, M.D., F.A.C.S.
Professor
Department of Otolaryngology
University of Iowa Health Center
Iowa City, IA

Karl L. Horn, M.D.
Medical Director
Presbyterian Ear Institute
Albuquerque, NM

Richard N. Hubbell, M.D.
Associate Professor of Surgery and Pediatrics
Department of Otolaryngology
University of Vermont
Fletcher Allen Health Care
Burlington, VT

Gordon B. Hughes, M.D., F.A.C.S.
Professor
Department of Otolaryngology and Communicative Disorders
Cleveland Clinic Foundation
Cleveland, OH

C. Gary Jackson, M.D.
Clinical Professor
Department of Otology and Neuro-otology
Vanderbilt University of North Carolina at Georgetown
Washington, DC

Jonas T. Johnson, M.D.
Professor
Departments of Otolaryngology and Radiation Oncology
University of Pittsburgh School of Medicine
The Eye and Ear Institute
Pittsburgh, PA

Jennifer Jordan, M.D.
Resident
Otolaryngology–Head and Neck Surgery
University of Texas Southwestern
Dallas, TX

Frank M. Kamer, M.D., F.A.C.S.
Clinical Professor
Division of Head and Neck Surgery
University of California
Los Angeles, CA

David W. Kennedy, M.D.
Professor and Chair
Otorhinolaryngology–Head and Neck Surgery
University of Pennsylvania Medical Center
Philadelphia, PA

Thomas J. Kereiakes, M.D.
Department of Otolaryngology
The Christ Hospital
Cincinnati, OH

Bradley W. Kesser, M.D.
Piedmont Ear, Nose, and Throat Associates
Piedmont Hospital
Atlanta, GA

Sam E. Kinney, M.D.
Head, Section of Otology and Neurotology
Department of Otolaryngology and Communicative Disorders
Cleveland Clinic Foundation
Cleveland, OH

Karen Iler Kirk, Ph.D.
Associate Professor and Psi Iota Xi Scholar
Otolaryngology–Head and Neck Surgery
Indiana School of Medicine
Indianapolis, IN

Douglas Kondziolka, M.D., F.A.C.S., F.R.C.S.(C.)
Professor of Neurological Surgery and Radiation Oncology
Department of Neurological Surgery
University of Pittsburgh
Pittsburgh, PA

Laura W. Kretschmer, Ed.D.
Professor of Audiology
Department of Communication Sciences and Disorders
University of Cincinnati
Cincinnati, OH

John F. Kveton, M.D.
Professor
Department of Surgery and Otolaryngology
Yale University School of Medicine
New Haven, CT

Paul R. Lambert, M.D.
Professor and Chairman
Otolaryngology–Head and Neck Surgery
Medical University of South Carolina
Charleston, SC

John P. Leonetti, M.D.
Professor
Otolaryngology–Head and Neck Surgery
Loyola University of Chicago
Maywood, IL

Paul A. Levine, M.D.
Professor and Chairman
Otolaryngology–Head and Neck Surgery
University of Virginia Health System
Charlottesville, VA

Thomas Linder, Ph.D., M.D.
Professor
Department of Ear, Nose, and Throat
Universitätsspital Zürich
Zürich, Switzerland

William H. Lippy, M.D.
Clinical Professor
Department of Ear, Nose, and Throat
Ohio State University
Columbus, OH

David B. Lovice, M.D.
Carolina Facial Plastic Surgery
Orangeburg, SC

L. Dade Lunsford, M.D., F.A.C.S.
Professor of Neurological Surgery, Radiation Oncology, and Radiology
Department of Neurological Surgery
University of Pittsburgh
Pittsburgh, PA

Rodney P. Lusk, M.D., F.A.C.S., F.A.A.P.
Professor of Otolaryngology
Department of Pediatric Otolaryngology
Washington University School of Medicine
St. Louis Children's Hospital
St. Louis, MO

Devinder S. Mangat, M.D.
Associate Clinical Professor
Otolaryngology–Head and Neck Surgery
University of Cincinnati
Cincinnati, OH

Douglas G. Mann, M.D.
Clinical Assistant Professor
Department of Otolaryngology
Thomas Jefferson University School of Medicine
Media, PA

Sam J. Marzo, M.D.
Assistant Professor
Otolaryngology–Head and Neck Surgery
Loyola University of Chicago
Maywood, IL

Jesus E. Medina, M.D.
Paul and Ruth Jonas Professor and Chair
Department of Otorhinolaryngology
University of Oklahoma Health Sciences Center
Oklahoma City, OK

Jon E. Mendelsohn, M.D.
Cinncinati, OH

William L. Meyerhoff, M.D., Ph.D.
Professor and Chair
Otolaryngology–Head and Neck Surgery
University of Texas Southwestern
Dallas, TX

Matthew D. Mingrone, M.D.
Los Gatos, CA

Sanchayeeta Mitra, M.D.
Attending Clinical Instructor
West Haven Veterans Administration Hospital
Otolaryngology
Yale University School of Medicine
New Haven, CT

Richard T. Miyamoto, M.D.
Arilla Spence DeVault Professor and Chairman
Otolaryngology–Head and Neck Surgery
Indiana School of Medicine
Indianapolis, IN

Charles M. Myer III, M.D.
Professor
Otolaryngology–Head and Neck Surgery
Children's Hospital Medical Center
University of Cincinnati
Cincinnati, OH

Eugene N. Myers, M.D.
Professor, Eye and Ear Foundation Chair
Department of Otolaryngology
University of Pittsburgh School of Medicine
The Eye and Ear Institute
Pittsburgh, PA

Joseph B. Nadol, Jr., M.D.
Walter Augustus Lecompte Professor and Chairman
Department of Otology and Laryngology
Harvard Medical School, *and*
Chief of Otolaryngology
Massachusetts Eye and Ear Infirmary
Boston, MA

Ajay Niranjan, M.B.B.S., M.S., M.Ch.
Assistant Professor
Department of Neurological Surgery
University of Pittsburgh
Pittsburgh, PA

Robert M. Owens, M.D.
Department of Otolaryngology and Neurotology
Baylor University Medical Center
Dallas, TX

Tapan A. Padhya, M.D.
Assistant Professor
Otolaryngology–Head and Neck Surgery
University of South Florida
Tampa, FL

William R. Panje, M.D., B.S., M.S., M.S.(Otolaryngology), F.A.C.S.
Professor of Otolaryngology
Director, Section of Skull Base and Reconstructive Surgery
Otolaryngology–Head and Neck Surgery
Rush University Medical College
Rush Presbyterian–St. Luke's Medical Center
Chicago, IL

Susan C. Pesznecker, R.N.
Research Coordinator
Neurotology Research
Legacy Clinical Research and Technology Center
Portland, OR

Harold C. Pillsbury, M.D.
Chief, Otolaryngology–Head and Neck Surgery
Department of Surgery
University of North Carolina
Chapel Hill, NC

Karen T. Pitman, M.D.
Assistant Professor
Otolaryngology–Head and Neck Surgery
St. Louis University
St. Louis, MO

Michael D. Poole, M.D., Ph.D.
Professor of Otolaryngology and Pediatrics
Chairman, Otolaryngology–Head and Neck Surgery
University of Texas Medical School
Houston, TX

Jack L. Pulec, M.D.
Clinical Professor of Otolaryngology–Head and Neck Surgery
Department of Otolaryngology
University of Southern California School of Medicine, *and*
Loma Linda University
Los Angeles, CA

K. Thomas Robbins, M.D.
Professor and Chair
Department of Otolaryngology
University of Florida
Shands Hospital
Gainesville, FL

Peter S. Roland, M.D.
Professor and Vice Chair
Otolaryngology–Head and Neck Surgery
University of Texas Southwestern Medical School
Dallas, TX

Michael J. Rutter, M.D., F.R.A.C.S.
Assistant Professor of Pediatric Otolaryngology
Pediatric Otolaryngology–Head and Neck Surgery
Children's Hospital Medical Center
University of Cincinnati College of Medicine
Cincinnati, OH

Abhay Sanan, M.D.
Clinical Assistant Professor of Surgery
Division of Neurosurgery
University of Arizona
Tucson, AZ

Clarence T. Sasaki, M.D.
Professor and Chief
Department of Otolaryngology
Yale University School of Medicine
New Haven, CT

Steven D. Schaefer, M.D., F.A.C.S.
Professor and Chair
Department of Otolaryngology
New York Eye and Ear Infirmary
New York Medical College
New York, NY

David E. Schuller, M.D.
Professor and Chair
Department of Otolaryngology
Ohio State University,
Arthur G. James Cancer Hospital, *and*
Richard J. Solove Research Institute
Columbus, OH

Mitchell K. Schwaber, M.D.
Attending Physician
St. Thomas Neuroscience Institute
St. Thomas Hospital
Nashville, TN

Samuel H. Selesnick, M.D.
Vice Chairman
Department of Otorhinolaryngology
Weill College of Medicine of Cornell University
New York, NY

Jatin P. Shah, M.D.
Attending Surgeon and Chief
Surgery–Head and Neck Service
Memorial Sloan-Kettering Cancer Center
New York, NY

Kerwin F. Shannon, M.B.B.S., F.R.A.C.S.
Visiting Medical Officer
Department of Head and Neck Surgery
Central Sydney Area Health Service
Royal Prince Alfred Hospital
Camperdown, NSW, Australia

John J. Shea, Jr., M.D.
Professor
Otolaryngology–Head and Neck Surgery
University of Tennessee College of Medicine
Memphis, TN

James L. Sheehy, M.D.
Clinical Professor
Department of Otolaryngology
University of Southern California
Los Angeles, CA

Maisie L. Shindo, M.D.
Associate Professor
Department of Surgery
Division of Otolaryngology
State University of New York
Stony Brook University Hospital
Stony Brook, NY

Kevin A. Shumrick, M.D.
Professor of Clinical Otolaryngology
Otolaryngology–Head and Neck Surgery
University of Cincinnati Medical Center
Cincinnati, OH

Leonard J. Singer, M.D., F.A.C.S.
Director, Division of Plastic Surgery
The Jewish Hospital of Cincinnati
Cincinnati, OH

Bhuvanesh Singh, M.D.
Assistant Attending Surgeon, Assistant Professor
Surgery–Head and Neck Service
Memorial Sloan-Kettering Cancer Center
New York, NY

Judith M. Skoner, M.D.
Resident
Department of Otolaryngology
University of South Carolina
Charleston, SC

Peter G. Smith, M.D., Ph.D.
Midwest Otologic Group
Saint Louis, MO

Russell B. Smith, M.D.
Resident Physician
Department of Surgery
Division of Otolaryngology
University of Missouri Health Care
Columbia, MO

Nancy L. Snyderman, M.D.
Associate Clinical Professor
Department of Otolaryngology
California-Pacific Medical Center
San Francisco, CA

John I. Song, M.D.
Assistant Professor
Otolaryngology–Head and Neck Surgery
H. Lee Moffitt Cancer Center
University of South Florida
Tampa, FL

William R. Spencer, M.D.
Chief Resident
Department of Otolaryngology
New York Eye and Ear Infirmary
New York Medical College
New York, NY

James A. Stankiewicz, M.D.
Professor
Otolaryngology–Head and Neck Surgery
Loyola University Medical Center
Maywood, IL

Joan St. Jean, M.S., M.N., B.N.
Balance and Hearing NW
Portland, OR

Marshall Strome, M.D., M.S.
Professor and Chairman
Department of Otolaryngology and Communicative Disorders
Cleveland Clinic Foundation
Cleveland, OH

James Y. Suen, M.D.
Professor and Chairman
Otolaryngology–Head and Neck Surgery
University of Arkansas for Medical Sciences
Little Rock, AR

Thomas A. Tami, M.D., F.A.C.S.
Professor
Otolaryngology–Head and Neck Surgery
University of Cincinnati
Cincinnati, OH

John M. Tew, Jr., M.D.
Professor and Chairman
Department of Neurosurgery
The Neuroscience Institute
University of Cincinnati
Cincinnati, OH

Howard A. Tobin, M.D.
Associate Clinical Professor of Surgery
University of Texas
Southwestern Medical Center
Dallas, TX

N. Wendell Todd, M.D.
Professor
Department of Otolaryngology and Pediatrics
Emory University School of Medicine
Children's Healthcare of Atlanta
Atlanta, GA

Dean M. Toriumi, M.D.
Professor
Otolaryngology–Head and Neck Surgery
Division of Facial Plastic and Reconstructive Surgery
University of Illinois at Chicago
Chicago, IL

LenhAnh P. Tran, M.D.
Chief, Pediatric Otolaryngology
Assistant Professor, Otolaryngology
Uniformed Services University of Health Sciences
Tripler Army Medical Center, HI

Mark L. Urken, M.D.
Mount Sinai Medical Center
New York, NY

Henry R. van Loveren, M.D.
Professor and Vice Chairman
Department of Neurosurgery
The Neuroscience Institute
University of Cincinnati
Cincinnati, OH

Douglas B. Villaret, M.D.
Assistant Professor
Department of Otolaryngology
University of Florida
Shands Hospital
Gainesville, FL

Everett E. Vokes, M.D.
Professor, Department of Medicine
Director, Section of Medical Hematology/Oncology
University of Chicago
Chicago, IL

Milton Waner, M.D.
Professor
Department of Otolaryngology
University of Arkansas for Medical Sciences
Little Rock, AR

Ernest A. Weymuller, M.D.
Professor and Chairman
Otolaryngology–Head and Neck Surgery
University of Washington
Seattle, WA

Brian J. Wiatrak, M.D., F.A.A.P., F.A.C.S.
Clinical Associate Professor of Surgery and Pediatrics
Department of Pediatric Otolaryngology
Children's Hospital of Alabama
Birmingham, AL

Erin D. Wright, M.D., C.M., F.R.C.S.C.
Assistant Professor
Department of Otolaryngology
University of Western Ontario
London, ON, Canada

George H. Zalzal, M.D., F.A.C.S., F.A.A.P.
Chairman and Professor of Otolaryngology and Pediatrics
Department of Otolaryngology
Children's National Medical Center
George Washington University School of Medicine
Washington, DC

Robert P. Zitsch III, M.D., F.A.C.S.
Associate Professor
Department of Surgery
Division of Otolaryngology
University of Missouri Health Care
Columbia, MO

PREFACE

As a medical student, I was initially introduced to the writings and aphorisms of the celebrated physician and scholar, William Osler. Returning not infrequently to his commentaries, I have been impressed as to how universal and timeless his observations were. Furthermore, not uncommonly, the citations recorded in his writings reflect prescient insights, as well as time-tested truths. Tucked within his 1904 *Aequanimitas* is the following passage:

> Every physician will make, and ought to make, observations from his own experience, but he will be able to make a better judgment and juster observations by comparing what he reads and what he sees together. It is neither an affront to any man's understanding, nor a cramp to his genius, to say that both the one and the other may be usefully employed, and happily improved in searching and examining into the opinions and methods of those who lived before him, especially considering that no one is tied up from judging for himself, or obliged to give into the notions of any author, any further than he finds them agreeable to reason, and reducible to practice. No one therefore need fear that his natural sagacity, whatever it is, should be perplexed or misled by reading. For there is as large and fruitful a field for sagacity and good judgment to display themselves in, by distinguishing between one author and another, and sometimes between the several parts and passages in the same author, as is to be found in the greatest extent and variety of practice... It has not usually been looked upon as an extraordinary mark of wisdom for a man to think himself too wise to be taught; and yet this seems to be the case of those who rely wholly upon their own experience, and despise all teachers but themselves.

It is with this background that, when I first encountered Dr. Jim Snow's 1983 text *Controversy in Otolaryngology*, I readily began to employ it as a source of reference on a regular basis. By choosing controversial areas of clinical practice, and offering the opinion of accomplished practitioners, I was able, as a student of our specialty, to foment and shape a management algorithm predicated upon distinguished experience and knowledge, tempered by the commentaries contained therein.

Because I valued the original text and found it to be unique amongst the many publications in our field, it seemed that a review and update would provide the contemporary practitioner with a valuable and portable source of information. Much to my delight, Dr. Snow and a number of my colleagues endorsed the project. Moreover, Jim has graciously written a broad-perspective introduction reflecting his unique experience as practitioner and former NIH Director. Not surprisingly, some of the "controversial topics" have been laid to rest and a general acceptance regarding management strategy has been adopted; however, several others remain fertile ground for difference of opinion, and as newer methodologies and management strategies have come into practice, new controversial issues have arisen.

Contributors to this text were chosen based upon their recognized clinical expertise, knowledge, and communicative skills. Each was charged with the task of addressing a given topic from a broad-perspective overview, establishing for the reader how a certain opinion was reached, citing relevant literature and experience, and providing a clearly articulated management algorithm that would enable the reader, in a relatively short period of time, to have a clear sense as to what particular viewpoint is being expressed and advocated, and why.

Ultimately, the goal of the book is to provide the contemporary practitioner with a focused discussion that allows for a critical comparison of what an individual practitioner is presently doing that parallels or disagrees with the approach advocated by an experienced colleague.

Acknowledgments

The Socratic method tests the student's ability to respond to challenging questions. During my career as an otolaryngologist, I have been fortunate in that a number of individuals have confronted me with controversial choices and demanded that I challenge my intellectual and surgical skills to formulate a management algorithm or technical strategy for dealing with a given problem. To these friends, mentors, teachers, and colleagues, I offer my heartfelt thanks.

FOREWORD

This book is a compilation of carefully articulated opinions on the best way to manage more than two dozen commonly encountered clinical problems in which there is uncertainty in otolaryngology—head and neck surgery. Indeed, if there were not, in some degree, a lack of fundamental knowledge about each of these problems, there probably would be a single management strategy agreed upon by all. Dr. Pensak has selected important problems in otology, rhinology, laryngology, facial plastic and reconstructive surgery, head and neck oncology, and skull base surgery. The problems are important because they are either life threatening or severely compromise the quality of life. Many represent substantial socioeconomic impact because of the number of individuals suffering from them. Each of these clinical problems confronts the thoughtful practitioner with alternative approaches that are theoretically appealing. There are no contrived or academic issues; each problem involves real life dilemmas or even a triad of choices.

Dr. Pensak has also selected some of the most distinguished intellectual leaders of their fields to present, based on their expertise and abundant experience, their preferred solutions to these problems. Each author has presented a reasoned advocacy of his or her approach based on the best data available at this time.

Twenty years ago, I edited a book on controversy in otolaryngology in which a similar number of difficult problems was addressed. It is not surprising that many of the problems are the same, but how great the differences in the solutions. These differences are a tribute to the clinical progress taking place in otolaryngology—head and neck surgery. They are also predicated on the amazing technological progress that has been applied by many of the authors of this book. Furthermore, diseases change over time. In the course of my career, many diseases affecting the practice of otolaryngology—head and neck surgery have been brought under control, including polio, rubella, measles, mumps, Wegener granulomatosis, and Haemophilus influenzae type B meningitis and epigiottitis, but unfortunately the diseases addressed in that book are still with us. Most of the progress in specific diseases is based on public health measures such as immunization, and much more can be accomplished in this way. A vaccine against otitis media should be available in less than a decade. Nevertheless, progress in the management of specific diseases such as Wegener granulomatosis with cyclophosphamide is based on careful clinical observations and the results of clinical trials like those cited in this book.

I am convinced that all disease is genetically determined or at least genetically predisposed. Even trauma may, in most instances, have a genetic basis in the psychological determination of risk taking. Certainly, the susceptibility to infectious diseases is genetically predisposed, and that susceptibility may range within a population from complete immunity to complete susceptibility with many gradations in between. In the case of hearing impediments, it is now being found that there is a genetic basis to forms of hearing loss that were formerly attributed solely to environmental factors. For example, it is now known that the ototoxicity of aminoglycoside antibiotics in some Asian populations is predisposed by a mutation in the *12S* RR,VA mitochon (Hal gene, A*I 555G*), and the individual variation in susceptibility to noise-induced hearing loss and presbyacusis may well be explained by mitochondrial mutations. The magnitude of the coming role of molecular genetics in clinical medicine is difficult to overestimate.

The remarkable progress in molecular biology related to otolaryngology—head and neck surgery will be the driving force providing the basis for the prevention and control of diseases in the future. For example, the discovery of a multitude of disease genes responsible for the autosomal dominant and recessive X-linked and mitochondrial modes of transmission of syndromic and nonsyndromic forms of hereditary hearing impairment will have a profound impact on the clinical management of hearing impairment. Already, many of these genes have been cloned and their protein products identified. Not only will these discoveries elucidate the development, normal structure and function, and maintenance of the various parts of the auditory and vestibular systems, they will provide the basis for rational therapeutic strategies of the next century and beyond.

The marvelous thing about molecular biologic research is that, for the first time, each discovery relates directly to the pathogenesis of the disease and suggests the strategy for intervention in the very pathogenesis of the disease.

These strategies will be tested in the clinical trials of the future. How fortunate is otolaryngology—head and neck surgery to have the financial resources of the National Institute on Deafness and Other Communication Disorders, the National Institute of Child Health and Human Development, the National Institute on Aging, the National Institute of Allergy and Infectious Diseases, the National Institute of Dental and Craniofacial Research, and the National Cancer Institute, as well as many private foundations and professional societies, to support basic and clinical research needed by our patients. From that research, a new millennium of progress in clinical otolaryngology–head and neck surgery will flow to the benefit of countless millions of individuals with disorders of human communication and other disabilities throughout the world.

This book presents fresh perspectives on an array of common clinical problems, and these perspectives can truly be characterized as cutting edge and innovative. Not only does it provide a stimulating intellectual journey through the land of the bêtes noires of clinical otolaryngology—head and neck surgery, it is filled with practical advice in the day-to-day practice of this fascinating field. The reader will be challenged to assess the evidence presented by each author supporting his or her point of view, and it is hoped that this process will be both enjoyable and informative.

James B. Snow, Jr., M.D., F.A.C.S.
Former Director
National Institute on Deafness and Other Communication Disorders,
National Institutes of Health;
Professor Emeritus,
University of Pennsylvania School of Medicine

This book is fondly dedicated to Joan Hock and Ruth Newman,
both of whom have encouraged and supported me these many years.

1

Role of Elective Neck Dissection for the N0 Neck

"Whether END provides a therapeutic benefit is more controversial. Intuitively it makes sense that removing microscopic metastases at the earliest opportunity would improve patient outcome. However, there are no prospective, randomized studies that carefully compare the outcome of patients managed with END to patients who are treated with therapeutic neck dissection for metastases that occur during observation."

Jonas T. Johnson

"Self-examination by the patient and reliable follow-up are essential for watchful waiting to succeed in the management of the N0 neck. Unfortunately, a significant number of the patients who do not undergo elective dissection can not be salvaged later, when they present with palpable metastases, because the disease is too far advanced."

Jesus E. Medina

"Elective treatment of lymph nodes at high risk for micrometastasis from upper aerodigestive tract cancers is warranted. Treatment should be undertaken when the risk for occult metastasis exceeds 10–15%. Effective treatment can be provided using either radiation therapy or surgery. Selective neck dissections are considered adequate for identifying lymph nodes with occult metastasis."

Jatin P. Shah

Role of Elective Neck Dissection for the N0 Neck

CHAPTER 1

Karen T. Pitman and Jonas T. Johnson

Management of the clinically negative neck (N0) in patients with head and neck squamous cell carcinoma (HNSCC) is controversial. In addition to the three treatment options available for the N0 patient, clinicians who advocate a surgical approach must be cognizant of controversies surrounding the use of elective neck dissection (END). The focus of this chapter is to discuss the role of END for patients who are clinically N0. Head and neck surgeons continue to evaluate several issues surrounding END, which are also discussed: (1) what are the indications for END?, (2) do selective neck dissections constitute adequate procedures for staging the N0 neck?, and (3) does neck dissection performed electively provide therapeutic benefit to patients with pathologic evidence of metastases?

END as a management strategy for the N0 neck has evolved because the status of the cervical lymphatics is the single most important prognostic factor in HNSCC. A subset of patients without clinical evidence of regional metastases are known to harbor occult metastases. Despite intensive research efforts to identify pathologic and molecular tumor markers that reliably predict the presence of occult cervical metastases, accurate biomarkers have not been characterized. Although tumor thickness,[1,2] perineural invasion,[3] lymphocytic infiltration,[4] and molecular tumor markers[5] are associated with occult metastases, they do not provide the accuracy required for therapeutic decision making. Examination of the neck contents after END provides pathologic staging and prognostic information, and accurately guides treatment decisions.

Definition of the N0 Neck

Clinical staging of the neck consists of physical examination and includes the results of imaging studies.[6] Computed tomography (CT) and magnetic resonance imaging (MRI) are commonly employed to evaluate the neck and can be helpful in patients whose necks are difficult to examine by palpation. The radiographic criteria that designate a lymph node as suspicious for metastases include size >1.0–1.5 cm, spherical shape, evidence of necrosis or soft tissue invasion, and groups of three or more nodes.[7,8]

Studies that have corroborated CT findings and pathologic staging data from N0 patients now question the accuracy of radiographic staging. An estimated 50% of cervical metastases are <5.0 mm.[9] Because micrometastases do not meet the size criteria, they are not considered suspicious on CT. Radiographic staging of the submandibular region in particular may be less accurate than physical examination because most (85%) level I metastases are <1.0 cm.[10,11] CT staging of the neck misses at least one-third of occult cervical metastases.[12,13] The sensitivity of CT staging is estimated to be 25%, and the specificity 77%.[14] Therefore, pathologic staging is the most accurate tool available to assess the status of the cervical lymphatics.

Alternatives for Therapy

An assessment of the risk of occult regional metastases is based on the site, stage, and pathologic characteristics of the primary tumor. Management of the N0 neck is typically addressed when this risk is estimated to be >20%.[15,16] With the exception of early-stage glottic tumors and very small superficial lesions, most primary tumors of the upper aerodigestive tract staged N0 probably warrant consideration of the neck.

Three management options exist for N0 patients who are determined to be at significant risk of occult metastases. A program of clinical observation reserves neck dissection for patients who develop regional metastases subsequent to treatment of the primary tumor. Elective neck irradiation (ENI) delivers a tumoricidal dose of radiation to the cervical lymphatics. END is the third option.

The salvage rate for patients who develop regional metastases during a program of clinical observation is estimated to be 50 to 59% after multimodal therapy.[16-18] Although a subset of truly pN0 managed with observation will not receive unnecessary surgery, those in whom cervical metastases do develop will have a poor outcome.

If the decision is to treat the N0 neck, radiation and surgery are options. For patients whose primary tumor is treated with irradiation, ENI is probably the treatment of choice. If the primary is treated surgically, one must decide whether to dissect or to radiate the neck.

As the regional recurrence rates after treatment of clinically N0 patients are 2.0 to 8.0% for ENI[19,20] and 2.0 to 11.0% for END, [21-24] other considerations are factored into the choice of treatment. Important differences include the length of time required for treatment, the comparative cost of treatments, and the increased morbidity associated with postirradiation surgery, if required.

If the primary tumor is resected, a policy of ENI will expose 60 to 70% of patients to the sequelae of irradiation unnecessarily. Radiation is not a benign form of therapy. Possible effects include xerostomia, fibrosis, and contracture, which confound the physical examination. Atherosclerosis and radiation-induced malignancy are also reported.[25,26] Patients who receive ENI will not get the prognostic information afforded by pathologic staging, and cervical irradiation will not be an option for recurrent or second primary disease.

The morbidity of neck dissection is an important factor in considering END. Compared with radical neck dissection, the routine use of selective procedures has decreased the impact of END on postoperative appearance and function. The main determinant of cost for END is surgical time; hospital stays are generally not lengthened if the primary tumor is resected.

Incidence of Occult Metastases

An estimate of the incidence of occult cervical metastases is available by reviewing studies that have reported the regional metastatic rate in patients who were observed clinically. Patients who develop cervical metastases subsequent to treatment of their primary tumor, and who have their primary site controlled, can be assumed to have had occult disease at the time of diagnosis. Table 1–1 presents the data reported for oral cavity lesions and suggests that the occult metastatic rate is 40 to 50%.[17,18,27,28]

Another way to assess the incidence of occult metastases is to review studies that have reported pathologic staging data on patients whose necks were dissected electively. Data from three studies[23,24,29] are shown in Table 1–2 and suggest that the occult metastatic rate is >20% for all sites examined. It is also important to note that up to 35% of microscopic metastases contain extracapsular spread (ECS),[12] a finding that has a significant impact on the regional recurrence and distant metastatic rate, and patient outcome.[30]

Patients who are staged pN+ after END have been shown to have a poorer prognosis than do those who do not harbor occult metastases.[24,30] Therefore, it may be advantageous to identify patients with occult disease.

TABLE 1–1

Regional Metastatic Rate: T1-T4 N0 Oral Cavity Squamous Cell Carcinoma-Neck Followed Clinically after Treatment of the Primary Tumor

Study/Reference	Regional Metastatic Rate (%)
Yuen et al. (1997)[18]	47
McGuirt et al. (1995)[17]	40
Fakih et al. (1989)[27]	66
Vandenbrouck et al. (1980)[28]	47

Potential Effects of END

The most immediate benefit of END is that the information obtained from pathologic staging of the neck contents can be used to target those patients who may benefit from combination therapy. Selectively targeting patients who will benefit from adjuvant therapy reduces overall the morbidity and cost of treatment.

Whether END provides a therapeutic benefit is more controversial. Intuitively, it makes sense that removing microscopic metastases at the earliest opportunity would improve patient outcome. However, no prospective randomized studies have been conducted to compare the outcome of patients managed with END with patients treated with therapeutic neck dissection for metastases that occur during observation. Retrospective studies have demonstrated a possible survival benefit for patients treated with END.

Figure 1–1 compares the results of four studies[15-18] that reported data comparing the survival rates of patients who were pN+ and who received END with the survival rates of patients who received therapeutic neck dissection for metastases that were clinically evident. These data suggest that survival is improved when patients receive END. Overall survival between studies cannot be compared because the two earlier studies included advanced lesions from many sites, whereas recent studies looked only at early oral cavity lesions. These retrospective studies suggest a therapeutic benefit for END, but they do not provide conclusive evidence that END in and of itself provides a survival advantage. To answer this question, prospective studies are required.

TABLE 1–2

Incidence of Occult Regional Metastases by Primary Site

Primary Site	pN+ (%)		
	UPMC[24]	Byers et al.[10]	Shah[29]
Oral cavity	41	45	34
Oropharynx	36	39	31
Hypopharynx	36	56	17
Larynx (supraglottic/advanced glottic)	30	26	37

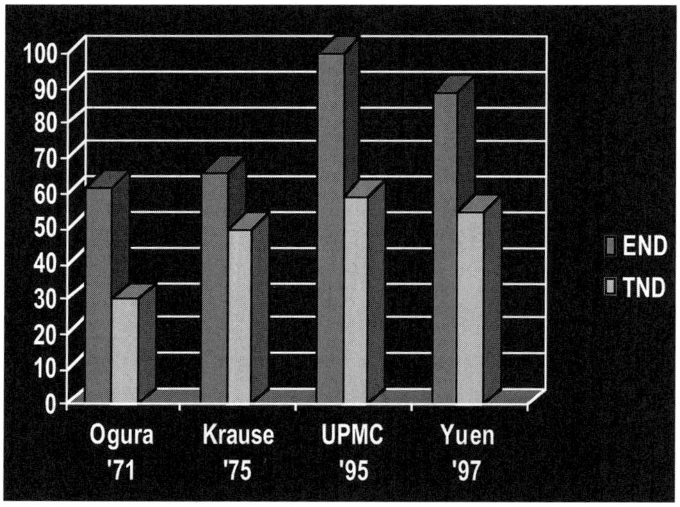

Figure 1–1 Patient survival with therapeutic neck dissection (TND) vs elective neck dissection (END) with pN+.

Extent of Surgery

In order for END to provide the most accurate staging information possible, the procedure must thoroughly remove the cervical lymphatics, which potentially harbor metastatic disease. Radical neck dissection (RND) was the procedure that was routinely employed for elective lymphadectomy when surgeons first began performing END. Careful examination of RND specimens according to the zone in the neck demonstrated that regional metastatic patterns could be predicted on the basis of the site and stage of the primary tumor.[23,29] Selective neck dissection (SND), which removes only the lymphatic zones at risk of the primary lesion and preserves major structures, has evolved as a result of these studies. By limiting the extent of surgery, selective procedures significantly decrease the morbidity and mortality, as compared with radical neck dissection.

Head and neck surgeons have examined regional recurrence rates and the location of regional recurrences in an effort to determine whether selective neck dissections constitute adequate procedures for staging the N0 neck.

Retrospective studies reporting the regional recurrence rate after selective and comprehensive procedures for END have shown that regional recurrences average approximately 5% for either procedure.[21,22,31,32] Comparisons between studies are difficult because of the time span over which they were performed. For instance, postoperative radiation therapy for the pN+ neck was not uniformly used in many of the early studies. Institutional differences in treatment philosophies also make comparisons between studies difficult. Studies that have directly compared comprehensive with selective procedures within the same institution confirm a similar regional recurrence rate between the two procedures.[24]

For selective procedures to achieve adequate nodal sampling and regional control, the zones at risk of occult metastases must be totally dissected. Critical assessment of the location of regional recurrences after SND has contributed to our understanding of the lymphatics considered to be at risk. Early experience with selective procedures led to understanding that the area posterior to the jugular vein and anterior to the cervical rootlets (level III to IVb) must be thoroughly dissected.[33,34] Other areas that merit consideration depending on the location of the primary tumor are the area surrounding the spinal accessory nerve at level II, level IV for oral cavity lesions,[35] and the subsites of the submandibular zone.[11] The retropharyngeal nodes may be at risk of some primary sites but are not routinely addressed by any standard procedure. The risk of metastases outside the zones at risk is probably extremely small. Therefore, selective procedures, if carefully performed, constitute adequate nodal sampling.

Indications for Adjuvant Therapy

One of the goals of END is to identify those patients who are at increased risk of regional recurrences and distant metastases, and who will potentially benefit from adjuvant therapy. Targeting high-risk patients will minimize the overall cost and morbidity of combined therapies. With this in mind, one must ask what pathologic findings are associated with an increased risk of recurrent disease.

In certain scenarios, the need for adjuvant therapy seems clear. Patients with ECS or with three or more occult nodes receive the recommendation for adjuvant therapy, regardless of whether a selective or comprehensive neck dissection has been performed. The situation is less clear if there are one or two lymph nodes without ECS. Whether a SND constitutes adequate therapy for very limited cervical disease remains unknown. Although the risk of additional occult metastases in the undissected zones after SND is very small, can irradiation therapy be withheld if all five zones have not been sampled? Many surgeons would be more confident recommending surgery alone as adequate therapy if a comprehensive procedure had been performed. In a small subset of patients with limited cervical disease, it is possible that comprehensive procedures performed electively may spare them combination therapy and the attendant sequelae.

Conclusion

Several controversies surround the use of END in the treatment of HNSCC. Included are the therapeutic effects of selective procedures and the indications for adjuvant therapies. Ongoing studies are attempting to define the role of SND for the treatment of limited cervical disease. END remains the most accurate tool currently available to stage the neck in HNSCC. Staging provides important prognostic information and targets patients who may benefit from combination therapy.

REFERENCES

Pitman and Johnson—CHAPTER 1

1. Baredes S, Leeman DJ, Chen TS, et al. Significance of tumor thickness in soft palate carcinoma. *Laryngoscope* 1993;103: 389–393
2. Fukano H, Matsuura H, Hasegawa, et al. Depth of invasion as a predictive factor for cervical lymph node metastasis in tongue carcinoma. *Head Neck* 1997;19:205–210
3. Fagan JJ, Collins B, Barnes L, et al. Perineural invasion in squamous cell carcinoma of the head and neck. *Arch Otolaryngol Head Neck Surg* 1998;124:637–640
4. Takes, RP, Baatenburg de Jong RJ, Schuuring E, et al. Markers for assessment of nodal metastasis in laryngeal carcinoma. *Arch Otolaryngol Head Neck Surg* 1997;123:412–418
5. Wolf GT, Fisher SG, Truelson JM, et al. DNA content and regional metastases in patients with advanced laryngeal squamous carcinoma. *Laryngoscope* 1994;104:479–483
6. American Joint Committee on Cancer. Manual for staging of cancer. 4th ed. Philadelphia: JB Lippincott, 1992
7. Friedman M, Roberts N, Kirshebaum G, et al. Nodal size of metastatic squamous cell carcinoma of the neck. *Laryngoscope* 1993;103:854–856
8. Moreau P, Goffart Y, Collignon J. Computed tomography of metastatic cervical lymph nodes. *Arch Otolaryngol Head Neck Surg* 1990;116:1190–1193
9. Don DM, Anzai Y, Lufkin RB, et al. Evaluation of cervical lymph node metastases in squamous cell carcinoma of the head and neck. *Laryngoscope* 1995;105:669–674
10. Byers RM, El-Naggar AK, Lee Y, et al. Can we detect or predict the presence of occult nodal metastases in patients with squamous carcinoma of the oral tongue. *Head Neck* 1998;20: 138–144
11. Dinardo LJ. Lymphatics of the submandibular space: an anatomic, clinical and pathologic study with applications to floor-of-mouth carcinoma. *Laryngoscope* 1998;108:206–214
12. van den Brekel MWM, van der Waal I, Meijer CJLM, et al. The incidence of micro metastases in neck dissection specimens obtained from elective neck dissections. *Laryngoscope* 1996;106:987–991
13. Woolgar JA. Carcinoma of the tongue: pathological consideration in management of the neck. *J R Soc Med* 1996; 89:611–615
14 Schuller DE, Bier-Lanning CM, Sharma PK, et al. Tissue-conserving surgery for prognosis, treatment, and function preservation. *Laryngoscope* 1998;108:1599–1604
15. Ogura JH, Biller HF, Wette R. Elective neck dissection for pharyngeal and laryngeal cancers. *Ann Otol* 1971;80:646–651
16. Lee JG, Krause CJ. Radical neck dissection: elective, therapeutic, and secondary. *Arch Otolaryngol* 1975;101:656–659.
17. McGuirt WF Jr, Johnson JT, Myers EN, et al. Floor of mouth carcinoma in management of the clinically negative neck. *Arch Otolaryngol Head Neck Surg* 1995;121:278–282
18. Yuen APW, Wei WI, Wong YM, et al. Elective neck dissection versus observation in the treatment of early oral tongue carcinoma. *Head Neck* 1997;19:583–588, *Ann Otolaryngol* 1980;89:578–581
19. Fletcher GH. Elective irradiation of subclinical disease in cancers of the head and neck. *Cancer* 1972;29:1450–1454
20. Mendenhall WM, Million RR. Elective irradiation for squamous cell carcinoma of the head and neck: analysis of dose related factors and causes of failure. *Int J Radiat Oncol Biol Phys* 1986;12:751
21. Bocca E, Pignataro O, Oldini C, Cappa C. Functional neck dissection: an evaluation and review of 843 cases. *Laryngoscope* 1984;94:942–945
22. Molinari R, Cantu G, Chiesa F, Grandi C. Retrospective comparison of conservative and radical neck dissection in laryngeal cancer. *Ann Otol Rhinol Laryngol* 1989;1980:578–581
23. Byers RM, Wolf PF, Ballantyne AJ. Rationale for elective modified neck dissection. *Head Neck Surg* 1988;10:160–167
24. Pitman KT, Johnson JT, Myers EN. Effectiveness of selective neck dissection for management of the clinical negative neck. *Arch Otolaryngol Head Neck Surg* 1997;123:917–922
25. Seydel HG. The risk of tumor induction in man following medical irradiation for malignant neoplasm. *Cancer* 1975; 35:1641–1645
26. van der Laan BF, Baris G, Gregor RT, et al. Oncology in focus: radiation-induced tumours of the head and neck. *J Laryngol Otol* 1995;109:346–349
27. Fakih AR, Rao RS, Patel AR. Prophylactic neck dissection in squamous cell carcinoma of oral tongue: a prospective randomized study. *Semin Surg Oncol* 1989;5:327–330
28. Vandenbrouck C, Sancho-Garnier H, Chassagen D, et al. Elective versus therapeutic radical neck dissection in epidermoid carcinoma of the oral cavity. *Cancer* 1980;46: 386–390
29. Shah JP. Patterns of cervical lymph node metastasis from squamous carcinomas of the upper aerodigestive tract. *Am J Surg* 1990;160:405–409
30. Alvi A, Johnson JT. Extracapsular spread in the clinically negative neck (N0): implications and outcome. *Otolaryngol Head Neck Surg* 1996;114:65–70
31. Spiro RH, Morgan GJ, Strong EW, et al. Supraomohyoid neck dissection. *Am J Surg* 1996;172:650–653
32. Medina J, Byers RM. Supraomohyoid neck dissection: rationale, indications and surgical technique. *Head Neck* 1989;11:111–112
33. Spiro RH, Gallo O, Shah JP. The jugular node dissection in patients with squamous carcinoma of the larynx or pharynx. *Am J Surg* 1993;166:399–402
34. Spiro JD, Spiro RH, Shah JP, Sesions RB, Strong EW. Critical assessment of supraomohyoid neck dissection. *Am J Surg* 1988;156:286–289
35. Byers RM, Weber RS, Andrews T, et al. Frequency and therapeutic implications of "skip metastases" in the neck from squamous carcinoma of the oral tongue. *Head Neck* 1997;19: 14–19

Role of Elective Neck Dissection for the N0 Neck

CHAPTER 2

Jesus E. Medina

"A topic ceases to be interesting when it is no longer controversial."

The choice of treatment of the neck in patients with cancer of the head and neck has been controversial for decades. In recent years, the focus of that controversy has shifted. The radical neck dissection is no longer the only operation performed when treatment of the neck nodes is necessary. In fact, today, it is the least commonly done type of neck dissection. Currently, one of the greatest controversies centers around the role of the selective neck dissections in the treatment of the N0 neck. Interestingly, alongside the decision to perform a selective neck dissection are a number of controversial issues regarding alternative, less invasive methods of staging the cervical lymph nodes, which include imaging studies. The discussion that follows addresses these controversies and analyzes the efficacy of the selective neck dissections.

Can Imaging of the Neck Preclude an Elective Neck Dissection?

One of the first controversies faced by the clinician during the process of determining whether to perform an elective neck dissection is the value of imaging studies of the neck. Admittedly, determination of the status of the lymph nodes of the neck by clinical examination is not always accurate in patients with cancer of the head and neck. Various imaging modalities have been shown to be more accurate in detecting minimal enlargement of lymph nodes in the neck.[1-3] A clinician may be more inclined to recommend elective treatment of the neck when one or more enlarged nodes are demonstrated by an imaging study, as the probability of an enlarged lymph node containing metastasis is higher. However, not all enlarged lymph nodes contain metastatic deposits. More importantly, a negative ultrasound, computed tomography (CT), or magnetic resonance imaging (MRI) scan cannot be relied on to withhold elective treatment of the neck, because none of these techniques can depict small tumor deposits within a lymph node. The presence of radiolucency within a lymph node, considered a very reliable criterion for the presence of metastasis, is not very useful in evaluating the N0 neck, because necrosis seldom occurs in micrometastases. Furthermore, the size criteria currently used to consider a node positive on CT or MRI (largest diameter >10 or 15 mm) are not optimal, especially for nodes in the submandibular triangle, a frequent site of metastases from cancers of the oral cavity. Recently, DiNardo[4] studied the lymph nodes of the submandibular triangle in patients with floor-of-mouth cancer. DiNardo found that 88% of the nodes harboring metastatic carcinoma were <10 mm in diameter. The UCLA group has reported a similar study of neck dissection specimens, which showed that 67% of lymph nodes containing metastasis were <10 mm in diameter.[5] Yuen et al.[6] recently studied neck dissection specimens by whole-organ sectioning at 3-mm intervals. Among 2826 lymph nodes examined, these investigators found that the median size of the metastatic foci was 3 mm and occupied a median of 6% of the cross-sectional area of the involved nodes. Clearly, ultrasound, CT, and MRI scans are unable to detect metastases of this size in a lymph node of any size, nor can they differentiate between reactive enlargement of a lymph node and enlargement caused by metastasis.

Multidirectional ultrasonography scanning has shown promise for improved preoperative evaluation of the N0 neck.[7] In experienced hands, this technique permits fine-needle aspiration of lymph nodes as small as 3 mm in diameter. Using this technique, Snow[8] and several other investigative groups in the Netherlands[1,9] have reportedly been able to identify 75 to 77% of patients with occult lymph node metastases. Despite the success reported by these groups and the results of a prospective multi-institutional study in the Netherlands, which showed that the results with ultrasound-guided fine-needle aspiration biopsy (FNAB) are not as investigator dependent as is often suggested,[9] this technique has not gained wide acceptance outside Europe. Perhaps it is because the technique is demanding in terms of equipment and personnel time. More importantly, long-term assessment of the outcome in patients deemed node-negative by ultrasonography and FNA cytology, in whom an elective neck dissection was not performed, has only recently been published. These results are not as encouraging as was hoped. In a study of 92 patients whose necks were staged N0, and which were cytologically negative, followed for 1 to 3 years, 19 (21%) subsequently developed a neck node metastasis. Six of these 19 patients (32%) died of distant metastases or of locoregional recurrence.[10]

It is hoped that positron emission tomography (PET) will be a more useful imaging technique for detecting metastases in the lymph nodes, without their removal and histopathologic examination. It relies on abnormal tissue metabolism to detect neoplasms. Myers and Wax[11] recently reported that PET permitted accurate determination of the presence or absence of metastasis in a small group of 11 patients with squamous cell carcinoma of the oral cavity. These patients were staged clinically N0 and underwent 19 neck dissections. PET scans were positive in all 7 instances in which the neck dissection had histologically confirmed metastasis and were negative in all 12 cases in which there was no histologic evidence of metastasis. Unfortunately, these investigators do not report examining the lymph nodes by more than one section. Although the results of this first study are encouraging, evaluation of this technique awaits studies of larger numbers of patients. These may not be forthcoming because of the limited accessibility to this technology and its prohibitive cost.[11]

Is Sentinel Node Biopsy a Substitute for Elective Neck Dissection?

Another controversy surrounding elective neck dissection concerns the value of sentinel node biopsy. Considering the experience with this technique in patients with melanoma and breast cancer, it is anticipated that gamma probe-directed biopsy of the sentinel node may be useful in the management of the N0 neck in patients with squamous cell carcinoma of the head and neck. To that end, a recent study of 5 patients conducted by Koch et al.[12] showed that identification and biopsy of the sentinel node are feasible in these patients. However, a number of substantial problems were identified: (1) the proximity of the primary tumor obscures the lymphoscintigram, particularly when the tumor is located in the oral cavity; (2) intramucosal injection of the radiolabeled material is more difficult than intradermal injections and the isotope often extrudes into the saliva; and (3) some sites in the head and neck are inaccessible, and the technique is limited in patients who have been previously irradiated. According to these investigators, their observations "cast doubt on the general applicability and utility of the technique" for squamous cell carcinoma of the head and neck.[12]

When Should the Neck Be Treated Electively?

The decision to recommend elective treatment of the neck nodes depends mainly on the location and stage of the primary tumor and on a few other potential factors.

ORAL CAVITY

Elective treatment of the neck is indicated in patients with T2, T3, and T4 cancers of the oral cavity, regardless of the site of origin. Possible exceptions are T2 tumors of the buccal mucosa, in which the associated rate of lymph node metastases is low,[13] and T1 tumors of the oral tongue, because some surgeons believe, as we do, that elective neck dissection is desirable in these patients,[14,15] particularly when the lesion is thicker than 1.5 to 2 mm.[16,17] An increasing number of clinical, histologic, biochemical, and genetic factors are under study as potential predictors of the propensity of a tumor to metastasize to the lymph nodes. Their role remains sufficiently unclear to recommend their use in routine treatment planning.

OROPHARYNX

Tumors of the oropharynx have a high propensity to metastasize to the regional lymph nodes even in early stages. Therefore, the regional lymph nodes should be treated electively, regardless of the stage of the primary tumor. With the exception of early, well-lateralized tumors, tumors of the oropharynx have a tendency to metastasize to both sides of the neck, often indicating treatment of both sides of the neck. Dissection of the retropharyngeal nodes should be considered particularly for tumors extending onto the pharyngeal walls, as retropharyngeal nodal metastasis occurred historically in up to 44% of cases.[18]

GLOTTIC CANCER

For glottic tumors staged T1 and T2, elective treatment of the neck is generally not indicated because the incidence of metastases is low. There are possibly two exceptions: (1) when tumor is found in a delphian node during the course of a partial laryngectomy, as the reported rate of lateral neck metastases in such cases is about 40%[19]; and (2) when treating recurrent T1–T2 tumors, because of the reported risk of occult metastases is about 20%. The need to dissect the neck in patients with T3 glottic tumors remains controversial. However, because lymph node metastases have been observed in 17 to 22% of cases, we believe that elective treatment of the neck is appropriate.[20,21] Elective dissection of the neck is clearly indicated in patients with T4 tumors.[22]

SUPRAGLOTTIC CANCER

Elective treatment is warranted in all stages of supraglottic cancer. A possible exception may be T1 tumors of the suprahyoid epiglottis. Furthermore, treatment of the neck should include the lymph nodes at risk on both sides of the neck, with as many as 75% of the recurrences in the neck occuring in the "undissected" contralateral side.[23]

SUBGLOTTIC CANCER

Elective treatment of the lateral compartments of the neck does not seem warranted in patients with subglottic cancer. The reported incidence of metastases to these nodes is only 10%.[24,25] By contrast, the paratracheal lymph nodes are involved more frequently and should be treated bilaterally.[26,27]

Is Elective Treatment Preferable to Observation and Therapeutic Neck Dissection?

The value of elective treatment of the neck is not universally accepted. The notion of watching the neck and treating it only when metastases become clinically apparent is allegedly supported by two prospective randomized studies.[28,29] In both studies, the survival of patients with cancer of the oral cavity who underwent "elective" neck dissection was not significantly better than the survival of patients who underwent a therapeutic neck dissection. Unfortunately, these studies have not resolved the controversy. In fact, they have been criticized because the number of patients studied was insufficient to arrive at a conclusive opinion.

The efficacy of elective treatment of the neck in patients with larynx cancer has been recently compared to that of therapeutic neck dissection at the time metastases become clinically apparent in an interesting retrospective study by Gallo et al.[30] From a population of 1808 patients with cancer of the larynx treated at the University of Florence, two groups of patients were selected for comparison. The first group of 76 patients had clinically an N0 neck, underwent elective neck dissection, and had histologically positive nodes. The second group consisted of 96 patients who were initially staged N0 but who subsequently developed lymph node metastases and underwent therapeutic neck dissection. Postoperative radiation to the neck was given to 11% of the patients in the first group and to 20.8% in the second group ($P = 0.178$). The criteria used to determine when patients were selected for one group or the other were not established a priori. However, Gallo and colleagues state that patients were "usually" selected to undergo elective neck dissection when they had an advanced tumor (T3–T4); had a fat, short, or muscular neck that was not easy to evaluate clinically; had a low educational level; and poor follow-up was anticipated. In this study, there was not a statistically significant difference between the two groups of patients in overall determinant and actuarial survival rates, with a minimum follow-up of 5 years. This is surprising because patients who underwent delayed therapeutic neck dissection had a significantly higher incidence of distant metastases, multiple positive nodes, and extracapsular tumor spread.[30] Other retrospective studies have found that elective neck dissection decreases the neck recurrence rates significantly in patients treated for N0 supraglottic carcinoma.[31]

Self-examination by the patient and reliable follow-up evaluation are essential for watchful waiting to succeed in the management of the N0 neck. Unfortunately, a significant number of the patients who do not undergo elective neck dissection cannot be salvaged later, when they present with palpable metastases, because the disease is too far advanced.[29] In a review of 122 patients with T3–T4 N0 cancers of the larynx who were treated by total laryngectomy and observation of the neck at the University of Hong Kong, 36% of the patients who later presented with palpable metastases had inoperable disease, amenable to palliative treatment only. Furthermore, of the patients who were operable, 42% eventually died of a neck recurrence. These observations, in combination with the idiosyncrasies of character and social background of many patients with larynx cancer, lead most head and neck surgeons to treat the neck electively, even though the impact of this decision on patient survival remains controversial.

Is Selective Neck Dissection Appropriate for the Treatment of the N0 Neck?

It is generally accepted today that a radical neck dissection is not indicated for surgical treatment of the N0 neck.[30] However, the preference between selective neck dissection and the modified radical neck dissection type III (MRND-III), in which the sternocleidomastoid muscle, the internal jugular vein, and the spinal accessory nerve are preserved, remains controversial. Some surgeons, particularly in Europe, advocate this type of MRND as the treatment of choice for the NO neck, whereas in North America many surgeons prefer a selective neck dissection. It is fitting to point out the differences between the two operations and to compare pertinent outcomes as they exist in the literature today.

MORBIDITY

One of the outcomes relevant to elective neck dissection is postoperative shoulder function. In this regard, two prospective nonrandomized studies have shown the superiority of the selective neck dissection in terms of objective measures of shoulder range of motion and postoperative electromyography (EMG) of the trapezius muscle.[33, 34]

The results of these studies are almost intuitive as dissection of the spinal accessory nerve is less extensive in a selective neck dissection. Interestingly, however, both studies showed abnormalities of trapezius function, albeit temporary and variably severe, in almost one-fourth (22%) of patients undergoing selective neck dissection and in almost two-thirds (65%) of patients undergoing modified radical neck dissection. These observations should remind us that shoulder function must be evaluated postoperatively in every patient who undergoes neck dissection. Early detection of functional deficits and prompt institution of measures to rehabilitate the shoulder will prevent further deterioration of function, particularly in elderly patients.

It was recently suggested that dissection of the "supraspinal recess" may not be necessary because the occurrence of metastases in this area of the neck is low.[35,36] This is the dissection of the fibrofatty tissues located medial to the upper end of the sternocleidomastoid muscle and above and behind the segment of the spinal accessory nerve located between the skull base and its entrance into the sternocleidomastoid muscle. Decreased morbidity in terms of function of the spinal accessory nerve has been cited as a reason to avoid dissection of this area. Future studies of shoulder function may be necessary to support such a contention.

TUMOR CONTROL

To date, only one prospective study has compared the efficacy of a selective neck dissection and the MRND-III. This prospective multi-institutional study, conducted by the Brazilian Head and Neck Cancer Study Group, has shown no significant difference in neck recurrence or survival between two groups of patients with cancer of the oral cavity stage N0. One group in the study received a "classic" modified radical neck dissection and the other a supraomohyoid neck dissection.[37] Unfortunately, the study was not randomized, and the investigators did not exclude patients with simultaneous recurrence at the primary site in calculating the recurrence rates in the neck. Furthermore, the results were not stratified according to the pathologic staging of the neck codes.

The effectiveness of the selective neck dissection for the treatment of the N0 neck is best analyzed according to the histopathologic staging of the treated side of the neck. This is because the false-positive and false-negative rates or the clinical examination of the neck is variable but generally as high as 20%.[38] It is also important to include a minimum follow-up evaluation of 2 years and to control the primary tumor in order to eliminate the possibility of reseeding of the neck by a recurrent tumor. The results can then be analyzed in the following categories.

Clinically N0/Pathologically N0 (cN0/pN0)

In a prospective analysis of our practice, the rate of recurrence in the neck in the category defined as clinically N0/pathologically N0 (cN0/pN0), at 2 years of follow-up, with the primary controlled, was 0% among 66 patients treated with surgery alone and 4.2% among 48 patients who also received postoperative radiation therapy. The latter treatment was given because of several characteristics of the primary tumor: close margins, perineural invasion, and advanced stage.[39] Almost identical recurrence rates for this category have been reported by other institutions that treat a large number of patients. These results are outlined in Table 2–1. Comparable results have been reported with the MRND-III, as shown in Table 2–2.

Clinically N0/Pathologically N+

In the category defined as clinically N0/pathologically N+, we must distinguish between those instances in which the histopathology of the surgical specimen shows a single positive

TABLE 2–1

Selective Neck Dissection, Pathologic Stage N0, Recurrence in the Neck

Type of Dissection	No. of Dissections	Follow-up (mo)	Recurrence Rate (%)
Pitman et al. (1997)[49]	103	24	4.9
Ambrosch et al. (1996)[50]	73	12	4.1
Kowalski et al. (1993)[53]	93	26	3.2
Pellitteri et al. (1997)[54]	33	24	3.0
Davidson et al. (1997)[55]	44	53	3.3
Kerrebijn et al. (1999)[56]	41	24	10.0

TABLE 2–2

Modified Radical Neck Dissection Type III, Pathologic Stage N0, Recurrence in the Neck

Type of Dissection	No. of Dissections	Follow-up (mo)	Recurrence Rate (%)
Calearo and Teatini (1983)[44]	154	36	3.25
Molinari et al. (1980)[43]	106	36	0.9
Suarez et al. (1993)[57]	258	60	2.0
Bocca et al. (1984)[58]	672		2.38
Gavilan and Gavilan (1995)[59]	169	60	8.9
Lingeman et al. (1977)[60]	60		0.9

TABLE 2–3
Modified Radical Neck Dissection Type III, Pathologic Stage N+, Recurrence in the Neck

Type of Dissection	No. of Dissections	Follow-up (mo)	Recurrence Rate (%)
Calearo and Teatini (1983)[44]	63	36	3.17
Molinari et al. (1980)[43]	22	36	4.5

node and those in which either multiple positive nodes or extracapsular spread of tumor are found. Byers,[40] Houck and Medina,[39] and Spiro et al.[41] and others have analyzed the results in this fashion. The recurrence rate among patients with either multiple positive nodes or extracapsular spread of tumor, with the primary controlled, at 2 years, varies between 9.5% and 15%. Treatment of these patients included selective neck dissection and postoperative radiation therapy. Leemans et al.[42] reported a recurrence rate of 11.3% among patients treated with a comprehensive MRND with preservation of the spinal accessory nerve and the SCMM, but with removal of the internal jugular vein, who received postoperative radiation and were followed up for a minimum of 2 years.

Unfortunately, there are no comparable reports for the MRND-III. The studies by Molinari et al.[43] and by Calearo and Teatini[44] (Table 2–3) report their results in all cases with histopathologically positive node metastases. At first glance, the figures reported suggest that the MRND-III yields better results for the neck with "histologically positive nodes." Some investigators have gone as far as performing a statistical analysis that compares the recurrence rates in these studies with the results reported by Byers[40] and Pellitteri et al.[45] for the selective neck dissection and have concluded that the results with the MRND-III are significantly better. These results are not comparable statistically for various reasons, however. First, the study by Molinari et al.[43] included only patients with cancer of the larynx, and they included patients with clinically N0 and N+ neck. Calearo and Teatini[44] studied 265 patients, 195 with cancer of the larynx and 30 with tumors of the thyroid, lower lip, salivary glands, and skin. Second, although these investigators report results for patients with histologically positive nodes, they do not stratify their analysis to indicate whether the metastases were single or multiple or whether there was extracapsular spread. By contrast, the selective neck dissection studies included patients with squamous cell carcinoma of different sites in the upper aerodigestive tract, and they report results for patients with single metastasis and for patients with multiple nodes or extracapsular spread. In any event, the fact that Molinari and colleagues observed a recurrence rate of 4.5% in a series of patients with histologically positive nodes treated with surgery only is remarkable.[43] Particularly because the reported recurrence rate observed in a similar series of patients treated with a radical neck dissection was 22%.[46]

Also pertinent today is the question recently posed by Johnson as to whether selective neck dissection is adequate therapy for patients with limited occult metastases, such as a single positive node (stage pN1). In a recent review of our experience the recurrence in the neck at 2 years in this category was 21%. A similar analysis performed by Ambrosch et al.[47] demonstrated a 16% recurrence rate, and data provided to us by Byers showed a 25% recurrence rate for this category in the MD Anderson experience.[48] There is no published detailed analysis of such cases trying to determine why the recurrence rates are so high. We can only speculate about possible causes and possible alternatives to decrease the rate of recurrence in these patients.

Perhaps the selective neck dissection is not extensive enough. Could these patients do better with a MRND? If we think in terms of the extent of the operation and compare the selective neck dissection with the MRND-III, it becomes apparent that the main difference between these operations is in the dissection of the lymph nodes in level V and level IV (Table 2–4). Is dissection of these levels expected to prove beneficial? An answer could be inferred by analyzing the incidence of metastases encountered in level V and the pattern of recurrences following selective neck dissection. The incidence of subclinical metastases in the lymph nodes of level V is low (Table 2–5). An analysis of the location of the neck recurrences among 142 selective neck dissections studied by Pitman et al.[49] showed that all recurrences developed in the regions predicted by the lymphatic drainage of the primary tumor site; none was outside the dissected levels. None was in level V. One recurrence was in the submandibular nodes (level I) from an oral cavity primary. The other 4 were at levels II and III from 3 laryngeal tumors and 1 oral cavity tumor. Similarly, in a study of 163 selective

TABLE 2–4
Selective versus Modified Radical Neck Dissection Type III

	Node Groups Removed
Selective:	
Supraomohyoid	I, II, III – –
Lateral	II, III, IV –
MRND-III	(I), II, III, IV, V

TABLE 2–5

Dissection of Level V N0 Neck: Incidence of Subclinical Metastases

	Primary Site	%
Skolnik (1976)[61]	Oral cavity	0
	Larynx	0
Shah et al. (1990)[62]	Oral cavity	2
	Oropharynx	7
	Hypopharynx	0
	Larynx	7
Moe et al. (1996)[63]	Larynx	0
Yang et al. (1998)[22]	Larynx, glottic	0

neck dissections reported by Ambrosch et al.[50] the recurrences in the neck, in the absence of recurrence at the primary site, developed in the dissected area of the ipsilateral neck (levels II and III). One patient with carcinoma of the uvula had a recurrence in the retropharyngeal nodes. Recurrences in level V were not observed.

In another recent study, Gui-yi Tu[51] performed dissection and frozen-section examination of the lymph nodes at level II in 155 patients with supraglottic carcinomas. In 13 patients, in whom the frozen section indicated metastatic carcinoma in the lymph nodes, a modified radical neck dissection was performed. In the remaining 142 patients, no additional surgery was performed in the neck. When postoperative radiation therapy was given to these patients for reasons related to the primary tumor, the fields encompassed only the upper and mid-jugular regions of the neck. All patients were followed for 5 years. The location of the recurrences in the neck is shown in Table 2–6. No recurrences were found in the lymph nodes of level V.

Because the cited analyses of the site of recurrence in selective neck dissections, and our experience, show that most recurrences develop in the dissected areas of the neck and not in level V, it is reasonable to speculate that dissection of levels II and III, where most recurrences take place, is not adequate or "radical" enough. It may be necessary to remove the jugular vein in these patients, as suggested and practiced by Leemans et al.[42] These investigators reported a recurrence rate of 9.1% in patients treated with a MRND in which the jugular vein and the sternocleidomastoid muscle were removed, whereas the spinal accessory nerve was preserved. Their patients did not receive postoperative radiation therapy when only one node was found to be positive. However, their report does not clarify whether some of these patients received radiation for reasons related to the primary tumor. An alternative has been suggested by Yuen et al.,[52] who observed that recurrence in the neck developed in 20% of patients with oral tongue cancer whose neck was staged pN1 and did not receive postoperative radiation therapy. By contrast, there were no recurrences among pN1 patients who received postoperative radiation. The observed difference could not be tested statistically because of the small size of the sample. A properly designed prospective multi-institutional study is clearly needed to elucidate the role of selective or MRND with or without radiation in treatment of the pN1 neck.

When Is Postoperative Radiation Recommended?

It is clear that postoperative radiation is not necessary when the histopathologic examination of a selective neck dissection shows no metastatic tumor in the lymph nodes. It also seems prudent to recommend postoperative radiation when extracapsular spread of the tumor is demonstrated in an elective neck dissection. It remains unclear whether radiation should be added to a selective neck dissection if there are one, two, or three histopathologically positive nodes.

TABLE 2–6

Supraglottic Carcinomas: Pattern of Recurrence in 142 Patients with Negative Level II Nodes (FS)[a]

	Node Group				
	II	III	IV	V	Total
Ipsilateral	3(30%)	6(60%)	1(10%)	0(0)	10 (100%)
Contralateral	1(20%)	2(40%)	2(40%)	0(0)	5 (100%)

SOURCE: Modified from Gui-yi T. Upper neck (level II) dissection for N0 neck supraglottic carcinoma. *Laryngoscope* 1999;109:467–470.[51]

[a] Frozen section.

REFERENCES

1. Close L, Merkel M, Vuitch MF, et al. Computed tomographic evaluation for regional lymph node involvement in cancer of the oral cavity and oropharynx. *Head Neck Surg* 1989;11:309–317
2. Friedman M, Mafee MF, Pacella BL, et al. Rationale for elective neck dissection in 1990. *Laryngoscope* 1990;100:54–59
3. Friedman M, Shelton VK, Mafee MM. Metastatic neck disease: evaluation by computed tomography. *Arch Otolaryngol Head Neck Surg* 1984;110:443–447
4. DiNardo LJ. Lymphatics of the submandibular space: an anatomic, clinical, and pathologic study with applications to floor-of-mouth carcinoma [see comments]. *Laryngoscope* 1998;108:206–214
5. Don DM, Anzai Y, Lufkin RB, et al. Evaluation of cervical lymph node metastases in squamous cell carcinoma of the head and neck. *Laryngoscope* 1995;105(7 Pt 1):669–674
6. Yuen AP, Lam KY, Chan AC, et al. Clinicopathological analysis of elective neck dissection for N0 neck of early oral tongue carcinoma. *Am J Surg* 1999;177:90–92
7. van den Brekel MW, Castelijns JA, Stel HV, et al. Modern imaging techniques and ultrasound guided aspiration cytology for the assessment of neck node metastases: a prospective comparative study. *Eur Arch Otorhinolaryngol* 1993;250:11–17
8. Snow GB. The N0 neck in head and neck cancer patients. *Eur Arch Otorhinolaryngol* 1993;250:423
9. Takes R, Knegt P, Manni J, et al. Regional metastasis in head and neck squamous cell carcinoma: revised value of US with US-guided FNAB. *Radiology* 1996;198:819–823
10. van den Brekel M, Reitsma LC, Snow G, et al. The outcome of a wait and see policy for the neck after negative ultrasound guided cytology results and follow-up with ultrasound guided cytology. *Br J Cancer* 1997;77(suppl 1):20
11. Myers LL, Wax MK. Positron emission tomographyin the evaluation of the negative neck in patients with oral cavity cancer. *J Otolaryngol* 1998;27:342–347
12. Koch W, Choti M, Civelek A, et al. Gamma probe–directed biopsy of the sentinel node in oral asquamous cell carcinoma. *Arch Otolaryngol* 1998;124:455–459
13. Dhawan IK, Verma K, Khazanchi RK, et al. Carcinoma of buccal mucosa: incidence of regional lymph node involvement. *Ind J Cancer* 1993;30:176–180
14. Lydiatt D, Robbins KT, Byers R, et al. Treatment of stage I and II oral tongue cancer. *Head Neck* 1993;15:308–312
15. Kerrebijn JD, Freeman JL, Irish JC, et al. Supraomohyoid neck dissection. Is it diagnostic or therapeutic? *Head Neck* 1999;21:39–42
16. Mohit-Tabatabai MA, Sobel HJ, Rush BF, et al. Relation of thickness of floor of mouth stage I and II cancers to regional metastasis. *Am J Surg* 1986;152:351–353
17. Spiro RH, Huvos AG, Wong GY, et al. Predictive value of tumor thickness in squamous cell carcinoma confined to the tongue and floor of the mouth. *Am J Surg* 1986;152:345–350
18. Ballantyne AJ. Significance of retropharyngeal nodes in cancer of the head and neck. *Am J Surg* 1964;108:500–503
19. Olsen K, DeSanto L, Pearson B. Positive delphian node: clinical significance in laryngeal cancer. *Laryngoscope* 1987;97: 1033–1037
20. T3 laryngeal cancer: the Dutch experience. 2nd World Congress on Laryngeal Cancer. Sydney, Australia: 1994
21. Hao SP, Myers E, Johnson J. T3 glottic carcinoma revisited. Transglottic vs. pure glottic carcinoma. *Arch Otolaryngol-Head Neck Surg* 1995;121:166–170
22. Yang CY, Andersen PE, Everts EC, et al. Nodal disease in purely glottic carcinoma: is elective neck treatment worthwhile? *Laryngoscope* 1998;108:1006–1008
23. Pillsbury H. A rationale for therapy of the N0 neck. *Laryngoscope* 1997;107:1294–1314
24. Lederman M. Cancer of the larynx. Part 1. Natural history in relation to treatment. *Br J Radiol* 1971;44:569–578
25. Martensson B, Fluur E, Jacobsson F. Aspects of treatment of cancer of the larynx. *Ann Otol Rhinol Laryngol* 1967;76:313
26. Hanna EY. Subglottic cancer [clinical conference]. *Am J Otolaryngol* 1994;15:322–328
27. Weber RS, Marvel J, Smith P, et al. Paratracheal lymph node dissection for carcinoma of the larynx, hypopharynx, and cervical esophagus. *Otolaryngol Head Neck Surg* 1993; 108:11–17
28. Vandenbrouck C, Sancho-Garnier H, Chassagne D. Elective versus therapeutic radical neck dissection in epidermoid carcinoma of the oral cavity: results of a randomized clinical trial. *Cancer* 1980;46:386
29. Fakih A, Rao R, Borges A, et al. Elective versus therapeutic neck dissection in early carcinoma of the oral tongue. *Am J Surg* 1989;158:309
30. Gallo O, Boddi V, Parrella F, et al. Treatment of the clinically negative neck in laryngeal cancer patients. *Head Neck* 1996;18:566–572
31. Ramadan HH, Allen GC. The influence of elective neck dissection on neck relapse in N0 supraglottic carcinoma. *Am J Otolaryngol* 1993;14:278–281
32. Bailey BJ. Selective neck dissection. The challenge of occult metastases. *Arch Otolaryngol* 1998;124:353
33. Sobol S, Jensen C, Sawyer W II, et al. Objective comparison of physical dysfunction after neck dissection. *Am J Surg* 1985; 150:503–509
34. Remmler D, Byers RM, Scheetz J. A prospective study of shoulder disability resulting from radical and modified neck dissections. *Head Neck Surg* 1986;8:280–286
35. Talmi YP, Hoffman HT, Horowitz Z, et al. Patterns of metastases to the upper jugular lymph nodes (the "submuscular recess"). *Head Neck* 1998;20:682–686
36. Kraus DH, Rosenberg DB, Davidson BJ, et al. Supraspinal accessory lymph node metastases in supraomohyoid neck dissection. *Am J Surg* 1996;172:646–649

37. Anonymous. Brazilian Head and Neck Cancer Study Group. The results of a prospective trial on elective modified radical classical versus supraomohyoid neck dissection in the management of oral squamous carcinoma. *Am J Surg* 1998; 176:422–427
38. Kowalski LP, Magrin J, Waksman G, et al. Supraomohyoid neck dissection in the treatment of head and neck tumors. Survival results in 212 cases. *Arch Otolaryngol Head Neck Surg* 1993;119:958–963
39. Houck JR, Medina JE. Management of cervical lymph nodes in squamous carcinomas of the head and neck. *Semin Surg Oncol* 1995;11:228–239
40. Byers RM. Modified neck dissection. A study of 967 cases from 1970 to 1980. *Am J Surg* 1986;150:414–421
41. Spiro JD, Spiro RH, Shah JP, et al. Critical assessment of supraomohyoid neck dissection. *Am J Surg* 1988;156:286–289
42. Leemans CR, Tiwari R, van der Wall I. The efficacy of comprehensive neck dissection with or without postoperative radiotherapy in nodal metastases of squamous cell carcinoma of the upper respiratory and digestive tracts. *Laryngoscope* 1990;100:1194–1198
43. Molinari R, Chiesa F, Cantu G, et al. Retrospective comparison of conservative and radical neck dissection in laryngeal cancer. *Ann Otol Rhinol Laryngol* 1980;89:578–581
44. Calearo CV, Teatini G. Functional neck dissection: anatomical grounds, surgical technique, clinical observations. *Ann Otol Rhinol Laryngol* 1983;89:215–222
45. Pellitteri PK, Robbins KT, Neuman T. Expanded application of selective neck dissection with regard to nodal status. *Head Neck* 1997;19:260–265
46. Farrar WB, Finkelmeier WR, McCabe DP, et al. Radical neck dissection: is it enough? *Am J Surg* 1988;156:173–176
47. Ambrosch P, Freudenberg L, Kron M, et al. Selective neck dissection in the management of squamous cell carcinoma of the upper digestive tract. *Eur Arch Otorhinolaryngol* 1996; 253:329–335
48. Houck JR, Medina JE. Management of cervical lymph nodes in squamous carcinomas of the head and neck. *Semin Surg Oncol* 1995;11:228–239
49. Pitman KT, Johnson JT, Myers EN. Effectiveness of selective neck dissection for management of the clinically negative neck. *Arch Otolaryngol Head Neck Surg* 1997;123:917–922
50. Ambrosch P, Freudenberg L, Kron M, et al. Selective neck dissection in the management of squamous cell carcinoma of the upper digestive tract. *Eur Arch Otorhinolaryngol* 1996; 253:329–335
51. Gui-yi T. Upper neck (level II) dissection for N0 neck supraglottic carcinoma. *Laryngoscope* 1999;108:467–470
52. Yuen AP, Lam KY, Chan AC, et al. Clinicopathological analysis of elective neck dissection for N0 neck of early oral tongue carcinoma. *Am J Surg* 1999;177:90–92
53. Kowalski LP, Magrin J, Waksman G, et al. Supraomohyoid neck dissection in the treatment of head and neck tumors. Survival results in 212 cases. *Arch Otolaryngol Head Neck Surg* 1993;119:958–963
54. Pellitteri PK, Robbins KT, Neuman T. Expanded application of selective neck dissection with regard to nodal status. *Head Neck* 1997;19:260–265
55. Davidson J, Khan Y, Gilbert R, et al. Is selective neck dissection sufficient treatment for the N0/Np+ neck? *J Otolaryngol* 1997;26:229–231
56. Kerrebijn JD, Freeman JL, Irish JC, et al. Supraomohyoid neck dissection. Is it diagnostic or therapeutic? *Head Neck* 1999;21:39–42
57. Suarez C, Llorente JL, Nunez F, et al. Neck dissection with or without postoperative radiotherapy in supraglottic carcinomas. *Otolaryngol Head Neck Surg* 1993;109:3–9
58. Bocca E, Pignataro O, Oldini C. Functional neck dissection: an evaluation and review of 843 cases. *Laryngoscope* 1984;94:942–945
59. Gavilan C, Gavilan J. Five-year results of functional neck dissection for cancer of the larynx. *Arch Otolaryngol Head Neck Surg* 1995;115:1193–1196
60. Lingeman RE, Stephens R, Helmus C, et al. Neck dissection: radical or conservative. *Ann Otol Rhinol Laryngol* 1977;86:737–744
61. Skolnik EM. The posterior triangle in radical neck surgery. *Arch Otolaryngol Head Neck Surg* 1976;102:1–4
62. Shah JP, Candela FC, Poddar AK. The patterns of cervical lymph node metastases from squamous carcinoma of the oral cavity. *Cancer* 1990;66:109–113
63. Moe K, Wolf G, Fisher S, et al. Regional metastases in patients with advanced laryngeal cancer. *Arch Otolaryngol Head Neck Surg* 1996;122:644–648

Role of Elective Neck Dissection for the N0 Neck

CHAPTER 3

Bhuvanesh Singh and Jatin P. Shah

The presence of regional lymph node metastasis at initial presentation is the single most important factor influencing the outcome of patients with upper aerodigestive tract squamous cell carcinomas.[1-4] Accordingly, an aggressive approach to the management of patients presenting with obvious lymphatic metastasis is advocated. However, the management of clinically occult dissemination of squamous cell carcinoma to regional lymph nodes is a topic of considerable debate.[5-11] The controversy focuses mainly on four issues: the need for elective treatment, selection of patients requiring intervention, the type of intervention to be used, and the benefit of such intervention to the patient.

Need for Elective Treatment

Several studies have shown a diminished survival rate in patients with occult lymphatic metastasis. Tulenko et al.[12] showed that the 5-year cure rate decrease from 79% in patients without any evidence of metastasis to 29% in those with occult disease detected on pathologic examination to 11% in those with clinically evident disease. Similarly, Alvi and Johnson[13] showed that disease control rates decreased from 82% for patients without metastasis to 47% for those with occult metastasis and to 31% when extracapsular spread was present in lymph nodes containing occult metastasis. Accordingly, identification and treatment of patients with occult metastasis appear warranted.

However, because there is no statistical difference in regional control rates or survival between patients undergoing elective neck dissection for micrometastasis compared with those undergoing therapeutic neck dissection for N1 disease, extrapolation suggests that patients with N0 necks can be followed until metastasis becomes clinically evident.[3] Unfortunately, patients at risk of micrometastasis to the cervical lymphatics do not absolutely progress in an orderly fashion.[3,9,14-17] A report by Anderson et al.[14] showed that most patients initially observed with N0 neck, have greater than N1 nodal involvement clinically at subsequent treatment, even under close follow-up (Fig. 3–1). In fact, most patients (77%) had metastatic disease greater than N1 or associated extracapsular spread on pathologic analysis. In addition, in patients with N0 necks, the rate of distant metastasis is higher in those who develop subsequent nodal recurrence (11%) as compared with patients who remain disease free (3%).[7,8] This suggests early intervention is warranted in patients at high risk of occult nodal involvement.

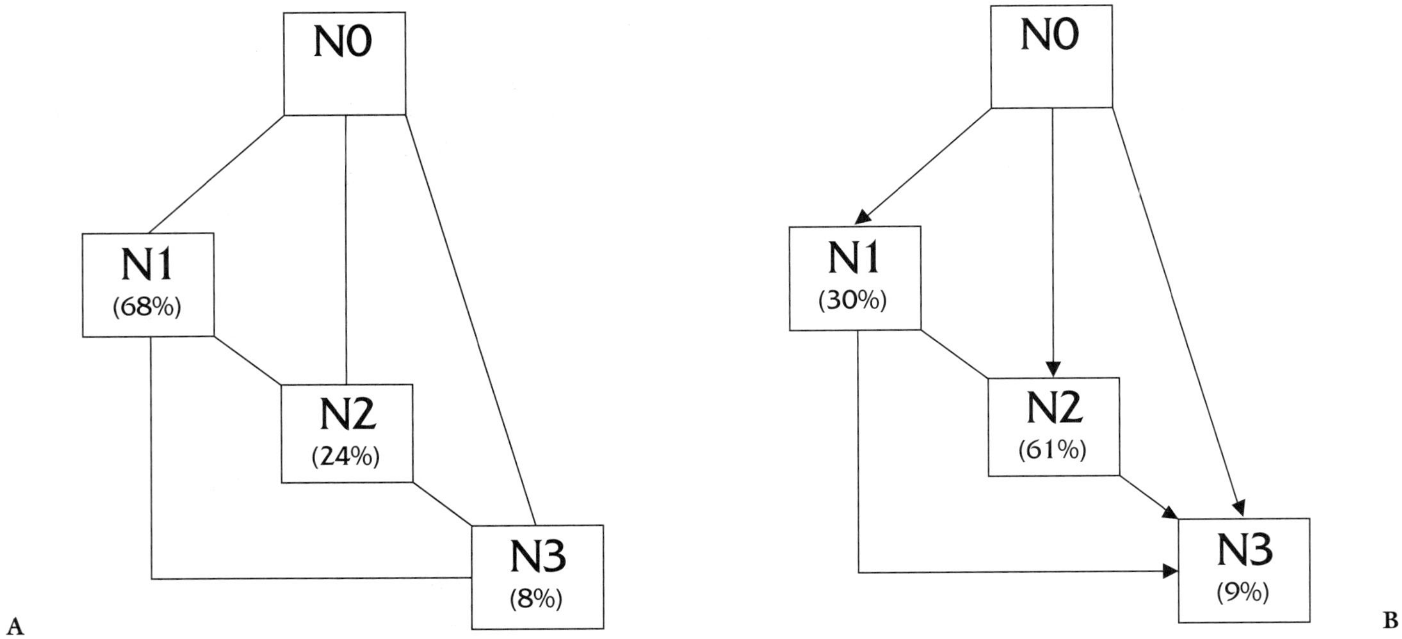

Figure 3–1 **(A)** Clinical findings in patients failing in the neck after observation for N0 neck. **(B)** Pathological findings in patients failing in the neck after observation for N0 neck.

Theoretically, the early identification and treatment of patients with metastatic squamous cell carcinoma to regional cervical lymph nodes will have a favorable impact on survival, but prospective studies have failed to confirm this association. However, improved disease-free survival has been observed in both prospective and retrospective analysis. Kligerman et al.[17] found that the disease-free survival increased from 49% to 72% with the addition of elective supraomohyoid neck dissection. Similarly, Fakih et al.[16] also reported increased disease-free survival with the addition of elective neck treatment (67% vs 47%). In summary, elective neck dissection helps in prognostication, identifies cases requiring adjuvant treatment, and improves initial disease control rates.

Selection of Patients Requiring Elective Treatment

No parameters have been established to identify patients reliably with clinically occult lymphatic metastasis. Most investigators have adopted an arbitrary cutoff of 10 to 15% incidence of occult nodal involvement to select patients requiring elective intervention. Decision analysis, based on the data from the available medical literature, suggests that a 20% risk should be the accepted threshold for providing treatment.[18]

The risk of occult regional lymphatic metastasis from primary squamous cell carcinomas of the upper aerodigestive tract can be assessed on the basis of anatomic location of the primary tumor, size, T stage, and histomorphologic characteristics (Table 3–1). In general, the risk of occult nodal metastasis increases from the anterior to posterior aspect of the upper aerodigestive tract (i.e. the lips, <5%; oral cavity, 19 to 50%; oropharynx, 22 to 66%; and hypopharynx, 38 to 77%.[1-3,19-22] For tumors of the larynx and pharynx, the risk of nodal metastasis increases as one progresses from the center of the laryngopharyngeal compartment to the periphery.[2,3,22,23] The risk of occult regional lymph node metastasis from carcinoma of the true vocal cord is exceedingly small, increasing as one progresses from the vocal cords to the false vocal cords, aryepiglottic fold (16 to 26%), pyriform sinus (38%), and pharyngeal wall (66%).[2,3,22,23] Within the oral cavity, a significantly higher risk of occult nodal metastases occurs in floor-of-mouth (40 to 50%), gingival (19%), and oral tongue cancers (25 to 54%) than those originating from the hard palate (<5%).[2,3,22,23] The risk of occult nodal metastases increases with increasing primary tumor burden at any site, as reflected by the T stage. The risk of nodal metastasis increases from <14% for T1 lesions to 30% for T2, 45% for T3, and 55 to 75% for T4 lesions. Occult involvement increases from 19% for T1 and T2 lesions to 26 to 32% of T3 and T4.[1-3,5,24]

Certain histomorphologic features of the primary tumor also predict an increased risk of nodal metastasis. Endophytic tumors are more inclined to metastasize than are exophytic tumors. It has been well documented that for tongue and floor-of-mouth cancers, tumor thickness is related to the risk of nodal metastases, with a 7.5% prevalence of occult metastasis for tumors <2 mm thick compared with 26% for 2–8 mm tumors and 42% for those >8 mm in thickness[25] (Table 3–2). Similarly, Fukano and his colleagues showed clinically negative necks turned out pathologically positive in 30% of cases with <5 mm depth of invasion, compared with 43% when the tumor depth was >5 mm.[26] Poorly differentiated carcinomas are associated with a higher risk of nodal metastasis compared with well-differentiated lesions. In addition, such factors as tumor–host interface have been suggested to be predictive of risk.[27]

Augmentation of clinical examination with various radiologic studies, including computed tomography (CT) (66%), magnetic resonance imaging (MRI) (75%), and ultrasound examination (68%), enhances the accuracy with which those patients who have nodal metastasis can be identified.[28-39] Although a 92% accuracy rate for identifying cervical metastasis is reported with the use of positron emission tomography (PET) scanning, it is tainted by sample size constraints.[38] The use of sentinel node biopsy and molecular assessment for occult metastasis also remains both limited and variable in efficacy.[40-43] The presence of metastasis that is missed on routine pathologic examination is confirmed in studies using supplemental subserial sectioning, immunohistochemistry, or molecular analysis.

An additional 8% of cases with metastasis in regional lymph nodes were identified by Ambroch and Brink[44] on serial sectioning of lymph nodes reported as negative on routine pathologic

TABLE 3–1

Risk Factors for Micrometastasis in Head and Neck Squamous Cell Carcinomas

Anatomic location
Size
T stage
Depth of invasion
Type of host–tumor interface
Endophytic growth pattern

TABLE 3–2

Relationship between Tumor Thickness and Development of Lymph Node Metastasis and Survival in Patients with T1 or T2 Oral, Tongue, and Floor-of-Mouth Carcinomas

	With Lymph Node Metastasis (%)	Dead of Disease (%)
<2 mm	13	3
2–9 mm	46	17
>9 mm	65	35

examination in N0 necks. Most strikingly, Brennan et al.[42] identified a 21% rate on missed lymphatic metastasis, using p53 mutation analysis. Finally, mathematical models, attempting to combine all available information, and molecular studies, attempting to identify patients at increased risk of occult metastasis, have also met with variable results.[19,45] Overall, even with the use of supplemental studies, no reliable methods have been identified for accurate prediction of the presence of nodal metastasis in individual patients with clinically undetectable disease. Accordingly, selection of patients for elective treatment continues to be made on the basis of arbitrary criteria.

Treatment Modality

Lymphatic basins at risk of metastasis can be managed effectively with either surgery or radiation therapy.[3,6,10,15-18,20,22,46-58] The selection of the appropriate modality should follow other tumor parameters. In patients with locally advanced lesions requiring adjunctive treatment, the neck can be effectively managed with radiation therapy alone. Studies have shown a >90% control rate of micrometastasis with the use of elective irradiation.[18,22,47-49,52-54,56,57] However, several questions remain regarding the use of radiation in this setting. Critics of the use of radiation therapy note that, in addition to the lack of valuable prognostic pathologic information, the reported failure rate of 10% in the setting of elective treatment for occult metastasis indicates a 33% failure rate, as only about 30% of cases treated in this manner actually have micrometastasis. Proponents of elective radiation therapy counter with the finding that the control rate with radiation in patients without recurrence at the primary site is 96 to 99%, extrapolating that radiation is highly effective in the setting of N0 necks.[22,53,54,56]

Surgical management of the neck should be considered in patients treated surgically for primary lesions that do not require adjunctive radiation. The extent of neck surgery should be guided by the location of the primary lesion. Given the significant functional and aesthetic morbidity after classic radical neck dissection, modifying the operation to reduce morbidity without compromising regional control rates or survival is indicated.[23] In the setting of elective treatment of the neck, it is seldom necessary to perform a comprehensive neck dissection to excise all five levels of lymph nodes.[1-5,23,24,52,59] Because cervical lymph node metastasis to the first echelon lymph nodes occurs in a predictable and sequential fashion, elective neck dissection can be limited to addressing only the lymph node groups at highest risk in a given primary site (Fig. 3–2). The use of selective neck dissections, instead of radical neck procedures, in the management of patients at risk of occult nodal metastasis achieves similar control rates, as confirmed in a prospective analysis. A prospective randomized study in Brazil, looking at 148 patients with oral cancers, found no differences in regional control (19 vs 16 neck failures) or survival (63% vs 67%) in patients treated with selective neck dissections as compared with those undergoing modified radical neck dissection.[46] In order to achieve comparable regional control rates, however, postoperative radiation therapy should be employed for the appropriate indications, including metastasis to multiple nodes and the presence of extracapsular spread. The dissection of lymph node levels in selective neck dissections is con-

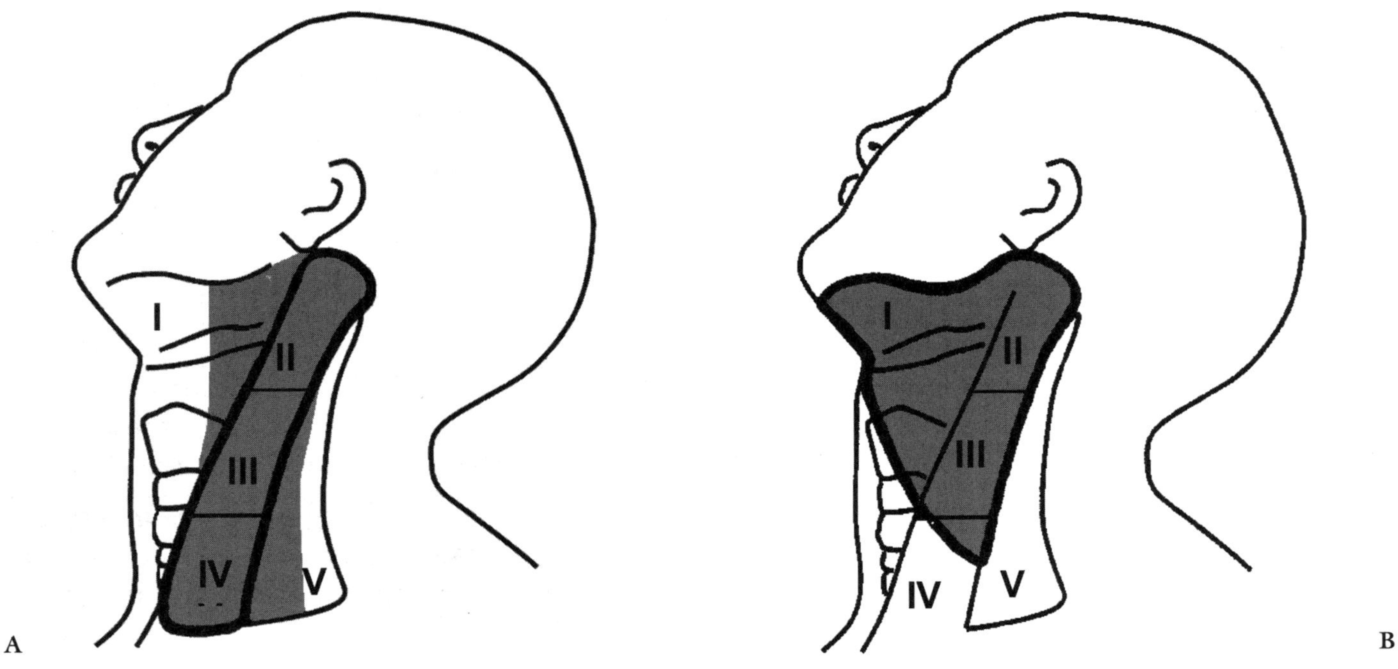

Figure 3–2 First echelon lymph nodes at risk for micrometastasis in head and neck squamous cell carcinomas. **(A)** Removed as part of a lateral neck dissection for laryngopharyngeal primaries. **(B)** Removed as part of a supraomohyoid neck dissection for oral cavity primaries.

sidered a staging procedure by most investigators, although some argue that selective neck dissections may be therapeutic in certain settings.[1-5,10,24,52,60] Nonetheless, the histologic information derived from the study of the excised lymph nodes facilitates selection of adjuvant therapy in patients at increased risk of neck failure, sparing the need for a morbid operation or adjuvant radiotherapy in others who are at reduced risk.

For primary tumors in the oral cavity, the regional lymph nodes at highest risk of early dissemination by metastatic cancer are limited to levels I, II, and III.[1,2,5,21,24,52,58,61] Anatomically, this translates into regional lymph node groups contained within the supraomohyoid triangle of the neck, including the submental, submandibular, prevascular facial, jugulodigastric, upper deep jugular, superior spinal accessory chain of lymph nodes, and mid-jugular lymph nodes. Skip metastasis to levels IV and V in the absence of metastatic disease at levels I, II, or III occurs in fewer than 5% of cases at the time of the initial procedure.[1,2,21,58] Therefore, if the neck is clinically negative, level IV and V lymph nodes are generally not at risk of harboring micrometastasis from primary squamous cells carcinomas of the oral cavity. The distribution of metastasis can be evaluated effectively by means of a supraomohyoid neck dissection.

Several investigators have questioned the true extent of nodal excision in a supraomohyoid neck dissection. One study questioned the benefit of dissection of the supraspinal accessory lymph nodes as part of the procedure, reporting only a single case in which metastasis was identified in this region, which also contained coexistent metastasis at level II of the neck.[62] Dissection and retraction along the accessory nerve can be minimized if the supraspinal accessory nodes do not require excision, but this limitation in dissection requires further corroboration. A study conducted by Byers et al.[63] reported a failure rate of 15% outside the traditional confines of a supraomohyoid neck dissection. These workers advocated the extension of the neck dissection to include level IV of the neck. The efficacy of this extension in limiting neck nodal recurrence needs to be confirmed.

For tumors on the lateral aspect of the oropharynx, hypopharynx, and larynx, the first echelon lymph nodes at highest risk of harboring micrometastasis in the clinically negative neck are the deep jugular lymph nodes at levels II, III, and IV on the ipsilateral side.[1,3,21] The lymph node groups in the deep jugular chain are jugulodigastric, highest spinal accessory chain of lymph nodes, mid-jugular lymph nodes, juguloomohyoid lymph nodes, and supraclavicular lymph nodes deep to the sternocleidomastoid muscle. Contiguous lymph nodes lateral to the internal jugular vein overlying the cutaneous roots of the cervical plexus are usually considered a component of levels II, III, and IV. In patients with primary carcinoma of the oropharynx with a clinically negative neck the risk of micrometastasis to levels I and V is exceedingly low. Skip metastasis to levels I and V in the absence of disease at levels II, III, or IV is usually not seen. Primary tumors that involve both sides of the midline have a potential of microscopic dissemination of metastatic disease to jugular lymph nodes on both sides of the neck. A jugular or lateral neck dissection, which encompasses the removal of all lymph nodes in levels II, III, and IV in the neck, is ideally suited for tumors in these anatomic locations.

Overall, selective neck dissections in patients with N0 neck provide accurate pathologic staging of the regional lymph nodes at risk of having micrometastasis and offer regional control rates comparable to those obtained with more radical operative procedures.

Conclusion

The advent of new diagnostic techniques, molecular analysis, and more accurate imaging may help identify patients with clinically undetectable lymphatic metastasis in the future. At present, however, elective treatment of lymph nodes at high risk of micrometastasis from upper aerodigestive tract cancers is warranted. Treatment should be undertaken when the risk of occult metastasis exceeds 10 to 15%. Effective treatment can be provided by means of either radiation therapy or surgery. Selective neck dissections are considered adequate for identifying lymph nodes with occult metastasis. Adjuvant radiotherapy is warranted in cases displaying the appropriate indications. The lack of improvement in survival in the patient population with occult nodal metastasis can be attributed to several factors, including false-negative pathologic examinations and inadequate adjuvant treatment. The inadequacy of currently available adjuvant treatment is shown by the lack of benefit of adjuvant chemotherapy in patients with extracapsular spread associated with lymphatic metastasis. The identification of the entire population of patients with occult metastasis and the use of directed novel adjuvant treatment, and thereby improvement in survival, remain high priorities in head and neck oncology.

REFERENCES

Singh and Shah—CHAPTER 3

1. Shah JP. Patterns of cervical lymph node metastasis from squamous carcinomas of the upper aerodigestive tract. *Am J Surg* 1990;160:405–409
2. Shah JP, Candela FC, Poddar AK. The patterns of cervical lymph node metastases from squamous carcinoma of the oral cavity. *Cancer* 1990;66:109–113
3. Shah JP, Medina JE, Shaha AR, et al. Cervical lymph node metastasis. *Curr Probl Surg* 1993;30:1–335
4. Byers RM. Neck dissection: concepts, controversies, and technique. *Semin Surg Oncol* 1991;7:9–13
5. Byers RM, Wolf PF, Ballantyne AJ. Rationale for elective modified neck dissection. *Head Neck Surg* 1988;10:160–167

6. Hughes CJ, Gallo O, Spiro RH, et al. Management of occult neck metastases in oral cavity squamous carcinoma. *Am J Surg* 1993;166:380–383
7. Jesse RH, Barkley HT Jr., Lindberg RD, et al. Cancer of the oral cavity. Is elective neck dissection beneficial? *Am J Surg* 1970;120:505–508
8. Traynor SJ, Cohen JI, Gray J, et al. Selective neck dissection and the management of the node-positive neck. *Am J Surg* 1996;172:654–657
9. Vandenbrouck C, Sancho-Garnier H, Chassagne D, et al. Elective versus therapeutic radical neck dissection in epidermoid carcinoma of the oral cavity: results of a randomized clinical trial. *Cancer* 1980;46:386–390
10. Pitman KT, Johnson JT, Myers EN. Effectiveness of selective neck dissection for management of the clinically negative neck. *Arch Otolaryngol Head Neck Surg* 1997;123:917–922
11. Breau RL, Suen JY. Management of the N0 neck. *Otolaryngol Clin North Am* 1998;31:657–669
12. Tulenko J, Priore RL, Hoffmeister FS. Cancer of the tongue. Comments on surgical treatment. *Am J Surg* 1966;112: 562–568
13. Alvi A, Johnson JT. Extracapsular spread in the clinically negative neck (N0): implications and outcome. *Otolaryngol Head Neck Surg* 1996;114:65–70
14. Andersen PE, Cambronero E, Shaha AR, et al. The extent of neck disease after regional failure during observation of the N0 neck. *Am J Surg* 1996;172:689–691
15. Fakih AR, Rao RS, Borges AM, et al. Elective versus therapeutic neck dissection in early carcinoma of the oral tongue. *Am J Surg* 1989;158:309–313
16. Fakih AR, Rao RS, Patel AR. Prophylactic neck dissection in squamous cell carcinoma of oral tongue: a prospective randomized study. *Semin Surg Oncol* 1989;5:327–330
17. Kligerman J, Lima RA, Soares JR, et al. Supraomohyoid neck dissection in the treatment of T1/T2 squamous cell carcinoma of oral cavity. *Am J Surg* 1994;168:391–394
18. Weiss MH, Harrison LB, Isaacs RS. Use of decision analysis in planning a management strategy for the stage N0 neck. *Arch Otolaryngol Head Neck Surg* 1994;120:699–702
19. Okamoto M, Ozeki S, Watanabe T, et al. Cervical lymph node metastasis in carcinoma of the tongue. Correlation between clinical and histopathological findings and metastasis. *J Craniomaxillofac Surg* 1988;16:31–34
20. McGuirt WF Jr, Johnson JT, Myers EN, et al. Floor of mouth carcinoma. The management of the clinically negative neck. *Arch Otolaryngol Head Neck Surg* 1995;121:278–282
21. Lindberg R. Distribution of cervical lymph node metastases from squamous cell carcinoma of the upper respiratory and digestive tracts. *Cancer* 1972;29:1446–1449
22. Mendenhall WM, Million RR, Cassisi NJ. Elective neck irradiation in squamous-cell carcinoma of the head and neck. *Head Neck Surg* 1980;3:15–20
23. Shah JP, Andersen PE. The impact of patterns of nodal metastasis on modifications of neck dissection. *Ann Surg Oncol* 1994;1:521–532
24. Byers RM. Modified neck dissection. A study of 967 cases from 1970 to 1980. *Am J Surg* 1985;150:414–421
25. Spiro RH, Huvos AG, Wong GY, et al. Predictive value of tumor thickness in squamous carcinoma confined to the tongue and floor of the mouth. *Am J Surg* 1986;152: 345–350
26. Fukano H, Matsuura H, Hasegawa Y, et al. Depth of invasion as a predictive factor for cervical lymph node metastasis in tongue carcinoma. *Head Neck* 1997;19:205–210
27. Yamamoto E, Miyakawa A, Kohama G. Mode of invasion and lymph node metastasis in squamous cell carcinoma of the oral cavity. *Head Neck Surg* 1984;6:938–947
28. van den Brekel MW, Castelijns JA, Stel HV, et al. Occult metastatic neck disease: detection with US and US-guided fine-needle aspiration cytology. *Radiology* 1991;180:457–461
29. Watkinson JC, Todd CE, Paskin L, et al. Metastatic carcinoma in the neck: a clinical, radiological, scintigraphic and pathological study. *Clin Otolaryngol* 1991;16:187–192
30. Feinmesser R, Freeman JL, Feinmesser M, et al. Role of modern imaging in decision-making for elective neck dissection. *Head Neck* 1992;14:173–176
31. Van Den Brekel MW, Snow GB, Castelijns JA. MRI in cervical lymph node staging. *J Otolaryngol* 1990;19:358–359
32. van den Brekel MW, Castelijns JA, Stel HV, et al. Detection and characterization of metastatic cervical adenopathy by MR imaging: comparison of different MR techniques. *J Comput Assist Tomogr* 1990;14:581–589
33. van den Brekel MW, Stel HV, Castelijns JA, et al. Lymph node staging in patients with clinically negative neck examinations by ultrasound and ultrasound-guided aspiration cytology. *Am J Surg* 1991;162:362–366
34. van den Brekel MW, Castelijns JA, Croll GA, et al. Magnetic resonance imaging vs palpation of cervical lymph node. *Arch Otolaryngol Head Neck Surg* 1991;117:663–673
35. van den Brekel MW, Castelijns JA, Stel HV, et al. Modern imaging techniques and ultrasound-guided aspiration cytology for the assessment of neck node metastases: a prospective comparative study. *Eur Arch Otorhinolaryngol* 1993;250:11–17
36. van den Brekel MW, Castelijns JA, Snow GB. Detection of lymph node metastases in the neck: radiologic criteria. *Radiology* 1994;192:617–618
37. van den Brekel MW, van der Waal I, Meijer CJ, et al. The incidence of micrometastases in neck dissection specimens obtained from elective neck dissections. *Laryngoscope* 1996;106:987–991
38. Myers LL, Wax MK, Nabi H, Simpson GT, Lamonica D. Positron emission tomography in the evaluation of the N0 neck. *Laryngoscope* 1998;108:232–236
39. Yucel T, Saatci I, Sennaroglu L, et al. MR imaging in squamous cell carcinoma of the head and neck with no palpable lymph nodes. *Acta Radiol* 1997;38:810–814
40. Pitman KT, Johnson JT, Edington H, et al. Lymphatic mapping with isosulfan blue dye in squamous cell carcinoma of the head and neck. *Arch Otolaryngol Head Neck Surg* 1998;124: 790–793
41. Koch WM, Choti MA, Civelek AC, et al. Gamma probe-directed biopsy of the sentinel node in oral squamous cell carcinoma. *Arch Otolaryngol Head Neck Surg* 1998;124: 455–459

42. Brennan JA, Mao L, Hruban RH, et al. Molecular assessment of histopathological staging in squamous-cell carcinoma of the head and neck. *N Engl J Med* 1995;332:429–435
43. Fortin A, Guerry M, Guerry R, et al. Chromosome 11q13 gene amplifications in oral and oropharyngeal carcinomas: no correlation with subclinical lymph node invasion and disease recurrence. *Clin Cancer Res* 1997;3:1609–1614
44. Ambroch P, Brink U. Detection of nodal micrometastasis in head and neck cancer by serial sectioning and immunostaining. *Oncology* 1996;10:1221–1226
45. Gray L, Robbins KT, Byers R. Multidimensional scaling of head and neck metastases. *Int J Biomed Comput* 1992;31:177–187
46. Brazilian Head and Neck Cancer Study Group. Results of a prospective trial on elective modified radical classical versus supraomohyoid neck dissection in the management of oral squamous carcinoma. *Am J Surg* 1998;176:422–427
47. Bataini JP. Radiotherapy in N0 head and neck cancer patients. *Eur Arch Otorhinolaryngol* 1993;250:442–445
48. Berger DS, Fletcher GH, Lindberg RD, et al. Elective irradiation of the neck lymphatics for squamous cell carcinomas of the nasopharynx and oropharynx. *AJR* 1971;111:66–72
49. Eschwege F, Bridier A, Luboinski B. Principles and techniques of irradiation for the N0 neck. *Eur Arch Otorhinolaryngol* 1993;250:439–441
50. Kligerman J, Olivatto LO, Lima RA, et al. Elective neck dissection in the treatment of T3/T4 N0 squamous cell carcinoma of the larynx. *Am J Surg* 1995;170:436–469
51. Lenz M, Kersting-Sommerhoff B, Gross M. Diagnosis and treatment of the N0 neck in carcinomas of the upper aerodigestive tract: current status of diagnostic procedures. *Eur Arch Otorhinolaryngol* 1993;250:432–438
52. Medina JE, Byers RM. Supraomohyoid neck dissection: rationale, indications, and surgical technique. *Head Neck* 1989;11:111–122
53. Mendenhall WM, Million RR. Elective neck irradiation for squamous cell carcinoma of the head and neck: analysis of time-dose factors and causes of failure. *Int J Radiat Oncol Biol Phys* 1986;12:741–746
54. Mendenhall WM, Parsons JT, Million RR. Elective lower neck irradiation: 5000 cGy/25 fractions versus 4050 cGy/15 fractions. *Int J Radiat Oncol Biol Phys* 1988;15:439–440
55. Mendenhall WM, Parsons JT, Brant TA, et al. Is elective neck treatment indicated for T2N0 squamous cell carcinoma of the glottic larynx? *Radiother Oncol* 1989;14:199–202
56. Million RR. Elective neck irradiation for TXN0 squamous carcinoma of the oral tongue and floor of mouth. *Cancer* 1974;34:149–155
57. Shasha D, Harrison LB. Elective irradiation of the N0 neck in squamous cell carcinoma of the upper aerodigestive tract. *Otolaryngol Clin North Am* 1998;31:803–813
58. Spiro RH, Morgan GJ, Strong EW, et al. Supraomohyoid neck dissection. *Am J Surg* 1996;172:650–653
59. Lingeman RE, Helmus C, Stephens R, et al. Neck dissection: radical or conservative. *Ann Otol Rhinol Laryngol* 1977;86:737–744
60. Davidson J, Khan Y, Gilbert R, et al. Is selective neck dissection sufficient treatment for the N0/Np+ neck? *J Otolaryngol* 1997;26:229–231
61. Byers RM, El-Naggar AK, Lee YY, et al. Can we detect or predict the presence of occult nodal metastases in patients with squamous carcinoma of the oral tongue? *Head Neck* 1998;20:138–144
62. Kraus DH, Rosenberg DB, Davidson BJ, et al. Supraspinal accessory lymph node metastases in supraomohyoid neck dissection. *Am J Surg* 1996;172:646–649
63. Byers RM, Weber RS, Andrews T, et al. Frequency and therapeutic implications of "skip metastases" in the neck from squamous carcinoma of the oral tongue. *Head Neck* 1997;19:14–19

2

Management of Inverting Papilloma

"Intranasal approaches have been fraught with recurrences because these tumors are usually bulky, creating a difficult exposure. However, otolaryngologists have been gradually extending the indications for minimally invasive intranasal operations, including endoscopic techniques. Does endoscopic sinus surgery have the potential to lower the high recurrence rate associated with the intranasal approach to that of external techniques, on a consistent basis?"

William R. Panje

"The only reason to change management philosophy depends on equivalent or improved management techniques. Endoscopic diagnosis and surgery can improve our management of inverted papilloma. The use of endoscopic sinus surgery by experienced surgeons expands the management of inverted papilloma and allows for individualization of treatment."

James A. Stankiewicz

"Many authors do not advocate conservative therapy for the treatment of any inverting papilloma because of the high risk of recurrence and the effectiveness of a medial maxillectomy/lateral rhinotomy."

Steven D. Schaefer

Management of Inverting Papilloma

CHAPTER 4

William R. Panje and Joseph P. Allegretti

The nasal neoplastic disease entity known as inverting papilloma (IP), also called inverted papilloma, has long been a topic of intense debate because of its recurrent, destructive, and malignant potential. Traditionally, these tumors are approached externally to ensure adequate margins of resection. Intranasal approaches have been fraught with recurrences because these tumors are usually bulky, creating a difficult exposure. However, otolaryngologists have been gradually extending the indications for minimally invasive intranasal operations, including endoscopic techniques. Does endoscopic sinus surgery have the potential to lower the high recurrence rate associated with the intranasal approach to that of external techniques, on a consistent basis? This chapter presents the controversy surrounding the management of IP.

Historical Aspects

In 1854, Ward[1] first described a nasal papilloma. Billroth reported on a recurring nasal papilloma 1 year later, which he called villiform cancer; many others began to look at this peculiar entity that appeared to invert,[1-6] as examined microscopically. In his landmark paper in 1971, Hyams[1] clarified the confusion regarding the characteristic growth behavior of IP by demonstrating the prognostic significance of certain histologic features. Hyams showed that increased mitotic activity, hypercellularity, pleomorphism, and atypia are associated with more aggressive and recurrent tumors. Furthermore, these histologic findings are associated with an increased tendency toward synchronous and metachronous carcinoma. When surface keratinization and dyskeratosis are found, there is increased suspicion for squamous cell carcinoma.[1]

Incidence

IP typically occurs within a peak age range of 50 to 70 years, although it has been found in children as young as 8 years old.[7] It has a male preponderance, as shown in one large series, in which 83% of patients were men. IP is typically unilateral, but it may be bilateral in less than 10% of cases.[8] The etiology of IP is unknown; nonetheless, both human papillomavirus (HPV) and Epstein-Barr virus (EBV) have been demonstrated in IP specimens.[9,10] Squamous cell carcinoma occurs in association with IP in less than 2 to 56% of cases, although no study with more than 50 cases had a greater than 30% incidence of carcinoma, and most had less than 15%.[8,11-17]

Malignancy is often associated with aggressive growth, including intracranial, orbital, or mastoid invasion.[18-20] Moreover, Cummings and Goodman[4] noted a few cases in which transitional cell carcinomas were reclassified as IP. Clearly, the marked atypia found in aggressive IP can be misleading with regard to the true incidence of carcinoma, with a falsely higher incidence reported in the cases. In addition, most institutions that report these cases are tertiary care referral centers; thus, unusual cases are selected out, whereas less aggressive cases may never get into the literature.[21] Lastly, histologic detection of a synchronous cancer during IP excision was reported at 4 to 11% in directed studies.[16,22] It may be even less common to find metachronous carcinoma.[21] Nonetheless, long-term follow-up in one study demonstrated a 16% (8/51) incidence, with cancer detected as late as 13 years after the diagnosis of IP.[16] Myers et al.[23] demonstrated a gradation in atypia from papilloma to malignancy in 4 of 6 synchronous carcinomas. This observation would support the theory that IP can undergo malignant transformation.[23] Several molecular genetics studies have shown a convincing association between tumor pathogenesis and either HPV or p53 tumor suppressor gene interaction, or both.[24-27]

Site of Origin

The middle turbinate and medial maxilllary sinus wall are the most common sites of origin of IP.[8] A single focus is the most likely source of the tumor. Multicentricity was documented in only 7 of 149 cases by Hyams[1] and in 10 of 29 cases by Norris.[3] These findings would support the conclusion that incomplete excision is the cause of recurrence, and not delayed development of IP at another site. As for the paranasal sinuses, the ethmoid and maxillary sinuses are the major sinuses involved. Only 1% of cases involve the frontal sinuses. In rare cases, the tumor can be isolated to the sphenoid sinus.[28] Paranasal sinus involvement has been linked to an increased recurrence rate.[29]

However, this adverse association has been demonstrated in recent small studies to be surmountable with endoscopic sinus surgery. Furthermore, the sinuses tend to become involved secondary to nasal cavity tumors. Suh et al.[12] showed that in 49 of 57 cases both the nasal cavity and paranasal sinuses were involved; in only 2 of 59 cases was the sinus involved exclusively.

Histology

IP occurs when the Schneiderian membrane of the nose and paranasal sinuses inverts into the stroma in a pattern of endophytic growth.[30,31] Microcysts are often trapped within the epithelium. The Schneiderian membrane is composed of ciliated pseudostratified columnar epithelium. It starts 1 to 2 cm posterior to the nares at the mucocutaneous junction and is found in the nasal cavity and paranasal sinuses. The membrane is of ectodermal origin, unlike the nasopharyngeal mucosa, which is endodermal, but similar in appearance. Fungiform (usually from the nasal septum) and cylindrical cell papillomas are histologic variants of Schneiderian papillomas, managed similarly to IP.[32] The data reported by Hyams[1] showed recurrence in roughly one-half of patients with IP, regardless of the type.

Evaluation and Diagnosis

The most frequent presenting symptoms of IP are nasal obstruction (64 to 78%), followed by headache, epistaxis, facial pain, periorbital swelling, purulent rhinorrhea, chronic sinusitis, allergy, hyposmia, visual changes, and meningitis. Some patients are even asymptomatic. These signs and symptoms make IP difficult to distinguish from inflammatory disease.[11,30,33,34] Office endoscopic examination and computed tomographic (CT) imaging of the nose and paranasal sinuses are the gold standards of evaluation.[8] In contrast to the more translucent bilateral inflammatory polyps, IP is usually unilateral (although in rare cases it is bilateral), vascular, and bulky. However, IP often arises along with nasal polyps, making the diagnosis difficult. The surgeon should always submit operative specimens according to their site of origin, rather than as a combined specimen. IP can display bone invasion on a CT scan, even to the extent that skull base erosion occurs; this finding requires craniofacial resection despite no evidence of cancer.[7,15,35] As a whole, intracranial invasion is rare, found in only 5 of 1468 cases reviewed.[18] Snyder and Perzin[5] demonstrated bone erosion in 5 of 34 nonmalignant IP cases. However, in patients with cancer, bone erosion occurred in all cases. By contrast, 3 cases of malignancy in Rothfield's study showed no erosion.[36] IP can also cause sinusitis, which can lead to radiographic bony sclerosis. If a lesion suspicious for IP is seen on examination and is accessible, office biopsy can be performed. If the differentiation between inflammatory disease and tumor cannot be made on CT scan, this distinction can often be made by T_2-weighted magnetic resonance imaging (MRI). Inflammatory disease or mucus has a high signal intensity on MRI, whereas tumor has a more intermediate intensity.[29,37]

Management

SIMPLE INTRANASAL APPROACH AND EXTERNAL TECHNIQUES

The recurrence rate for IP has been reported to be as high as 35 to 78% for simple intranasal excision.[8,15,23,38] The average time to recurrence is relatively rapid, averaging 10 months in one series.[23] However, it has been shown to recur as much as 24 years later.[23] The widest exposure for complete excision is through an external approach. Some investigators have proposed the midfacial degloving approach, or the sublabial septal translocation.[39-41] Myers et al.[23] stated that the "lateral rhinotomy and en bloc excision of the lateral nasal wall, followed by meticulous removal of all additional mucosa in the ipsilateral paranasal sinuses, remains the standard therapy." This approach removes most of the Schneiderian membrane to which IP can extend. Bilateral rhinotomy naturally follows as the approach for bilateral IP.[42] These external resection methods have displayed recurrence rates within the range of 3 to 17%.[8,11,12,23,38] However, simple intranasal procedures with or without transantral sinusotomy have been advocated for "limited" tumors (see next section) that involve the turbinates and more accessible aspects of the ethmoid and sphenoid sinuses. This approach has not been advocated for tumors involving the maxillary or frontal sinus, where direct or microscopic anterior rhinoscopy has poor visualization.[15,43] In a recent update reviewing 112 patients, Lawson et al.[35] continue to support this approach.

ENDOSCOPIC TECHNIQUES

The introduction of endoscopic sinus surgery with angled telescopes and specialized instrumentation has further refined the intranasal approach and has been shown to have recurrence rate comparable to external methods of resection.[30,33,44-46] The endoscopic technique permits safe exposure of the entire maxillary sinus, and thus the possibility of complete IP excision. The endoscopic resection of IP can be performed on limited and select recurrent lesions, even when the prior procedure was a lateral rhinotomy approach. Microscopic verification of negative margins free of both IP and metaplasia should be obtained.[44] These indications are in contrast to those reported by Lawson et al.,[15] who stated that intranasal surgery should be performed only on nonrecurrent limited lesions of the lateral nasal wall with minimal extension into the ethmoid labyrinth. Waitz and Wigand[33] proposed the use of a diamond burr to sterilize the bone margins from the infiltrative edges of IP tumors. This endoscopic transnasal technique includes resection of the middle turbinate, making a wide middle meatal antrostomy, ethmoidectomy, and sphenoidotomy, if indicated. Moreover, the definition of limited lesions has been broadened with endoscopic capabilities, to include varying degrees of maxillary sinus involvement. Kamel[35,44] has proposed a transnasal endoscopic medial maxillectomy in which an extremely wide antrostomy is performed. The entire medial maxillary wall is removed, including the posterior two-thirds of the inferior turbinate and inferior meatus, and potentially the area anterior to the nasal lacrimal duct. The lamina papracea and medial orbital wall can be preserved.[44,47] If frozen section endoscopic biopsy detects carcinoma, depending on the extent of the tumor, an external technique is warranted, employing a lateral rhinotomy and possible maxillectomy. This procedure can be followed by radiation therapy.

Stereotactic computer-aided endoscopic sinus surgery should further improve safety, completeness of endoscopic resection, and operative time.[48] Fried et al.[49] introduced a new electromagnetic localizer in the InstaTrak System (Visualization Technologies, Inc., Wilmington, MA), which has become increasingly commonplace for difficult endoscopic sinus procedures. Endoscopic approaches generally avoid the complications of external operations, including external facial scars, nasal collapse, epiphora, dacryocystitis, transient blepharitis, lid edema, diplopia, nasocutaneous fistula, longer hospitalization, and more blood loss.[7,44,47] The endoscopic sinus surgery approach has been shown to have recurrence rates comparable to those of external techniques (<25%). Long-term follow-up evaluation is needed to confirm this finding. Kamel[44] reported no recurrences after endoscopic removal in 17 cases. His study was followed up for 43 months in the nasal cavity–exclusive group, but for only 28 months for the maxillary sinus–inclusive patients. Nonetheless, these results are impressive. Waitz and Wigand reported a 17% recurrence rate in 35 endoscopic surgical cases, with an average follow-up of 46 months.[33] Stankiewicz and Girgis[45] performed endoscopic procedures in 15 cases without maxillary sinus involvement; the recurrence rate was 20% over an average follow-up period of 36 months. Thus, the three recent endoscopic resection studies with 17, 35, and 15 patients, respectively, had a combined recurrence rate of 13% (9/67) with an average follow-up range of 28 to 46 months.[33,44,45]

When the frontal sinus shows tumor involvement, endoscopic resection alone is generally not indicated, for fear of incomplete resection. Several articles in the literature mention an external approach to IP in the frontal sinus.[5,13,15,23,29,35,50] In two cases, Shohet and Duncavage[29] specifically proposed performing an osteoplastic flap with mucosal resection and drill sterilization. In their approach, the sinus is not obliterated, in order to permit follow-up imaging and endoscopic examinations. The nasofrontal ducts are opened with a mastoid drill. A 14 Fr polyethylene suction catheter is then left in place in the ducts for 2 weeks. Evaluation at 11 months and 24 months for each case, respectively, demonstrated no evidence of disease on follow-up CT scan.[29]

In following IP patients after resection, frequent nasal endoscopy is indicated for early detection of recurrence. Either CT or MRI, or both, are helpful in determining the extent of recurrence. Follow-up management of the patient on a continuing basis is recommended.

Finally, some investigators have proposed the use of radiation therapy for patients with aggressive recurrent IP or for those with medically inoperative health status. Follow-up of patients for 4.5 to 20 years after treatment consisting of radiation therapy alone (3 of 7 patients) or in combination with surgery after positive margins (4 of 7), was encouraging, with recurrence in only 1 patient.[51]

Conclusion

The endoscopic approach to IP management appears to offer an alternative to direct visual or external ablative techniques. Regardless of the approach, the experience of the surgeon plays a major role in successful outcome. Recurrence after initial endoscopic removal of IP warrants strong consideration for an external approach. The use of irradiation in the treatment of IP should be reserved for recurrent aggressive tumors, including multiple recurrences and squamous cell cancer changes. Perhaps in the future, molecular markers such as HPV type–specific primers and p53 detected on biopsies and margins will help guide the aggressiveness of our treatment.

REFERENCES

Panje and Allegretti—CHAPTER 4

1. Hyams VJ. Papillomas of the nasal cavity and paranasal sinuses: a clinicopathologic study of 315 cases. *Ann Otol Rhinol Laryngol* 1971;80:192–206
2. Skolnik EM, Loewy A, Friedman JE. Inverted papilloma of the nasal cavity. *Arch Otolaryngol* 1966;84:61–67
3. Norris HJ. Papillary lesions of the nasal cavity and paranasal sinuses. Part II: Inverting papillomas. A study of 29 cases. *Laryngoscope* 1963;73:1–17
4. Cummings CW, Goodman M. Inverting papilloma of the nose and paranasal sinuses: report of 20 cases. *Arch Otolaryngol* 1970;92:445–449
5. Snyder RN, Perzin KH. Papillomatosis of nasal cavity and paranasal sinuses (inverted papilloma, squamous papilloma): a clinicopathologic study. *Cancer* 1972;30:668–690
6. Calcaterra TC, Thompson JW, Paglia DE. Inverting papilloma of the nose and paranasal sinuses. *Laryngoscope* 1980;90:53–60
7. Graham SM, Gross CW, Manning SC. Management of inverted papilloma. *Head Neck* 1995;March/April:148–151
8. Momose KJ, Weber AL, Goodman M et al. Radiological aspects of inverted papilloma. *Radiology* 1980;134:73–79
9. MacDonald MR, Le KT, Freeman JL, et al. A majority of inverted sinonasal papillomas carries Epstein-Barr virus. *Cancer* 1995;75:2307–2312
10. Harris MO, Beck JC, Terrell JE, et al. Expression of human papillomavirus 6 in inverted papilloma arising in a renal transplant recipient. *Laryngoscope* 1998;108:115–119
11. Phillips PP, Gustafson RO, Facer, GW. The clinical behavior of inverting papilloma of the nose and paranasal sinuses: report

of 112 cases and review of the literature. *Laryngoscope* 1990;100:463–469
12. Suh KW, Facer GW, Devine KD, et al. Inverting papilloma of the nose and paranasal sinuses. *Laryngoscope* 1977;87:35–46
13. Vrabec DP. The inverted Schneiderian papilloma: a clinical and pathological entity. *Laryngoscope* 1975;85:186–220
14. Fechner RE, Alford DO. Inverted papilloma and squamous cell carcinoma. *Arch Otolaryngol* 1968;88:507–512
15. Lawson W, Biller HF, Jacobson A, et al. The role of conservative surgery in the management of inverted papilloma. *Laryngoscope* 1983;93:148–155
16. Lesperance MM, Esclamado RM. Squamous cell carcinoma arising in inverted papilloma. *Laryngoscope* 1995;105:178–183
17. Buchwald C, Franzmann MB, Tos M. Sinonasal papillomas: a report of 82 cases in Copenhagen county, including a longitudinal epidemiological and clinical study. *Laryngoscope* 1995;105:72–79
18. Miller PJ, Jacobs J, Roland JT Jr, et al. Intracranial inverting papilloma. *Head Neck* 1996;18:450–454
19. Elner VM, Burnstine MA, Goodman ML, et al. Inverted papillomas that invade the orbit. *Arch Ophthalmol* 1995;113: 1178–1183
20. Seshul MJ, Eby TL, Crowe DR, et al. Nasal inverted papilloma with involvement of middle ear and mastoid. *Arch Otolaryngol* 1995;121:1045–1048
21. Woodson GE, Robbins KT, Michaels L. Inverted papilloma. *Arch Otolaryngol* 1985;111:806–811
22. Osborn DA. Nature and behavior of transitional tumors in the upper respiratory tract. *Cancer* 1970;25:50–60
23. Myers EN, Schramm VL, Barnes EL. Management of inverted papilloma of the nose and paranasal sinuses. *Laryngoscope* 1981;91:2071–2084
24. Harris MO, Beck JC, Lancaster W, et al. The HPV 6 E6/E7 transforming genes are expressed in inverted papilloma. *Otolaryngol Head Neck Surg* 1998;118:312–318
25 Mirza N, Montone K, Sato Y, et al. Identification of p53 and human papilloma virus in Schneiderian papillomas. *Laryngoscope* 1998;108:497–501
26 Franzmann MB, Buchwald C, Jacobsen GK, et al. Expression of p53 in normal nasal mucosa and in sinonasal papillomas with and without associated carcinoma and the relation to human papillomavirus (HPV). *Cancer Lett* 1998;128: 161–164
27. Beck JC, McClatchey KD, Lesperance MM, et al. Human papillomavirus types important in progression of inverted papilloma. *Otolaryngol Head Neck Surg* 1995;113:558–563
28. Peters BW, O'Reilly RC, Wilcox TO Jr, et al. Inverted papilloma isolated to the sphenoid sinus. *Otolaryngol Head Neck Surg* 1995;113:771–777
29. Shohet JA, Duncavage JA. Management of the frontal sinus with inverted papilloma. *Otolaryngol Head Neck Surg* 1996; 114:649–652
30. McCary WS, Gross CW, Reibel JF, et al. Preliminary report: endoscopic versus external surgery in the management of inverted papilloma. *Laryngoscope* 1994;104:415–419
31. Batsakis JG. Nasal (Schneiderian) papillomas. *Ann Otol Rhinol Laryngol* 1981;90:190–191
32. Wenig BM. *Atlas of Head and Neck Pathology*. Philadelphia: WB Saunders; 1993:29–34
33. Waitz G, Wigand ME. Results of endoscopic sinus surgery for the treatment of inverted papillomas. *Laryngoscope* 1992;102: 917–922
34. Granet KM, Movva SR, Jaeger J. Inverting papilloma presenting with meningitis. *Laryngoscope*1996;106:688
35. Lawson W, Ho BT, Biller HF. Inverted papilloma: a report of 112 cases. *Laryngoscope* 1985;105:282–288
36. Rothfield P, Shapiro R, Lasser A, et al. Epithelial (inverted) papilloma—a correlated radiological, histological study. *Clin Radiol* 1977;28:539–544
37. Roobottom CA, Jewell FM, Kabala J. Primary and recurrent inverting papilloma: appearances with magnetic resonance imaging. *Clin Radiol* 1995;50:472–475
38. Ridolfi RL, Lieberman PH, Erlandson RA, et al. Schneiderian papillomas: a clinicopathologic study of 30 cases. *Am J Clin Pathol* 1977;1:43–53
39. Sacks ME, Conley J, Rabuzzi DD, et al. Degloving approach for total excision of inverted papilloma. *Laryngoscope* 1984;94: 1595–1598
40. Sofferman RA. The septal translocation procedure: an alternative to lateral rhinotomy. *Otolaryngol Head Neck Surg* 1988;98:18–25
41. Maniglia AJ, Phillips DA. Midfacial degloving for the management of nasal, sinus, and skull-base neoplasms. *Otolaryngol Clin North Am* 1995;28:1127–1143
42. Hosal SA, Freeman JL. Bilateral lateral rhinotomy for resection of bilateral inverted papilloma. *Otolaryngol Head Neck Surg* 1996;114:103–105
43. Outzen KE, Grontveld A, Jorgensen K, et al. Inverted papilloma: incidence and late results of surgical treatment. *Rhinology* 1996;34:114–118
44. Kamel RH. Transnasal endoscopic medial maxillectomy in inverted papilloma. *Laryngoscope* 1995;105:847–853
45. Stankiewicz JA, Girgis SJ. Endoscopic surgical treatment of nasal and paranasal sinus inverted papilloma. *Otolaryngol Head Neck Surg* 1993;109:988–995
46. Stammberger H. Zum invertierten Papillom der Nasenschleimhaut. *Head Neck Otolaryngol* 1981;29:128–133
47. Kamel RH. Conservative endoscopic surgery in inverted papilloma. *Arch Otolaryngol Head Neck Surg* 1992;118:649–653
48. Anon JB. Computer-aided endoscopic sinus surgery. *Laryngoscope* 1998;108:949–961
49. Fried MP, Kleefield J, Gopal H, et al. Image-guided endoscopic surgery: results of accuracy and performance in a multicenter clinical study using an electromagnetic tracking system. *Laryngoscope* 1997;107:594–601
50. Vrabec DP. The inverted Schneiderian papilloma: a 25-year study. *Laryngoscope* 1994;104:582–605
51. Guedia F, Mendenhall W, Parsons J, et al. The role of radiation therapy in inverted papilloma of the nasal cavity and paranasal sinuses. *Int J Radiat Oncol* 1991;220:777–880

Management of Inverting Papilloma*

CHAPTER 5

James A. Stankiewicz

Inverting papilloma is a benign tumor of the nose and paranasal sinuses, which in a small percentage of patients can convert into or hide an associated squamous cell carcinoma. If not completely removed, inverting papilloma will recur and long-term tumor control may become a problem. This lesion has a tendency to move from one sinus to another, requiring that adjacent sinuses be checked for spread of tumor. Therefore, inverting papilloma must be completely removed using surgical principles of tumor removal. The "gold standard" for the treatment of inverting papilloma affecting the maxillary and ethmoid sinuses is the extranasal medial maxillectomy. This standard was largely established before the advent of endoscopic nasal and sinus surgery. However, considering the improved lighting and visualization provided by the endoscope, along with current state-of-the-art imaging techniques, it can be argued that there is a role for endoscopic diagnosis and treatment in the management of inverting papilloma, hence the controversy—gold standard extranasal medial maxillectomy versus endoscopic techniques for intranasal excision of inverting papilloma.

Background

Several articles have showed the benefit of extranasal medial maxillectomy versus intranasal removal of inverted papilloma affecting either the ethmoid or maxillary sinuses, or both.[1-6] Before the advent of the use of endoscopes for nasal and sinus diagnosis and surgery, there was no better way to control inverting papilloma, hence the need for extranasal medial maxillectomy. Treatment trials using a Caldwell–Luc operation and intranasal removal were not as successful as the extranasal medial maxillectomy.[7,8] Extranasal medial maxillectomy recurrence rates were 9 to 42% versus 10 to 100% intranasally.[2-10] Adding to the problem was information from Vrabec[6] that a follow-up of at least 6 years was necessary to ensure local control. These data led to reflection on why extranasal surgery recurrences in some cases were as low as 10% and as high as 42% and on why intranasal surgery recurrences were as low as 10% and as high as 100%. The answers lie in the location of tumor, the surgeries done, and the control of disease. What one learns in reviewing these various studies is that optimal management of nasal and sinus inverting papilloma requires a number of considerations:

1. Inverting papilloma is not multicentric, as opposed to noninverting papilloma, and will usually arise from one area (unifocal) and spreads sinus to sinus.[6,7,11] This tumor can destroy bone, and it can be aggressive.
2. The most common site of inverting papilloma is the ethmoid sinus.[6,7,11]
3. Spread into the maxillary sinus is through the antrostomy and usually is limited to the medial wall.[7,11] Spread can also occur through the fontanelle, with aggressive progression into the maxillary sinus.[6]
4. Disease spread or extension, or disease primarily occurring in the maxillary sinus away from the medial wall, in most cases cannot be cured by an intranasal surgery.[1-3,6]
5. Limited disease in the nose, turbinate, septum, or ethmoid sinus with a clean maxillary sinus on radiologic evaluation should be considered for intranasal removal.[1,3,4-8]
6. Contiguous sinuses to areas of tumor location require surgical evaluation to rule out spread of disease into those sinuses, with upper ethmoid tumor requiring frontal recess evaluation and biopsy,[6,7,11] posterior ethmoid tumor requiring sphenoid sinus evaluation and possible biopsy,[6,7,11] and anterior ethmoid tumor requiring evaluation and possible biopsy of maxillary sinus.[6,7,11]
7. The use of advanced radiographic studies such as computed tomography (CT) scanning with contrast and magnetic resonance imaging (MRI) with contrast can help identify tumor extent, allowing for better surgical planning.[3,12,13] This is especially helpful in finding tumor extending into the frontal, sphenoid, or maxillary sinus as opposed to fluid or sinusitis secondary to ostia blockage.[1]
8. For the average practitioner, any inverting papilloma involving the ethmoid and maxillary sinus requires an extranasal ethmoidectomy and medial maxillectomy for optimum results.[2,3,6]
9. Endoscopy can offer excellent intranasal visualization, allowing for earlier diagnosis of inverting papilloma resulting in less extensive surgery in specific cases.[1,4,5,14]
10. Tumor limited to the nose and ethmoid sinus is amenable to precise endoscopic removal in experienced hands.[1,3-5,8,14,15]
11. Tumor limited to the ethmoid sinus or medial wall of the maxillary sinus, or both, is amenable to endoscopic ethmoidectomy and medial maxillectomy in experienced hands.[14]
12. Tumor extensively involving the maxillary sinus requires removal of all mucosa. This tumor requires an extranasal lateral rhinotomy or degloving approach to medial maxillectomy with possible Caldwell–Luc procedure.[2,3,6,16] Performed by a surgeon experienced with endoscopy, the endoscopic medial maxillectomy can be used with the Caldwell–Luc.[1,14]
13. The use of computerized stereotaxic endoscopic technique improves tumor removal and control.[17]

*Thanks are due to Ms. Susan Whelton for her assistance in manuscript preparation.

Discussion

Extranasal lateral rhinotomy or maxillary degloving with ethmoidectomy and medial maxillectomy are the gold standard operations for extensive inverting papilloma involving the ethmoid and maxillary sinuses. These procedures and the positive results reported in treating inverting papilloma were developed after years of inadequate intranasal and extranasal procedures. The only reason to change management philosophy depends on equivalent or improved management techniques. Endoscopic diagnosis and surgery can improve our management of inverting papilloma. The use of endoscopic sinus surgery by experienced surgeons expands the management of inverting papilloma and allows for individualization of treatment. The management philosophy described below is safe, effective, and consistent with cutting-edge treatment of inverting papilloma.

The differential diagnosis of any unilateral nasal lesion should consider tumor first. The most common benign nasal tumor is inverting papilloma. Once endoscopic examination and/or CT scanning indicates that the tumor is limited to the nose or sinuses, or both, an endoscopic examination can often pinpoint the precise origin of the tumor, permitting more precise surgical planning. This possiblity was unavailable before endoscopy and is one of the reasons intranasal removal under direct vision failed. Tumors were usually detected only when large and bulky, requiring extensive surgery for removal. Also, the advent of endoscopic diagnosis with CT scanning for sinusitis has resulted in earlier diagnosis of sinusitis and sinus tumors—again, less surgery. Once the diagnosis is made, further radiologic evaluation to determine the extent of tumor may be necessary. Small localized tumors require only a CT scan. Large tumors affecting the nose and ethmoid sinus with evidence of sinusitis or opacification in contiguous sinuses such as the frontal, sphenoid, or maxillary sinus require an MRI with contrast to determine whether inverting papilloma is present in those sinuses. Tumor extending into other sinuses in addition to the ethmoid requires specific planning for removal. Biopsy of unilateral nasal lesions can be performed in the clinic, provided that pre-biopsy radiologic evaluation (CT scanning) shows that the lesion is limited to the nose and sinuses and does not include the brain or skull base. For postoperative follow-up, the endoscope has a valuable role in diagnosis and treatment, which will be discussed later.

For primary tumors limited to the septum, middle, or superior turbinate or to the ethmoid sinus, endoscopic surgery is much more advantageous than direct headlight or microscope visualization and certainly superior to any type of external removal procedure. Carefully planned endoscopic procedures with complete control of inverting papilloma is the rule in most of these cases. Tumor origins can be nicely seen and tumor with safe margins removed. Ethmoidectomy for inverting papilloma should require not only tumor removal and ethmoidectomy, but also mucous membrane removal to lamina papyracea. In some instances, such as with bony erosion or involvement, the lamina papyracea requires removal. Removal of mucous membrane can be enhanced using a diamond drill burr or a microdebrider; removal of the lamina papyracea in the tumor area can be enhanced under endoscopic guidance. Inferior, middle, or superior turbinate inverting papilloma requires partial or total turbinectomy, depending on the extent of the tumor. Septal tumor necessitates mucosa removal to cartilage or bone for control. I have removed several localized tumors in this fashion, as have others, with good success.[1-5,14]

Removal of tumors in the ethmoid area with extent into the maxillary sinus requires an ethmoidectomy and a medial maxillectomy, which can be performed extranasally or endoscopically, but this should be performed by experienced surgeons only[4,14] (Fig. 5–1). The procedures for extranasal medial maxillectomy and ethmoidectomy have been nicely documented. The intranasal endoscopic procedures require ethmoidectomy with removal of mucosa, possible removal of

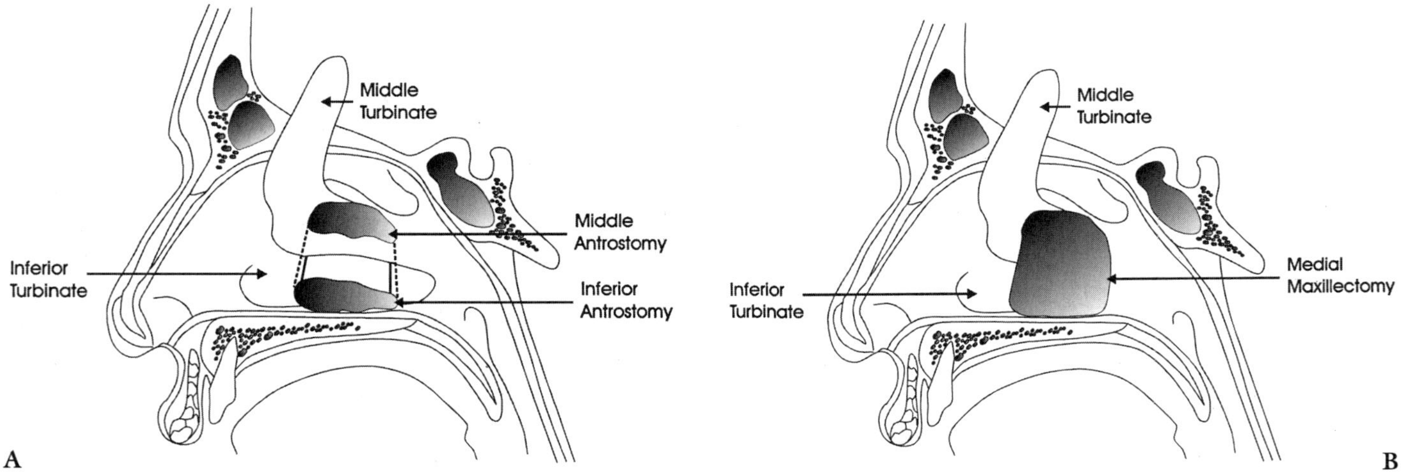

Figure 5–1 Incisions for endoscopic medial maxillectomy. (The middle turbinate is retracted upward for the illustration.) **(A)** The dotted line represents the incision between antrostomies. The solid line represents the turbinate (inferior) incisions. **(B)** Completed endoscopic medial maxillectomy.

lamina papyracea, and possible excision of middle turbinate, if affected with tumor. The medial maxillectomy is performed by removing the inferior turbinate just posterior to the nasolacrimal duct along with the medial maxillary sinus wall. This is done with medial and inferior meatus antrostomies, followed by bone cuts made with through-cut punch forceps through the anterior inferior turbinate, punch cuts vertically through the anterior fontanelle joining the antrostomies, punch cuts inferiorly moving posteriorly to the posterior wall of the maxillary sinus, and a vertical cut between the medial and inferior antrostomies posteriorly releasing the specimen. Disease extending into the maxillary sinus is removed down to bone, by means of angled telescopes and special instrumentation. Frozen-section biopsies can aid in achieving good tumor margins. Any tumor occurring laterally, anteriorly, or posterolaterally may require an anterior maxillary sinusotomy or a Caldwell–Luc to gain tumor control. In practice, the tumor is limited primarily to the medial wall, with most of the remaining thickened mucosa caused by associated sinusitis. Close follow-up management is necessary in all these patients. In my early experience with inverting papilloma in the maxillary sinus, I automatically converted to an external medial maxillectomy. As I gained endoscopic surgical experience and a better feel for inverting papilloma, I have been able to resect these tumors using endoscopic intranasal techniques only, as supported by the literature.[1,14]

Inverted papilloma occurs in rare cases in the sphenoid or frontal sinuses. This occurs from either extension from the ethmoid sinuses superiorly or posteriorly or direct involvement. A treatment dilemma occurs due to exposure and tumor removal. Should the frontal sinus be obliterated? Should all the mucosa be removed from the sphenoid given that the carotid artery may be dehiscent? Certainly, an osteoplastic flap may need consideration. Whether to obliterate or not is a judgment decision. Many surgeons have concern about placing fat into a sinus where tumor was present. I have concern about leaving tumor in the frontal recess, which is a difficult area to obliterate. Alternatives include a frontal floor sinusotomy (Lothrop procedure) through an osteoplastic flap, endoscopic frontal osteoplasty with trephination, external frontoethmoidectomy (Lynch procedure), or endoscopic frontal osteoplasty with sinusotomy (endoscopic Lothrop procedure). This is a rare occurrence and, therefore, it is difficult to recommend one procedure over another. Each case should be treated individually with the paramount consideration being removal of all tumor. For sphenoid inverting papilloma, a wide sphenoidotomy should be made, with removal of tumor mucosa guided by frozen section. Posterolateral dissection should be performed with great caution to avoid injury to the carotid artery. The carotid is dehiscent in up to 20% of patients, the optic nerve in 5%. Computerized stereotactic surgery may be very helpful in identifying key anatomy, to avoid complications, and in aiding tumor removal, particularly in the frontal or sphenoid sinuses.[17]

For patients failing primary inverting papilloma surgery, endoscopic diagnosis and surgery can help identify recurrence, salvage small recurrences, and help debride and reduce tumor bulk in large recurrences not amenable to further surgery; this approach can also aid in the diagnosis via biopsy showing benign inverted papilloma changing into or harboring squamous cell carcinoma. The endoscope can be a powerful weapon in all of these cases, as verified by my own personal experience. Recurrent disease in the maxillary sinus not treated initially by medial maxillectomy warrants consideration for this procedure. Endoscopic medial maxillectomy should only be considered by expert endoscopic surgeons familiar with the technique and the principles of tumor surgery. The important point is that the goal is to achieve control of inverting papilloma at the first surgery. The best procedure to accomplish complete removal should be used.

Radiation therapy for uncontrolled inverting papilloma changing to carcinoma is an effective treatment. For an uncontrolled tumor not changing to carcinoma, radiation therapy has been used in a few cases for control of the tumor.[18] I prefer close observation and timely biopsy as a better alternative for localized tumor, as there are concerns about the possibility that radiation therapy can induce inverting papilloma to change into carcinoma. Widespread uncontrolled tumor should be considered for radiation therapy.

Conclusion

For most surgeons, the treatment of inverting papilloma affecting the ethmoid and maxillary sinuses is not controversial. The treatment is ethmoidectomy with medial maxillectomy. The extranasal approach is the safest and surest way to accomplish total tumor removal. For a handful of skilled surgeons, the ethmoidectomy and medial maxillectomy can be accomplished endoscopically. Both approaches should be guided by frozen-section biopsy.

Tumor can hide laterally, anteriorly, or posteriorly in the maxillary sinus and may be missed even with extranasal medial maxillectomy, leading to recurrence. These areas need to be visualized with direct vision via a Caldwell–Luc operation or with angled telescopes at the end of surgery to ensure that all tumor has been removed. Endoscopic observation used during and after surgery can often identify precisely where inverting papilloma originated, ensuring complete removal. Endoscopic follow-up can identify recurrent disease that may be amenable to an endoscopic salvage if medial maxillectomy has already been performed. Tumor uncontrolled with proper extensive surgery can be followed, biopsied, debulked, and debrided using endoscopic techniques. Inverting papilloma that does not involve the maxillary sinus is amenable to endoscopic removal. Any ethmoidectomy must be accompanied by mucous membrane removal to bone or even lamina papyracea removal. State-of-the-art imaging using CT and MRI scanning can identify tumor extension into contiguous sinuses, aiding in surgical planning. Computerized stereotactic surgery can precisely identify all pockets of disease as well as orbit, skull base, optic nerve, and carotid artery, assisting with tumor removal in hazardous anatomic sites. Radiation therapy should be reserved for inverted papilloma with frank carcinoma, carcinoma in situ that cannot be removed, and diffuse uncontrolled inverting papilloma.

REFERENCES

1. Stankiewicz JA, Girgis SJ. Endoscopic surgical treatment of nasal and paranasal sinus inverted papilloma. *Otolaryngol Head Neck Surg* 1993;109:988–995
2. Lawson W, Ho BT, Shaari CM, Biller HF. Inverted papilloma: a report of 112 cases. *Laryngoscope* 1995;105:282–288
3. Bielamowicz S, Calcaterra TC, Watson D. Inverted papilloma of the head and neck: UCLA update. *Otolaryngol Head Neck Surg* 1993;109:71–76
4. Waitz G, Wigand M. Results of endoscopic sinus surgery for the treatment of inverted papilloma. *Laryngoscope* 1992;102:917–922
5. Kamel RH. Conservative endoscopic surgery in inverted papilloma. *Otolaryngol Head Neck Surg* 1992;118:649–653
6. Vrabec DP. The inverted Schneiderian papilloma: a 25-year study. *Laryngoscope* 1994;104:582–605
7. Buchwald C, Franzmann MB, Tos M. Sinonasal papillomas: a report of 82 cases in Copenhagen county. *Laryngoscope.* 1995;105:72–79
8. Ravel E, Feinmesser R, Shpitzer T, Yaniv E, Segal K. Inverted papilloma of the nose and paranasal sinuses: a study of 56 cases and review of the literature. *Israel J Med Sci* 1996;32: 1163–1167
9. Siegel R, Atar E, Mor C. Inverted papilloma of the nose and paranasal sinuses. *Laryngoscope* 1986;96:358–394
10. Suh K, Facer G, Device K. Inverted papilloma of the nose and paranasal sinuses. *Laryngoscope* 1977;87:35–46
11. Hyams V. Papillomas of the nasal cavity and paranasal sinuses: a clinicopathological study of 315 cases. *Ann Rhinol Laryngol* 1971;80:192–206
12. Woodson J, Robbins K, Michael L. Inverted papilloma. *Arch Otolaryngol* 1985;111:806–811
13. Woodruff WW, Vrabec DP. Inverted papilloma of the nasal vault and paranasal sinuses: a spectrum of CT findings. *AJR* 1994;161:419–423
14. Kamel RH. Transnasal endoscopic medial maxillectomy in inverted papilloma. *Laryngoscope* 1995;105:847–853
15. Ouzen KE, Grontveld A, Jorgensen K, Clausen PP, Lodeforged C. Inverted papilloma: in advanced and late results of surgical treatment. *Rhinology* 1996;34:114–118
16. Krause DH. Lateral rhinotomy approach to inverted papilloma. *Am J Rhinol* 1995;9:77–80
17. Petruzzelli G, Origitano TC, Stankiewicz, JA, McSherry D, Anderson DE. Frameless stereotactic localization in cranial base surgery. *Skull Base Surgery* 2000;10:125–129
18. Guedea F, Mendenhall WM, Parsons J. The role of radiation therapy in inverted papilloma of a nasal cavity and paranasal sinuses. *Int J Radiat Oncol* 1991;20:777–780

Management of Inverting Papilloma

William R. Spencer and Steven D. Schaefer

CHAPTER 6

The inverting Schneiderian papilloma has been recorded in the medical literature for more than a century and remains a topic of controversy.[1] It is generally accepted that inverting papilloma is a benign tumor of the sinonasal tract mucosa that is locally aggressive and has significant malignant potential. It is an uncommon lesion in which proliferated epithelial reserve cells invert into the underlying stroma rather than growing outwardly from the surface.[2] Inverting papilloma is derived from sinonasal (Schneiderian) mucosa, formed from the invaginating ectoderm of the olfactory plates at the end of the fourth week of embryonic life.[1] The neoplastic epithelium may be of a respiratory, transitional, or squamous type. Inverting papillomas most often arise from the lateral nasal wall in the area of the middle turbinate and may extend into the maxillary and ethmoid sinuses. In most cases, this slow-growing tumor is unilateral.[3]

Inverting papillomas are unique, characterized by their capacity to destroy bone by pressure erosion.[4] They are also associated with squamous cell carcinoma and have a tendency to recur if incompletely excised. Lesperance and Esclamado[5] retrospectively found squamous cell carcinoma with inverting papillomas in 27% of cases in their study.

Questions that remain unanswered regarding inverting papilloma include its etiology, malignant potential, and appropriate management.

Background

Inverting papilloma was first described by Ward in 1854 and by Billroth in 1855. Kramer and Som in 1935[6] distinguished the disease from inflammatory polyps.

Because of the infrequent occurrence of the lesion, an appropriate name has not yet been agreed upon. At least 20 different terms have been used in referring to this lesion.[7] Such terms as *papillary sinusitis* or *epithelial papilloma* do not reflect the seriousness of the lesion. Conversely, such expressions as *papillary carcinoma* or *villous cancer* are perhaps overly threatening and can lead to overly aggressive treatment measures.[8]

Epidemiology

The overall incidence of inverting papillomas varies from 0.5% to 4% of all primary nasal tumors.[1] They are three times more common in men than in women. Whites have a higher incidence than blacks. Papillomas are rarely found in childhood and adolescence and are seen primarily in the 40- to 70-year-old age group, with a peak incidence during the sixth and seventh decades of life.[8]

Etiology

The etiology of the lesion is uncertain. Chronic infection, allergy, tobacco, and occupational exposures are unlikely etiologic factors, as inverting papillomas are usually unilateral.[1] Several studies using in situ hybridization have demonstrated the presence of human papillomavirus (HPV) DNA. Types 6b and 11 were isolated in inverting papillomas in 76% of cases in a study conducted by Weber et al.[9] Epstein-Barr virus (EBV) has also been implicated.

Diagnosis

Patients with inverting papilloma usually present with unilateral nasal obstruction, sinusitis, epistaxis, and rhinorrhea. Physical examination shows a unilateral mass, which frequently resembles a bleeding inflammatory polyp. Inflammatory polyps are usually bilateral; consequently, the presence of a unilateral polyp raises suspicion of the presence of an inverting papilloma. The diagnostic workup includes computed tomography (CT) or magnetic resonance imaging (MRI) of the sinuses as well as biopsy. CT delineates whether there is septal deviation, bone erosion, intracranial extension, or opacification of the nasal cavity and sinuses. MRI is useful for distinguishing tumor from mucosal inflammation and mucus secretions. Imaging studies should precede biopsy in patients suspected to have encephaloceles. Although clinical and radiologic suspicion of an inverting papilloma may be high, an adequate biopsy for tissue diagnosis must be obtained before proceeding with definitive management. Biopsy serves not only to confirm the diagnosis, but also to rule out associated squamous cell carcinoma.

Treatment

The tendency of the tumor to recur, its destructive capacity, and its propensity to be associated with malignancy have led to controversy regarding the management of inverting papillomas. Some clinicians view them as benign, some classify them as premalignant, and others regard them as malignant.[1] This confusion regarding the clinical features and projected behavior has resulted in a poorly defined clinical approach to the management of these tumors. Some clinicians promote initial conservative procedures for smaller lesions, reserving more radical procedures for large or recurrent lesions.[8] The method of surgical management should be dictated by the extent and location of the disease.[10]

Discussion

Intranasal endoscopic resections that avoid external incisions and bony resections are considered conservative and are associated with recurrence rates as high as 74%, as reported by Beilamowicz et al.[6] By contrast, with careful case selection, Myers et al.[1] had no recurrences using conservative approaches. Lesions amenable to conservative management are those limited to the inferior and middle turbinates or middle meatal region with minimal extension into the anterior ethmoids or antrum. Lesions that involve the supraorbital air cells, perilacrimal cells, frontal sinus, and cribriform plate preclude the use of conservative surgery because of poor visualization and subsequent incomplete resection.[10]

Many investigators do not advocate conservative therapy for the treatment of any inverting papilloma because of the high risk of recurrence and because of the effectiveness of a medial maxillectomy/lateral rhinotomy. Stankiewicz and Girgis[11] believe that endoscopic treatment is feasible because of the pathology of the tumor. In 1971, Hyams demonstrated that inverting papilloma is primarily a lateral wall disease, and most commonly involves the ethmoid sinus and maxillary antrum. Endoscopic excision should be biopsy-controlled to ensure complete excision, as opposed to limited transnasal excision.[11] During endoscopic excision, if any unreachable areas of tumor are observed, the procedure should be converted to a medial maxillectomy. Endoscopic resections had an overall recurrence rate of 17% in the Waitz and Wigand[12] series of papillomas limited to the nasal cavity and maxillary antrum. Endoscopes have a role in the diagnosis and postoperative follow-up evaluation of all inverting papillomas, but their place in management should be limited to lesions involving the ethmoid sinuses, face of the sphenoid sinus, and lateral nasal wall.[11]

Mid-face degloving offers an acceptable alternative for small lesions that extend into the maxillary sinus. Sacks et al.[13] reported the use of this approach in 46 cases in 1984. This approach consists of making a sublabial incison and elevating the soft tissues of the mid-face, gaining exposure to the piriform aperture and lateral nasal wall.[1] At this point, a lateral rhinotomy and limited medial maxillectomy is performed. Advocates believe that this procedure offers excellent exposure to the mid-face, nasal cavity, and maxillary and anterior sphenoid sinuses, while avoiding a facial scar. Consequently, exposure is limited to the frontal and supraorbital ethmoids and lacrimal fossa. The mid-face degloving approach is best reserved for small to moderate lesions that extend into the maxillary sinus and that are not amenable to endoscopic excision.

Lateral rhinotomy and medial maxillectomy is the procedure of choice for patients with bulky polypoid lesions not amenable to more limited resection.[12] En bloc resection of the lateral nasal wall removes areas into which the tumor normally extends and affords access to the anterior sphenoid sinus, supraorbital ethmoids, and frontal sinus, which are areas of local spread of the tumor.[12] In some instances, an external frontoethmoidectomy or osteoplastic flap may be needed for additional exposure. Clinicians have criticized this operation because the large mid-facial Weber-Fergusen incision required for this approach is considered cosmetically unacceptable. Our experience has been that a meticulous wound closure will produce minimal postoperative scarring. Variations to the Weber-Fergusen incision include not transecting the upper lip, thereby improving the cosmetic results. Lateral rhinotomy/medial maxillectomy has a recurrence rate of 0 to 14%.[14] Recurrences after these procedures may be the result of tumor seeding to nondiseased mucosa or insufficient resection.

Craniofacial resection may be required for tumors that erode into the skull base. Unfortunately, current radiographic imaging techniques poorly differentiate between benign and malignant disease, making it difficult to determine whether craniofacial resection is warranted.[11] The decision to proceed with resection should be made intraoperatively after biopsy confirmation in these cases.

Radiation therapy is reserved for cases of advanced inverting papilloma with intracranial extension or associated with squamous cell carcinoma. The possibility of malignant transformation must be considered when giving radiation therapy. Mayberry et al.[15] reported 4 of 14 tumors with malignant transformation after radiation treatment. Other studies show that radiation can effectively control locally advanced inverting papilloma after multiple recurrences from incomplete resections.

Conclusion

The appropriate management of inverting papilloma depends on the size and location of the lesion. The presence of squamous cell carcinoma, skull base erosion, or intracranial extension or distant metastasis mandates more aggressive therapy. Using biopsy-controlled resection, there is a role for endoscopic management of limited lesions. Recurrent lesions have a higher incidence of associated carcinoma. Thus, the procedure selected should permit complete resection of the tumor at the first attempt. We have developed an algorithm to provide an organized approach for managing inverting papillomas (Figure 6–1). Whenever there is a question in the clinician's mind, the next higher approach should be selected.

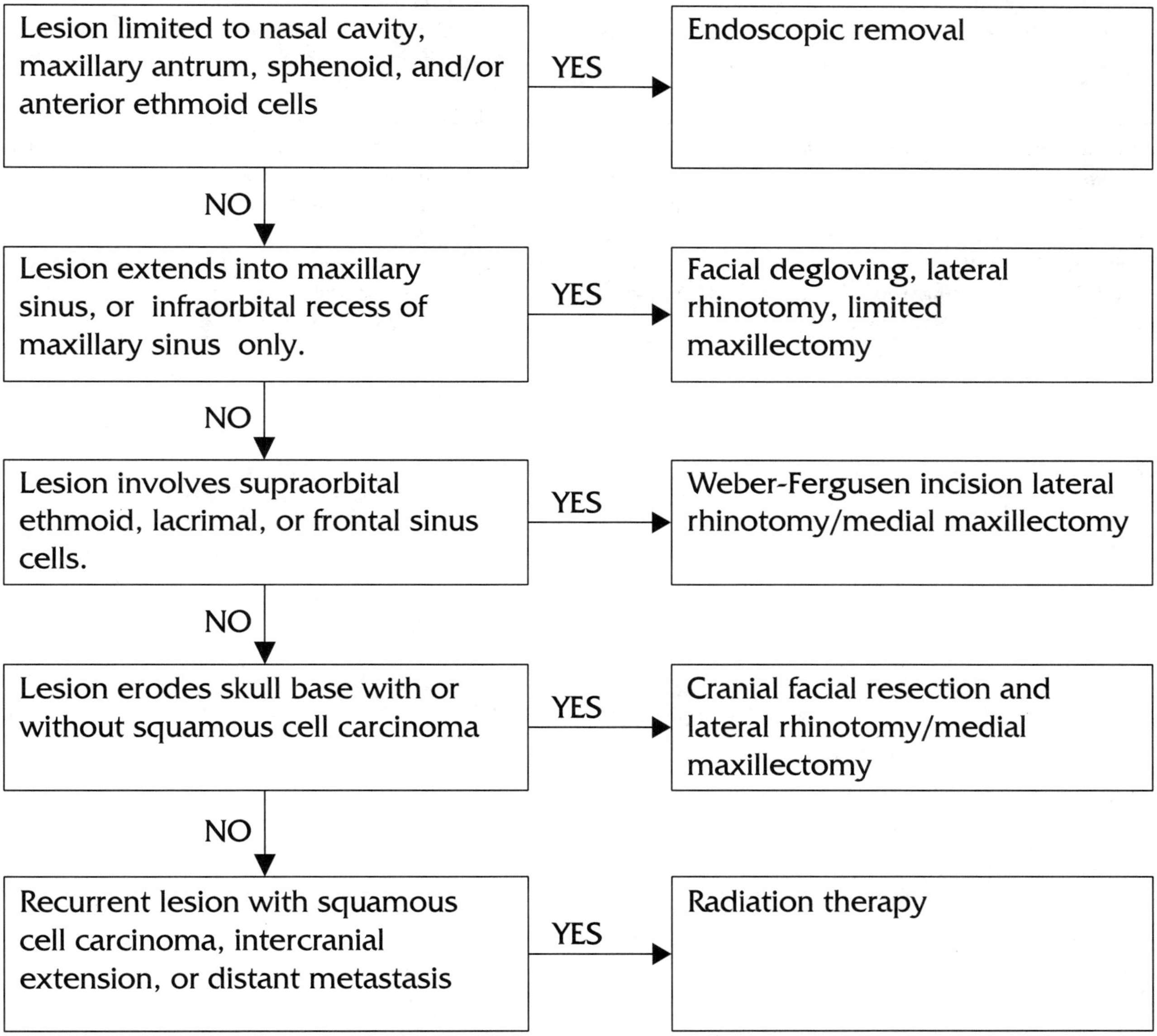

Figure 6–1 Management algorithm for inverting papillomas.

REFERENCES

1. Myers EN, Fernau JL, Johnson JT, Tabet JC, Barnes EL. Management of inverting papilloma. *Laryngoscope* 1990;100:481–490
2. Bailey BJ. *Head and Neck Surgery-Otolaryngology*. Vol 1. Philadelphia: JB Lippincott; 1993:335
3. Ballenger JJ, Snow JB. *Otorhinolaryngology: Head and Neck Surgery*. 15th ed. Baltimore: Williams & Wilkins, 1996:200
4. Wenig BM. *Atlas of Head and Neck Pathology*. Philadelphia: WB Saunders; 1994:29
5. Lesperance MM, Esclamado RM. Squamous cell carcinoma arising in inverting papilloma. *Laryngoscope* 1995;105: 178–183
6. Beilamowicz S, Calcaterra TC, Watson D. Inverting papilloma of the head and neck: the UCLA update. *Otolaryngol Head Neck Surg* 1993;109:71–76
7. Million RR, Cassisi NJ. *Management of Head and Neck Cancer: A Multidisciplinary Approach*. 2nd ed. Philadelphia: JB Lippincott; 1994:559
8. Vrabec DP. The inverting Schneiderian papilloma: a 25-year study. *Laryngoscope* 1994;104:582–605
9. Weber RS, Shillitoe EJ, Robbins KT. Prevalence of human papilloma virus in inverted nasal papillomas. *Arch Otolaryngol Head Neck Surg* 1988;114:23–26
10. Lawson W, Ho BT, Shaari CM, Biller HF. Inverting papilloma: a report of 112 cases. *Laryngoscope* 1995;105:282–288
11. Stankiewicz JA, Girgis SJ. Endoscopic surgical treatment of nasal and paranasal sinus inverting papilloma. *Otolaryngol Head Neck Surg* 1993;109:988–995
12. Waitz G, Wigand ME. Results of endoscopic sinus surgery for the treatment of inverted papillomas. *Laryngoscope* 1992;102: 917–922
13. Sacks ME, Conley J, Rabuzzi DD. Degloving approach for total excision of inverted papilloma. *Laryngoscope* 1984;94:1595–1598
14. Myers EM, Schramm VL, Barnes EL. Management of inverted papilloma of the nose and paranasal sinuses. *Laryngoscope* 1981;91:2071–2084
15. Mayberry GW, Devine KD, Harrison EG. The problem of malignant transformation in a nasal papilloma. Report of a case. *Arch Otolaryngol* 1965;82:296–300

3

The Role of Chemotherapy in Head and Neck Cancer

"The use of chemotherapy to treat patients with incurable metastatic or recurrent HNSCC is well established. The median survival for these patients is approximately 6 months, and chemotherapy has had little impact on overall survival. The goal of this treatment is the palliation of cancer-related symptoms attributable to a reduction in tumor burden."

Everett E. Vokes

"Previously treated cancer responds much differently than naive tumors, and unresectable tumors may respond differently than resectable tumors."

Ernest A. Weymuller, Jr.

"Researchers still struggle to demonstrate a clear survival benefit, but the secondary goal of preserving function of the larynx and pharynx without compromising survival can now be successfully achieved."

K. Thomas Robbins

The Role of Chemotherapy in Head and Neck Cancer

CHAPTER 7

Gary S. Gordon and Everett E. Vokes

Over the past 20 years, there has been a gradual evolution in the treatments offered to patients with head and neck squamous cell cancer (HNSCC). Although 60 to 80% of patients with early-stage I and II HNSCC can be cured with surgery and/or radiation therapy, the cure rate falls to 30% or less for patients with locally advanced stage III and IV disease. Local and regional relapse accounts for most of the failures observed in patients treated with surgery and radiation therapy. A few patients experience distant tumor spread. Chemotherapy, historically used for palliation in patients with recurrent and/or metastatic disease, has been investigated in several experimental multimodality primary treatment regimens. These investigations have attempted to improve survival, locoregional control, and organ preservation. Distant failure rates and quality of life have also been evaluated. Although surgery and radiotherapy are the most accepted primary treatments for patients with locally advanced HNSCC, recent literature, including meta-analyses of randomized studies, suggests that concomitant chemo- and radiotherapy, with or without surgery, has become the new standard. This chapter briefly reviews the traditional role of chemotherapy for the palliation of recurrent and/or metastatic disease and then describes the recent studies that show a role for chemotherapy in the front-line treatment of patients with locally advanced disease.

TABLE 7–1
Single Chemotherapeutic Agents with Activity in Head and Neck Squamous Cell Cancer

Chemotherapy	Pooled Response Rate (%)[a]
Methotrexate	31
Cisplatin	28
Carboplatin	22
Bleomycin	21
Paclitaxel	40
Docetaxel	31
5-Fluorouracil	15
Ifosfamide	26
Topotecan	22
Vinorelbine	22
Gemcitabine	13

[a] Includes both complete remission (CR) and partial remission (PR).

Background

TREATMENT OF RECURRENT OR METASTATIC DISEASE

The use of chemotherapy to treat patients with incurable metastatic or recurrent HNSCC is well established. The median survival for these patients is approximately 6 months, and chemotherapy has had little impact on overall survival. The goal of this treatment is palliation of cancer-related symptoms attributable to a reduction in tumor burden. Multiple chemotherapeutic regimens using single agents and combinations of effective drugs have been investigated. Tumor response, time to progression, and overall survival time are the endpoints most frequently reported. Tumor responses include complete responses (CR, i.e., the disappearance of all measurable disease) and partial responses (PR, i.e., 50% reduction in measurable disease). Quality of life is becoming an additional valued endpoint.

Single-Agent Chemotherapy

Multiple single agents have efficacy in the treatment of HNSCC (Table 7–1). Methotrexate is frequently listed as the standard treatment for metastatic and recurrent HNSCC. The drug is given weekly by intravenous infusion, with mucositis and myelosuppression the dose-limiting toxicities. Although initial response rates of 30% were reported, a large multi-institutional randomized study reported a response rate of only 10%.

Cisplatin is one of the most active agents used in the treatment of HNSCC. Response rates of 14 to 41% and a pooled average response rate of 28% have been reported. Nephrotoxicity, neurotoxicity, and ototoxicity, coupled with significant nausea and vomiting, are the major toxicities associated with cisplatin. The cisplatin analogue, carboplatin, may have less toxicity. Response rates for carboplatin are 14 to 30%, with a pooled average of 22%.

The taxanes, paclitaxel (Taxol) and docetaxel (Taxotere), have shown impressive response rates of 30 to 40% in patients with recurrent HNSCC. The major toxicities of these agents include myelosuppression, peripheral neuropathy, mucositis, and hypersensitivity.

5-FU has been studied extensively in a variety of doses and schedules. Mucositis is the primary dose-limiting toxicity. Although it has a significant role in combination chemotherapy for HNSCC, the pooled single-agent response rate by continuous infusion is only 15%.

TABLE 7–2

Selected Randomized Trials of Chemotherapy in Recurrent/Metastatic HNSCC*

Study/ Chemotherapy	Patients	CR +PR (%)	CR (%)	Median Survival (mo)
Stanford[a]	249			
Cisplatin/5-FU	79	32	5	5.5
Cisplatin	83	17	3	5.0
5-FU	83	13	2	6.1
SWOG Study[b]	277			
Cisplatin/5-FU	87	32	6	6.6
Carboplatin/5-FU	86	21	2	5.0
Methotrexate	88	10	2	5.6
EORTC study[c]	365			
CABO	127	37	10	(6.5 for all patients)
Cisplatin/5-FU	116	34	2	
Cisplatin	122	13	3	
Liverpool study[d]	200			
Cisplatin/5-FU	50	12	3	
Cisplatin/methotrexate	50	11	0	Not available
Cisplatin	50	14	1	
Methotrexate	50	6	0	

*5-FU, 5-fluorouracil; CABO, cisplatin, methotrexate, bleomycin, vincristine; CR, complete remission; PR, partial remission.

SOURCE: Vokes EE, Athanasidis I. Chemotherapy for squamous cell carcinoma of head and neck: the future is now. *Ann Oncol* 1996;7:15–29.

[a]Jacobs C, Lyman G, Velez-Garcia E, et al. A phase III randomized study comparing cisplatin and fluorouracil as single agents in combination for advanced squamous cell carcinoma of the head and neck. *J Clin Oncol* 1992;10:257–263.

[b]Forastiere AA, Metch B, Schuller DE, et al. Randomized comparison of cisplatin plus fluorouracil and carboplatin plus fluorouracil versus methotrexate in advanced squamous-cell carcinoma of the head and neck: a Southwest Oncology Group Study. *J Clin Oncol* 1992;10:1245–1251.

[c]Clavel M, Vermorken JB, Cognetti F, et al. Randomized comparison of cisplatin, methotrexate, bleomycin and vincristine (CABO) versus cisplatin and 5-fluorouracil (CF) versus cisplatin (C) in recurrent or metastatic squamous cell carcinoma of the head and neck. A phase III study of the EORTC Head and Neck Cancer Cooperative Group. *Ann Oncol* 1994;5:521–526.

[d]Liverpool Head and Neck Oncology Group. A phase III randomized trial of cisplatinum, methotrexate, cisplatinum + methotrexate and cisplatinum + 5-FU in end stage squamous carcinoma of the head and neck. *Br J Cancer* 1992;61:311–315.

Other single agents that have activity in HNSCC are ifosfamide, vinorelbine, and gemcitabine.

Combination Chemotherapy

Combination chemotherapy for metastatic and recurrent HNSCC has been studied extensively. The combination of cisplatin and 4 to 5 days of continuous infusion of 5-FU (PF) has been shown in single-institution trials to produce response rates as high as 70%. Four large randomized studies [1, 2, 3, 4] (Table 7–2) have compared this regimen with single-agent and alternative combination therapies. The response rates from these studies were approximately 30%. Although early studies suggested that the addition of interferon-α_{2b} (IFN-α_{2b}) to PF might lead to improved response, a randomized study demonstrated increased toxicity without improvement in response or survival.

A 1994 study of standard chemotherapy for metastatic and recurrent HNSCC analyzed 15 randomized studies of single-agent and combination therapy.[5] The authors concluded that although the combination of cisplatin and 5-FU produced a higher response rate and a possible limited improvement in survival, this came at the expense of significant additional toxicity.

Recently, single-institution taxane-based combination therapy has yielded encouraging responses rates. A phase II study of paclitaxel, ifosfamide, and cisplatin (TIP)[6] in patients with recurrent or metastatic disease reported an overall response rate of 58% with a 17% complete response rate, and a median survival of 8.8 months. These newer drug combinations will have to be compared in multi-institution randomized studies before any firm conclusions can be reached.

TREATMENT OF INITIAL LOCOREGIONALLY ADVANCED DISEASE

The use of chemotherapy in the front-line treatment of locally advanced HNSCC has been studied extensively over the past three decades. Induction chemotherapy has been given before definitive surgery and/or radiotherapy to reduce tumor bulk and possibly to treat subclinical micrometastatic disease. Concomitant chemotherapy has been given with radiotherapy to achieve synergistic improvement in the efficacy of radiotherapy. Adjuvant chemotherapy has been given after definitive surgery or radiation to help maintain remission and decrease the appearance of distant disease relapse. Studies of adjuvant chemotherapy have typically occurred in the setting of prior induction or concomitant chemotherapy, making independent analysis of this treatment approach difficult.

Induction Chemotherapy

The rationale for induction chemotherapy is based on the high overall response rates that could be achieved with combination chemotherapy. A significant decrease in tumor bulk would theoretically lead to tumor downstaging and the greater ability of surgery and radiation to eradicate remaining disease. Early studies that reported response rates to chemotherapy in excess of 80% were encouraging. As many as 50% of patients in some studies had histologically confirmed complete remissions before undergoing either surgery or radiation, or both. Unfortunately, subsequent randomized studies failed to identify improved survival for patients compared with patients who had received no induction chemotherapy. Although several studies showed a decrease in relapse of distant disease, chemotherapy did not appear to have an impact on locoregional control, and therefore did not significantly affect overall survival.

Although survival has not been increased by induction chemotherapy to date, organ preservation may be achieved. The Department of Veterans Affairs (VA) Laryngeal Cancer Study Group[7] published its results in 1991. The study showed that organ preservation could be achieved without a decrease in survival. Patients with previously untreated stage III and IV resectable cancers were randomly assigned to either three cycles of induction chemotherapy (cisplatin/5-FU) followed by radiotherapy, or surgery followed by radiotherapy. Those patients who had a clinical tumor response after two cycles of chemotherapy were given a third cycle of chemotherapy, followed by definitive radiation. Patients who had no tumor response after two cycles of chemotherapy or who had recurrent disease after chemotherapy and radiation were treated with laryngectomy. Overall survival at 2-year follow-up was 68% in both groups. Distant metastatic relapse was significantly less likely in the induction chemotherapy arm (11% vs 17%, $P = 0.001$). The larynx was preserved in 64% of the patients who had chemotherapy, and at a median follow-up of 33 months, 39% of patients remained alive and disease free with a functioning larynx. Although the study has been criticized for the lack of a radiation-only treatment arm, this study and a subsequent European study[8] established organ preservation induction chemotherapy as a standard option for patients with locally advanced laryngeal cancer.

Concomitant Chemo- and Radiotherapy

Chemotherapy has been given with radiotherapy in an effort to improve the efficacy of radiation, and in turn to improve locoregional disease control. Both in theory and in practice, specific chemotherapies can act as radiation enhancers by interfering with the cancer cell's ability to repair radiation-induced damage. This approach has proved effective in the treatment of lung cancer, anal cancer, cervical cancer, and esophageal cancer. Although the goal of improved survival is mainly dependent on locoregional control, chemotherapy given in systemically effective dosages may also lead to the eradication of subclinical micrometastatic disease. Organ preservation is an additional goal of treatment.

Over the past three decades, multiple randomized studies have been published in an effort to define the efficacy of concomitant chemo- and radiotherapy. Two general approaches have been described. One approach involves the addition of chemotherapy to a standard radiation schedule. This approach is attractive because it preserves the standard of care while adding experimental chemotherapy. Chemotherapy is frequently given in dosages below the level of systemic activity, with the drugs acting mainly as radiation enhancers. A second approach uses higher dosages of systemically active chemotherapy along with an altered radiation schedule. This change in the radiation schedule is required to offset the additional toxicity of the treatment. Despite the intensity of this treatment approach, many worry that the prolongation of the radiotherapy may decrease its efficacy.

Dozens of single-arm and randomized studies of concomitant chemo- and radiotherapy for HNSCC have been published. Studies have compared concomitant chemo- and radiotherapy with surgery or radiotherapy, or both. Many studies lack the statistical power required to show a difference in outcome. Several large studies of 5-FU and cisplatin-based concomitant chemo- and radiotherapy have yielded positive results. Most recently, investigators from Duke University published their results of a multicenter randomized study of hyperfractionated irradiation with or without concurrent chemotherapy for locally advanced head and neck cancer. These investigators noted improvement in locoregional disease control at 3 years for the concurrent chemotherapy arm (70% vs 44%, $P = 0.01$), as well as a strong trend toward improvement in overall survival (55% vs 34%, $P = 0.07$). The principal toxicities of concomitant chemo- and radiotherapy are mucositis, dermatitis, myelosuppression, xerostomia, and weight loss. Many patients require temporary gastric feeding tubes in order to complete treatment.

Recently, three independent meta-analyses[9-11] of published randomized studies of chemo- and radiotherapy for locally advanced HNSCC have reported a statistical improvement in survival for patients who have received concomitant chemo- and radiotherapy. Two studies used data as described in the initial publications, whereas the MACH-NC collaborative group used updated individual patient data. For the MACH-NC study, researchers updated survival data for 10,717 patients treated in 63 randomized trials from 1965 until 1993. The median follow-up period was 6 years; with an overall 8% survival benefit at 5 years for patients who had received concomitant chemo- and radiotherapy.

NASOPHARYNGEAL CANCER

Early studies of head and neck cancer treatment frequently included small numbers of patients with nasopharyngeal cancer (NPC). NPC differs from other HNSCC in histopathology, epidemiology, and natural history. These cancers have a greater propensity for early systemic metastasis and appear to be more responsive to chemotherapy. Subgroup analyses of larger studies of multimodality treatment suggested a survival advantage for patients with NPC treated with either induction chemotherapy or concomitant chemo- and radiotherapy, or both. A recent intergroup study[12] randomized patients with locally advanced NPC to concomitant chemo- and radiotherapy, followed by adjuvant chemotherapy or radiation alone. Patients in the chemotherapy arm received cisplatin on days 1, 22, and 43 of standard radiotherapy, followed by adjuvant cisplatin and infusional 5-FU monthly for three cycles. The study was terminated early due to a significant survival advantage in the experimental arm. The 3-year survival rate was 46% for patients treated with radiotherapy and 76% ($P < 0.001$) for patients treated with chemo- and radiotherapy. This study should help establish a new standard of care for patients with locally advanced NPC.

ONGOING INVESTIGATIONS

Investigators are currently evaluating the efficacy of alternative radiation schedules along with concomitant chemotherapy. Researchers at the University of Chicago have developed a regimen of hyperfractionated radiation and concomitant chemotherapy. This novel treatment schedule consists of cisplatin, continuous-infusion 5-FU, and hydroxyurea, along with concomitant b.i.d. radiation (150 cGy/fraction) given on days 1 to 5 of each 14-day treatment cycle. Five cycles are given over a 10-week period. A recent analysis of 76 patients treated with this regimen showed a 3-year progression-free survival rate of 69%. Major toxicities included mucositis, dermatitis, and myelosuppression. Investigators have attempted to decrease toxicity and improve efficacy by substituting paclitaxel for cisplatin.

The treatment of patients with recurrent locoregional disease after definitive radiation therapy remains problematic. Although the standard of care is systemic chemotherapy, the feasibility of reirradiation along with concomitant chemo- and radiotherapy has been evaluated at the University of Chicago. Small preliminary investigations indicate that as many as 30% of patients with locally recurrent disease may be cured with this approach.

Discussion

Patients with metastatic disease should receive chemotherapy in an effort to reduce the symptoms of the disease. Cure is not a realistic goal, and the prolongation of survival is frequently no more than a few months. Although several agents have been shown to reduce tumor burden, there is no single clear standard regimen. Combination cisplatin and 5-FU can lead to greater tumor responses at the price of increased toxicity. Therefore, this regimen should be reserved for patients with adequate performance. Whenever possible, patients should be referred for enrollment in ongoing clinical trials of newer agents and schedules.

The treatment of locally advanced HNSCC is an area of active clinical investigation. Treatment should be given with curative intent. Several studies and three meta-analyses indicate that patients with locally advanced disease benefit from initial treatment with concomitant chemo- and radiotherapy. The best specific treatment protocol has not yet been identified. Therefore, whenever possible, patients with locally advanced HNSCC should be referred for treatment on clinical trials. If a patient with locally advanced

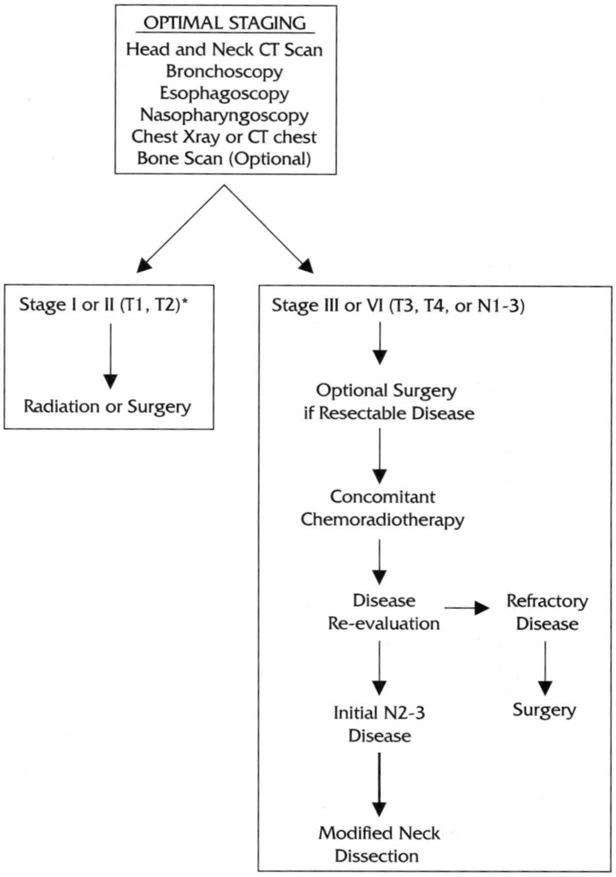

Figure 7–1 University of Chicago treatment algorithm for patients with head and neck squamous cell carcinoma. *Patients with early stage unresectable tumors (i.e., base-of-tongue cancers) may benefit from treatment with concomitant chemo- and radiotherapy (chemoradiotherapy).

HNSCC cannot be referred for an investigational protocol, treatment may be given by a multidisciplinary team according to one of the larger randomized regimens of concomitant chemo- and radiotherapy. In cases of locally advanced disease, surgery should be performed either for salvage of persistent disease after chemoradiotherapy or for modified neck dissection after chemoradiotherapy in patients with initial bulky lymphadenopathy (N2–N3 disease). The University of Chicago general algorithm for the treatment of locally advanced disease is illustrated in Figure 7–1.

Conclusion

Three decades of investigation have led to a gradual change in the treatments offered to patients with HNSCC. Whereas single modality surgery or radiation, or both, may cure most patients with early-stage disease, patients with locoregionally advanced disease require more aggressive multimodality treatment. Recent analyses show a significant role for the use of concomitant chemo- and radiotherapy in the initial treatment of locally advanced HNSCC. Further investigations are required to define the best treatment protocol.

REFERENCES

1. Forastiere AA, Metch B, Schuller DE, et al. Randomized comparison of cisplatin plus fluorouracil and carboplatin plus fluorouracil versus methotrexate in advanced squamous-cell carcinoma of the head and neck: a Southwest Oncology Group Study. *J Clin Oncol* 1992;10:1245–1251
2. Jacobs C, Lyman G, Velez-Garcia E, et al. A phase III randomized study comparing cisplatin and fluorouracil as single agents in combination for advanced squamous cell carcinoma of the head and neck. *J Clin Oncol* 1992;10:257–263
3. Liverpool Head and Neck Oncology Group. A phase III randomized trial of cisplatinum, methotrexate, cisplatinum + methotrexate and cisplatinum + 5-FU in end stage squamous carcinoma of the head and neck. *Br J Cancer* 1992;61: 311–315
4. Schrijvers D, Johnson J, Jiminez U, et al. Phase III trial of modulation of cisplatin/flurouracil chemotherapy by interferon alpha-2b in patients with recurrent or metastatic head and neck cancer. *J Clin Oncol* 1998;16:1054–1059
5. Clavel M, Vermorken JB, Cognetti F, et al. Randomized comparison of cisplatin, methotrexate, bleomycin and vincristine (CABO) versus cisplatin and 5-fluorouracil (CF) versus cisplatin (C) in recurrent or metastatic squamous cell carcinoma of the head and neck. A phase III study of the EORTC Head and Neck Cancer Cooperative Group. *Ann Oncol* 1994;5: 521–526
6. Shin D, Glisson B, Khuri F, et al. Phase II trial of paclitaxel, ifosfamide, and cisplatin in patients with recurrent head and neck squamous cell carcinoma. *J Clin Oncol* 1998;16: 1325–1330
7. The Department of Veterans Affairs Laryngeal Cancer Study Group. Induction chemotherapy plus radiation compared with surgery plus radiation in patients with advanced laryngeal cancer. *N Engl J Med* 1991;324:1685–1690
8. Brizel DM, Albers ME, Fisher SR, et al. Hyperfractionated irradiation with or without concurrent chemotherapy for locally advanced head and neck cancer. *N Engl J Med* 1998; 338:1798–1804
9. Munro AJ. An overview of randomized controlled trials of adjuvant chemotherapy in head and neck cancer. *Br J Cancer* 1995;71:83–91
10. El-Sayed S, Nelson N. Adjuvant and adjunctive chemotherapy in the management of squamous cell carcinoma of the head and neck region: a meta-analysis of prospective and randomized trials. *J Clin Oncol* 1996;14:838–847
11. Bourhis J, Pignon JP, Designe M, et al. Meta-analysis of chemotherapy in head and neck cancer (MACH-NC):(1) loco-regional treatment vs same treatment + chemotherapy. *Proc Am Soc Clin Oncol* 1998;17:386a
12. Al-Sarraf M, LeBlanc M, Shanker Giri PG, et al. Chemoradiotherapy versus radiotherapy in patients with advanced nasopharyngeal cancer: phase III randomized intergroup study 0099. *J Clin Oncol* 1998;16:1310–1317
13. Vokes EE, Weichselbaum RR, Lippman S, Hong WK. Head and neck cancer. *N Engl J Med* 1993;328:184–194
14. Vokes EE, Athanasiadis I. Chemotherapy for squamous cell carcinoma of head and neck: the future is now. *Ann Oncol* 1996;7:15–29
15. Smith R, Thornton D, Allen J. A phase II trial of paclitaxel in squamous cell carcinoma of the head and neck with correlative laboratory studies. *Semin Oncol* 1995;22(3 suppl 6):41–46
16. Forastiere A, Shank D, Neuberg D, et al. Final report of a phase II evaluation of paclitaxel in patients with advanced squamous cell carcinoma of the head and neck: an Eastern Cooperative Oncology Group Trial (PA390). *Cancer* 1998; 82:2270–2274
17. Catimel G, Verweij J, Mattijssen V, et al. Docetaxel (Taxotere®): an active drug for the treatment of patients with advanced squamous cell carcinoma of the head and neck. *Ann Oncol* 1994; 5:533–537
18. Dreyfuss A, Clark J, Norris CM, et al. Docetaxel: an active drug for squamous cell carcinoma of the head and neck. *J Clin Oncol* 1996;14:1672–1678
19. Couteau C, Chouaki N, Leyvraz S, et al. A phase II study of docetaxel in patients with metastatic squamous cell carcinoma of the head and neck. *Br J Cancer* 1999;81:457–462
20. Browman PB, Cronin L. Standard chemotherapy in squamous cell head and neck cancer: what have we learned from randomized trials. *Semin Oncol* 1994;21:311–319
21. Brockstein BE, Vokes EE. Chemoradiotherapy for head and neck cancer. *PPO Updates* 1996;10:1–19

The Role of Chemotherapy in Head and Neck Cancer

CHAPTER 8

Douglas B. Villaret and Ernest A. Weymuller, Jr.

The addition of chemotherapy to the treatment of advanced head and neck cancer is a controversial subject, with vocal opponents and proponents. Clinical trials have been devised to elucidate the role of treating squamous cell carcinoma in the head and neck with chemotherapeutic drugs. There are many difficulties, however, in interpreting the results from these studies: (1) the heterogeneous sites of the head and neck seem to respond differently to similar treatments; (2) the effectiveness of a drug depends not only on its intrinsic properties, but also on the dose used, the schedule in which it is delivered, and the subsites treated; duplication of all these events is difficult, hence the limited number of corroboratory studies; (3) drugs are often used in combination to take advantage of the different modes of action, with widely diverse combinations; (4) previously treated cancer responds much differently than naive tumors, and nonresectable tumors may respond differently than resectable tumors; (5) patients themselves vary widely and should be stratified according to well-known criteria, such as performance, alcohol, and nutritional status; and (6) many trials are not randomized, making their evaluation difficult, as even prospective studies must then use historical controls, which may or may not be relevant.

This chapter collates some of the data and presents a case for the use of chemotherapy for the management of squamous cell carcinoma in certain clinical settings.

The Drugs

For a complete understanding of the use of individual and combination regimens, a brief description of the more commonly used drugs is presented. Cisplatin (P) and carboplatin are platinum-based compounds. These agents differ in that carboplatin has fewer side effects (especially renal failure and hematogenesis) and is slightly less efficacious. Their mechanism of action is by binding to DNA strands and causing multiple chain breaks in dividing cells, eventually leading to cell death. Major toxicities include acute renal failure, neuropathy, ototoxicity, severe emesis, and occasional myelosuppression.[1,2]

The antimetabolites include methotrexate (a folate antagonist), 5-fluorouracil (5-FU), and gemcitabine (pyrimidine analogues), and 6-mercaptopurine (a purine analogue). They exert their action by disrupting DNA chain elongation, either by directly incorporating into the chain or by depleting the cells of necessary enzymes. Toxicities include myelosuppression, thrombocytopenia, nausea and vomiting, and mucositis.[1,2]

The most commonly used antibiotics (anthracyclines) are doxorubicin (Adriamycin), bleomycin (B), and mitomycin C (Mito). These agents act by producing intracellular free radicals (requiring a well-oxygenated tumor), damaging the DNA chain in association with topoisomerase. Cardiac and pulmonary side effects predominate, particularly pulmonary fibrosis and arrhythmias and, with larger doses, congestive heart failure.[1,2]

Vincristine, vinblastine, and the newer agent, vinorelbine, are plant alkaloids that bind to tubulin, interrupting the mitotic spindle and preventing the cell from completing meiosis. Partially irreversible peripheral neuropathy, gastrointestinal cramping, and mild myelosuppression are side effects noted with these agents.[1,2]

The newest group is the taxoid family, consisting of paclitaxel (Taxol) and docetaxol (Taxotere). In contrast with the vinca alkaloids, these drugs stabilize the microtubules, eventually causing the cells to accumulate arrays of disorganized microtubules, leading to cell death. As with the vinca alkaloids, they are active during the S phase of the cell cycle. Myelosuppression is the most common side effect, and irreversible toxicity may be seen with doses above 250 mg/m^2.[3]

Palliative Chemotherapy

CHEMOTHERAPY TRIALS: SINGLE AGENTS AND COMBINATION THERAPY

Chemotherapy as the sole modality of treatment for head and neck cancer has been limited to almost exclusively recurrent or persistent disease after failure of primary locoregional therapy. In this setting, the goal of treatment is limited to palliation, as no improvement has been demonstrated for either disease-specific or overall survival.[1,4-10] Treating recurrent or metastatic head and neck cancer is much different than treating a naive tumor. Previous therapy usually diminishes the effectiveness of chemotherapy by 30 to 50%.[11] Theories to explain this include more hypoxic cells, decreased blood flow to the tumor, and chemical resistance.[1,5,11,12] The difference in effectiveness can easily be seen when comparing the complete and partial responses achieved with induction (neoadjuvant) chemotherapy (30 to 92%)[12-17] to the response rate of palliative treatment for recurrences (10 to 40%).[4-10,13] This section discusses chemotherapy only as it applies to recurrent or metastatic head and neck cancer.

Deciding on which therapeutic endpoint to use in clinical trials becomes important, as the "gold standard" of increased survival is no longer applicable. The most easily and objectively measured

TABLE 8–1
Efficacy of Single Agent Chemotherapy

Drug	Average Response (range)
Methotrexate	30% (16 to 58%)
Cisplatin	30% (8 to 46%)
Carboplatin	21% (14 to 27%)
Fluorouracil	15% (0 to 33%)
Bleomycin	20% (6 to 46%)
Vinblastine	29%
Hydroxyurea	25%
Paclitaxel	22% (20 to 45%)

Modified from Catimel,[1] Stupp,[2] and Schrivers.[3]

outcome is tumor response (Table 8–1). Most trials measuring the benefit from chemotherapy use this as their main index of effectiveness, making the assumption that a decrease in tumor size will directly benefit the patient. For painful or obstructing lesions, as is often the case, this argument probably holds merit. However, a major concern relates to the toxicity of the treatment itself, as this group of patients receive no survival benefit. If the side effect profile of the treatment causes considerable discomfort, a few months of reduced tumor burden will not be worthwhile.

A counterargument is that an increase in side effects is acceptable if the probability of a complete response (CR) is increased, as a longer survival time has been associated with CR.[18-20] However, as Adelstein[11] and Fu[12] point out, this association may simply reflect selection of those patients who have a better prognosis to begin with. Response to chemotherapy and improved survival are linked, both occurring in those patients with a better performance status, less prior treatment, and certain head and neck subsites (larynx, mobile tongue). This same selection bias has been used as the basis for the organ preservation strategy (as explained later). Other measurements of therapeutic improvement include an increase in quality-of-life scores and time to progression and, for those achieving a CR, time until recurrence.

SINGLE AGENTS

Does chemotherapy add any benefit beyond providing pain control? In one of the few randomized studies with a "no-treatment" control arm, Morton et al.[21] compared the use of cisplatin, bleomycin, and the combination of cisplatin plus bleomycin. They found a statistically significant increased survival in the platinum arms (4.0 to 4.2 months) as compared with the control arm (2.1 months). The population in this study was relatively small, with about 24 patients in each treatment arm, and survival was relatively short, but this does provide some evidence that chemotherapy can have an impact on survival. Most trials, however, show that there is no survival advantage to chemotherapy over historical controls.[1,4-10]

Methotrexate (M) has been the standard therapy for palliation of advanced tumors for three decades. The dose is 40 to 60 mg/m^2/week given intravenously (IV). The average response rate is 30% with a range of 8 to 57% (CR range from 6 to 26%).[22,23] Toxicities are tolerable, with mild to moderate leukopenia, anemia, mucositis, and diarrhea the most commonly cited.[5] The duration of the response is approximately 4 months.

Cisplatin has been used extensively with response rates of 8 to 41%, also averaging around 30% (0 to 8% CR).[21,24,25] Additional side effects of nephrotoxicity, neuropathy, and ototoxicity must be accounted for when choosing this drug over methotrexate. Carboplatin has fewer side effects than cisplatin, but the response rate is also decreased to around 21% (14 to 26%).

Three randomized studies have conducted direct comparison of cisplatin with methotrexate. In the first two studies, consisting of 144 patients, no difference was seen in response rate, response duration, or survival.[24,26] The larger of these studies showed a low response rate to cisplatin (8%) and methotrexate (16%), with an overall survival of only 4.5 to 5 months. A third trial from the group in Liverpool showed a significantly higher response rate of the tumors to cisplatin (26% vs 12%) and, again, no improvement in survival.[27]

Bleomycin also produces a 21% response rate (6 to 45%) in refractory tumors, with the effects lasting 1 to 3 months.[5] The standard dose is 15 U IV on a weekly schedule. Pulmonary toxicity is the main drawback, especially once a total dose of 200 to 400 U is reached.

5-FU is not often used alone to treat head and neck cancer, but response rates average 15% (0 to 33%).[28] The optimal administration is a 5-day continuous infusion, rather than bolus treatment.[20,29] Side effects include bone marrow suppression, cardiac toxicity, and mucositis.

The taxoids are generating some interest, with one phase II report showing a 40% response rate and another a 32% response.[30,31] Hematologic toxicity was severe, however, even with the use of granulocyte-colony-stimulating factor (G-CSF).

Other less frequently used agents are hydroxyurea (25%); alkylating agents, including cyclophosphamide and ifosfamide (36%); vinblastine (29%); gemcitabine (13%); and the anthracyclines (5 to 8%)[1] (Table 8–1).

SINGLE AGENTS VERSUS COMBINATIONS

Combination chemotherapy takes advantage of two characteristics of chemotherapeutic drugs. The first is their mechanism of action. The rationale is that the addition of drugs that target different areas of the cell might overcome the selection pressure causing resistance to the agents. Also, separate subpopulations might be better targeted (mitomycin C and hypoxic cells). The second purpose of combining drugs is to take advantage of the different toxicity profiles and to reduce the severity of side effects experienced by the patient.

Do combination regimens improve tumor responsiveness as compared with single agents? In two studies comparing single-agent methotrexate with cisplatin plus 5-FU in recurrent or metastatic head and neck cancer, one showed a significantly higher response rate in the combination therapy arm, and the other showed a trend toward significance in the combination therapy arm.[27,32] Two other studies compared the single-agent approach of cisplatin and 5-FU with the combination and again found a significantly improved response rate to the combination but no change in survival rate.[33,34]

A meta-analysis was undertaken by Browman and Cronin[7] in 1994 to evaluate single-agent versus combination chemotherapy. These investigators analyzed 15 trials that included 1916 patients and 17 different treatment regimens. Single-agent methotrexate was less effective at reducing tumor size than was found in the pooled combination studies. The odds ratio (OR) was used to define statistical significance, with an OR of >1 favoring comparison treatment); the OR was 1.71 with a 95% confidence interval (CI) of 1.28–2.31. Pooled combination treatments were also statistically better at achieving tumor regression than were the pooled single agents (M, P, B, 5-FU), with OR-1.59 and 95% CI-1.28–2.01. The combination of cisplatin and 5-FU was found to be the most efficacious. The side effects of the different regimens were also evaluated showing that the combinations have a greatly increased risk of nausea and vomiting. It appears that combination chemotherapy should be used for those patients with end-stage metastatic or recurrent squamous cell cancer if they have a life expectancy of more than 4 to 5 months and a good performance score and can tolerate the treatment.

Therapeutic Chemotherapy

COMBINED-MODALITY THERAPY

Radiotherapy has proved effective in head and neck cancer. Its mechanism of cell killing is postulated to be mediated by the direct interaction of superoxide radicals with cellular enzymes and DNA, indicating that adequate oxygen content of the tumor is necessary for efficacy of this treatment.[35] In addition, radiotherapy has been found to be most effective during the G2 and M stages of the cell cycle. Adding chemotherapy to radiation has several theoretical benefits. Chemotherapy can prevent the repair of sublethal damage inflicted by ionizing radiation. Certain drugs act as sensitizers (e.g., 5-FU) and improve the effect of radiation on tumors. Some drugs are particularly toxic to hypoxic cells (mitomycin C) and thus can target a population that is radioresistant. Both cause apoptosis, probably by different mechanisms, so each potentiates the other.[12] Chemotherapy often causes growth arrest of cells at a certain part of the cell cycle, allowing them to be more sensitive to radiation.[35]

One of the difficulties of combining the two treatment modalities has been in determining the appropriate timing of each. The schedule for adding chemotherapy to radiation has traditionally been divided into three groups: induction or neoadjuvant, concomitant (including alternating), and adjuvant (posttreatment) administration.

NEOADJUVANT CHEMOTHERAPY

Giving chemotherapy before radiation has theoretical benefits and risks. By reducing the size of the tumor without interrupting the blood supply, the oxygen content of the mass should be higher, leading to greater sensitivity to radiation. In addition, responders to chemotherapy may be treated effectively with a single modality treatment, usually radiation, and thus spared surgery (at least as a primary modality). On the downside, Toohill et al.[36] reported a worse survival rate with the neoadjuvant arm than with the standard (radiotherapy) arm. This raises the possibility that delaying definitive therapy may allow the tumor to become further disseminated and reduce survival.

A large number of trials have been designed to evaluate the benefit of neoadjuvant chemotherapy.[1,13-17,36-41] Many show high response rates, up to 98% in operable laryngeal cancer.[17] But survival data show no statistically significant change in overall or (where available) disease-specific survival (Table 8–2). Many of these studies have been criticized with respect to low patient numbers, inadequate drug dosages, and variable "standard" treatment arms, but several well-controlled studies have been completed.

Is there a role for induction chemotherapy? Several trials have looked at this specific question, especially in light of the organ-preservation protocols. According to this concept, an increase in survival might not be a realistic goal, but improved quality of life by retaining organs such as the larynx might be obtainable. To this end, the Veteran's Affairs Laryngeal Cancer Cooperative Study (VALCS) was designed.[16] It included 332 patients who were randomized to receive either surgery and postoperative radiotherapy or neoadjuvant chemotherapy (cisplatin and 5-FU) and definitive locoregional therapy. In the chemotherapy arm, the patient was evaluated after two cycles. If the tumor response was greater than 50%, a third dose of chemotherapy was administered, followed by definitive radiotherapy. For those patients who failed to respond, surgery was perfomed (usually total laryngectomy), followed by postoperative radiation. Of those patients who received chemotherapy, 85% showed a major response (31% CR) and 64% retained their larynx. The 2-year survival data showed no difference compared with the control arm. In a follow-up study, the 4-year evaluation showed that 31% of the 166 patients randomized to the chemotherapy arm were alive and retained their larynx.[17] Their overall survival rate was 46% for the chemotherapy group and 43% for the control group.

A similar study was performed by the European Organization for Research and Treatment of Cancer (EORTC), except that eligible patients had T2-4, N0-2b squamous cell carcinoma of the aryepiglottic fold or piriform sinus.[37] Another difference was that only those patients showing a complete response to chemotherapy were allowed to progress to radiotherapy. In this study, 43% of patients required a laryngectomy for lack of

TABLE 8–2
Randomized Neoadjuvant Trials

First Author, Year	*N*	Drugs	Response Rate (%)	Survival Benefit
Taylor,[42] 1985	82	Methotrexate	40	NS*
Toohill,[36] 1987	60	Cisplatin 5-fluorouracil	85	NS
HNCP,[†40] 1987	443	Cisplatin Bleomycin	37	NS
Schuller,[43] 1988	158	Cisplatin Methotrexate Bleomycin Vincristine	70	NS
DVALCSG,[‡16] 1991	332	Cisplatin 5-fluorouracil	85	NS
Dalley,[44] 1995	280	Cisplatin 5-fluorouracil	80	NS
Lefebvre,[37] 1996	194	Cisplatin 5-fluorouracil	86	NS
Lewin,[15] 1997	461	Cisplatin 5-fluorouracil	71	NS
Salvajoli,[45] 1997	60	Vinblastine Mitomycin-C Cisplatin Bleomycin	60	NS

*Not significant
† Head and Neck Contracts Program
‡ The Department of Veterans Affairs Laryngeal Cancer Study Group

response or salvage after radiation (as compared to 38% in the VALCS trial). The EORTC trial also showed that 28% of patients could be expected to be alive with a functioning larynx at 3 years. No difference was found in overall survival.

These reports and others, including the noncontrolled trial from M.D. Anderson, show that induction chemotherapy can be used to retain a functioning larynx without compromising survival.[13] A major question raised from these studies is whether the neoadjuvant chemotherapy is really any benefit or is simply a selection marker for those who will respond to radiation. To help answer this question, the Head and Neck Intergroup is conducting a study that will accrue 546 patients divided into three groups: (1) induction chemotherapy (similar to the VALCS protocol) followed by radiotherapy for responders, and salvage surgery with postoperative radiation for nonresponders; (2) radiotherapy with concomitant chemotherapy (cisplatin alone); and (3) radiotherapy alone.[46] The goal of this study is to determine the true benefit of induction chemotherapy over radiotherapy alone for organ preservation, as well as to evaluate the efficacy of concomitant chemo- and radiotherapy. There is still the question of selecting out the responders to radiation. Laboratory tests may be able to make this prediction independent of having the patient undergo the toxicity of chemotherapy. Bradford et al.[47] looked at the p53 status of 178 of the tumors from the VALCS study and found a significant correlation with overexpression of p53 and response to radiotherapy, but no correlation with overall survival. Neoadjuvant chemotherapy for advanced, previously untreated, laryngeal cancers is generally the accepted regimen.

CONCOMITANT CHEMO- AND RADIOTHERAPY

Is concomitant chemo- and radiotherapy better than radiation alone? Early concomitant trials employed single-agent chemotherapy with simultaneous radiotherapy. Agents included methotrexate, hydroxyurea, bleomycin, 5-FU, and cisplatin.[48-50] Except for a few trials, one each with methotrexate, bleomycin, and 5-FU, all results showed no significant difference over radiation alone. Recent trials have more often used combination chemotherapy in conjunction with various delivery schedules of radiation.[45, 51-56] The subjects are varied, but most trials concentrate on previously untreated patients with or without resectable disease. The locoregional control and survival statistics of the combined-modality arms of these trials are improved from their predecessors (Table 8–3).

TABLE 8–3

Randomized Concomitant Chemo- and Radiotherapy Trials†

First Author, Year	N	Chemo‡	Resectable	H&N sites§	LRC#	Overall Survival	Dz. Free survival	Comments
Lo,[50] 1976	136	F	Y	OC OP HP L	<0.05	<0.05	NA	
Shanta,[57] 1980	157	B	Y	OC OP L	0.05	<0.05	<0.05	Used IV, IM, and IA delivery of chemo
Stefani,[58] 1980	150	Hu	Y	OC OP HP L	NS	NS	NA	Median survival better in control
Vermund,[59] 1985	222	B	Y	OC NP S OP HP L	NS	NS	NS	Trend for control to live longer
Gupta,[60] 1987	313	M	Y	OC NP OP HP L	0.016	NS	NA	OP only has significant survival difference
Fu,[49] 1987	96	B	N	OC NP OP HP L	0.001	NS	0.043	Adjuvant chemo also
Weissberg,[61] 1989	117	Mito	Y	OC NP OP HP L	<0.02	NS	<0.07	
Sanchiz,[62] 1990	577	F	Y	OC NP S OP HP L	NA	<0.001	<0.001	3rd arm of hyperfraction XRT equal to comb tx
Weissler,[51] 1992	58	P-F	Y N	OC OP HP L E	NA NA	NS 0.013	NS 0.002	radiation hyperfractionated
Salvajoli,[45] 1992	60	B-P	Y	OC OP HP	NS	NS	NA	3rd arm neoadjuvant also NS
Merlano,[52] 1992	157	P-F	N	OC NP OP HP L	<0.05	0.01	0.008	Alternating schedule
Herskovic,[63] 1992	123	P-F	Y	E	0.01	<0.0001	0.0003	Early closure of study, adjuvant P-F
Keane,[55] 1992	212	F-Mito	Y	HP L	NS	NS	NS	Split course radiation
Browman,[64] 1994	175	F	Y	OC OP HP L	NS	NS	NS (0.06)	Trend for increased survival in combination
Smid,[56] 1994	49	B-Mito	N	OC OP HP	<0.001	NA	0.001	Median follow-up 18 months
Bachaud,[65] 1996	83	P	Y	OC OP HP L	0.08	<0.01	<0.02	Treatment delivered postoperatively
Adelstein,[53] 1997	100	P-F	Y	OC OP HP L	0.03	NS	0.03	Excluded T4 with bone involvement
Haffty,[66] 1997	203	Mito	Y	OC NP S OP HP L	0.002	NS	0.002	Disease-specific survival p0.005, post-op treatment
Jeremic,[67] 1997	159	P CP	N	OC NP OP HP L	0.018* 0.04*	0.011 0.019	0.018 0.040	* local control only, regional control = NS
Al-Sarraf,[68] 1998	147	P	Y	NP	<0.01	0.005	<0.001	Early closure of study, adjuvant P-F
Brizel,[69] 1998	116	P	Y	OC NP S OP HP L	0.01	0.07	0.08	Radiation hyperfractionated
Wendt,[54] 1998	270	P-F-LV	N	OC OP HP L	<0.004	0.003	NA	4-year survival 49% vs 24%

† Results are p values comparing radiation alone to concomitant therapy ($p<0.05$ favors concomitant).

‡ B = bleomycin, F = fluorouracil, Hu = hydroxyurea, LV = leucovorin, M = methotrexate, Mito = mitomycin-C, P = cisplatin

§ E = esophagus, HP = hypopharynx, L = larynx, NP = nasopharynx, OC = oral cavity, OP = oropharynx, S = sinus

LRC = Loco-Regional Control

Of interest are five trials employing cisplatin and 5-FU with different radiation regimens. Using a hyperfractionation scheme with 150 centigray (cGy) twice a day (b.i.d.) with a 2-week scheduled break after the first 10 treatments, Weissler et al.[51] found a significant difference in locoregional control and overall survival rate only in those patients who were deemed to be unresectable. Merlano et al.[52] used alternating radiotherapy and chemotherapy in unresectable patients and also found a significant difference between the treatment and control arms in several areas, including progression-free survival (25% vs 7%, respectively). Adelstein's group[53] used standard daily radiation with 4 days of chemotherapy initiated on days 1 and 28; nonresponders underwent surgical salvage. Relapse-free survival was better in the treatment arm (67 to 52%). All these trials used cisplatin at a dose of 100 mg/m^2. In 1998, Wendt et al.[54] reported on a trial of unresectable patients using accelerated fractionated radiation (1.8 cGy b.i.d.). They used only 60 mg/m^2 of cisplatin, but leucovorin was added to the combination. A 3-year overall survival rate difference of 48 to 24% was found in favor of the combined therapy. An important Intergroup trial focusing on esophageal cancer was first reported in 1992 and updated in 1997.[63, 70] This trial included both squamous cell carcinoma and adenocarcinoma of the esophagus. Patients were stratified on the basis of histopathologic status, tumor size, and weight loss. They were randomly divided between concomitant chemo- and radiotherapy with cisplatin (75 mg/m^2) and 5-FU, also receiving two courses of adjuvant therapy with the same agents, and with radiotherapy alone. Surgical resection was reserved for those failing the primary therapy. The trial stopped accruing patients at the interim analysis, when investigators noted a 2-year survival difference of 38 to 10% ($P < 0.0001$) favoring the combined modality group. The follow-up report showed that none of the patients who received radiotherapy alone was alive at 3 years, whereas the 3- and 5-year survival rates for the combined group were 30% and 27%, respectively ($P < 0.0001$). A similar survival rate was found for other patients treated with this regimen since the conclusion of the trial. So, despite certain differences, all these trials of cisplatin-based concomitant chemo- and radiotherapy demonstrated improved survival, as compared with the control (radiotherapy-only) arm of each study.

A meta-analysis evaluated 25 prospective randomized studies. A control arm was included for definitive locoregional control, to which chemotherapy was added as a treatment arm.[71] When all reports were summated, there was no difference in survival rates. However, when only those trials that used concomitant chemo- and radiotherapy were evaluated, a 0.78 reduction in mortality rate from the radiotherapy-only control group was observed.

While the great majority of trials show no difference between standard radiotherapy and concomitant chemo- and radiotherapy, the newer trials have often shown differences in survival.[42, 45, 51-56, 58-69, 72-74] These longer survival rates come at the expense of increased short-term morbidity, mostly in the form of grade 3 and 4 mucositis. But there is evidence that chemotherapy is having an impact not only on tumor regression, but on both disease-free and, occasionally, overall survival, as well.

ADJUVANT CHEMOTHERAPY

The idea behind adjuvant treatment is to eliminate any micrometastatic disease left behind after locoregional treatment. One benefit of administering chemotherapy after surgery or radiation, or both, is that the tumor is addressed with definitive therapy first, unlike neoadjuvant therapy, where it is delayed. Also, as no chemotherapy is given preoperatively, there is no decrease in the patient's nutritional, immunologic, hematologic, or general health status. The disadvantages are that the vascularity has been interrupted, so theoretically less of the drug will get to the residual cancer. Also, these patients have already been disabled by the initial treatment and are unlikely to be compliant with a further decrease in their performance status.

Two trials have shown a significant improvement in survival rates for those who underwent adjuvant therapy.[49,68] Unfortunately, these patients also had concomitant chemo- and radiotherapy, so no definite conclusion can be made. Of the many other trials performed using definitive treatment with or without adjuvant chemotherapy, no survival benefit has been seen.[40,75,76] Distant metastases have been seen to decrease in some trials, but this has not had an impact on overall survival. Finally, the Head and Neck Contracts Program trial exemplifies the difficulties in getting patients to be compliant: only 9% of the 151 patients scheduled to receive adjuvant therapy completed all six courses.[40]

Special Issues

NASOPHARYNGEAL CANCER

Nasopharyngeal cancer is a highly radioresponsive tumor. This is especially true for the World Health Organization (WHO) class II and III (nonkeratinizing and undifferentiated squamous cell carcinoma). In the United States, however, 30 to 50% of patients will have WHO class I (keratinized squamous cell carcinoma), which is associated with alcohol and tobacco use and is much less radiosensitive.[77] Advanced-stage disease is associated with poor 5-year survival rates, within a range of 10 to 40% when treatment is with radiotherapy alone. For this reason, adding chemotherapy to the treatment protocol has been investigated.

Several trials have evaluated the use of neoadjuvant chemotherapy in this disease. In a noncontrolled study from Israel, 27 patients treated with induction cisplatin and 5-FU achieved a 93% response rate (37% CR).[78] The 5-year actuarial survival was 66%. Again, those patients achieving a CR did significantly better, with all patients in this subgroup alive at the end of the follow-up period. Investigators from M.D. Anderson reported on a randomized trial comparing neoadjuvant cisplatin and 5-FU with radiation alone. This study showed a significantly improved 5-year survival rate in the neoadjuvant group, 69 to 48%. Another trial used neoadjuvant and adjuvant treatment, both using cisplatin and 5-FU. In this study, all patients were WHO stage III. No significant difference was found in either the 2-year disease-free survival or the overall survival rates.

A landmark article was reported by Al-Sarraf for the Intergroup Study 0099. This trial reported on 147 patients randomized to receive either 70 gray (Gy) of external beam radiation or the same radiation treatment with the addition of three doses of concomitant cisplatin (100 mg/m^2) and three courses of adjuvant treatment with cisplatin and 5-FU. The patients had stage III and IV disease and were stratified by tumor and nodal stage, WHO histologic category, and performance status. The trial was closed before accrual of the pre-specified 270 patients, as there was a highly significant difference in the two groups at the interim analysis. The progression-free survival rates were 24% and 69%, respectively, for radiotherapy versus chemo- and radiotherapy ($P < 0.001$). Overall survival was also highly significant, with rates of 47% and 78%, respectively ($P = 0.005$). Although this treatment response may not be reflective of results achievable for groups in whom WHO type III tumors predominate, this trial has reset the standard therapy for nasopharyngeal carcinoma in the United States.

INTRA-ARTERIAL CHEMOTHERAPY

An exciting prospect in the delivery of chemotherapy is the intra-arterial route. The advantages include directly perfusing the tumor with the drug, thereby not losing efficacy to the first-pass effect. Also, when cisplatin is used, sodium thiosulfate can be given systemically to neutralize the cisplatin by covalently binding to it once it has passed out of the tumor vascular bed. This should allow decreased side effects, including mucositis and nephrotoxicity. The additional risks revolve around the arterial puncture and possible vascular and cerebrovascular events.

Robbins et al.[78] evaluated a cohort of 57 patients with stage III (27%) and stage IV (73%) squamous cell carcinoma of the head and neck in a noncontrolled study. These investigators achieved a 75% complete response (CR) rate in the primary tumor and regional neck disease. The treatment includes a femoral artery puncture with arteriography to select the feeding blood vessels to the tumor before administration of the "supradose" cisplatin (150 mg/m^2). This is repeated weekly for a total of four doses. The thiosulfate is given intravenously concomitant with the cisplatin. Radiation is delivered using 1.8- to 2.0-Gy fractions daily. Their follow-up time is short, averaging 18 months, but the results are impressive. They report a 91% CR rate of the primary tumor. Fifty-two percent of their patients are alive with no evidence of disease, 25% have died with disease, and 17% died of other causes.

The main argument against intra-arterial chemotherapy is the increase in complication rates without a significant benefit in survival rates. With the addition of the neutralizing agent, the severe grade 3 and 4 mucositis has decreased, as well as nephrotoxicity. Two transient ischemic attacks and two cerebrovascular attacks were reported, with no permanent disability. One patient had deep venous thrombosis, and three patients had pulmonary embolisms, one of whom died.

The results of this trial are encouraging. Only 4% of patients showed a recurrence above the clavicles; 23% failed with distant metastases. Although some complications were serious, the relatively low morbidity of this procedure appears to be highly dependent on the skill of the interventional radiologists, and this may be a limiting factor. In addition, longer survival and disease-free rates need to be reported. The protocol has been expanded to a multi-institutional trial, an important step in verifing the reproducibility of the Memphis trial experience.

Conclusion

The logic behind the delivery of chemotherapeutic drugs to head and neck cancer patients is complex. When these agents are given without locoregional treatment, the goal is palliation; in these cases, tumor response and toxicity alone are important considerations. Neoadjuvant therapy has proved a good predictor of response to radiation; an excellent organ-sparing approach without a decrement in survival. However, substituting laboratory studies, such as p53 overexpression, for the toxic induction treatment is a real possibility that warrants evaluation. Concomitant chemo- and radiotherapy has recently shown great promise, with several studies demonstrating an improvement in survival, the most notable being the Intergroup Study 0099 of the nasopharynx. The future holds several challenges:

1. *Defining the appropriate drugs:* Several newer drugs, including the taxols and gemcitabine, hold promise and need to be studied further to define their role in the treatment of head and neck cancer.
2. *Defining the appropriate radiation schedule:* The more toxic hyperfractionation and accelerated fractionation schemes may be more efficacious than the "standard" 1.8- to 2.0-Gy daily dose.
3. *Defining the appropriate chemotherapy schedule:* Will there be a role for sequential administration of the drugs or for concomitant delivery methods (simultaneous, split course, or alternating)?
4. *Adding other adjunctive medicines:* Will such agents as hematopoietic growth factors (G-CSF) and cytoprotectants (amifostine) decrease the toxicity of treatment?[79-82]
5. *Defining the tumors and the patient cohort with greater accuracy:* Trials need to be designed so that their results can be more accurately compared and evaluated.

The treatment of head and neck cancer with chemotherapy does hold promise. The challenge is in scientifically proving its effectiveness in prolonging survival.

REFERENCES

1. Catimel G. Head and neck cancer: guidelines for chemotherapy. Drugs 1996;51:73–88
2. Stupp R, Vokes EE. Chemotherapy of head and neck tumors. In: Thawley SE, Panje WR, Batsakis JG, Lindberg RD, eds. *Comprehensive Management of Head and Neck Tumors.* Philadelphia: WB Saunders; 1998:141–156
3. Schrivers D, Vermorken JB. Update on the taxoids and other new agents in head and neck cancer therapy. *Curr Opin Oncol* 1998;10:233–241
4. Wheeler RH. Chemotherapy of patients with recurrent head and neck cancers. In: Jacobs C, ed. *Carcinomas of the Head and Neck: Evaluation, Management.* Boston: Kluwer Academic; 1990:171–193
5. Pinto HA, Jacobs C. Chemotherapy for recurrent and metastatic head and neck cancer. *Hematol Oncol Clin North Am* 1991;5:667–686
6. Wittes RE, Cvitkovic E, Shah J, et al. *cis*-Dichlorodiammineplatinum(II) in the treatment of epidermoid carcinoma of the head and neck. *Cancer Treat Rep* 1977;61:359–366
7. Browman GP, Cronin L. Standard chemotherapy in squamous cell head and neck cancer: what we have learned from randomized trials. *Semin Oncol* 1994;3:311–319
8. Al-Sarraf M. Clinical trials with fluorinated pyrimidines in patients with head and neck cancer. *Invest New Drugs* 1985;7: 71–81
9. Eisenberger MA, Hornedo J, Silva H, et al. Carboplatin (NSC-241-240), an active platinum analog for the treatment of squamous cell carcinoma of the head and neck. *J Clin Oncol* 1986;4:1506–1509
10. Forastiere AA. Chemotherapy of head and neck cancer. *Ann Oncol* 1992;3(suppl 3):S11–S14
11. Adelstein DJ. The community approach to salvage therapy for advanced head and neck cancer. *Semin Oncol* 1994;21:52–57
12. Fu KK. Combined-modality therapy for head and neck cancer. *Oncology* 1997;11:1781–1791
13. Shirinian MH, Weber RS, Lippman SM, et al. Laryngeal preservation by induction chemotherapy plus radiotherapy in locally advanced head and neck cancer: the M.D. Anderson Cancer Center experience. *Head Neck* 1994;16:39–44
14. Vokes EE, Panje WR, Mick R, et al. A randomized study comparing two regimens of neoadjuvant and adjuvant chemotherapy in multimodal therapy for locally advanced head and neck cancer. *Cancer* 1990;66:206–213
15. Lewin F, Damber L, Jonsson H, et al. Neoadjuvant chemotherapy with cisplatin and 5–fluorouracil in advanced squamous cell carcinoma of the head and neck: a randomized Phase III study. *Radiother Oncol* 1997;43:23–28
16. The Department of Veterans Affairs Laryngeal Cancer Study Group. Induction chemotherapy plus radiation compared with surgery plus radiation in patients with advanced laryngeal cancer. *N Engl J Med* 1991;324:1685–1690
17. Wolfe GT, Hong WK, Fisher SG. Neoadjuvant chemotherapy for organ preservation: current status. In: Shah JP, Johnson JT, eds. In: *International Conference on Head and Neck Cancer,* Toronto, Canada. The Society of Head and Neck Surgeons and American Society of Head and Neck Surgery; 1996:89–97
18. Al-Sarraf M. Head and neck cancer: chemotherapy concepts. *Semin Oncol* 1988;15:70–85
19. Forastiere AA. Management of advanced stage squamous cell carcinoma of the head and neck. *Am J Med Sci* 1986;291:405–415
20. Kish JA, Ensley JF, Jacobs J, et al. A randomized trial of cisplatin (CACP) + 5-fluorouracil (5-FU) infusion and CACP + 5-FU bolus for recurrent and advanced squamous cell carcinoma of the head and neck. *Cancer* 1985;56: 2740–2744
21. Morton RP, Rugman RF, Dorman EB, et al. Cisplatinum and bleomycin for advanced or recurrent squamous cell carcinoma of the head and neck: a randomized factorial phase III controlled trial. *Cancer Chemother Pharmacol* 1985;15:283–289
22. Vogler WR, Jacobs J, Moffitt S, et al. Methotrexate therapy with or without citovorum factor in carcinoma of the head and neck, breast, and colon cancer. *Cancer Clin Trials* 1979; 2:227–236
23. Priestman TJ. Results in fifty cases of advanced squamous cell carcinoma of the head and neck treated by intravenous methotrexate. *Br J Cancer* 1973;27:400–405
24. Grose WE, Lehane DE, Dixon DO, et al. Comparison of methotrexate and cisplatinum for patients with advanced squamous cell carcinoma of the head and neck region: a Southwest Oncology Group study. *Cancer Treat Rep* 1985;69: 577–581
25. Stephens R, Coltman C, Rossof A, et al. Cis-dichlorodiammineplatinum in adult patients: Southwest Oncology Group studies. *Cancer Treat Rep* 1979;63:1609–1610
26. Hong WK, Schaefer S, Issell B, et al. A prospective randomized trial of methotrexate versus cisplatin in the treatment of recurrent squamous cell carcinoma of the head and neck. *Cancer* 1983;52:206–210
27. Liverpool Head and Neck Oncology Group. A phase III randomized trial of cisplatinum, methotrexate, cisplatinum + methotrexate and cisplatinum + 5-FU in end stage squamous cell carcinoma of the head and neck. *Br J Cancer* 1990;61: 311–315
28. Al-Sarraf M. Chemotherapeutic management of head and neck cancer. *Cancer Metast Rev* 1987;6:191–198
29. Tapazoglou E, Kish J, Ensley J, et al. The activity of a single-agent 5-fluorouracil infusion in advanced and recurrent head and neck cancer. *Cancer* 1986;57:1105–1109
30. Forastiere A. Use of paclitaxel ("Taxol") in squamous cell carcinoma of the head and neck. *Semin Oncol* 1993;20(suppl 3): 56–60

31. Catimel G, Verwij J, Mattijssen V, et al. Docetaxel ("Taxotere"): an active drug for the treatment of patients with advanced squamous cell carcinoma of the head and neck. *Ann Oncol* 1994;5:533–537
32. Campbell JB, Dorman EB, McCormick J, et al. A randomized phase III trial of cisplatinum, methotrexate, cisplatinum + methotrexate, and cisplatinum + fluorouracil in end-stage head and neck cancer. *Acta Otolaryngol (Stockh)* 1987;103: 519–528
33. Clavel M, Vermorken JB, Cognetti F, et al. Randomized comparison of cisplatin, methotrexate, bleomycin and vincristine (CABO) versus cisplatin and 5–fluorouracil (CF) versus cisplatin (C) in recurrent or metastatic squamous cell carcinoma of the head and neck: a phase III study of the EORTC Head and Neck Cooperative Group. *Ann Oncol* 1994;5:521–526
34. Jacobs C, Lyman G, Velez-Garcia E, et al. A phase II randomized study comparing cisplatin and fluorouracil as single agents and in combination for advanced squamous cell carcinoma of the head and neck. *J Clin Oncol* 1992;10:257–263
35. Mulcahy RT, Sutherland RM, Siemann DW. Basic principles of radiobiology. In: Rubin P, ed. *Clinical Oncology: A Multidisciplinary Approach for Physicians and Students.* 7th ed. Philadelphia: WB Saunders; 1993
36. Toohill RJ, Anderson T, Byhard RW, et al. Cisplatin and fluorouracil as neoadjuvant therapy in head and neck cancer: a preliminary report. *Arch Otolaryngol Head Neck Surg* 1987;113:758–761
37. Lefebvre JL, Chevalier D, Luboinski B, et al. Larynx preservation in pyriform sinus cancer: preliminary results of a European Organization for Research and Treatment of Cancer phase III trial: EORTC Head and Neck Cancer Cooperative Group. *J Natl Cancer Inst* 1996;88:890–899
38. Depondt J, Gehanno P, Martin M, et al. Neoadjuvant chemotherapy with carboplatin/5-fluorouracil in head and neck cancer. *Oncology* 1993;50:23–27
39. Fazekas J, Sommer C, Kramer S, et al. Adjuvant intravenous methotrexate or definitive radiotherapy alone for advanced squamous cancers of the oral cavity, oropharynx, supraglottic larynx, or hypopharynx. Concluding reports of an RTOG randomized trial on 638 patients. *Int J Radiat Oncol Biol Phys* 1980;6:533–541
40. Head and Neck Contracts Program. Adjuvant chemotherapy for advanced head and neck squamous cell carcinoma. Final report of the Head and Neck Contracts Program. *Cancer* 1987;60:301–311
41. International Nasopharynx Study Group. Preliminary results of a randomized trial comparing neoadjuvant chemotherapy (cisplatin, epirubicin, bleomycin) plus radiotherapy vs. radiotherapy alone in Stage IV (≥N2,M0) undifferentiated nasopharyngeal carcinoma: a positive effect on progression-free survival: VUMCA I trial. *Int J Radiat Oncol Biol Phys* 1996; 35:463–469
42. Taylor SG, Murthy AK, Vannetzel J-M, et al. Randomized comparison of neoadjuvant cisplatin and fluorouracil infusion followed by radiation versus concomitant treatment in advanced head and neck cancer. *J Clin Oncol* 1994;12: 385–395
43. Schuller DE, Metch B, Stein DW, et al. Preoperative chemotherapy in advanced resectable head and neck cancer: final report of the Southwest Oncology Group. *Laryngoscope* 1988;98:1205–1211
44. Dalley D, Beller E, Aroney R, et al. The value of chemotherapy (CT) prior to definitive local therapy (DLT) in patients with locally advanced squamous cell carcinoma (SCC) of the head and neck (HN) [abstract]. *Proc Am Soc Clin Oncol* 1995;14:297
45. Salvajoli JV, Morioka H, Trippe N, et al. A randomized trial of neoadjuvant vs concomitant chemotherapy vs radiotherapy alone in the treatment of stage IV head and neck squamous cell carcinoma. *Eur Arch Otorhinolaryngol* 1992;249:211–215
46. Fu KK, Cooper JS, Marcial VA, et al. Evolution of the Radiation Therapy Oncology Group clinical trials for head and neck cancer. *Int J Radiat Oncol Biol Phys* 1996;35:425–438
47. Bradford CR, Zhu S, Wolf GT, et al. Overexpression of p53 predicts organ preservation using induction chemotherapy and radiation in patients with advanced laryngeal cancer. *Otolaryngol Head Neck Surg* 1995;113:408–412
48. Archangeli G, Nervi C, Righini R, et al. Combined radiation and drugs: the effect of intra-arterial chemotherapy followed by radiotherapy in head and neck cancer. *Radiother Oncol* 1983;1:101–107
49. Fu KK, Phillips TL, Silverberg IJ, et al. Combined radiotherapy and chemotherapy with bleomycin and methotrexate for advanced inoperable head and neck cancer: update of a northern California oncology group randomized trial. *J Clin Oncol* 1987;5:1410–1418
50. Lo TC, Wiley AL Jr, Ansfield FJ, et al. Combined radiation therapy and 5–fluorouracil for advanced squamous cell carcinoma of the oral cavity and oropharynx: a randomized study. *AJR* 1976;126:229–235
51. Weissler MC, Melin S, Sailer SL, et al. Simultaneous chemoradiation in the treatment of advanced head and neck cancer. *Arch Otol Head Neck Surg* 1992;118:806–810
52. Merlano M, Vitale V, Rosso R, et al. Treatment of advanced squamous-cell carcinoma of the head and neck with alternating chemotherapy and radiotherapy. *N Engl J Med* 1992;327: 1115–1121
53. Adelstein DJ, Saxton JP, Lavertu P, et al. A phase III randomized trial comparing concurrent chemotherapy and radiotherapy with radiotherapy alone in resectable stage III and IV squamous cell head and neck cancer: preliminary results. *Head Neck* 1996;18:567–574
54. Wendt TG, Grabenbauer GG, Rodel CM, et al. Simultaneous radiochemotherapy versus radiotherapy alone in advanced head and neck cancer: a randomized multicenter study. *J Clin Oncol* 1998;16:1318–1324
55. Keane TJ, Cummings BJ, O'Sullivan B, et al. A randomized trial of radiation therapy compared to split course radiation therapy combined with mitomycin C and 5–fluorouracil as initial treatment for advanced laryngeal and hypopharyngeal squamous carcinoma. *Int J Radiat Oncol Biol Phys* 1993;25:613–618
56. Smid L, Lesnicar H, Zakotnik B, et al. Radiotherapy, combined with simultaneous chemotherapy with mitomycin C and

bleomycin for inoperable head and neck cancer—preliminary report. *Int J Radiat Oncol Biol Phys* 1995;32:769–775
57. Shanta V, Krishnamurthi S. Combined bleomycin and radiotherapy in oral cancer. *Clin Radiol* 1980;31:617–620
58. Stefani S, Chung TS. Hydroxyurea and radiotherapy in head and neck cancer: long term results of a double blind randomized prospective study [abstract]. *Int J Radiat Oncol Biol Phys* 1980;6:1398
59. Vermund H, Kaalhus O, Winther F, et al. Bleomycin and radiation therapy in squamous cell carcinoma of the upper aerodigestive track: a phase III clinical trial. *Int J Radiat Oncol Biol Phys* 1985;11:1877–1886
60. Gupta NK, Pointon RCS, Wilkinson PM. A randomized clinical trial to contrast radiotherapy with radiotherapy and methotrexate given synchronously in head and neck cancer. *Clin Radiol* 1987;38:575–581
61. Weissberg JB, Son YH, Papac RJ, et al. Randomized clinical trial of mitomycin C as an adjunct to radiotherapy in head and neck cancer. *Int J Radiat Oncol Biol Phys* 1989;17:3–9
62. Sanchiz F, Milla A, Torner J, et al. Single fraction per day versus two fractions per day versus radiochemotherapy in the treatment of head and neck cancer. *Int J Radiat Oncol Biol Phys* 1990;19:1347–1350
63. Herskovic A, Martz K, Al-Sarraf M, et al. Combined chemotherapy and radiotherapy compared with radiotherapy alone in patients with cancer of the esophagus. *N Engl J Med* 1992;326:1593–1598
64. Browman GP, Cripps C, Hodson DI, et al. Placebo-controlled randomized trial of infusional fluorouracil during standard radiotherapy in locally advanced head and neck cancer. *J Clin Oncol* 1994;12:2648–2653
65. Bachaud JM, Cohen-Jonathan E, Alzieu C, et al. Combined postoperative radiotherapy and weekly cisplatin infusion for locally advanced head and neck carcinoma: final report of a randomized trial. *Int J Radiat Oncol Biol Phys* 1996;36:999–1004
66. Haffty BG, Son YH, Papac R, et al. Chemotherapy as an adjunct to radiation in the treatment of squamous cell carcinoma of the head and neck: results of the Yale Mitomycin Randomized Trials. *J Clin Oncol* 1997;15:268–276
67. Jeremic B, Shibamoto Y, Stanisavljevic B, et al. Radiation therapy alone or with concurrent low-dose daily either cisplatin or carboplatin in locally advanced unresectable squamous cell carcinoma of the head and neck: a prospective randomized trial. *Radiother Oncol* 1997;43:29–37
68. Al-Sarraf M, LeBlanc M, Giri S, et al. Chemoradiotherapy versus radiotherapy in patients with advanced nasopharyngeal cancer: phase III randomized Intergroup Study 0099. *J Clin Oncol* 1998;16:1310–1317
69. Brizel DM, Albers ME, Fisher SR, et al. Hyperfractionated irradiation with or without concurrent chemotherapy for locally advanced head and neck cancer. *N Engl J Med* 1998;338:1798–1804
70. Al-Sarraf M, Martz K, Herskovic A, et al. Progress report of combined chemotherapy versus radiotherapy alone in patients with esophageal cancer: an Intergroup study. *J Clin Oncol* 1997;15:277–285.
71. El-Sayed S, Nelson N. Adjuvant and adjunctive chemotherapy in the management of squamous cell carcinoma of the head and neck region: a meta-analysis of prospective and randomized trials. *J Clin Oncol* 1996;14:838–847
72. Kies MS, Haraf DJ, Athanasiadis I, et al. Induction chemotherapy followed by concurrent chemoradiation for advanced head and neck cancer: improved disease control and survival. *J Clin Oncol* 1998;16:2715–2721
73. Merlano M, Corvo R, Margarino G, et al. Combined chemotherapy and radiation therapy in advanced inoperable squamous cell carcinoma of the head and neck. *Cancer* 1991;67:915–921
74. Merlano M. Chemotherapy trials in head and neck cancer. *Head Neck* 1995;17:266–267
75. Taylor SG, Applebaum E, Showel JL, et al. A randomized trial of adjuvant chemotherapy in head and neck cancer. *J Clin Oncol* 1985;3:672–679
76. Laramore GE, Scott CB, Al-Sarraf M, et al. Adjuvant chemotherapy for resectable squamous cell carcinomas of the head and neck: report on Intergroup Study 0034. *Int J Radiat Oncol Biol Phys* 1992;23:705–713
77. Chan AT, Teo PM, Johnson PJ. Controversies in the management of locoregionally advanced nasopharyngeal carcinoma. *Curr Opin Oncol* 1998;10:219–225
78. Robbins KT, Kumar P, Regine WF, et al. Efficacy of targeted supradose cisplatin and concomitant radiation therapy for advanced head and neck cancer: the Memphis experience. *Int J Radiat Oncol Biol Phys* 1997;38:263–271
79. Vokes EE, Pajak TF. Enhancing the therapeutic index of concomitant chemoradiotherapy for head and neck cancer. *Ann Oncol* 1998;9:471–473. Editorial
80. Griggs JJ. Reducing the toxicity of anticancer therapy: new strategies. *Leukemia Res* 1998;22(suppl 1):S27–S33
81. Gabrilove JL, Jakubowski A, Scher H, et al. Effect of granulocyte colony stimulating factor on neutropenia and associated morbidity due to chemotherapy for transitional cell carcinoma of the urothelium. *N Engl J Med* 1988;318:1414–1422
82. Buntzel J, Kuttner K, Frohlich D, Glatzel M. Selective cytoprotection with amifostine in concurrent radiochemo-therapy for head and neck cancer. *Ann Oncol* 1998;9:505–509

The Role of Chemotherapy in Head and Neck Cancer

CHAPTER 9

Kerwin F. Shannon and K. Thomas Robbins

Despite advances in surgical technique, head and neck reconstruction, and the delivery of radiotherapy, outcomes for people suffering from head and neck cancer have generally remained poor. With early tumors, a single modality of therapy results in a high rate of cure but with advanced disease, the rates of locoregional recurrence and the development of systemic metastases are unacceptably high despite the use of multimodality therapy.[1,2] Chemotherapy has been used for head and neck cancer for several decades, but its use has yet to find a universally accepted role. Early experience showed encouraging response rates, but these were short-lived in the setting of advanced disease, and large trials failed to show a survival benefit when chemotherapy was used in the adjuvant setting. Researchers still struggle to demonstrate a clear survival benefit, but the secondary goal of preserving function of the larynx and pharynx without compromising survival can now be successfully achieved. The advent of new drug types, novel ways of combining therapies, and new methods of drug delivery are now producing high rates of organ preservation and are beginning to provide survival benefits in some groups of patients.

Chemotherapy for Recurrent or Metastatic Disease

Chemotherapy was initially used for palliation of advanced, unresectable tumors, and systemic disease. Numerous agents have been found to have activity in this setting, including methotrexate, bleomycin, 5-fluorouracil (5-FU), cisplatin, and carboplatin, with response rates ranging from 10% to 35%. Most of these responses are partial, and few are lasting, with median duration of only 4 to 6 months.[3,4] Methotrexate has been used most extensively and despite numerous phase II trials, no other single agent has demonstrated a clear superiority over this drug. One trial has reported an improved response and survival benefit using cisplatin, but the numbers treated and the improvement in overall survival (approximately 2 months) were small.[5] Newer agents being investigated include the topoisomerase inhibitor, topotecan, and the pyrimidine antimetabolite, gemcitabine. Trials to date have reported modest response rates. Some encouraging results have been seen with the taxanes, paclitaxel and docetaxel, with response rates reported as high as 50%. These drugs may prove useful in combination therapies or as adjuncts to radiotherapy.

It was hoped that the use of drugs in combination would provide a better outcome. Numerous phase II and III trials have been performed using a variety of combinations, but the results have been disappointing. Four multi-institutional trials large enough to detect a significant difference between combination and single-agent chemotherapy have been reported.[6-9] These were all able to demonstrate an improvement in response rates with multiagent treatments, but this was achieved at the cost of greater toxicity without any improvement in median survival. A meta-analysis of trials of combination chemotherapy conducted during the early 1990s found cisplatin to be the most effective single agent, and that the combination of cisplatin and 5-FU was more efficacious than any other single agent or combination.[10] This combination remains the gold standard to which all new combinations are compared. However, even with this combination, responses are seen in about one-third of patients, no more than one-half of which are complete. What is still unknown is whether this group of patients with advanced disease would fare better with good supportive care than with toxic therapies producing responses that are infrequent and of brief duration. One subset of this group in which cisplatin-based combination chemotherapy has produced lasting responses is patients with recurrent undifferentiated nasopharyngeal carcinoma. Higher response rates than at other sites, both complete and partial, are usually reported, and long-term disease-free survival has been reported in a few.[11-13] At most subsites of the head and neck, the role of chemotherapy cannot be considered part of standard management even in its traditional use in incurable disease, outside the context of trials designed to evaluate new therapies.

Chemotherapy for Advanced Resectable Disease

Although the success of chemotherapy in unresectable disease has been modest, encouraging results have been achieved in the setting of locally advanced primary disease. Although the primary goal of cancer therapy remains cure or prolonged survival, an important secondary goal of the use of chemotherapy is the reduction of the morbidity of treatment. In the head and neck, this takes the form of preservation of the organs of speech and swallowing. Three general approaches have been used, alone or in combination: induction therapy, adjuvant therapy, or chemotherapy concomitant with primary radiation.

INDUCTION CHEMOTHERAPY

Induction chemotherapy is given before definitive local therapy in an attempt to downstage local disease and make it more amenable to local therapy, to improve both local recurrence rates, and to treat microscopic systemic disease. This approach is attractive in that the drug is delivered to the tumor bed before it has been interfered with by surgery or radiotherapy and is delivered before the cells have had the chance to develop resistance to therapy. Preliminary studies from single institutions using this approach reported response rates as high as 90% with cisplatin-based regimens, with 40% complete response (CR) rates. Two-thirds of these had a pathologic CR. When followed with definitive radiotherapy, it was found that the response to induction chemotherapy was predictive of the subsequent response to radiation, and ultimately with survival.

Several randomized controlled trials of chemotherapy given before surgery[14-18] and before radiation[19,20] have been reported. The first of these large multi-institutional studies reported was the Head and Neck Contracts Program. The three arms of this study compared standard surgery and postoperative radiotherapy, induction chemotherapy with a single course of cisplatin and bleomycin before standard treatment, and induction chemotherapy plus standard treatment plus maintenance cisplatin.[14] The overall response rate to the chemotherapy was only 37%, and no survival benefit was demonstrated; however, lower rates of distant metastasis were obtained with chemotherapy, and the disease-free interval was prolonged in those who received maintenance therapy.

The Southwest Oncology Group investigated three preoperative cycles of cisplatin, bleomycin, methotrexate, and vincristine. No significant difference in survival rate was demonstrated with survival favoring the standard arm, but the rate of distant metastases was lower in those receiving chemotherapy.[16]

Perhaps the most successful trial of neoadjuvant therapy was reported by the Veterans' Affairs (VA) Laryngeal Cancer Study Group.[19] This trial compared intravenous cisplatin and 5-FU given before definitive radiotherapy with total laryngectomy. Patients were assessed after two courses of chemotherapy. If a significant response was not seen, the patient underwent total laryngectomy. If a good response was seen, the patient received a third cycle of chemotherapy and then underwent definitive radiotherapy. No difference in survival was seen between the two groups. Significantly, the survival was not compromised in the group receiving chemotherapy, yet two-thirds of patients surviving in this group retained a functioning larynx. Again, there was a reduction in the rate of systemic metastases in the chemotherapy group. It remains debatable as to whether this effect is durable, with some believing that the differences in the rates of distant metastases in the two groups become more similar with more prolonged follow-up.[21,22] The VA study did establish induction chemotherapy followed by definitive radiotherapy as a standard treatment option in advanced carcinoma of the larynx.

Positive findings in these studies were that high response rates to induction chemotherapy could be achieved, a significant proportion of which were complete, and that survival times were increased in those that did respond. Chemotherapy response predicted response to subsequent radiotherapy, and rates of distant metastases were significantly lowered in the groups receiving chemotherapy. The induction chemotherapy did not increase complications from subsequent surgery or radiotherapy. Perhaps most importantly, laryngeal preservation could be achieved without compromising survival. Despite this good evidence of the drugs' activity, the trials were disappointing because the responses were translated neither into an increase in locoregional control, nor an increase in overall survival. A subset analysis of the Head and Neck Contracts Program study did, however, demonstrate an improvement in survival in oral cavity carcinomas and in those with limited neck disease.[23] Concerns have been raised about the adverse effects of delaying definitive therapy in those who do not respond.[24,25] A meta-analysis of early trials showed a nonsignificant trend to the harmful effects of the addition of chemotherapy.[26]

Organ Preservation

The success of the VA Laryngeal Cancer Study has established induction chemotherapy and definitive radiotherapy as a standard treatment option in laryngeal cancer, allowing preservation of laryngeal speech in most patients. This approach has been applied to advanced primary tumors of the oropharynx and hypopharynx in which total laryngectomy would be required as part of standard therapy. A large randomized trial by the European Organization for Research and Treatment of Cancer (EORTC) applied the VA protocol to patients with piriform sinus cancer. As with the laryngeal experience, survival was not compromised by a trial of induction chemotherapy, and 42% of patients in the experimental arm had a functioning larynx at 3 years.[27] This protocol is now considered the standard therapy arm in ongoing EORTC trials. The addition of chemotherapy to other forms of definitive therapy comes at the cost of significant morbidity. Despite the success of organ preservation studies, chemotherapy is used as part of initial definitive therapy of head and neck cancer in only about 6% of cases in the United States, although its use appears to be increasing in the treatment of advanced cancer.[28] The actual contribution made by chemotherapy in these trials is controversial. Large studies employing radiation alone have yielded disease specific survival rates similar to those achieved in induction chemotherapy trials[29,30] and improved survival of induction chemotherapy over radiation alone has yet to be established in a randomized trial.

ADJUVANT CHEMOTHERAPY

The use of chemotherapy as an adjuvant after definitive local therapy has some theoretical advantage over induction chemotherapy in that definitive therapy is not delayed and the potential to underestimate tumor margins after a clinical response is avoided. Two large trials evaluated the effects of adjuvant chemotherapy and again no differences in survival have been demonstrated.[31,32] In the first study,[31] a longer survival was reported in the control arm. The study conducted by Rossi et al.[32] of nasopharyngeal carcinoma reported no difference in survival with the addition of vincristine, cyclophosphamide, and doxorubicin after definitive radiotherapy.

A large intergroup study compared the addition of cisplatin and 5-FU after resection, but before radiotherapy.[20] No survival difference was observed, but the pattern of failure was different between the two groups, with the patients receiving chemotherapy showing a lower incidence of distant metastases. An interesting finding was that a group with high-risk pathologic findings seemed to benefit from the systemic therapy. Induction chemotherapy trials have also included adjuvant arms. The Head and Neck Contracts Program[14] included an arm with adjuvant cisplatin for 6 months. There was no difference in survival and very poor compliance with the chemotherapy. There was again a decrease in the rate of distant metastases.

In another induction trial, by Ervin et al.,[33] patients who responded to induction chemotherapy were randomized to receive maintenance therapy or not. Disease-free survival on the maintenance arm was significantly greater at 3 years (88% vs 57%). A significant improvement in survival was demonstrated in only one small trial of patients with oral cavity carcinoma.[34] The results suggest that chemotherapy can affect the rate of distant metastases, and survival may be improved. Problems with adjuvant trials are that it is difficult to administer therapy after surgery or radiotherapy because of greater toxicity of drugs after local treatment and lack of motivation in patients who have no clinical evidence of disease. There may be a role for adjuvant therapy in patients with high-risk pathologic features who are well motivated, but the overall disappointing results and high toxicity prevent this approach from becoming a standard therapy.

CONCOMITANT CHEMO- AND RADIOTHERAPY

Although chemotherapy has been demonstrated to have systemic activity against metastatic disease, improvements in overall survival are unlikely to be seen without improvements in rates of local and regional control.[35] Changes in surgical technique are unlikely to produce such an improvement. New techniques of radiation delivery, such as accelerated fractionation, may contribute. In addition to their direct antitumor effects, several chemotherapy agents, including cisplatin, have been noted to have effects as radiation sensitizers.[36,37] The concomitant use of chemotherapy and radiation is therefore a very attractive approach to the treatment of advanced disease. It has been the only primary chemotherapeutic approach that has consistently shown improved disease-free and overall survival in comparison with local therapy and sequential chemotherapy.

Two recent meta-analyses of randomized trials of chemotherapy for head and neck cancer have shown that the modest improvement in overall survival that can be demonstrated is confined to regimens in which the chemotherapy is given simultaneously with the definitive therapy. El-Sayed and Nelson[38] analyzed 42 prospective randomized trials of chemotherapy for squamous cell carcinoma of the head and neck region until 1990. These investigators found that chemotherapy did increase the chance of initial tumor response and local control, but at the cost of a significant increase in the morbidity of treatment. A significant increase in survival was found when the chemotherapy and the definitive treatment were used simultaneously, although this improvement was modest. A similar finding was reported by Bourhis et al.[39] for the MACH-NC Collaborative group in France. A meta-analysis was performed. On 63 prospective randomized trials performed by this group between 1965 and 1993. No significant difference in survival was found if chemotherapy was given in an adjuvant or neoadjuvant setting, but an 8% improvement in survival was noted at 5 years for concomitant therapy.[39]

Trials of concurrent chemotherapy and radiation have been undertaken using methotrexate, hydroxyurea, bleomycin, mitomycin C, 5-FU, and cisplatin. Phase III studies with methotrexate, hydroxyurea, and mitomycin have been largely negative, some survival benefit has been demonstrated with single-agent bleomycin, and encouraging results have been seen with 5-FU and cisplatin. Concomitant multiagent chemotherapy has been compared with radiation alone in five trials, with most reporting a modest survival benefit in the chemotherapy arm. Because drug combinations tend to enhance toxicity, several trials employing split-course radiotherapy have been used.[40] An Italian study demonstrated a small but significant improvement in survival alternating radiotherapy with cisplatin and 5-FU.[41,42]

A clear survival benefit was recently shown for concomitant chemo- and radiotherapy in the treatment of nasopharyngeal carcinoma.[43] This Intergroup study randomized patients to receive radiotherapy alone, or radiotherapy and synchronous intravenous cisplatin and 5-FU followed by adjuvant chemotherapy after the completion of radiotherapy. Despite relatively poor compliance with the adjuvant portion of the therapy, significant differences in relapse-free survival (24% vs 69%) and overall survival (46% vs 76% at 3 years) were seen, such that the trial was closed early after an interim analysis. Although this has redefined standard treatment of nasopharyngeal carcinoma in the United States, workers in areas where nasopharyngeal carcinoma is endemic question the findings of this study, citing the poor overall response rates in the radiation-only arm.[44]

Trials of adjuvant concomitant chemo- and radiotherapy have been reported. Haffty et al.,[45] demonstrated an improvement in locoregional control adding mitomycin C to postoperative radiotherapy, whereas improvement in survival was shown by Bachaud et al.[46] with the use of weekly cisplatin. An ongoing Radiation Therapy Oncology Group (RTOG) protocol is examining postoperative cisplatin chemo- and radiotherapy. Several recent prospective studies have demonstrated the efficacy of concomitant radiotherapy and cisplatin-based chemotherapy. The Cleveland Clinic Group demonstrated improved relapse-free survival with primary site preservation, but overall survival was not improved in a randomized study comparing concurrent cisplatin and 5-FU and continuous-course radiotherapy with radiotherapy alone in patients with resectable laryngeal and pharyngeal tumors.[47,48] The protocol was also shown to be beneficial for some T4 laryngeal tumors, a subgroup that does poorly from radiation alone.[49] A study from Duke University compared hyperfractionated radiotherapy with and without concurrent chemotherapy and demonstrated improved local control and a trend toward improved survival at 3 years.[50] Two studies looked at concurrent chemo- and radiotherapy in patients with unresectable disease and demonstrated improved local control and survival, despite problems with acute toxicity.[51,52] The French Group of Radiation Oncology for Head and Neck Cancer recently presented preliminary results of a randomized study comparing radiation with and without concomitant carboplatin and 5-FU in patients with advanced oropharyngeal carcinoma. These investigators reported a significant improvement in locoregional control and disease-free and overall survival, although two-thirds of patients receiving chemotherapy had significant mucositis.[53] A further interesting study from Europe used intravenous carboplatin with each treatment fraction of a hyperfractionated radiation schedule and observed a 96% CR rate and 72% local control rate at 52 months for advanced tumors at nonlaryngeal sites.[54] In the setting of unresectable recurrent disease, the Gustave-Roussy Institute reported the feasibility of concomitant chemotherapy and reirradiation.[55] Combinations used included 5-FU and hydroxyurea or mitomycin C, 5-FU, and cisplatin. Median survival was improved over palliative chemotherapy alone, and a small proportion of patients were long-term survivors.

Although the results of pilot and randomized studies suggest that improved survival is possible using concomitant chemotherapy, the benefit comes at the expense of considerable toxicity. Further randomized studies are ongoing to help determine optimal drug doses and radiation schedules. RTOG 97-03 is examining three chemo- and radiotherapy schedules, whereas a follow-up study to the VA Laryngeal Cancer Study is comparing its induction protocol with concurrent chemo- and radiotherapy and with radiation alone.

INTRA-ARTERIAL CHEMOTHERAPY

In the treatment of advanced tumors, higher rates of complete tumor response are difficult to achieve because of dose-limiting toxicity. In theory, much higher drug concentrations within a tumor can be achieved by delivering the drug directly to the tumor through its arterial blood supply. The theoretical advantage of intra-arterial chemotherapy over standard intravenous (IV) chemotherapy is that a higher concentration of the drug can be delivered directly to the tumor bed than to other organs, potentially allowing for greater tumor cell killing with lower toxicity. Depending on the amount of drug uptake by the tumor during this first pass, it is also possible to deliver to the tumor cells themselves a greater amount of drug using this route than can be achieved by the IV route. Dynamic vascular flow studies indicate that head and neck lesions are suited to the pharmacodynamic advantages of intra-arterial chemotherapy.[56]

The use of intra-arterial chemotherapy for head and neck cancer is not new but, despite good tumor responses, this form of therapy failed to become popular because of catheter-related complications and outcomes not significantly different from those achieved with chemotherapy administered systemically. When it has been used, intra-arterial chemotherapy has produced response rates in the head and neck exceeding 70%.[57,58] Methotrexate, bleomycin, 5-FU, and cisplatin have been used with success. One subsite of the head and neck ideally suited for regional chemotherapy is the paranasal sinuses. Using combinations of intra-arterial cisplatin and bleomycin and systemic doxorubicin or 5-FU, a 91 % response rate was seen in 24 patients with advanced paranasal sinus tumors. One-third avoided craniofacial resection as a result.[59] A novel approach has been pioneered by Robbins et al.[60] using intra-arterial cisplatin at a dose intensity five times greater than what is generally achieved with intravenous therapy. This dose is achieved by giving the chemotherapy by weekly intra-arterial infusion, while simultaneously administering a cisplatin antagonist (sodium thiosulfate) intravenously to remove the drug from the systemic circulation. Because the relative advantage of an intra-arterial infusion is directly proportional to the plasma clearance of the drug and inversely proportional to the tumor plasma flow,[61] this approach optimizes drug delivery. The cisplatin is delivered selectively to small vessels, and the thiosulfate effectively increases the plasma clearance of the drug.

Response rates greater than 85% were seen in a pilot study in advanced disease.[61,62] When delivered with synchronous radiotherapy in standard fractionation, CR rates greater than 90% are seen, and overall response rates approach 100% in those completing therapy.[63] Laryngeal preservation rates are high using this approach in advanced laryngeal and hypopharyngeal carcinomas.[64] Early experience with this approach in advanced sinonasal tumors has produced a high rate of local control.[65] The protocol is the subject of a multi-institutional study of patients with T4 primary tumors.

Chemoprevention of Squamous Cancer

Although the improvements in local control may benefit overall survival, this form of targeted therapy is still a locoregional treatment, and a high proportion of distant failures and second primary cancers occur. Given that adjuvant systemic therapy has not generally been found to improve outcomes, significant advances in survival improvement are only likely to be achieved if systemic disease can similarly be targeted. Drug delivery systems that are selectively taken up and retained by tumor cells will be required. Such methods are not yet available but are the subject of intensive research. Drugs to reduce the incidence of second primary cancers are also being investigated. Numerous agents have been investigated, and the most successful to date have been retinoic acid and its derivatives. Concerns of toxicity and the temporary nature of the responses have prevented the widespread use of chemopreventive agents. No standard approach exists for control of high-risk premalignant lesions. New treatments using agents such as cyclooxygenase inhibitors and biomodulation of retinoids are under investigation.

Conclusion

Despite more than three decades of experience with chemotherapy, no undisputed role for its use has been established. In metastatic disease, the role is purely palliative, but chemotherapy benefits a small minority, and only for a brief duration. Whether the use of multiple agents is more beneficial than the use of single agents alone remains controversial, and until higher and more lasting response rates can be achieved, its widespread use is hard to justify outside the context of clinical trials.

Some cures are possible, however, with the use of concomitant chemotherapy and radiation for advanced, unresectable locoregional disease at initial presentation or when recurrent. In this setting, superiority over either palliative chemotherapy or radiation alone has recently been demonstrated in randomized trials, but ideal protocols have yet to be established. In primary resectable disease, there is a definite indication for the use of chemotherapy as a neoadjuvant therapy in organ preservation protocols.

Although not yet standard therapy, induction chemotherapy for organ preservation should at least be considered a standard treatment option. This use is still not widespread, and an answer to the debate over whether the benefits seen can be attributed to radiotherapy alone is still pending. Induction chemotherapy has not achieved the important goal of improved survival. With the current therapies available, the best hope for improved survival is by improving rates of locoregional disease. The greatest promise has been achieved using concomitant chemo- and radiotherapy, with benefits repeatedly demonstrated in both primary and recurrent disease. Whether this approach is superior to neoadjuvant chemotherapy is the subject of ongoing multicenter studies.

The use of intra-arterial drug delivery also shows promise in the improvement of locoregional control, but whether long-term survival is improved by this approach remains to be established.

A need to control systemic disease and the development of second primary tumors also exists. Success depends not so much on the development of new agents, but on the development of new methods of delivering effective drugs selectively to systemic tumor in such a way that normal tissues are minimally affected. Such targeted systemic therapy will depend on advances in tumor genetics and immunology, which are currently the subject of intensive research.

A final controversy that remains, when success with chemotherapy is achieved, is whether complicated protocols from specialized cancer centers can be made available in settings outside such centers, to benefit larger numbers of patients.

REFERENCES

Shannon and Robbins—CHAPTER 9

1. Vikram B, Strong EW, Shah JP, et al. Failure at distant sites following multimodality therapy for advanced head and neck cancer. *Head Neck Surg* 1984;6:730–733
2. Kramer S, Gelber RD, Snow JB, et al. Combined radiation therapy and surgery in the management of advanced head and neck cancer: final report of study 73-03 of the Radiation Therapy Oncology Group. *Head Neck Surg* 1987;10:49–55
3. Hong WK, Bromer R. Chemotherapy in head and neck cancer. *N Engl J Med* 1984;308:75–79
4. Vokes EE, Weichselbaum RR, Lippman SM, Hong WK. Head and neck cancer. *N Engl J Med* 1993;328:184–194
5. Morton RP, Fugman F, Dorman EB, et al. Cisplatin and bleomycin for advanced or recurrent squamous cell carcinoma of the head and neck: a randomized factorial phase III controlled trial. *Cancer Chemother Pharmacol* 1985;15:283–289
6. Vogl SE, Schonfeld DA, Kaplan BH, et al. A randomized prospective comparison of methotrexate with a combination of methotrexate, bleomycin and cisplatin in head and neck cancer. *Cancer* 1985;56:432–442
7. Forastiere AA, Metch B, Schuller DE, et al. Randomized comparison of cisplatin plus fluorouracil versus carboplatin plus fluorouracil versus methotrexate in advanced squamous cell carcinoma of the head and neck: a Southwest Oncology Group study. *J Clin Oncol* 1992;10:1245–1251
8. Jacobs C, Lyman G, Velez-Garcia E, et al. A phase III randomized study comparing cisplatin and fluorouracil as single agents and in combination for advanced squamous cell carcinoma of the head and neck. *J Clin Oncol* 1992;10:257–263
9. Clavel M, Vermorken JB, Cognetti F, et al. Randomized comparison of cisplatin, methotrexate, bleomycin, and vincristine versus cisplatin and 5-fluorouracil versus cisplatin in recurrent or metastatic squamous cell cancer of the head and neck. *Ann Oncol* 1994;5:521–526
10. Browman GP, Cronin L. Standard chemotherapy in squamous cell head and neck cancer: what we have learned from randomized trials. *Semin Oncol* 1994;21:311–319
11. Boussen H, Cvitkovic E, Wendting JL, et al. Chemotherapy of metastatic and/or recurrent undifferentiated nasopharyngeal carcinoma with cisplatin, bleomycin and fluorouracil. *J Clin Oncol* 1991;9:1675–1681
12. Choo R, Tannock I. Chemotherapy for recurrent or metastatic carcinoma of the nasopharynx: a review of the Princess Margaret Hospital experience. *Cancer* 1991;68:2120–2124
13. Fandi A, Altun M, Azli N, et al. Nasopharyngeal cancer: epidemiology, staging, and treatment. *Semin Oncol* 1994;21:382–397
14. Head and Neck Contracts Program. Adjuvant chemotherapy for advanced head and neck squamous carcinoma: final report of the Head and Neck Contracts Program. *Cancer* 1987;60:301–311
15. Rentschler RE, Wilbur DW, Petti GH, et al. Adjuvant methotrexate escalated to toxicity for resectable stage III and

IV squamous head and neck carcinomas: a prospective randomized study. *J Clin Oncol* 1987;5:278–275
16. Schuller DE, Wilson HE, Smith RE, et al. Preoperative chemotherapy in advanced resectable head and neck cancer: final report of the Southwest Oncology Group. *Laryngoscope* 1988;98:1205–1211
17. Jortay A, Demard F, Dalesio O, et al. A randomized EORTC study on the effect of preoperative polychemotherapy in pyriform sinus carcinoma treated by pharyngolaryngectomy and irradiation: results from 5 to 10 years. *Acta Chir Belg* 1990;90: 115–122
18. Richard JM, Kramar A, Molinari R, et al. Randomised EORTC head and neck cooperative group trial of preoperative intra-arterial chemotherapy in oral cavity and oropharynx carcinomas. *Eur J Cancer* 1991;27:821–827
19. The Department of Veterans Affairs Laryngeal Cancer Study Group. Induction chemotherapy plus radiation compared with surgery plus radiation in patients with advanced laryngeal cancer. *N Engl J Med* 1991;324:1685–1690
20. Laramore GE, Scott CB, Al-Sarraf M, et al. Adjuvant chemotherapy for resectable squamous cell carcinomas of the head and neck: report of the Intergroup study 0034. *Int J Radiat Oncol Biol Phys* 1992;23:705–713
21. Hong WK, Lippman SM, Wolf GT. Recent advances in head and neck cancer—larynx preservation and cancer chemoprevention: the seventeenth annual Richard and Hinda Rosenthal Foundation award lecture. *Cancer Res* 1993;53:5113–5120
22. Wolf GT, Hong WK. Induction chemotherapy for organ preservation in advanced laryngeal cancer: is there a role? *Head Neck* 1995;17:279–283
23. Jacobs C, Makuch R. Efficacy of adjuvant chemotherapy for patients with resectable head and neck cancer: a subset analysis of the Head and Neck Contracts Program. *J Clin Oncol* 1990;8:838–847
24. Toohill RJ, Duncavage JA, Grossman TW, et al. The effects of delay in standard treatment due to induction chemotherapy in two randomized prospective studies. *Laryngoscope* 1987;97: 407–412
25. Okura M, Hiranuma T, Adachi T, et al. Induction chemotherapy is associated with an increase in the incidence of locoregional recurrence in patients with carcinoma of the oral cavity: results from a single institution. *Cancer* 1998;82:804–815
26. Stell PM, Dalby JE, Stisckland P, et al. Sequential chemotherapy and radiotherapy in advanced head and neck cancer. *Clin Radiol* 1983;34:463
27. Lefebvre J-L, Chevalier D, Luboinski B, et al. Larynx preservation in pyriform sinus cancer: preliminary results of a European Organization for Research and Treatment of Cancer phase III trial. *J Natl Cancer Inst* 1996;88:890–899
28. Shah JP, Karnell LH, Hoffman HT, et al. Patterns of care for cancer of the larynx in the United States. *Arch Otolaryngol Head Neck Surg* 1997;123:475–483
29. Harwood AR, Hawkins NV, Beale FA, et al. Management of advanced glottic cancer: a 10-year review of the Toronto experience. *Int J Radiat Oncol Biol Phys* 1979;5(6):899–904
30. Mendenhall WM, Parsons JT, Stringer SP, et al. Stage T3 squamous cell carcinoma of the glottic larynx: a comparison of laryngectomy and irradiation. *Int J Radiat Oncol Biol Phys* 1992;23:725–732
31. Domenge C, Marandas P, Vignoud J, et al. Post-surgical adjuvant chemotherapy in extracapsular spread invaded lymph node (N+ R+) of epidermoid carcinoma of the head and neck: a randomized multicentric trial. In: *Second International Conference on Head and Neck Cancer* 1988:74
32. Rossi A, Molinari R, Boracchi P, et al. Adjuvant chemotherapy with vincristine, cyclophosphamide, and doxorubicin after radiotherapy in local-regional nasopharyngeal cancer: results of a 4-year multicenter randomized study. *J Clin Oncol* 1988; 6:1401–1410
33. Ervin TJ, Clark JR, Weichselbaum RR, et al. An analysis of induction and adjuvant chemotherapy in the multidisciplinary treatment of squamous cell cancers of the head and neck. *J Clin Oncol* 1987;5:10–20
34. Bitter K. Postoperative chemotherapy versus postoperative cobalt 60 radiation in patients with advanced oral cavity carcinoma: report on a randomized study. *Head Neck Surg* 1981;3:264
35. Forastiere AA. Randomized trials of induction chemotherapy. A critical review. *Hematol Oncol Clin North Am* 1991;5:725–736
36. Steel GG, Peckham MJ. Exploitable mechanisms in combined radiotherapy–chemotherapy: the concept of additivity. *Int J Radiat Oncol Biol Phys* 1979;5:85–91
37. Fu KK. Biological basis for the interaction of chemotherapeutic agents and radiation therapy. *Cancer* 1985;55:2123–2130
38. El-Sayed S, Nelson N. Adjuvant and adjunctive chemotherapy in the management of squamous cell carcinoma of the head and neck region: a meta-analysis of prospective and randomized trials. *J Clin Oncol* 1996;14:838–847
39. Bourhis J, Pignon JP, Designe L, et al. Meta-analysis of chemotherapy in head and neck cancer: locoregional treatment vs same treatment plus chemotherapy. In: *American Society of Clinical Oncology Thirty-fourth Annual Meeting* 1998:386a
40. Taylor SG. Integration of chemotherapy into the combined modality therapy of head and neck squamous cancer. *Int J Radiat Oncol Biol Phys* 1987;13:779–783
41. Merlano M, Grimaldi A, Bernasso M, et al. Alternating cisplatin-5-fluorouracil and radiotherapy in head and neck cancer. *Am J Clin Oncol* 1988;11:538–542
42. Merlano M, Vitale V, Rosso R, et al. Treatment of advanced squamous cell carcinoma of the head and neck with alternating chemotherapy and radiotherapy. *N Engl J Med* 1992;327: 1115–1121
43. Al-Sarraf M, LeBlanc M, Shanker Giri PG, et al. Chemotherapy versus radiotherapy in patients with advanced nasopharyngeal cancer: phase III randomized Intergroup study 0099. *J Clin Oncol* 1998;16:1310–1317
44. Chan ATC, Teo PML, Leung TWC, Johnson PJ. The role of chemotherapy in the management of nasopharyngeal carcinoma. *Cancer* 1998;82:1003–1012
45. Haffty BG, Son YH, Sasaki CT, et al. Mitomycin C as an adjunct to postoperative radiotherapy in squamous cell carci-

noma of the head and neck: results from two randomized clinical trials. *Int J Radiat Oncol Biol Phys* 1993;27:241–250
46. Bachaud JM, Cohen-Jonathon E, Alzieu C, et al. Combined postoperative radiotherapy and weekly cisplatin infusion for locally advanced head and neck cancer: final report of a randomized trial. *Int J Radiat Oncol Biol Phys* 1996;36:999–1004
47. Adelstein DJ, Rice TW, Becker M, et al. Use of concurrent chemotherapy, accelerated fractionation radiation, and surgery for patients with esophageal carcinoma. *Cancer* 1997;80:1011–1120
48. Adelstein DJ, Lavertu P, Saxton JP, et al. Mature results of a phase III randomized trial comparing concurrent chemoradiotherapy with radiotherapy alone in resectable stage III and IV squamous cell head and neck cancer. *Cancer* 2000;88:876–883
49. Adelstein DJ, Lavertu P, Saxton JP, Wood BG, Eliachar I, Larto MA. Is organ preservation appropriate for T4 larynx cancer? *Head Neck* 1998;20:444
50. Brizel DM, Albers ME, Fisher SR, et al. Hyperfractionated irradiation with or without concurrent chemotherapy for locally advanced head and neck cancer. *N Engl J Med* 1998;338:1798–1804
51. Wendt TG, Grabenbauer GG, Rodel CM, et al. Simultaneous radiochemotherapy versus radiotherapy alone in advanced head and neck cancer: a randomized multicenter study. *J Clin Oncol* 1998;16:1318–1324
52. Harrison LB, Raben A, Pfister DG, et al. A prospective phase II trial of concomitant chemotherapy and radiotherapy with delayed accelerated fractionation in unresectable tumors of the head and neck. *Head Neck* 1998;20:497–503
53. Calais G, Alfonsi M, Bardet E, et al. Randomized study comparing radiation alone (RT) versus RT with concomitant chemotherapy (CT) in stages III and IV oropharynx carcinoma. Preliminary results of the 94.01 study from the *French Group of Radiation Oncology for Head and Neck Cancer.* American Society of Clinical Oncology 1998:1484
54. de Serdio JL, Villar A, Martinez JC, et al. Chemotherapy as part of each treatment fraction in a twice-a-day hyperfractionated schedule: a new chemoradiotherapy approach for advanced head and neck cancer. *Head Neck* 1998;20:489–496
55. De Crevoisier R, Bourhis J, Domenge C, et al. Full-dose reirradiation for unresectable head and neck carcinoma: experience at the Gustave-Roussy Institute in a series of 169 patients. *J Clin Oncol* 1998;16:3556–3562
56. Wheeler RH, Ziessman HA, Medvec BR, et al. Tumor blood flow and systemic shunting in patients receiving intraarterial chemotherapy for head and neck cancer. *Cancer Res* 1986;46:4200–4204
57. Grigoletto G, et al. Intra-arterial cisplatin in head and neck cancer: a phase I–II study. *Proc Am Soc Clin Oncol* 1982;23:198
58. Mortimer JE, Taylor ME, Schulman S, et al. Feasibility and efficacy of weekly intra-arterial cisplatin in locally advanced (stage III and IV) head and neck cancers. *J Clin Oncol* 1988;6:969–975
59. Lee YY, Dimery IW, Van Tassel P, et al. Superselective intra-arterial chemotherapy of advanced paranasal sinus tumors. *Arch Otolaryngol Head Neck Surg* 1989;115:503–511
60. Robbins KT, Storniolo AM, Kerber C, et al. Phase I study of highly selective supradose cisplatin infusions for advanced head and neck cancer. *J Clin Oncol* 1994;12:2113–2120
61. Eckman WW, Patlak CS, Fenstermacher JD. A critical evaluation of the principles governing the advantages of intra-arterial infusions. *J Pharmacokinet Biopharm* 1974;2:257–285
62. Robbins KT, Storniolo AM, Kerber C, et al. Rapid superselective high-dose cisplatin infusion for advanced head and neck malignancies. *Head Neck* 1992;14:364–371
63. Robbins KT, Vicario D, Seagren S, et al. A targeted supradose cisplatin chemoradiation protocol for advanced head and neck cancer. *Am J Surg* 1994;168:419–422
64. Robbins KT, Fontanesi J, Wong FSH, et al. A novel organ preservation protocol for advanced carcinoma of the larynx and pharynx. *Arch Otolaryngol Head Neck Surg* 1996;122:853–857
65. Shannon KF, Robertson J, Kumar P, Robbins KT. Targeted intra-arterial cisplatin and concurrent radiotherapy in the treatment of paranasal sinus cancer. *Aust NZ J Surg* 1998;68(suppl):A83

4

Indications for UPPP in Snoring and Sleep Apnea

"The risk of palatal insufficiency following uvulopalatopharyngoplasty, with resultant hypernasal speech or regurgitation of liquids or foods into the nasopharynx, is often used to discourage the surgery. This author has found this to be completely without merit"

Thomas J. Kereiakes

"Although the response rate is less than ideal, UPPP remains the first line surgical therapy for patients with OSA who fail to tolerate nasal CPAP."

Harold C. Pillsbury

"Although once considered the panacea for managing OSA, the UPPP has clear and distinct limitations. While it still has a therapeutic role in the surgical management of OSA, its effectiveness is often over-estimated by patient and physician alike."

Thomas A. Tami

Indications for UPPP in Snoring and Sleep Apnea

CHAPTER 10

Thomas J. Kereiakes

Controversies in Surgical Management of Sleep Apnea

One of the more controversial issues in otolaryngology deals with the sleep-obstructive patient. This spectrum ranges from patients with the noise-only snore, to patients who frequently awaken with sleep interruption disorder of snoring, to patients with full-blown apnea with documented obstruction and desaturation. Several standards are established for the criteria for apnea, on the basis of frequency of pauses and degree of oxygen desaturation stated as the clinical parameters of sleepiness. It remains puzzling that when one compares symptoms of sleepiness with research data, patients who are frequently awakened by their own snoring, or who awaken from nocturnal restless periods, are often more fatigued and symptomatic than are patients with mild to moderate apnea. I find the best parameters to follow are persistent fatigue after sleep and daytime fatigue with sleepiness.

This chapter compares clinical assessment and patient counseling regarding continuous positive airway pressure (CPAP) with the results achieved with palatal surgery or dental appliances. Office-based palatal reduction and tongue base reduction remain either unproven for true sleep apnea patients or somewhat experimental.[1]

The initial controversy faced by many of us is the value of CPAP and its effectiveness in the long-term management of sleep apnea. The trend of managed care has been to require patients to use CPAP as first-line therapy before considering surgery. CPAP has proved the most effective and safest form of therapy, but compliance and patient acceptance are usually dismal, with the patient often remaining untreated with the machine at the bedside.[1,2]

Patients I do not consider candidates for CPAP, and who I do not feel obliged to have fail this modality before surgery, are those with nasal obstruction[3] or significant tonsil hypertrophy. These patients have obstruction that can be dealt with by time-proven surgical techniques, with a high potential for cure. In the overweight patient with no significant nasal obstruction, CPAP is by far the most effective and possibly only effective treatment other than tracheostomy. Unfortunately, even this population is reticent to accept the lifelong commitment to CPAP. In addition, nasal tip instability or tip collapse may often be worsened by CPAP, making this modality a non-option requiring tip-lift rhinoplasty or tip reconstruction as well.

The effectiveness of surgery as successful treatment of apnea has been established.[4] The larger issue is identifying the limiting factors of patient characteristics that lead to unsuccessful surgery. Clearly, weight is the most limiting factor for success. As people become extremely obese, the posterior oronasal aperture narrows. This decrease in cross-sectional area limits the maximum dimension that can be obtained by surgery. Therefore, I tend to recommend against surgery for uvulopalatopharyngoplasty (UPPP) unless large tonsils are involved. Removal of these with UPPP may still effect a cure or may allow a reduced pressure CPAP utilization, increasing compliance.

Tonsillar hypertrophy is a positive factor in determining surgical outcome. If a patient has large obstructive tonsils, this alone or in conjunction with UPPP often creates a surgical cure. I consider significant tonsillar hypertrophy a contraindication for CPAP, because surgical intervention can create a cure and will not require patient compliance for the use of CPAP in the future. Conversely, in a patient with a long palate or a large uvula with normal tonsils (not beyond the anterior pillar), or both, I do not recommend tonsillectomy. Postoperative constriction of the tonsillar fossa with loss of lateral dimension often replaces a lost volume of tonsillar tissue. In addition, the superior-to-inferior contraction of the fossa with the loss of a tonsillar lingual sulcus pulls the tongue base superiorly, limiting the oropharyngeal opening somewhat as well. The risk of postoperative hemorrhage and airway swelling is not justified unless the tonsils are enlarged and the overall net gain of space, considering the postoperative fossa contractions, results in an overall opening of the airway.

Nasal obstruction is a positive factor in sleep apnea when considering recommendations for surgery. The more obstructed the nose, considering both the septum and turbinate involvement, the more likely a positive outcome will be obtained with surgery. Certainly evaluation of the nasopharynx for adenoid hypertrophy or other obstructive masses is mandatory. The turbinates are usually surgically reduced in size in the sleep apnea patient. The increased obstructive effect in the nighttime airway due to the venous enlargement of the turbinates in the recumbent patient often makes the nighttime airway worse than the patient's daytime baseline. Significant nasal tip droop in the elderly patient or nasal tip instability is a positive factor for recommending surgery as well. CPAP including the use of CPAP pillows often does not prove beneficial in patients with tip collapse.

Age is a relative limiting factor. Certainly the tissue laxity of aging causes palatal collapse. Tongue base and cervical tissue collapse seem worse as well. However, correction of these obstructions in the nonobese patient may yield a rewarding result. When not severe, retrognathia may also be a relative limiting factor. Cephalometrics (normal anteroposterior dimensions of the tongue base to posterior wall) may be helpful predictors. I have found sleep fluoroscopy helpful as a predictor of epiglottic or tongue base collapse, but it is prohibitively cumbersome to set up and accomplish from a practical standpoint. Surgery may be beneficial in the nonobese patient with moderate retrognathia with nasal obstruction and large tonsils. I do not believe that mild retrognathia limits surgical recommendations. In order to use a mandibular advancement splint adequately, the nasal and pharyngeal airway needs to be opened.

The risk of palatal insufficiency after UPPP with resultant hypernasal speech or regurgitation of liquids or foods into the nasopharynx is often used to argue against the surgery. I have found this to be completely without merit. An accurate choice of the level of dissection below the point of muscular closure will avoid this problem in all surgical cases.

The technique is simple and effective. At surgery, before induction of the anesthetic, the patient is asked to sit upright on the surgical table. The palate is visualized, and the patient is asked to say "ah" and "K." The concavity of the palate where it closes against the nasopharyngeal wall is visualized. This is termed "the palatal buckle." A point at 0.75 cm below the palatal buckle is chosen and marked with a spinal needle and with Methylene Blue. This is considered the highest point of resection for the palate. This is based not on arbitrary measurements from the posterior wall or from the bony palate but anatomically, on the point of palate closure. This approach not only limits the amount of palate taken to avoid overresection, but also ensures maximal removal of collapsible tissue for optimal results. It is based on the individual patient's muscular closure, and not on an arbitrary measurement. I have observed no palatal insufficiency in any patient undergoing this technique.

In summary, the highest success with surgery will be achieved in the younger nonobese patient with large tonsils, a long palate and large uvula, and normal mandibular anatomy. Obese patients generally do poorly unless there is a relatively overwhelming factor, such as tonsil hypertrophy or nasal obstruction. Surgery may still be useful in these patients, as a means of lessening their symptoms, the number and length of apnea pauses, and the overall reduction of time spent under a 90% saturation of oxygen. The surgical approach may be an adjunct in the successful management of the CPAP at lower pressures while weight loss measures are attempted.

REFERENCES

Kereiakes—CHAPTER 10

1. Barthel SW, Stome M. Snoring, obstructive sleep apnea, and surgery. *Med Clin North Am* 1999;83:85–96
2. McArdle N, Devereux G, Heidarnejad H, et al. Long-term use of CPAP therapy for sleep apnea/hypopnea syndrome. *Am J Respir Crit Care Med* 1999;159(pt 1):1108–1114
3. Hester TO, Phillips B, Aracher SM. Surgery for obstructive sleep apnea: effects on sleep, breathing, and oxygenation. *South Med J* 1995;88:907–910
4. Lojander J, Maasilta P, Partinen M. Nasal-CPAP, surgery, and conservative management for treatment of obstructive sleep apnea syndrome. A randomized study. *Chest* 1996;110:114–119

Indications for UPPP in Snoring and Sleep Apnea

CHAPTER 11

Harold C. Pillsbury and Steven S. Ball

Uvulopalatopharyngoplasty (UPPP), first introduced in 1981 by Fujita[1] for the treatment of obstructive sleep apnea (OSA), is now the most frequently performed surgical procedure for this disorder. Despite its widespread use, it is effective in less than 50% of patients with OSA. According to the American Sleep Disorders Association meta-analysis, only 40.7% of patients with OSA respond to UPPP; response was defined as a 50% decrease in apnea index (AI) or respiratory disturbance index (RDI) and the resultant achievement of an RDI of <20 or an AI of <10.[2] This definition is loosely based on limited mortality data; patients with an AI of >20 have much higher mortality.[3]

To improve success rates, a number of methods have been proposed to select patients who will respond favorably to UPPP: somnofluoroscopy, pharyngeal computed tomography (CT) scan, awake fiberoptic endoscopy with and without Muller's maneuver, asleep endoscopy with continuous positive airway pressure (CPAP), airway manometry, and cephalometry.[2] Two of these methods—fiberoptic endoscopy with Muller's maneuver (FEMM) and lateral cephalometry—are relatively inexpensive and readily accessible to the clinician. Initial studies concluded that they were useful for predicting UPPP success.[4-6]

Early cephalometric studies suggested that those who fail to benefit from UPPP have narrow retrolingual airways. Riley et al[4] and Gislason et al.[5] found that nonresponders have a narrow posterior airway space (distance between the base of the tongue and posterior pharyngeal wall), an inferiorly positioned hyoid, and macroglossia. In contrast, Ryan et al.[7] demonstrated that patients with a narrow posterior airway space are actually more likely to respond to UPPP. More recent studies have not shown a significant difference between responders and nonresponders.[8-10] Therefore, the value of traditional cephalometric analysis in predicting response to UPPP is low. Despite its low predictive efficacy, cephalometry continues to be studied intensively. In a recent study, cephalometric analysis was useful for selecting UPPP responders when OSA patients were stratified by skeletal type.[11] Such studies hold promise that cephalometry may reliably be used to predict response to UPPP in the future.

Awake FEMM has also been proposed to help identify good UPPP candidates. Sher et al.[6] introduced fiberoptic endoscopy for the preoperative evaluation of patients with OSA. Sher found the predictive value of FEMM to be high; 87% of patients with collapse confined to the velopharynx during FEMM had greater than 50% reduction in AI. In contrast, Katsantonis et al.[12] and Aboussouan et al.[13] were unable to predict success for patients with velopharyngeal collapse. However, these investigators found that FEMM has a high negative predictive value; in other words, they were able to predict failure for those with hypopharyngeal collapse. They concluded that FEMM may be useful in identifying poor UPPP candidates, that is, patients with hypopharyngeal collapse. Still other workers have concluded that FEMM has no predictive value.[10,14]

Lateral cephalometry and FEMM have not been universally accepted or validated for selecting OSA patients who will respond to UPPP. Although objective, easily accessible, and relatively inexpensive, the predictive value of both techniques is low, as they may not localize the critical obstructive pathophysiology that occurs in OSA patients during sleep. It is also possible that these methods may identify the site of obstruction, but that UPPP surgery does not reliably alleviate the abnormality that causes OSA. Several studies have demonstrated that in most UPPP failures the level of obstruction is retropalatal.[15-17] Persistent obstruction at the level of the palate may account for the low predictive efficacy of techniques such as fiberoptic endoscopy and lateral cephalemetry.

A thorough history and physical examination are extremely important in evaluating patients for OSA. Patients with OSA frequently complain of snoring, restless and fragmented sleep, excessive daytime sleepiness, morning headaches and confusion, and poor work performance. The typical patient is overweight with a short, fat neck. Examination of the oral cavity, nose, and pharynx is critical. Patients often have an elongated soft palate and uvula associated with laxity of the posterior and lateral pharyngeal walls and tonsillar pillars. The tonsils may be enlarged, although tonsils of normal size may contribute to airway obstruction as a result of oropharyngeal size or ptosis. In addition, mandibular size, height and shape of the hard palate, and tongue size and position are assessed. Nasal examination is important to rule out nasal obstructive lesions such as septal deviation, nasal polyposis, turbinate hypertrophy, and adenoid hypertrophy. To examine the pharynx, flexible fiberoptic endoscopy is performed; thus, specific space-occupying lesions are identified. Approximately 3 in 200 adult patients with OSA have such a lesion.[2] Surgical removal will correct OSA. Finally, medical disorders such as hypothyroidism, amyloidosis, and other matabolic storage disorders that may contribute to upper airway obstruction must be ruled out if appropriate.

All patients suspected of having OSA on the basis of history and physical examination are evaluated with polysomnography (PSG). Patients diagnosed with OSA by PSG are first treated medically. They are counseled to avoid alcohol and sedative medication, to lose weight, and to alter sleep position if the apnea is position related. However, behavior modifications alone are rarely successful. Mechanical devices that affect oral and pharyngeal mechanics benefit some patients. Most with

OSA require nasal CPAP, the mainstay of medical therapy. It is highly effective for treating OSA when properly and consistently used.[18] In addition, CPAP, unlike UPPP, has been shown to reduce mortality.[3] CPAP, however, is often poorly tolerated, making long-term compliance a problem.

Patients who fail to tolerate nasal CPAP are surgical candidates. A select few are treated with procedures other than UPPP. Patients with significant sequelae of OSA, including cardiac arrhythmias, cor pulmonale, and disabling somnolence, are encouraged to have a tracheostomy. Tracheostomy, like nasal CPAP, is highly effective at resolving OSA and its complications and has been shown to reduce mortality.[2] In a select group with mild OSA, nasal obstruction, and normal oral and pharyngeal anatomy, nasal surgery alone may be successful.[19] Finally, patients with specific craniofacial abnormalities are evaluated by our craniofacial team and treated appropriately.

All other individuals are first offered UPPP. Patients are not selected on the basis of lateral cephalometry, FEMM, or other techniques. Although patients with milder OSA are more likely to respond to UPPP,[2] all patients with OSA, regardless of severity, are offered UPPP. Even though more patients with severe OSA may not respond as defined, many will, and, for those who do not, improvement in their OSA may allow them to decrease their CPAP pressures to tolerable levels. For patients with OSA and nasal obstruction, nasal surgery is performed at the time of UPPP, except in the cases noted previously.

After UPPP, PSG should be repeated. On the basis of these results, nasal CPAP may be adjusted or terminated. Patients with persistent OSA and who are unable to tolerate CPAP are evaluated for other maxillofacial procedures, including geniotubercle advancement, hyoid fixation, and maxillomandibular advancement. Success rates of 65 to 97% with these procedures have been reported.[20-22] However, the number of studies evaluating such procedures is limited, and the preoperative selection of patients is frequently confusing and complex.

Indications for UPPP in Snoring

UPPP is highly effective for the treatment of snoring. The success rate of this technique has ranged from 76% to 94%, and, in most series, is greater than 90%.[23] Although highly efficacious, UPPP is associated with considerable morbidity and thus is frequently unacceptable to many patients. It requires a general anesthetic and hospital admission, often to the intensive care unit. Postoperative pain is moderate to intense and often unremitting for days; in most cases, a narcotic is required for days, and often weeks. Complications can be significant and include death secondary to airway obstruction, hemorrhage, velopharyngeal insufficiency, voice change, and foreign-body sensation.[1]

The significant morbidity associated with UPPP has led to attempts to develop procedures that are as effective as UPPP at alleviating snoring, but with fewer side effects and less postoperative discomfort. One procedure, laser-assisted uvulopalatoplasty (LAUP), was introduced in 1993 as a treatment for snoring; intensely publicized, its use proliferated rapidly. Response rates appear to be comparable to those for UPPP.[23] LAUP has a number of advantages over UPPP. It is an office-based procedure, performed without general anesthesia. Patients are not hospitalized and usually can return to work the same day as the procedure. It is safer than UPPP, with no cases of airway obstruction or death having been reported, to our knowledge. The risk of postoperative hemorrhage and palatal insufficiency is lower.[24]

Despite these advantages, LAUP is not without controversy. The standard LAUP requires multiple procedures to stiffen the palate and, as a result, the cost advantage over UPPP is marginal. However, one-stage LAUP is now being performed and preliminary studies report success rates comparable to those of standard LAUP.[25] Furthermore, although LAUP was initially publicized as much less painful than UPPP, in our experience, patients who undergo LAUP experience moderate levels of pain and often require a narcotic for several days. Another novel procedure, somnoplasty or radiofrequency ablation of the soft palate, appears to be much less painful than UPPP and even LAUP. Preliminary studies suggest that somnoplasty is as efficacious as LAUP for snoring and may have a lower incidence of palatal incompetence.[26]

Finally, many patients with severe antisocial snoring may suffer from more serious sleep-related disorders and, if not correctly diagnosed, may be inadequately treated with LAUP. As many as 40% of patients with OSA documented by PSG report snoring as their only symptom.[27] These patients are at risk of being misdiagnosed as nonapneic snorers. As a result, they may be offered a procedure such as LAUP that is highly efficacious for snoring, but of questionable benefit for OSA. Only a few studies have evaluated the efficacy of LAUP for treating OSA. In the largest trial of LAUP patients, in which pre- and post-treatment PSG were compared, Laurentano et al.[28] demonstrated that mild to moderate OSA worsened and that severe OSA persisted after LAUP. Thus, patients with OSA who complain only of snoring may be inappropriately treated with LAUP. LAUP may delay the diagnosis of OSA by masking the only symptom and, in some patients, may worsen OSA.

Surgery for snoring has followed national trends in our department. Increasing numbers of patients are electing to undergo LAUP and somnoplasty, rather than traditional UPPP. All patients requesting surgery for snoring have a thorough preoperative clinical evaluation similar to that for OSA. Patients with marked tonsillar hypertrophy, redundant pharyngeal mucosa, or nasal obstruction requiring correction under general anesthesia are encouraged to undergo UPPP. All others are considered candidates for LAUP or somnoplasty. Although the American Sleep Disorders Association recommends that all surgical candidates for snoring procedures such as LAUP undergo PSG to screen for OSA, we do not believe that it is cost effective. However, all our candidates for LAUP or somnoplasty are informed of the risks of missing the diagnosis of OSA, and patients suspected of suffering from OSA based on the information obtained from the history and physical examination are encouraged to undergo PSG.

Conclusion

UPPP is used to treat both OSA and snoring. It is effective in less than one-half of patients with OSA. To improve success rates, a number of techniques have been proposed to select patients that will respond favorably to UPPP. However, no technique has been universally validated or accepted. Although the response rate is less than ideal, UPPP remains the first-line surgical therapy for patients with OSA who fail to tolerate nasal CPAP. In contrast, UPPP is highly effective for snoring. However, it is not acceptable to many patients because it is associated with significant morbidity. As a result, less morbid procedures, such as LAUP and somnoplasty, are becoming extremely popular. Although reportedly as effective as UPPP for the treatment of snoring, these techniques may be used inappropriately to treat snorers who have more serious sleep-related disorders.

REFERENCES

1. Fujita S, Conway W, Zorick F. Surgical correction of anatomic abnormalities in obstructive sleep apnea syndrome: uvulopalatopharyngoplasty. *Otolaryngol Head Neck Surg* 1981;89: 923–934
2. Sher AE, Schechtman KB, Piccirillo JF. The efficacy of surgical modification of the upper airway in adults with obstructive sleep apnea syndrome. *Sleep* 1996;19:156–177
3. He J, Kryger MH, Zorick FJ, et al. Mortality and apnea index in obstructive sleep apnea. *Chest* 1988;94:9–14
4. Riley R, Guilleminault C, Powell N, Simmons FB. Palatopharyngoplasty failure, cephalometric roentgenograms, and obstructive sleep apnea. *Otolaryngol Head Neck Surg* 1985;93:240–243
5. Gislason T, Lindholm CE, Almqvist M, et al. Uvulopalatopharyngoplasty in the sleep apnea syndrome. *Arch Otolaryngol Head Neck Surg* 1988;114:45–51
6. Sher AE, Thorpy MJ, Shprintzen RJ, et al. Predictive value of Muller maneuver in selection of patients for uvulopharyngopalatoplasty. *Laryngoscope* 1985;95:1483–1487
7. Ryan CF, Dickson RI, Lowe AA, et al. Upper airway measurements predict response to uvulopalatopharyngoplasty in obstructive sleep apnea. *Laryngoscope* 1990;100:248–253
8. Woodson BT, Conley SF, Dohse A, et al. Posterior cephalometric radiographic analysis in obstructive sleep apnea. *Ann Otol Rhinol Layngol* 1997;106:310–313
9. Yao M, Utley DS, Terris DJ. Cephalometric parameters after multilevel pharyngeal surgery for patients with obstructive sleep apnea. *Laryngoscope* 1998;108:789–795
10. Doghramji K, Jabourian ZH, Pilla M, et al. Predictors of outcome for uvulopalatopharyngoplasty. *Laryngoscope* 1995;105:311–314
11. Woodson BT, Conley SF. Prediction of uvulopalatopharyngoplasty response using cephalometric radiographs. *Am J Otolaryngol* 1997;18:179–184
12. Katsantonis GP, Maas CS, Walsh JK. The predictive efficacy of the Muller maneuver in uvulopalatopharyngoplasty. *Laryngoscope* 1989;99:677–680
13. Aboussouan LS, Golish JA, Wood BG, et al. Dynamic pharyngoscopy in predicting outcome of uvulopalatopharyngoplasty for moderate and severe obstructive sleep apnea. *Chest* 1995; 107:946–951
14. Wittig R, Fujita S, Fortier J. Results of uvulopalatopharyngoplasty (UPPP) in patients with both oropharyngeal and hypopharyngeal collapse Muller maneuver. *Sleep Res* 1987;17:269
15. Shepard JW, Thawley SE. Localization of upper airway collapse during sleep in patients with obstructive sleep apnea. *Am Rev Respir Dis* 1990;141:1350–1355
16. Woodson BT, Wooten MR. Manometric and endoscopic localization of ariway obstruction after uvulopalatopharyngoplasty. *Otolaryngol Head Neck Surg* 1994;111:38–43
17. Skatvedt O. Continuous pressure measurements during sleep to localize obstructions in the upper airways in heavy snorers and patients with obstructive sleep apnea syndrome. *Eur Arch Otorhinolayngol* 1995;252;11–14
18. Anand VK, Ferguson PW, Schoen LS. Obstructive sleep apnea: a comparison of continuous positive airway pressure and surgical treatment. *Otolaryngol Head Neck Surg* 1991; 105:382–390
19. Series F, St Pierre S, Carrier G. Surgical correction of nasal obstruction in the treatment of mild sleep apnea: importance of cephalometry in predicting outcome. *Thorax* 1993;48: 360–363
20. Riley RW, Powell NB, Guilleminault C. Obstructive sleep apnea syndrome: a review of 306 consecutively treated surgical patients. *Otolaryngol Head Neck Surg* 1993;108:117–125
21. Waite PD, Wooten V, Lachner JH. Maxillomandibular advancement surgery in 23 patients with obstructive sleep apnea syndrome. *J Oral Maxillofacial Surg* 1989;47: 1256–1261
22. Hochban W, Brandenburg U, Peter JH. Surgical treatment of obstructive sleep apnea by maxillomandibular advancement. *Sleep* 1994;17:624–629
23. An American Sleep Disorders Association Report. Practice parameters for the use of laser-assisted uvulopalatoplasty. *Sleep* 1994;17:744–748
24. Walker RP, Gopalsami C. Laser-assisted uvulopalatoplasty: postoperative complications. *Laryngoscope* 1996;106:834–838
25. Dickson RI, Mintz DR. One-stage laser-assisted uvulopalatoplasty. *J Otolaryngol* 1996;25:155–161
26. Powell NB, Riley RW, Troell RJ, et al. Radiofrequency volumetric tissue reduction of the palate in subjects with sleep-disordered breathing. *Chest* 1998;113:1163–1174
27. Hoffstein V, Szalia JP. Predictive value of clinical features in diagnosing obstructive sleep apnea. *Sleep* 1993:16:118–122
28. Laurentano AM, Khosla RK, Richardson G. Efficacy of laser-assisted uvulopalatoplasty. *Lasers Surg Med* 1997;21:109–116

Indications for UPPP in Snoring and Sleep Apnea

Thomas A. Tami

CHAPTER 12

The field of sleep medicine, especially as it relates to obstructive sleep apnea (OSA) is in its infancy. Before 1980, only a handful of published reports described this condition. A distinct clinical subspecialty has since developed around this condition. In fact, a cottage industry was born, consisting of surgical supply and diagnostic companies, to service the needs of this medical diagnosis.

Otolaryngologists first became interested in OSA after early reports of a simple surgical procedure purported to offer a cure in many patients. The uvulopalatopharyngoplasty (UPPP) described by Fujita in 1981[1] created a stir in the otolaryngologic as well as in the sleep disorders medical community. This procedure was soon heralded as a safe, quick, and permanent solution to this difficult medical condition.

As might have been predicted, not everyone who underwent this procedure benefited. Snoring was relieved in most instances (usually providing a measure of satisfaction for the sleeping partner), but the clinical success of UPPP for OSA was only within the range of 50 to 60%. Although upper airway obstruction often results from narrowing in the region of the oropharynx and velum, anatomic collapse in the hypopharynx, larynx, and tongue base can also produce OSA. It became clear that if patients could be classified according to anatomic site of narrowing and collapse, UPPP could be more appropriately and, perhaps, more successfully applied only to those patients found to have narrowing in the region of the oropharynx and velum.[2,3]

Many techniques have been used to help establish this possible anatomic relationship. Cephalometric measurements, anatomic descriptions of the oropharyngeal and hypopharyngeal anatomy, cine-computed tomography (CT) evaluation of the dynamic airway, and nasopharyngeal fiberoptic examination at rest and during obstructed inspiration (Muller maneuver) have all been tried to preselect patients who would benefit from UPPP. At best, these techniques for predicting surgical success have produced mixed results. One of the only groups to claim success in predicting surgical outcomes based on preoperative parameters is the Stanford University group. Riley et al.[4] reported that the use of extensive preoperative data analysis, including physical examination, fiberoptic nasopharyngoscopy with the Muller maneuver, and lateral cephalometric analysis to determine the site of obstruction resulted in a surgical success rate of 61%, defined as a reduction of the apnea/hypopnea index (AHI) to < 20. Clearly, even in this, the best case of clinical situations, the ability to predict the surgical success of UPPP is barely acceptable.

Medical Implications of OSA

What, then, should be the clinical approach to patients with OSA? Which patients should be offered UPPP as a therapeutic alternative? To come to grips with this question, the medical implications of OSA must be clearly understood and appreciated. Both patient and physician must appreciate that this is a serious medical problem. Whereas snoring alone is generally considered a social issue, albeit often a considerable one, OSA is associated with significant health implications. The cycle of frequent nighttime arousals that accompanies OSA is rarely reported by patients. However, because these frequent interruptions in sleep disrupt normal sleep patterns, patients with OSA are often sleep deprived. This constant sleep fragmentation results in hypersomnolence and interferes substantially with the performance of routine activities and cognitive tasks.[5-8] Regulatory agencies now also recognize the danger of OSA-related hypersomnolence in the workplace and on highways. Guidelines are being developed to restrict the activities of severely affected individuals.[9]

Severe cardiovascular disease is also common in patients with OSA. Hypertension, cardiac arrhythmia, left ventricular dysfunction, myocardial infarction, pulmonary hypertension, stroke, and sudden death are all more common in patients with this condition.[10] Systemic hypertension has been reported in up to 50% of patients with OSA, and one report implicated undiagnosed OSA in as many as 40% of patients with essential systemic hypertension.[11] In an often quoted study by He et al.[12] in 1988, a large cohort of patients with OSA were evaluated at the Henry Ford Hospital Sleep Disorders Center and followed for up to 9 years. Untreated subjects with an AHI of >20 had significantly increased mortality compared with those with less severe AHI scores. Aggressive treatment with nasal continuous positive airway pressure (CPAP) appeared to reverse this trend, clearly implicating OSA for the increased mortality.

Nonsurgical Treatment Options

Many otolaryngologists fail to recognize that UPPP is by no means the only treatment alternative for OSA, and it is far from the most clinically effective. Treatment options must include simple nonsurgical alternatives as well. Eliminating associated risk factors for OSA can often produce dramatic results. Because the use of sedative medications and alcohol is clearly associated with OSA, their use must be avoided. Obesity also has a clear relationship to OSA, however combating this problem is fraught with patient resistance and therapeutic failures.[13,14] Nevertheless, both simple interventions must be included in the treatment algorithm.

Orthodontic devices have also been developed to alter the upper airway by changing the tongue–jaw anatomic relationship. Schmidt-Nowara et al.[15] reviewed the effectiveness of several of these currently available devices. In an examination of 21 publications, these investigators concluded that snoring was improved or eliminated in most patients fitted with these devices; however, OSA as measured by the AHI was sometimes reduced but rarely brought to within the normal range. Although limited controlled data support the efficacy of these various devices for the treatment of OSA, their use continues to be widespread, largely because they offer a nonsurgical, relatively nonintrusive technique to manage this problem.

Nasal CPAP was first introduced in 1981 as a nonsurgical treatment for OSA and has since become widely used for this condition.[16] Nasal CPAP delivers positive airway pressure through a tightly sealed nasal mask, which, when titrated appropriately, produces a constant pneumatic splint to prevent upper airway collapse during nocturnal respiration. Excessive daytime somnolence and other neuropsychological symptoms associated with OSA are quickly reversed by means of this device. The cardiovascular sequelae and mortality associated with this disorder can also be dramatically reduced.

The impressive clinical effectiveness of nasal CPAP is often overshadowed by poor patient acceptance and low compliance. Early studies designed to quantify self-reported patient compliance reported rates ranging from 47% to 91%; however, these studies relied on patient reporting and contained built-in bias toward higher reported compliance rates. Several subsequent studies have looked more objectively at this issue by using covert digital microprocessor monitoring devices within the CPAP unit. As expected, these studies disclosed much lower rates of continuous usage.[17-19] Because patient compliance appears to be correlated with the patient's understanding of the medical condition, patient education about OSA and nasal CPAP is vital if this treatment is to be successful.

Surgical Management

Surgical management also includes several options other than UPPP. Tracheotomy is an extremely effective surgical tool for the management of OSA. Although this technique provides an absolute solution to the problem, it is usually associated with both patient and physician resistance. In general, only the most severely affected patients with severe daytime somnolence or cardiovascular disease are offered this treatment option.

Nasal obstruction is often grouped with other traditional causes of OSA, and nasal surgery is often recommended as part of the treatment of patients who snore or who suffer OSA. The evidence to implicate nasal obstruction in the pathophysiology of this condition is minimal. One recent study that systematically evaluated the effects of surgical correction of nasal obstruction failed to demonstrate any meaningful postoperative reduction in sleep-disordered breathing in patients with OSA.[20] Interestingly, several patients in this group had very mild apnea preoperatively and no other obvious upper airway structural abnormalities; among this patient group, the AHI normalized postoperatively. These findings suggest that nasal obstruction plays a role in only a small subpopulation of patients with mild OSA.

Recent excitement has accompanied the introduction of laser-assisted uvulopalatoplasty (LAUP). This procedure was initially introduced as an outpatient alternative for snoring, but its similarity to the widely used UPPP made it an enticing alternative for managing OSA. LAUP appears to be highly successful in decreasing or eliminating socially unacceptable snoring; however, there are limited data to support its use for OSA. Several recent studies have suggested that LAUP can improve OSA in certain mild cases of the disorder, among properly selected patients. Nevertheless, the efficacy of LAUP has not been established in this setting.[21-24]

Surgical procedures aimed primarily at the hypopharynx and tongue base have also been developed. Among these are the mandibular osteotomy/genioglossus advancement with hyoid myotomy/suspension (GAHM) and the more aggressive maxillary and mandibular osteotomies (MMO) with mandibular and midfacial advancement.[4] These more invasive procedures may provide improved airway stabilization in selected cases; however, other than the studies provided by the Stanford University group, their effectiveness is unknown. Other more recent attempts to address the tongue base problem include various suture suspension and tongue base radiofrequency ablation techniques. Although theoretically sound, these newer procedures remain to prove their clinical efficacy.

Role of UPPP

Given the currently available technology for OSA and considering the significant health implications of this disorder, I tend to use the algorithm shown in Figure 12–1 to provide a basis for managing these patients. In general, after a thorough discussion of OSA and its clinical implications, the success rate and nonsurgical nature of nasal CPAP is emphasized to the patient. I encourage all patients to seriously consider this alternative. However, many patients cannot or will not use the nasal CPAP alternative, citing that they are frequent business travelers or are claustrophobic or that they simply do not want to be bothered with a mechanical device every night. The importance of altering lifestyle factors such as alcohol or sedative drug intake and body mass index (obesity) should be reemphasized at every opportunity. Dental orthodontic appliances and UPPP should be discussed. Most patients favor the surgical approach because, if it is successful, it has the potential of a one-time treatment. The poor success of this procedure must be honestly discussed with the patient before the patient makes the decision to

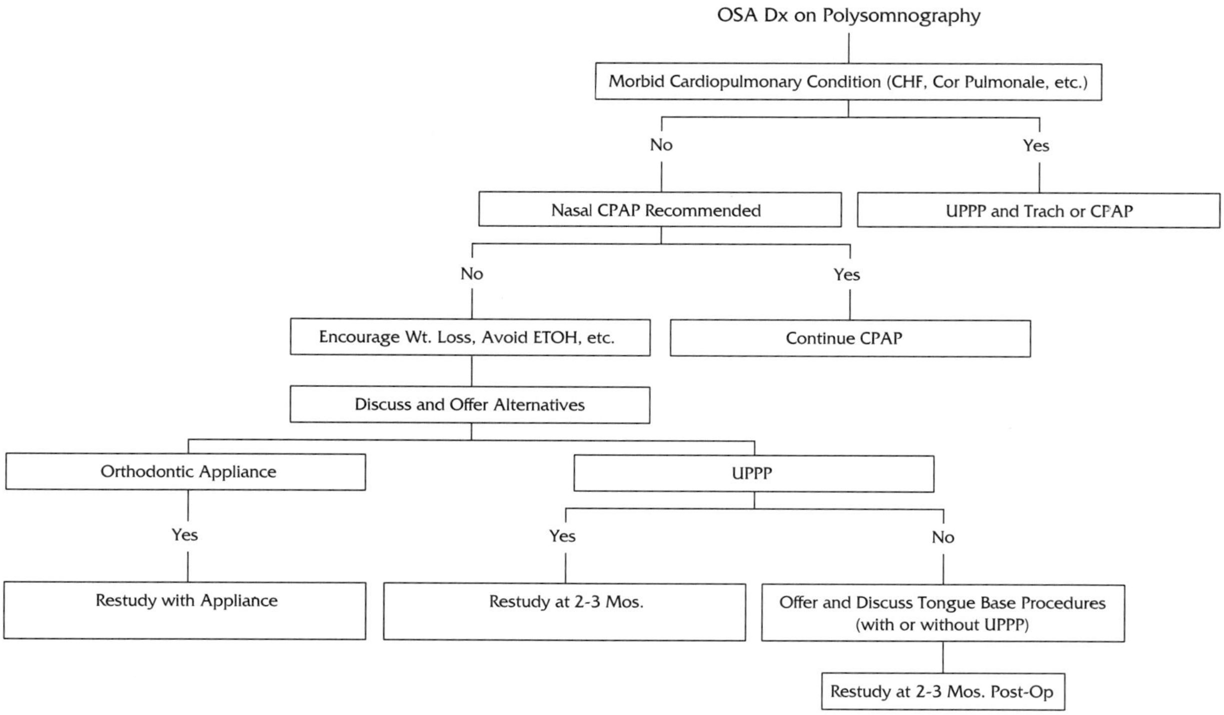

Figure 12–1 Patient diagnosed with obstructive sleep apnea (OSA).

proceed. Although patients often report dramatic symptomatic improvement after undergoing UPPP, a postoperative polysomnographic study is essential for clear documentation of its success or failure. If the procedure has failed to deliver the patient within a normal AHI range, the need for further treatment (preferably nasal CPAP) must be strongly recommended.

Once considered the panacea for managing OSA, UPPP has clear and distinct limitations. Although it continues to have a therapeutic role in the surgical management of OSA, its effectiveness is often overestimated both by patients and by physicians. Otolaryngologists must constantly be reminded of the limitations of UPPP and of the significant health implications of inadequately managed OSA when discussing treatment options and making recommendations to patients with this condition.

REFERENCES

Tami—CHAPTER 12

1. Fujita S, Conway W, Zorick F. Surgical correction of anatomic abnormalities in obstructive sleep apnea syndrome: uvulopalatopharyngoplasty. *Otolaryngol Head Neck Surg* 1981; 89:923–934
2. Schechtman KB, Sher AE, Piccirillo JF. Methodological and statistical problems in sleep apnea research: the literature on uvulopalatopharyngoplasty. *Sleep* 1995;18:659–666
3. Sher AE, Schechtman KB, Piccirillo JF. The efficacy of surgical modifications of the upper airway in adults with obstructive sleep apnea syndrome. *Sleep* 1996;19:156–177
4. Riley RW, Powell NB, Guilleminault C. Obstructive sleep apnea syndrome: a review of 306 consecutively treated surgical patients. *Otolaryngol Head Neck Surg* 1993;108:117–125
5. Findley LJ, Unverzagt ME, Suratt PM. Automobile accidents involving patients with obstructive sleep apnea. *Am Rev Respir Dis* 1988;138:337–340
6. Findley L, Unverzagt M, Guchu R, et al. Vigilance and automobile accidents in patients with sleep apnea or narcolepsy. *Chest* 1995;108:619–624
7. Mitler MM. Daytime sleepiness and cognitive functioning in sleep apnea. *Sleep* 1993;16(8 suppl):S68–70
8. Pack AI. The prevalence of work-related sleep problems [editorial]. *J Gen Intern Med* 1995;10:57
9. Pakola SJ, Dinges DF, Pack AI. Review of regulations and guidelines for commercial and noncommercial drivers with sleep apnea and narcolepsy. *Sleep* 1995;18:787–796
10. Shepard JWJ. Hypertension, cardiac arrhythmias, myocardial infarction, and stroke in relation to obstructive sleep apnea. *Clin Chest Med* 1992;13:437–458
11. Millman RP, Redline S, Carlisle CC, et al. Daytime hypertension in obstructive sleep apnea. Prevalence and contributing risk factors. *Chest* 1991;99:861–866

12. He J, Kryger MH, Zorick FJ, et al. Mortality and apnea index in obstructive sleep apnea. Experience in 385 male patients. *Chest* 1988;94:9–14
13. Riley RW, Powell NB, Guilleminault C, et al. Obstructive sleep apnea. Trends in therapy [see comments]. *West J Med* 1995;162:143–148
14. Smith PL, Gold AR, Meyers DA, et al. Weight loss in mildly to moderately obese patients with obstructive sleep apnea. *Ann Intern Med* 1985;103(pt 1):850–855
15. Schmidt-Nowara W, Lowe A, Wiegand L, et al. Oral appliances for the treatment of snoring and obstructive sleep apnea: a review. *Sleep* 1995;18:501–510
16. Sullivan CE, Issa FG, Berthon-Jones M, Eves L. Reversal of obstructive sleep apnoea by continuous positive airway pressure applied through the nares. *Lancet* 1981;1:862–865
17. Kribbs NB, Pack AI, Kline LR, et al. Objective measurement of patterns of nasal CPAP use by patients with obstructive sleep apnea [see comments]. *Am Rev Respir Dis* 1993; 147:887–895
18. Reeves-Hoche MK, Meck R, Zwillich CW. Nasal CPAP: an objective evaluation of patient compliance. *Am J Respir Crit Care Med* 1994;149:149–154
19. Rauscher H, Formanek D, Popp W, Zwick H. Self-reported vs measured compliance with nasal CPAP for obstructive sleep apnea. *Chest* 1993;103:1675–1680
20. Series F, St. Pierre S, Carrier G. Effects of surgical correction of nasal obstruction in the treatment of obstructive sleep apnea. *Am Rev Respir Dis* 1992;146(pt 1):1261–1265
21. Kamami YV. Outpatient treatment of snoring with CO_2 laser: laser-assisted UPPP. *J Otolaryngol* 1994;23:391–394
22. Macdougald I. Sleep apnoea. Laser therapy for OSAS. *Nurs Times* 1994;90:32–34
23. Mickelson SA. Laser-assisted uvulopalatoplasty for obstructive sleep apnea. *Laryngoscope* 1996;106:10–13
24. Walker RP, Grigg-Damberger MM, Gopalsami C, Totten MC. Laser-assisted uvulopalatoplasty for snoring and obstructive sleep apnea: results in 170 patients. *Laryngoscope* 1995; 105(pt 1):938–943

5

The Role of Free Flaps in Head and Neck Reconstruction

"Irrespective of the donor site, the main objective of cranial base reconstruction is to separate the CNS from the sinonasal cavity. When compared with local and pedicled flaps, free flap reconstruction has been demonstrated to be the safest and most economical method for skull base reconstruction offering the best outcomes after extensive surgical resections."

Mark L. Urken

"In our current cost-conscious medical environment, many have questioned whether complex surgical procedures such as free flaps would be supported in an era where the cost of care plays a major role in determining patient treatment."

Eugene N. Myers

"Depending on the selection of free flap, it is possible to transfer skin and subcutaneous tissue as a single entity, muscle, fascia, bone, and even nerve–muscle combinations to achieve goals of re-animation. This flexibility to transfer a combination of different types of tissue facilitates surgical creativity to precisely tailor the reconstruction to the defect by replacing the type of tissue that has been destroyed by cancer or trauma."

David E. Schuller

The Role of Free Flaps in Head and Neck Reconstruction

CHAPTER 13

Eric M. Genden and Mark L. Urken

The role of free flap surgery in contemporary head and neck reconstruction is the culmination of several decades of trying to solve a select group of reconstructive challenges, using conventional local and regional flaps, as well as an evolution in technique and technology that have enhanced the safety and reliability of this method of reconstruction. Although the first successful free flap in humans was performed in 1959, it took several decades before free tissue transfer surgery became a widely accepted method of head and neck reconstruction.[1] Initially, it was the problem of the pharyngoesophageal defect and the segmental mandibulectomy defect that provided the impetus for applying microvascular surgery to the head and neck region. Over the past decade, advances in skull base surgery have led to new reconstructive demands for reliable soft tissue flaps, in order to permit the safe application of new surgical techniques to remove benign and malignant neoplasms located at the cranial base. The role of free flaps in contemporary head and neck reconstruction has become much broader than for these three defects. Reinnervated flaps have been used to restore dynamic activity for patients with facial paralysis and to restore sensation to the lining of the upper aerodigestive tract. However, a discussion of the history and of the requirements for successful restoration of circumferential pharyngoesophageal defects, segmental mandibular defects, and extensive skull base defects serves as the focus of this chapter on the role of free tissue transfer in head and neck reconstruction.

Before 1963, postablative surgical defects were either closed primarily or with random pattern or axial pattern skin flaps. As a result, functional and cosmetic outcomes were often quite poor. Limited mobility and reliability restricted the use of such donor sites as the nape of neck, acromial thoracic, and forehead flaps. These donor sites supplied a small area of cutaneous tissue with a limited arc of rotation and little or no bulk. The reconstructive techniques available at the time often limited the extent of an ablative surgical resection, compromising curative surgical therapy. Free tissue transfer in the head and neck was first reported in 1959 by Seidenberg et al.,[1] who, without the benefit of an operating microscope, transferred a free jejunal segment for reconstruction of a circumferential mucosal defect after a laryngopharyngectomy. Although free tissue transfer was a novel reconstructive approach, limited donor sites, as well as extensive, often exhaustive, intraoperative time requirements, and technical limitations, prevented its widespread acceptance.

The introduction of the pedicled latissimus dorsi myocutaneous flap by Olivari,[2] in 1976, led the way for the next reconstructive technologic breakthrough, the myocutaneous flap. Along with the latissimus flap, the pectoralis flap, introduced by Ariyan in 1979,[3] and the trapezius flap[4] described shortly thereafter, composed the vast majority of the head and neck reconstructive armamentarium. These flaps were reliable and easy to harvest and served to reconstruct a wide range of soft tissue defects of the head and neck. The rich vascular supply of the muscle component of these myocutaneous flaps served to protect the carotid artery, while providing the reconstructive surgeon with a one-stage reconstruction that was relatively simple to harvest. However, it soon became apparent that complex hard and soft tissue defects of the pharyngoesophagus, mandible, and skull base were poorly managed by pedicled flap reconstruction. Attempts at tubing myocutaneous flaps were often fraught with complications. Similarly, mandibular reconstruction by transferring rib with pectoralis muscle led to limited success.[5] Although regional myocutaneous flaps were thought to be the panacea, it became evident that predictable reconstruction of the mandibular, pharyngoesophageal, and skull base defects required a more sophisticated form of reconstruction. Furthermore, the impetus for an improved functional outcome in these areas encouraged the development of reliable free tissue transfer. During the mid- and late 1970s, when most head and neck surgeons relied on pedicled myocutaneous flaps, Taylor et al.[6] and others[7] identified a series of free tissue donor sites with longer and larger-diameter vascular pedicles, which resulted in a dramatic improvement in reliability and applicability. In addition to soft tissue donor sites, several composite bone flaps were described. All head and neck reconstruction has benefited from these developments in free tissue transfer, but reconstruction of the pharyngoesophagus, mandible, and the skull base have shown the most profound improvements.

Pharyngoesophageal Reconstruction

Early reconstruction of circumferential pharyngoesophageal defects represented one of the most challenging dilemmas for the reconstructive head and neck surgeon. The inability to reestablish continuity of the cervical esophagus resulted in a chronic pharyngocutaneous fistula often leading to infection and a poor outcome. Early attempts to remedy this problem led Czerny[8] Mikulicz,[9] and Trotter[10] to use cervical skin flaps in a staged reconstruction. This approach proved unreliable, requiring multiple stages and prolonged hospitalization; it was commonly associated with a high rate of morbidity as a result of flap necrosis and eventual wound breakdown. Nearly a half-century later, Wookey reintroduced this technique, redesigning the cervical flaps with a wide pedicle, which resulted in a more reliable two-stage reconstruction. Although this was an improvement, a review of 148 patients reconstructed in this fashion, demonstrated that these patients required prolonged hospitalization ranging from 6 to 16 weeks, and 94% sustained some form of postoperative complication related to the reconstruction.[11] Complications, including stenosis, fistula, or flap necrosis, required an average of three corrective procedures prior to successful resumption of deglutition. The limitations associated with random pattern skin flaps led to the application of the deltopectoral and, soon thereafter, the pectoralis major myocutaneous flap.

The deltopectoral flap offered reconstructive surgeons a source of reliable, well-vascularized tissue from a regional site, which was particularly useful in irradiated patients. Although this technique was an improvement over prior reconstructive methods, there were disadvantages of a staged procedure with the mandatory creation of a pharyngostome, as well as an unacceptably high complication rate (56%).[11] The drive to reconstruct the pharyngoesophagus primarily, influenced Withers et al.[12] and Baek et al.[13] to report on the use of a tubed pectoralis major flap as a method of "immediate" reconstruction of circumferential defects of the pharynx and cervical esophagus. The pectoralis major flap offered the advantage of introducing nonirradiated muscle to the reconstruction site. However, the bulky nature of the flap lacked the necessary pliability to comfortably create a circumferencial skin tube and thereby hindered the reconstruction in many patients. As a result, most tube-shaped pectoralis major pharyngoesophageal reconstructions required the formation of a controlled fistula, either at the time of primary reconstruction or as a result of an often inevitable postoperative wound dehiscence.

In an effort to address the problems associated with delayed reconstruction, and the requirement for thin, pliable tissue, a variety of pedicled visceral flaps were introduced.[14-16] The theoretical advantages of the gastric pull-up include a single anastomosis and hence less potential for anastomotic failure, a source of thin, pliable, nonirradiated tissue, and the opportunity for immediate reconstruction. Unfortunately, these advantages did not translate into a reliable method of reconstruction. Surkin et al.[11] found mortality to range from 10% to 15%, and 50% of patients sustained major abdominal, medical, or thoracic complications. Although anastomotic stenosis is uncommon, patients often suffer from an uncontrolled regurgitation of gastric contents, or a "dumping syndrome," as a result of the atonic gastric segment. Although the gastric pull-up still plays a role in contemporary reconstruction of the thoracic esophagus, its routine use in cervicoesophageal reconstruction has been limited because of the unacceptably high complication rate and the introduction of less morbid and more reliable alternatives.

Microvascular free tissue transfer has been widely applied in contemporary head and neck reconstruction, and its impact on the primary reconstruction of the pharyngoesophagus has been profound. The drive to circumvent the morbidity associated with delayed reconstruction led to the application of free tissue transfer for pharyngoesophageal reconstruction. Seidenberg et al.[1] first introduced free jejunal transfer in 1959, but this technique lay dormant for many years until 1975, when free jejunal reconstruction became increasingly popular as reported in the head and neck literature. Since then, a host of donor sites have been described for the reconstitution of circumferential defects, including visceral flaps such as the tubed gastro-omental free flap[17] and free colon segments, as well as tubed cutaneous free flaps.[18] Harii et al.[19] were the first to report their success in using tube-shaped cutaneous radial forearm flaps. This approach offered an attractive alternative to the necessity for a laparotomy, with its attendant morbidity, to harvest a visceral flap.[19] Several different cutaneous flaps have since been applied in a similar manner, including the lateral thigh[20] and ulnar forearm flaps.[21]

Colonic segments have been used as free flaps based on the ileocolic, middle colic, and sigmoid arteries. Although this donor site is no longer the primary choice for reconstruction of the pharyngoesophagus, the mucosa-lined colon offers an inner lining similar to the native pharynx. Its large diameter facilitates the pharyngeal anastomosis, but it can present some difficulty at the distal esophageal anastomotic site.

Free jejunal autografts offer several advantages over the free colon transfer, including the ability to harvest large segments of jejunum with little or no functional gastrointestinal disturbance. The popularity of the free jejunal autograft in head and neck reconstruction[22] stemmed from its diversity as a reconstructive tool. The mucosal tube can be split to reconstruct a defect in the posterior pharyngeal wall, or it can be used as a circumferential mucosal tube for primary reconstruction of the cervical esophagus and hypopharynx. Splitting the jejunal segment along its antemesenteric border can facilitate the resurfacing of defects that extend to the oral cavity. Furthermore, a jejunal harvest does not require preoperative bowel preparation and has less potential for postoperative complications as compared with the colon donor site. Similar to the colon, the jejunum offers the advantage of providing a mucosa-lined conduit; however, the diameter of the jejunum more closely approximates that of the pharyngoesophagus. The distant harvest site permits a two-team approach. The harvest itself is technically easy, usually requiring less than 1 hour to perform.

Tube-shaped cutaneous free flaps offer a source of thin and pliable tissue ideal for the primary reconstruction of the pharyngoesophagus. The enhanced pliability and vascularity of the radial forearm, lateral thigh, ulnar forearm,[21] and lateral arm donor sites avoid the high rates of fistulization and stenosis associated with myocutanoeus and locoregional flaps.[18,2320] All three donor sites permit a two-team harvest, as well as the decreased risk of donor site morbidity and the flexibility in design. The potential morbidity associated with a laparotomy has led many head and neck surgeons to use tube-shaped cutaneous free flaps as a first choice of reconstruction. The notable exception is when the inferior cervical esophageal margin is below the sternum, resulting in difficult distal exposure. In the case of a technically difficult anastomosis between a tube-shaped skin flap and the esophagus, an enteric stapling device enables a safe and reliable anastomosis, using a free jejunal autograft. The harvest of the radial forearm, lateral thigh, or lateral arm flaps may be closed primarily or with a split-thickness skin graft, resulting in limited donor site morbidity. Limitations may exist when the patient is obese and excessive subcutaneous fat prevents the tubing of the flap. Under these circumstances, a visceral free flap would be a more suitable option.

Microvascular free tissue transfer offers a reliable single-staged reconstruction of the pharyngoesophageal segment with low donor site morbidity. Tube-shaped cutaneous free flaps provide an excellent first-line tool, as they are associated with excellent functional results with respect to swallowing and speech, very low donor site morbidity, and an acceptably low complication rate.[60]

Mandibular Reconstruction

Since the late nineteenth century, many reconstructive techniques have been used for mandibular restoration after extirpation of oral cavity malignancies or traumatic injury. The challenge of achieving oromandibular rehabilitation is a formidable task involving soft tissue restoration as well as bone in most cases. Ideally, the aim of the reconstruction is to achieve both a functional and aesthetic restoration, addressing specific functions related to the oral cavity, including salivary continence, aspiration, mastication, deglutition, and speech. Prior exposure to irradiation and chemotherapy may further complicate the success of a restoration.

The complex issues related to restoration of the oromandibular defect are best highlighted by work done during World War II, when traumatic mandibular injuries were treated with static splints. Patients were often left with severe contractures and, as oral cripples, were unable to maintain oral competency.[24] The sequelae related to delayed mandibular reconstruction were observed quite early in history. In an effort to prevent these sequelae, nonvascularized rib, tibia, clavicle, and iliac bone were all used to primarily reconstruct the mandible during the early 1900s.[24,25] Progressive resorption and the inability of the bone to withstand the axial stress associated with mastication led to poor results.[26] To address this problem, Snyder et al.[27] and Conley[28] reported on the use of pedicled osteocutaneous flaps for mandibular reconstruction. A decade later, Barnes et al.[29] pedicled clavicle on sternocleidomastoid muscle and Biller et al.[5] reported on the use of rib pedicled on pectoralis major muscle. The success rate of these techniques, however, was quite poor, largely because the bone stock and vascular supply were inadequate.[30] The introduction of bone plating systems during the mid-1970s seemed to fulfill many of the requirements for successful mandibular reconstruction. Early results reported by Klotch and Prein[31] appeared promising; however, complications, including plate extrusion, fistula formation, delayed plate fractures, and poor functional results, limited the success of reconstruction plates.[61] The complications associated with reconstruction plates were exacerbated by the use of adjuvant external beam irradiation, which had been used more frequently since the early 1980s. Although other concerns such as radiation scatter associated with the presence of metal plates were poorly defined at this time, the most significant drawback to this system was the inability to achieve lasting functional oral rehabilitation in these patients. Because the insertion of osseointegrated dental implants was not possible with metal plate reconstruction, the retention and stability of functional dentures could not be achieved.[32]

Free tissue transfer for mandibular reconstruction was first introduced in 1974 by Ostrup and Fredrickson,[33] who used revascularized rib in the canine model. Shortly thereafter, McKee[34] and Daniel[35] applied this technology in humans and, although revascularized rib is no longer used clinically, this pioneering work revolutionized mandibular reconstruction. Composite defects involving the mandible and its adjacent soft tissue could now be reliably reconstructed with vascularized bone as well as adjacent vascularized soft tissue, obviating the need for a second soft tissue flap. Using fluorochrome markers, Ariyan[36] demonstrated the role of the periosteal blood supply and the ability to safely perform contouring osteotomies. Baker and Sullivan[37] demonstrated that transferred bone formed a strong union with the adjacent native mandible after 6 to 8 weeks, even in irradiated patients.

As the advantages of vascularized bone became evident, a number of new donor sites for composite flaps were described. The fibula,[38] iliac crest,[39] and scapula[40] donor sites have become the most popular sources of vascularized bone. Inherent differences in each donor site, with regard to bone stock, soft tissue quality, potential for sensory reinnervation, and pedicle geometry, dictate the best choice for reconstruction. The fibula, iliac, and scapula donor sites all provide bone stock sufficient for dental implants in most patients,[41] which Urken et al.[42] have demonstrated, is an essential factor for optimal oral rehabilitation. Successful reconstruction of the oral complex requires control of salivary continence, prevention of aspiration, functional mastication, and speech. Vascularized bone flaps permit primary reconstruction of the oromandibular complex, avoiding contractures and scarring which often complicate secondary reconstruction.[42,43] Although the recipient bed is often compromised by salivary contamination and prior irradiation, vascularized bone grafts remain capable of healing to the adjacent native mandible such that they may withstand the loading forces associated with mastication.[44,45] Furthermore, the soft tissue components harvested with each of these three composite flap donor sites serve as useful sources of tissue for either intraoral lining or extraoral coverage.[46]

It has become clear that mandibular reconstruction can now be achieved in the primary setting in a safe and reliable manner with minimal donor site morbidity.[47,48] It remains a complex challenge, the results of which greatly influence the patient's postoperative quality of life.[49] In addition, primary oromandibular reconstruction has had a significant impact on disease management. This procedure has eliminated some of the guesswork for the surgeon in deciding whether a marginal mandibulectomy was a safe oncologic procedure. Because of reduced concern for the impact of a larger bony defect in the mandible, it has enhanced our ability to obtain clear margins at the time of resection.[48] Finally, it has greatly affected the management of osteoradionecrosis of the mandible and maxilla, where the resection of the diseased bone can be followed by immediate replacement. The use of vascularized bone in this hostile recipient bed is a critical factor in achieving a successful result.

Skull Base Reconstruction

Advances in imaging for tumor mapping as well as the introduction of new techniques for safe surgical access during the last decade have had a significant impact on skull base surgery. The reconstruction of most anterior and lateral skull base defects was dependent on vascularized pedicled tissue such as local pericranial flaps, temporalis muscle, or nonvascularized fat. Although pedicled myocutaneous flaps have also been used, an inherent restriction in reach limited their applicability. Surgical extirpation of lesions located in the central skull base or those resulting in an extensive defect were often associated with a high morbidity, and hence, were considered surgically unresectable. Partitioning the contaminated sinonasal compartment from the brain remained a reconstructive problem that limited the use of surgical extirpation as a treatment for extensive tumors involving the cranial base. With the institution of free tissue transfer, vascularized tissue could, for the first time, be reliably transferred to the central skull base for the closure of complex defects.

A number of different free flap donor sites[50] have been used for the closure of skull base defects, with the rectus abdominis probably the most frequently used. Urken et al.[51] demonstrated its reliability while others have reported on its versatility for complex cranial base defects.[52] The bulk associated with this myocutaneous flap is ideal for large central defects with extensive "dead space." In contrast, smaller, centrally located basicranial defects may be addressed with a deepithelialized radial forearm free flap. The thin, more pliable tissue characteristic of the forearm free flap provides an excellent source of vascularized soft tissue to repair dural defects, and its long vascular pedicle facilitates central skull base reconstruction requiring a distant vascular anastomosis. Irrespective of the donor site, the main objective of cranial base reconstruction is to separate the central nervous system (CNS) from the sinonasal cavity. When compared with local and pedicled flaps, free flap reconstruction has been demonstrated to be the safest and most economical method for skull base reconstruction,[53] offering the best outcomes after extensive surgical resections.[54]

Conclusion

Although the authors have highlighted the impact of free tissue transfer on three reconstructive problems in the head and neck, it is evident that the management of many other defects has been greatly effected. Reinnervated free muscle flaps have been shown to restore mimetic activity to the paralyzed face.[55,56] Sensate flaps have provided valuable information to the patient to avert the effects of relining the upper aerodigestive tract with anesthetic tissue.[57,58] Vascularized bone-containing flaps have been applied to the midface region to reconstruct the palate in a manner similar to that which has been achieved in the mandible.[59] The use of free tissue transfer has pushed the envelope of partial laryngectomy surgery to the next level.

However, despite these advances, which have occurred over the past decade, the goal of these efforts has been to use the entire body as the source of tissue to most closely match the characteristics of the missing part in the head and neck. With the first successful laryngeal transplantation having been achieved in a human subject by Marshal Strome and his colleagues, the ability to match missing parts with comparable tissues from a different donor has now been realized. At Mount Sinai, we have been working on the reconstruction of long segment tracheal defects with a tracheal transplant. It is evident that the ability to transplant organs in the head and neck successfully is now possible. The return of function when dynamic activity and sensory feedback are important factors in functional recovery of such organs as the larynx and the tongue remains a major issue, as do issues related to immunosuppression. However, it is clear that head and neck reconstruction will take a new direction in the new millennium.

REFERENCES

Genden and Urken—CHAPTER 13

1. Seidenberg B, Rosenak S, Hurwitt ES, et al. Immediate reconstruction of the cervical esophagus by revascularized isolated jejunal segment. *Ann Surg* 1959;142:162
2. Olivari N. The latissimus flap. *Br J Plast Surg* 1976;29:126–128
3. Ariyan S. The pectoralis major myocutaneous flap. A versatile flap for reconstruction in the head and neck. *Plast Reconstr Surg* 1979;63:73–81
4. Baek SM, Biller HF, Krespi YP, Lawson W. The lower trapezius island myocutaneous flap. *Ann Plast Surg* 1980;5:108–114
5. Biller HF, Baek SM, Lawson W, Krespi YP, Blaugrund SM. Pectoralis major myocutaneous island flap in head and neck surgery: analysis of complications in 42 cases. *Arch Otolaryngol* 1981;107:23–26
6. Taylor GI, Miller GD, Ham FJ. The free vascularized bone graft. A clinical extension of microvascular techniques. *Plast Reconstr Surg* 1975;55:533–544
7. Soutar DS, Shaeker LR, Tanner NS, McGregor IA. The radial forearm flap: a versatile method for intra-oral reconstruction. *Br J Plast Surg* 1983; 36:1–8
8. Czerny F. Neue Operationen. *Zentralbl Chir* 1877;4: 433–434
9. Mikulicz J. Ein fall von resection des carcinomatosen esophagos mit platichem ersatz des excidirten stuckes. *Prag Med Wochenschr* 1886;11:93–97
10. Trotter, W. Operative treatment of diseases of the mouth and pharynx. *Lancet* 1913;1:1075–1081

11. Surkin MI, Lawson W, Biller HF. Analysis of the methods of pharyngoesophageal reconstruction. *Head Neck Surg* 1984;6: 953–970
12. Withers EH, Franklin JD, Madden JJ, Lynch JB. Immediate reconstruction of the pharynx and cervical esophagus with the pectoralis major myocutaneous flap following laryngopharyngectomy. *Plast Reconstr Surg* 1981;68:898–904
13. Baek SM, Lawson W, Biller HF. Reconstruction of hypopharynx and cervical esophagus with pectoralis major island myocutaneous flap. *Ann Plast Surg* 1981;7:18–24
14. Heimlich HJ. Reversed gastric tube (RGT) esophagoplasty for failure of colon, jejunum and prosthetic interpositions. *Ann Surg* 1975;182:154–160
15. Mes G. A new method of esophagoplasty. *J Int Coll Surg* 1948;11:270
16. Leonard J, Maran AG. Reconstruction of the cervical esophagus using esophagus via gastric anastomosis. *Laryngoscope* 1970;80:849
17. Hiebert C, Cummings GO. Successful replacement of the cervical esophagus by transplantation and revascularization of a free graft of gastric antrum. *Ann Surg* 1961;154:103–106
18. Harii K, Ebihara S, Ono I, Saito H, Terui S, Takato T. Pharyngoesophageal reconstruction using a fabricated forearm free flap. *Plast Reconstr Surg* 1985;75: 463–476
19. Harii K, Iwaya T, Kawaguchi N. Combination myocutaneous flap and microvascular free flap. *Plast Reconstr Surg* 1981;68:700–711
20. Hayden R. Reconstruction of the hypopharynx and the cervical esophagus. In: Cummings C, Harker LA, et al., eds. *Otolaryngology–Head and Neck Surgery.* St. Louis: CV Mosby; 1993
21. Li KK, Salibian AH, Allison GR, et al. Pharyngoesophageal reconstruction with the ulnar forearm flap. *Arch Otolaryngol Head Neck Surg* 1998;124:1146–1151
22. McDonough JJ, Gluckman JL. Microvascular reconstruction of the pharyngoesophagus with free jejunal graft. *Microsurgery* 1988;9:116–127
23. Takato T, Harii K, Ebihara S, Ono I, Yoshizumi T, Nakatsuka T. Oral and pharyngeal reconstruction using the free forearm flap. *Arch Otolaryngol Head Neck Surg* 1987;113:873–879
24. Blocker TS, Stout RA. Mandibular reconstruction during World War II: a review of the literature. *Plast Reconstr Surg* 1949; 4:153–156
25. Parel SM, Drane JB, Williams EO. Mandibular replacements: a review of the literature. *J Am Dent Assoc* 1977;94:120–129
26. Conley J. A technique for immediate bone grafting in the treatment of benign and malignant tumors of the mandible and the review of 17 consecutive cases. *Cancer* 1953;6:568–577
27. Snyder C, Bateman JM, Davis CW, et al. Mandibulaofacial restoration with live osteocutaneous flaps. *Plast Reconstr Surg* 1970;45:14–19
28. Conley J. The use of composite flaps containing bone for major repairs in the head and the neck. *Plast Reconstr Surg* 1972;49:522–526
29. Barnes DR, Ossoff RH, Pecaro B, Sisson GA. Immediate reconstruction of mandibular defects with a composite sternocleidomastoid musculoclavicular graft. *Arch Otolaryngol* 1981;107:711–714
30. Gullane PJ, Holmes H. Mandibular reconstruction. New concepts. *Arch Otolaryngol Head Neck Surg* 1986;112:714–719
31. Klotch DW, Prein J. Mandibular reconstruction using AO plates. *Am J Surg* 1987;154:384–388
32. Gullane PJ. Primary mandibular reconstruction: analysis of 64 cases and evaluation of interface radiation dosimetry on bridging plates. *Laryngoscope* 1991;101(pt 2):1–24
33. Ostrup LT, Fredrickson JM. Reconstruction of mandibular defects after radiation, using a free, living bone graft transferred by microvascular anastomose. An experimental study. *Plast Reconstr Surg* 1975;55:563–572
34. McKee DM. Microvascular bone transplantation. *Clin Plast Surg* 1978;5:283–292
35. Daniel RK. Free rib transfer by microvascular anastomoses [letter]. *Plast Reconstr Surg* 1977;59:737–738
36. Ariyan S. The viability of rib grafts transplanted with the periosteal blood supply. *Plast Reconstr Surg* 1980;65:140–151
37. Baker SR, Sullivan MJ. Osteocutaneous free scapular flap for one-stage mandibular reconstruction. *Arch Otolaryngol Head Neck Surg* 1988;114:267–277
38. Hidalgo DA. Fibula free flap: a new method of mandible reconstruction. *Plast Reconstr Surg* 1989;84:71–79
39. Daniel RK. Mandibular reconstruction with free tissue transfers. *Ann Plast Surg* 1978;1:346–371
40. Swartz WM, Banis JC, Newton ED, Ramasastry SS, Jones NF, Acland R. The osteocutaneous scapular flap for mandibular and maxillary reconstruction. *Plast Reconstr Surg* 1986;77:530–545
41. Moscoso JF, Keller J, Genden E, et al. Vascularized bone flaps in oromandibular reconstruction. A comparative anatomic study of bone stock from various donor sites to assess suitability for enosseous dental implants. *Arch Otolaryngol Head Neck Surg* 1994;120: 36–43
42. Urken ML, Buchbinder D, Weinberg H, et al. Functional evaluation following microvascular oromandibular reconstruction of the oral cancer patient: a comparative study of reconstructed and nonreconstructed patients [see comments]. *Laryngoscope* 1991;101:935–950
43. Lawson W, Baek S, Loscalzo L, et al. Experience with immediate and delayed mandibular reconstruction. *Laryngoscope* 1988;92:5–10
44. Duncan MJ, Manktelow RT, Zuker RM, Rosen IB. Mandibular reconstruction in the radiated patient: the role of osteocutaneous free tissue transfers. *Plast Reconstr Surg* 1985;76:829–840
45. Urken ML. Composite free flaps in oromandibular reconstruction. Review of the literature. *Arch Otolaryngol Head Neck Surg* 1991;117:724–732
46. Urken ML, Buchbinder D, Weinberg H, Vickery C, Lawson W, Biller HF. The internal oblique–iliac crest free flap in composite defects of the oral cavity involving bone, skin, and mucosa. *Laryngoscope* 1991;101:257–270
47. Moscoso JF, Urken ML. The iliac crest composite flap for oromandibular reconstruction. *Otolaryngol Clin North Am* 1994; 27:1097–1117
48. Urken ML, Buchbinder D, Costantino PD, et al. Oromandibular reconstruction using microvascular composite flaps: report of 210 cases. *Arch Otolaryngol Head Neck Surg* 1998;124:46–55

49. Wilson KM, Rizk NM, Armstrong SL, Gluckman JL. Effects of hemimandibulectomy on quality of life. *Laryngoscope* 1998; 108:1574–1577
50. Basteiro J, Aki FE, Ferreira MC, et al. Free flap reconstruction of tumors involving the cranial base. *Microsurgery* 1994;15:9–13
51. Urken ML, Turk JB, Weinberg H, Vickery C, Biller HF. The rectus abdominis free flap in head and neck reconstruction [comment]. *Arch Otolaryngol Head Neck Surg* 1991;117:1031
52. Izquierdo R, Leonetti JP, Origitano TC, al-Mefty O, Anderson DE, Reichman OH. Refinements using free-tissue transfer for complex cranial base reconstruction. *Plast Reconstr Surg* 1993;92:567–574; discussion 575
53. Neligan PC, Mulholland S, Irish J, et al. Flap selection in cranial base reconstruction. *Plast Reconstr Surg* 1996;98:1159–1166; discussion 1167–1168
54. Clayman GL, DeMonte F, Jaffe DM, et al. Outcome and complications of extended cranial-base resection requiring microvascular free-tissue transfer. *Arch Otolaryngol Head Neck Surg* 1995;121: 1253–1257
55. Rubin L. *Reanimation of the Paralyzed Face.* St. Louis: CV Mosby; 1977
56. Aviv JE, Urken ML. Management of the paralyzed face with microneurovascular free muscle transfer. *Arch Otolaryngol Head Neck Surg* 1992;118:909–912
57. Urken ML. The restoration or preservation of sensation in the oral cavity following ablative surgery. *Arch Otolaryngol Head Neck Surg* 1995;121:607–612
58. Urken ML, Weinberg H, Vickery C, Biller HF. The neurofasciocutaneous radial forearm flap in head and neck reconstruction: a preliminary report. *Laryngoscope* 1990;100(pt 1): 161–173
59. Urken ML, Weinberg H, Buchbinder D, et al. Microvascular free flaps in head and neck reconstruction. Report of 200 cases and review of complications. *Arch Otolaryngol Head Neck Surg* 1994;120: 633–640
60. Deschler DG, Doherty ET, Reed CG, Anthony JP, Singer MI. Tracheoesophageal voice following tubed free radial forearm flap reconstruction of the neopharynx. *Ann Otol Rhinol Laryngol* 1994;103:929–936
61. Blackwell KE, Buchbinder D, Urken ML. Lateral mandibular reconstruction using soft-tissue free flaps and plates. *Arch Otolaryngol Head Neck Surg* 1996;122:672–678

The Role of Free Flaps in Head and Neck Reconstruction

CHAPTER 14

John I. Song and Eugene N. Myers

The goals of head and neck reconstruction have been to ensure primary wound healing and to maximize functional restoration while minimizing patient morbidity. During the past two decades, the use of modern microvascular free-tissue transfer has revolutionized the reconstruction of large defects in the head and neck. By enabling reliable one-stage reconstruction, microvascular free-tissue transfer has expanded the limits to which extirpative techniques can reasonably be applied in the head and neck.[1] Although, in expert hands, the success of these free flaps is greater than 95% with low morbidity,[2-13] questions regarding their suitability in older patients,[14-18] as well as their cost-effectiveness[19,20] and superiority over conventional techniques,[21-28] continue to be raised.

At the Department of Otolaryngology, University of Pittsburgh School of Medicine, we have amassed extensive experience with the use of microvascular free-flap reconstructions of deficits in the head and neck. Our published experience of more than 300 free flaps was one of the largest in the English literature with a greater than 90% success rate and described the factors responsible for the success of free flaps in our institution.[2] Some of the keys to the consistent success of free flaps in our experience have been appropriate patient selection, choosing the most appropriate flap for each defect, meticulous preoperative and postoperative management, and a close working relationship between the oncologic and reconstructive surgical teams. Although we do not use free flaps in all cases, microvascular free-tissue transfer, when used appropriately, represents the most reliable, cost-effective, and functional state-of-the-art technique for reconstruction of defects in the head and neck.

Flap Selection in the Head and Neck

Distinguishing between patients whose defects can be reconstructed by more conventional techniques and those who would benefit from free-tissue transfer is critical in achieving a successful outcome. Such factors as the size and location of the defect, its complexity, and compromised wound situations attributable to preoperative radiation therapy and infection may predispose to the use of free flaps.[1] For example, we now consider free flaps the most reliable technique for reconstruction of the mandible and full circumferential pharyngeal defects. It is the technique of choice in our department. In other cases, when selecting a method of reconstruction, we give careful consideration to preoperative functional status and to the patient's expectations. For some patients, the use of skin grafts and regional muscle pedicle flaps continues to play an important role in reconstruction of defects in the head and neck. In each case, success depends on understanding the functional and cosmetic aspects of the defect that will be created and selecting the flap most appropriate for the given site in the head and neck.

ORAL CAVITY

Successful reconstruction in the oral cavity is measured by the ability to restore speech, swallowing, and airway function.[29] The ultimate functional outcome is generally influenced more by the volume of soft tissue loss and its reconstruction than by the reconstruction of the mandible.[30] The surface of the oral cavity and oropharynx consists of thin, pliable, sensate, lubricated tissue; it should be replaced by similar tissue whenever possible. Bulky tissue is needed only in the area of the base of tongue, where it aids in the oral phase of swallowing.[30] The anterior and lateral regions of the floor of mouth are vitally important because of their effect on tongue mobility and in maintaining salivary flow. Studies indicate that as the percentage of oral tongue and base of tongue resected increased, the efficiency of swallowing decreased.[31]

Split-thickness skin grafts are well suited for the reconstruction of defects in the oral cavity and oropharynx unless the resection involves extensive areas of the base of the tongue or mandible. In a recent study of relatively limited resections of the oral tongue (< 30%) and base of the tongue (< 60%), patients in whom primary closure or skin grafting was used had more efficient swallowing of liquids, less pharyngeal residue, and shorter pharyngeal delay times than were noted in similarly matched patients whose reconstruction involved a free flap.[31] In our department, split-thickness skin grafting is the technique most often used for reconstructing surgical defects of the tongue, floor of mouth, and buccal and oropharyngeal defects, as well as for re-creating the alveolar sulcus.

For larger defects in the oral cavity, our preferred alternative is the radial forearm flap. This flap is thin and pliable enough to be used in the oral cavity. The radial artery and its venae comitantes are relatively straightforward to harvest and, as the arm is out of the field, the reconstructive team can harvest the flap simultaneously with the resection. Bulky flaps such as the pectoralis myocutaneous (PMC) flap often interfere with mobility of the tongue and flow of saliva, and reliability is variable. In a study of 211 patients who underwent immediate reconstruction with a PMC flap, 63% developed flap-related complications and 26% required reoperation.[24] In contrast, the radial forearm flap has had a greater than 90% success rate when used at our department and at other institutions.[2-6] Donor site morbidity with the radial forearm flap consists mainly of partial loss of the skin graft with exposure of the flexor carpi radialis tendon, numbness in the distribution of the radial nerve, and dissatisfaction with the appearance of the skin graft.[11] The radial forearm has become the most frequently used flap for reconstruction of the oral cavity at our institution despite these problems.

MANDIBLE

The goals of mandibular reconstruction are to reconstitute the mandibular arch and to allow for dental restoration. The bone available with pedicled flaps, such as the trapezius or scapular spine, is inadequate for dental implantation; moreover, nonvascularized bone heals by slow substitution of bone stock and is not suitable for patients who will need radiation within 6 weeks of surgery.[29] For lateral mandible defects that do not involve the symphysis, the criterion for reconstruction with bone remains unclear. Provided that good mobility of the tongue is present, most patients can swallow effectively after segmental resection, even with mandibular drift and malocclusion. In these patients, an expedient option entails either no reconstruction of the mandible or a reconstruction plate covered with a radial forearm flap to stabilize the mandible.[2,29] Using this technique, exposure of the plate has been noted in 5% of patients with lateral and posterior defects. In anterior defects, the exposure rate increases to 20%, probably due to the resection of the depressor muscles of the mandible, which permit unopposed retraction of the plate superiorly through the flap.[33]

Patients with more extensive resection of the mandible, particularly the anterior segment, must undergo reconstruction in order to restore contour, swallow effectively, and avoid the problems of salivary incontinence. Several flaps have been described for mandibular reconstruction; in our experience, the fibular osteocutaneous flap and the radial forearm osteocutaneous flap have advantages over the iliac crest and scapular flap.[2] The radial forearm osteocutaneous flap has a more reliable skin paddle than the fibular osteocutaneous flap, but only 30% of the radius can be harvested for bone, and osseointegrated implants are not possible, owing to a lack of adequate bone stock. The radial flap is an excellent choice for straight segmental resections of the posterior body of the mandible and for lateral defects requiring only one osteotomy to reconstruct the posterior body and inferior portion of the ascending ramus.[2] It is our flap of choice where soft tissue sacrifice in the retromolar trigone, tonsillar fossa, lateral floor of mouth, and hypopharyngeal areas requires reconstruction and bone replacement is desired. The fibular osteocutaneous flap offers up to 25 cm of bone of sufficient height and is specifically indicated for reconstruction of anterior defects, for large defects from parasymphysis to ascending ramus, and for patients requiring eventual osseointegration.[29] The major drawback of this flap is the questionable reliability of the overlying skin paddle, which depends on small perforating branches lying in the septum between the peroneal and soleus muscles. The flap has been modified to include a cuff of soleus muscle to improve the reliability of the skin paddle. The major advantage of using free microvascular bone flaps for oral cavity reconstruction is that the chances for bone healing and tolerating radiation therapy are far better than with conventional bone grafts.

PHARYNX AND CERVICAL ESOPHAGUS

Reconstruction of circumferential defects of the pharynx and esophagus has been revolutionized through the use of free flaps. As in other defects of the head and neck, the extent and location of the defect will determine the need for free flap reconstruction. Small defects of the pharynx that spare the larynx can be closed primarily if adequate mucosa is saved. Some defects in the lateral pharyngeal wall may be closed with a pectoralis flap, but swallowing is generally compromised. Defects of the posterior pharyngeal wall usually require a radial forearm or a split jejunal flap, which are not too bulky for closure.[30] When the entire circumference of the pharynx and esophagus is resected, the defect is best repaired using a gastric pull-up or free flap to prevent stricture and fistula formation. For circumferential defects below the thoracic inlet, a gastric pull-up is indicated because of the potential for a distal anastomotic leak into the mediastinum if a free flap is used. Contraindications to a gastric pull-up include severe pulmonary disease (because the procedure requires traversing the mediastinum) and hepatobiliary disease. The mortality from gastric pull-up procedures remains significant at 8 to 12%.[30]

An absolute indication for the use of a free flap includes circumferential defects that extend more superiorly into the nasopharynx. We prefer either the free jejunum or radial forearm flap for defects above the thoracic inlet. The free jejunal transfer has the advantage of almost unlimited length for reconstruction; because mucosal tissue is sutured to mucosal tissue, the problem of anastomotic stricture is reduced. In our department, free jejunal transfer has an overall success of 95%, with successful swallowing achieved in 88% of patients with an average interval until swallowing of 10.6 days.[1] The most common complication has been fistula formation, which has occurred in 15% of patients;[1] however, most of the fistulae healed spontaneously. The mortality rate after a free jejunal transfer is about 5%, which is considerably less than that for a gastric pull-up procedure.[30] A consideration in using this flap is that, unlike patients who successfully undergo reconstruction with a gastric pull-up, the large lumen of the jejunal segment may not allow sufficient air for neo-esophageal speech.[29] We have routinely performed a tracheoesophageal puncture (TEP) in our jejunal flaps, which has resulted in remarkably good quality of speech despite these concerns. Another consideration is the increased morbidity with laparotomy in obese or elderly patients or in patients who have undergone previous abdominal surgery. In these cases, a fasciocutaneous flap such as a radial forearm or lateral thigh flap should be considered. We prefer the tubed radial forearm flap, as ≤ 20 cm can be harvested with minimal morbidity. Disadvantages of this flap include the presence of hair-bearing skin and a higher incidence of fistula formation than is associated with the jejunal flap, presumably due to the additional longitudinal suture line required to tube the flap. Although the radial forearm flap obviates the need for a laparotomy in medically compromised patients, the jejunal graft remains the gold standard for defects of extensive length.

MIDFACE

Most maxillectomy defects can be managed conventionally without the use of free flaps. A split-thickness skin graft and palatal obturator are adequate to maintain coverage and contour of the midface; functionally restore mastication, speech, and swallowing; and allow for detection of recurrent tumor. However, when not enough palate remains to support a prosthesis, autologous tissue is needed for reconstruction. In these patients, we prefer the use of the pedicled temporalis flap for reconstructing total palatal defects. The advantages of the temporalis include immediate restoration of oral-nasal separation and fast healing; however, the flap does not permit placement of dentures or an obturator and thus limits dental rehabilitation. We have not found swallowing to be significantly affected in these patients. Indications for free flaps in this area include full-thickness defects of the midface, which require complex three-dimensional volume and multi-surface coverage requirements. Although a pedicled flap such as the pectoralis myocutaneous (PMC) may be used in the midface, it is limited in its superior extent and arc of rotation by its pedicle. The combined effect of the pedicle and weight of the PMC can place tension at the suture line, resulting in dehiscence. The large muscle bulk can cross functional areas interfering with mastication, speech, and swallowing. For these reasons, we do not favor the use of pedicled flaps in the midface unless the patient is not a candidate for free-flap reconstruction.

Many different flaps, including the radial forearm, rectus abdominis, scapular, and latissimus dorsi, can be used with multiple skin paddles designed to reconstruct the palate and external skin defect.[29] We prefer the subscapular system for reconstruction, as it provides multiple flaps that can be tailored independently and inset in a three-dimensional manner. The ribs or lateral edge of the scapula provide vascularized bone.[30] The thicker edge of the scapula is an ideal buttress for the infraorbital rim, zygomaticomaxillary buttress, and alveolar ridge; the thin portion is useful for the orbital floor or orbit.[29] For obliterating the paranasal sinus cavity, we prefer the latissimus dorsi or serratus anterior muscles, which can be harvested with other components of the subscapular system with a common vascular pedicle. These muscle flaps can then be rolled to provide multiple skin paddles for lining the intraoral and external skin defects and to provide adequate contour to the midface.

CRANIAL BASE

The goal in reconstructing the cranial base is reliable separation of saliva from the meninges and neurovascular structures. Because of the aggressive nature of many tumors of the cranial base, arguments have been made to delay reconstruction until permanent sections have confirmed tumor clearance and to cover the defects temporarily with a skin graft, to facilitate detection of recurrence.[34] Although these are real concerns, in most instances, exposed vessels or tenuous dural closures mandate immediate flap coverage. Multiple frozen sections are used in our department in order to secure microscopically clear margins. Magnetic resonance imaging scans are used to detect recurrence under the flap. Local flap options (e.g., temporalis flap, galeal, and pericranial flaps) and regional flaps (e.g., pectoralis major, sternocleidomastoid muscle, or latissimus dorsi flaps) are usually sufficient for most small to moderate cranial base defects. In extensive resections, however, the pericranial and temporalis flaps may be devascularized, and a regional flap may be limited by its arc of rotation. The temporalis muscle flap is also less reliable in its ability to cover medial and posterior cranial base defects.[1]

The rectus abdominis flap has been the free flap used most frequently in our department for cranial base defects. The flap can be harvested simultaneously with the resection, saving operative time. It has a long and large-diameter vascular pedicle and a large muscle volume that can be transferred with or without varying amounts of skin and vascularized fat to accommodate most defects.[29] The latissimus dorsi can be used as a free flap in this area, but the patient must be repositioned so that the flap can be harvested simultaneously with the resection. The serratus anterior flap can also be used, but it is a smaller muscle flap than the latissimus dorsi, with all its disadvantages. Other flaps include the omentum which is soft and pliable with a long vascular pedicle; and there is no functional defect secondary to flap harvest.[34] Although we have no personal experience with omentum, the main disadvantages are said to include the need for intra-abdominal surgery, the possibility for peritoneal bleeding, and respiratory compromise secondary to abdominal pain.[34]

Whether to reconstruct the bony cranial base remains a controversial issue. Proponents argue that reconstruction with bone is especially important in the anterior cranial base, in order to prevent herniation of cranial contents. Opponents state that the absence of bony reconstruction causes minimal if any herniation of the brain, reduces the risks of infection of the bone fragments, and gives a better chance for skin grafts to take.[35] In one study of 16 cranial base resections without reconstruction of the bone, only one herniation occurred through an absent orbital roof in a patient who had five previous surgeries and previous radiation therapy.[36] The authors concluded that, in their experience, the presence of a defects in the bony cranial base did not predispose to an increased risk of complications. Our own experience supports these findings, as we have not seen any increased complications or herniations in those patients in whom the bony cranial base has not been reestablished. As long as adequate separation of the intradural and extradural spaces can be accomplished by local, regional, or free flaps, we do not recommend additional bony reconstruction for the cranial base.

Other Considerations in the Use of Free Flaps

ELDERLY PATIENTS

A common criticism of free flap reconstruction is that the techniques are complex and time consuming, and some clinicians are reluctant to subject elderly patients to free flap reconstruction for fear of a higher potential complication rate attributable to prolonged anesthesia. Many studies in recent years have shown no relationship between age and increased complication rates in patients undergoing free flap reconstruction.[14-18] A study completed at our institution did not find significant differences in major surgical and medical complications in patients <50 and >50 years of age undergoing free flap reconstruction. The overall flap survival was 99%, and the authors concluded that advanced chronologic age alone does not play a significant role in surgical outcome and should not preclude free tissue transfer.[14] A similar study by Urken et al., in patients older than 70 years of age undergoing free flap reconstruction did not find any differences in complications rates when stratified for premorbid factors including age; overall flap survival was 94% in this group.[15] This is not to state that all free flaps in older patients are without risk; chronologic age, however, is not as important as biologic or physiologic age, as determined by the American Society of Anesthesiologists (ASA) classification of physical status, in predicting the risk of postoperative morbidity and mortality.[14-16]

The risk of major medical complications is highest for those patients judged to be ASA classes 3 or 4, with bronchopulmonary and cardiovascular events predominating.[14,15,18] Postoperative pulmonary complications increased with age for all patients with head and neck cancer.[37] Aging is associated with decreased vital capacity and increased alveolar–arterial oxygen gradient; compounding this is the decreased ability of head and neck cancer patients to protect the airway due to tumor or extirpative surgery.[7,15] A history of smoking was found to be the most significant risk factor for the development of postoperative pulmonary complications in the head and neck surgery patient: the relative risk was calculated as 24 times the risk for nonsmokers with risk increasing 3.6 times with each division of increased smoking history.[7] The age of the patient, as it relates to the physiologic changes of the bronchopulmonary system and length of smoking, does appear to increase the risk of postoperative pulmonary complications. These facts, rather than precluding older patients from free flap reconstruction, should encourage strict protocols that minimize risks and maximize flap survival. At our institution, for all elderly patients scheduled for flap surgery, an electrocardiogram, chest radiograph, pulmonary function test, and hematologic and biochemical tests are performed and an ASA grade assigned. We have a dedicated expert in anesthesia as a member of our team managing head and neck patients. Invasive monitoring, careful intraoperative fluid management, and measures to ensure a warm, vasodilated patient are other key ingredients for flap success. Postoperatively, meticulous fluid and electrolyte balance, aggressive pulmonary toilet, and vigilant monitoring of the flap in special care units ensure against avoidable complications.

COST-EFFECTIVENESS

In our current cost-conscious medical environment, many have questioned whether complex surgical procedures such as free flaps would be supported in an era in which the cost of care plays a major role in determining patient treatment.[20] Some investigators have pointed to the added operative time for free flaps, equating longer operative times with added postoperative complications. On the contrary, many studies have not supported this assumption.[2-9] Comparative studies actually demonstrate lower postoperative complication rates in free flaps relative to pedicled flaps.[4,5,21] In one study, the rate of fistula formation was significantly lower in the free flap group versus the pedicled flap group (4% vs 21%)[19]; overall surgical intensive care unit and hospital stay were shorter in the free flap group, resulting in a net reduction in the consumption of hospital resources.[19] Another study found the mean resource cost associated with PMC flaps to be $48,917 versus $37,314 for free flaps despite the fact the free flap group had higher initial costs due to longer operative times.[20] Complications such as wound infection, oropharyngeal fistula, and partial flap necrosis are all more common in patients reconstructed with a pedicle flap.[20] These complications lead to longer hospitalization and higher ultimate costs for these patients. By choosing free flaps and initially investing more time and money, major wound complications are avoided, hospital stays shortened, and resource consumption reduced, making free flaps more cost-effective in the long-term.[19]

PRIOR RADIOTHERAPY

Radiotherapy and chemoradiotherapy are increasingly used in the treatment of locally advanced head and neck cancer in an attempt to preserve organ function or to control persistent or recurrent disease. Previous radiotherapy can cause thickening and perivascular fibrosis in the irradiated field. The vascular changes induced by radiation include transmural fibrosis, formation of microthrombi, atheromatous plaque deposition, and endarteritis obliterans.[38-40] Because of these changes, irradiated vessels can have lower flow rates than nonirradiated vessels of similar diameter and may be more susceptible to spasm. These findings have led some investigators to conclude that irradiated vessels are not well suited for microvascular surgery. Despite these changes, studies have not shown detrimental effects of previous irradiation on anastomotic patency rates or postoperative free flap complications.[38,40-42]

In a study of 42 patients undergoing free flap reconstruction, Kiener et al.[41] noted no differences in total flap loss or major complications between groups of previously irradiated and nonirradiated patients. A larger study by Bengtson et al.[42] of 354 free flap patients also showed no differences in total flap loss (5.3% vs 5%), partial flap loss, or major wound complications (16% vs 11%) between previously irradiated and nonirradiated patients. The overall complication rates of free flaps in this study were still significantly less than for PMC flap reconstruction in similarly irradiated fields (16% vs 35%).[43] Unlike regional flaps, free flaps, with their independent blood supply, do not have any limitations on the amount of well-vascularized tissue that can be brought into an irradiated area.

These and other studies confirm our own experience that previous radiation in and of itself does not increase failure rates of free flaps and should not be a contraindication to reconstruction with a free flap. Our approach has been to perform anastomoses into the largest available vessels (usually the external carotid and internal jugular vein) which have the greatest flow and are least prone to spasms, thus minimizing the effects of radiation on flap survival. Meticulous technique in performing the anastomosis is even more important in the irradiated field as our experience confirms the finding of others that any acute intraoperative complications (thrombosis, kinking, length discrepancy) requiring revision significantly increases flap failure.[42]

NECK DISSECTION

Vessel thrombosis rates for head and neck free flaps are lower than for any other anatomic site due to in part to the abundance of accessible recipient vessels.[2] However, potential recipient vessels, such as the external and internal jugular veins and their tributaries, may be sacrificed in an extensive neck dissection or may be damaged due to radiation or inflammatory changes. In these cases, local veins of small caliber can be used, but the risk of thrombosis is increased. We prefer to use the undamaged contralateral veins if ipsilateral veins are not available, by using an interpositional vein graft. A cephalic vein can be readily harvested either by itself or in conjunction with the pedicle if a radial forearm flap is being used. A theoretical disadvantage of an interpositional vein graft is the increased risk of thrombosis due to two anastomoses, but we have not found this to be a significant problem. Alternatively, a cephalic vein transposition whereby the vein is harvested as distally as possible and transposed to the head and neck with its proximal origin at the subclavian vessels left intact has been described.[44] Although we have not had experience with this technique, there are several reported advantages to this technique: (1) only one anastomosis is needed, (2) the cephalic-subclavian system is a relatively high flow system, (3) the vein is usually outside the surgical and radiation fields, and (4) the pedicle is long enough to reach the midface or contralateral neck without tension.[44]

Even in cases of modified radical neck dissections (MRND), in which the internal jugular system is spared, the incidence of thrombosis of the internal jugular vein has been reported to range between 15% and 33%.[45] The presence of salivary fistula, abscess, or wound dehiscence in the vicinity of the internal jugular can increase the rate of thrombosis of the internal jugular vein to 29.6%.[46] Although oncologic considerations are paramount in our therapeutic and prophylactic neck dissection, we advocate surgical techniques that will optimize the patency of the internal jugular system, which include: (1) ligation of side branches far enough from the vein to prevent constriction, (2) avoiding the use of an electrocautery, (3) avoiding desiccation of the vein once it has been dissected, and (4) atraumatic manipulation of the vein.[42]

Future Directions

The development of free flap reconstruction for the head and neck began with skepticism regarding the safety and reproducibility of transferring tissue to the head and neck. We are now in a second phase in which questions regarding the true value of these techniques in changing the quality of a patient's life are being raised.[5] The future success of free flaps seems secure as we gain greater understanding of the pathophysiology of small vessel thrombosis, improvements in instrumentation, and utilization of flaps with longer vascular pedicles. We must continue to ensure that the high level of flap success continues as the techniques become more popular and widely disseminated. Increasingly, otolaryngologists are being exposed to microvascular techniques at both the residency and fellowship levels. One study identified 27 fellowships per year offering some microvascular training within the field of otolaryngology-head and neck surgery.[47] Close cooperation between head and neck cancer surgeons, microvascular head and neck surgeons, and plastic and reconstructive surgeons is imperative as we move into the second era of free flap evolution. Future studies in this field need to consider cosmetic, functional, and quality-of-life outcomes as more meaningful interpretations of free flap reconstruction, rather than flap survival alone.[47] There are relatively few objective reports in this area, especially in head- and neck-specific quality-of-life measures for free flap reconstruction. As we become more capable of extirpating larger tumor volumes and more sophisticated in our reconstructive techniques, we must not lose sight of the impact of these procedures on the lives of our patients.

REFERENCES

1. Shestak KC, Myers EN, Ramasastry SS, et al. Vascularized free-tissue transfer in head and neck surgery. *Am J Otolaryngol* 1993;14:148–154
2. Jones NF, Johnson JT, Shestak KC, et al. Microsurgical reconstruction of the head and neck: interdisciplinary collaboration between head and neck surgeons and plastic surgeons in 305 cases. *Ann Plast Surg* 1996;36:37–43
3. Schusterman MA, Horndeski G. Analysis of the morbidity associated with immediate microvascular reconstruction in head and neck cancer patients. *Head Neck* 1991;13: 51–55
4. Qattan MM, Boyd BJ. Complications in head and neck microsurgery. *Microsurgery* 1993;14:187–195
5. Urken ML, Weinberg H, Buchbinder D, et al. Microvascular free flaps in head and neck reconstruction. *Arch Otolaryngol Head Neck Surg* 1994;120:633–640
6. Truelson JM, Leach JL, Close LG. Reliability of microvascular free flaps in head and neck reconstruction. *Otolaryngol Head Neck* 1994;111:557–559
7. McCulloch TM, Jensen NF, Girod DA, et al. Risk factors for pulmonary complications in the postoperative head and neck surgery patient. *Head Neck* 1997;19:372–377

8. Brown MT, Cheney ML, Gliklich RL, et al. Assessment of functional morbidity in the radial forearm free flap donor site. *Arch Otolaryngol Head Neck Surg* 1996;122:991–994
9. Mahoney J. Complications of free flap donor sites. *Microsurgery* 1995;16:437–444
10. Haughey BH, Frederickson JM. The latissimus dorsi donor site. *Arch Otolaryngol Head Neck Surg* 1991;117:1129–1134
11. Swanson E, Boyd JB, Manktelow RT. The radial forearm flap: reconstructive applications and donor-site defects in 35 consecutive patients. *Plast Reconstr Surg* 1990;85:258–266
12. Schusterman MA, Miller MJ, Reece GP, et al. A single center's experience with 308 free flaps for repair of head and neck cancer defects. *Plast Reconstr Surg* 1994;93:472–478
13. Clayman GL, DeMonte F, Jaffe DM, et al. Outcome and complications of extended cranial-base resection requiring microvascular free-tissue transfer. *Arch Otolaryngol Head Neck Surg* 1995;121:1253–1257
14. Shestak KC, Jones NF, Wu W, et al. Effect of advanced age and medical disease on the outcome of microvascular reconstruction for head and neck defects. *Head Neck* 1992;14:14–18
15. Shaari CM, Buchbinder D, Costantino PD, et al. Complications of microvascular head and neck surgery in the elderly. *Arch Otolaryngol Head Neck Surg* 1998;124:407–411
16. Bridger AG, O'Brien CJ, Lee KK. Advanced patient age should not preclude the use of free-flap reconstruction for head and neck cancer. *Am J Surg* 1994;168:425–428
17. Peters GE, Grotting JC. Free-flap reconstruction of large head and neck defects in the elderly. *Microsurgery* 1989;10:325–328
18. Malata CM, Cooter RD, Batchelor AGG, et al. Microvascular free-tissue transfer in elderly patients: the Leeds experience. *Plast Reconstr Surg* 1996;98:1234–1241
19. Brown MR, McCulloch TM, Funk GF, et al. Resource utilization and patient morbidity in head and neck reconstruction. *Laryngoscope* 1997;107:1028–1031
20. Kroll SS, Evans GR, Goldberg D. A comparison of resource costs for head and neck reconstruction with free and pectoralis major flaps. *Plast Reconstr Surg* 1997;99:1282–1286
21. Kroll SS, Reece GP, Miller MJ, et al. Comparison of the rectus abdominis free flap with the pectoralis major myocutaneous flap for reconstructions in the head and neck. *Am J Surg* 1992;164:615–618
22. Righi PD, Weisberger EC, Slakes SR, et al. The pectoralis major myofascial flap: clinical applications in head and neck reconstruction. *Am J Otolaryngol* 1998;19:96–101
23. Keidan RD, Kusiak JF. Complications following reconstruction with the pectoralis major myocutaneous flap: the effect of prior radiation therapy. *Laryngoscope* 1992;102:521–524
24. Shah JP, Haribhakti V, Loree TR, et al. Complications of the pectoralis myocutaneous flap in head and neck reconstruction. *Am J Surg* 1990;160:352–355
25. Fabian RL. Pectoralis major myocutaneous flap reconstruction of the laryngopharynx and cervical esophagus. *Laryngoscope* 1988;98:1227–1231
26. Zbar RI, Funk GF, McCulloch TM, et al. Pectoralis major myocutaneous flap: a valuable tool in contemporary head and neck reconstruction. *Head Neck* 1997;19:412–418
27. Ord RA. The pectoralis major myocutaneous flap in oral and maxillofacial reconstruction: a retrospective analysis of 50 cases. *J Oral Maxillofac Surg* 1996;54:1292–1295
28. Shaha A. A long term follow-up of pectoralis osteomyocutaneous flaps. *J Surg Oncol* 1992:49:49–51
29. Rassekh CH. Free flap options for common head and neck defects. *Facial Plast Surg* 1996:12:97–100
30. Jones TR, Jones NF. Advances in reconstruction of the upper aerodigestive tract and cranial base with free tissue transfer. *Clin Plast Surg* 1992;19:819–831
31. McConnel FMS, Pauloski BR, Logemann JA, et al. Functional results of primary closure vs flaps in oropharyngeal reconstruction. *Arch Otolaryngol Head Neck Surg* 1998;124:625–630
32. Martin PJ, O'Leary MJ, Hayden RE. Free tissue transfer in oromandibular reconstruction: necessity or extravagance? *Otolaryngol Clin North Am* 1994;27:1141–1150
33. Wells MD, Edwards AL, Luce EA. Intraoral reconstructive techniques. *Clin Plast Surg* 1995;22:91–108
34. Thomson JG, Restifo RJ. Microsurgery for cranial base tumors. *Clin Plast Surg* 1995;22:563–572
35. Schramm V, Myers E, Maroon J. Anterior skull base surgery for benign and malignant disease. *Laryngoscope* 1979;89: 1077–1091
36. Spirelli HM, Irizarry D, McCarthy JG. An analysis of extradural dead space after fronto-orbital surgery. *Plast Reconstr Surg* 1994;93:1372–1377
37. McGuirt WF, Davis SP. Demographic portrayal and outcome analysis of head and neck cancer surgery in the elderly. *Arch Otolaryngol Head Neck Surg* 1995;121:150–154
38. Fried MP. The effects of radiation therapy in microvascular anastomosis. *Laryngoscope* 1985;37(suppl):1–33
39. Cunningham BL, Shons AR. Free tissue transfer in rats using an irradiated recipient site. *Br J Plast Surg* 1979;32:137–140
40. DeWilde RL, Donders G. Scanning electron micrographic study of microvascular anastomoses on irradiated vessels: long-term effects of radiation. *Microsurgery* 1986;7:156–157
41. Kiener JL, Hoffman WY, Mathes SJ. Influence of prior radiotherapy on microvascular reconstruction in the head and neck region. *Am J Surg* 1991;162:404–407
42. Bengtson BP, Schusterman MA, Baldwin BJ, et al. Influence of prior radiotherapy on the development of postoperative complications and success of free tissue transfer in head and neck cancer reconstruction. *Am J Surg* 1993;166:326–330
43. Keidan RD, Kusiak JF. Complications following reconstruction with the pectoralis myocutaneous flap: the effect of prior radiation therapy. *Laryngoscope* 1992;102:521–524
44. Kim KA, Chandrasekhar BS. Cephalic vein in salvage microsurgical reconstruction in the head and neck. *Br J Plast Surg* 1998;51:2–7
45. Brown DH, Mulholland S, Yoo JHH, et al. Internal jugular vein thrombosis following modified neck dissection: implications for head and neck reconstruction. *Head Neck* 1998;20:169–174
46. Leontsinis TG, Currie AR, Mannell A. Internal jugular vein thrombosis following functional neck dissection. *Laryngoscope* 1995;105:169–173
47. Blackwell KE, Brown MR, Gonzalez D. Overcoming the learning curve in microvascular head and neck reconstruction. *Arch Otolaryngol Head Neck Surg* 1997;123:1332–1335

The Role of Free Flaps in Head and Neck Reconstruction

CHAPTER 15

David E. Schuller, L. Arick Forrest, and Amit Agrawal

Since the publication of the first successful transfer of a free flap for oral cavity reconstruction by Panje et al.,[1] the use of microvascular surgery for tissue transfer to reconstruct defects within the head and neck has flourished. The initial reports primarily involved discussions of the feasibility and reliability of this highly specialized tissue transferring technique.[2-4] Other publications included descriptions of the type of reconstructions that could be successfully accomplished with free flap transfer.[5-8]

The objectives of any reconstructive technique are to preserve function and reestablish form. The refinements of head and neck reconstructive techniques over the past 20 years have enhanced the ability of the otolaryngologist–head and neck surgeon to achieve these goals in many cases, but there continue to be times when both cannot be achieved. When a variety of techniques are available that are reported to achieve the same goal, there is the potential for confusion and controversy as to which is the most appropriate technique. That is certainly the case with the array of tissue transfer approaches that are currently available to contemporary otolaryngologist–head and neck surgeons involved in facial reconstruction. This book deals with controversies, as well as a discussion of the topic of the role of free flaps in head and neck reconstruction within that theme.

It is the goal of this chapter to identify those issues that are relevant to the controversies concerning the role of free flaps in head and neck surgery, in an effort to help the reader identify the issues. Thus, decisions about utilization can be made in an objective fashion based on factual information. The chapter includes discussions of the advantages and disadvantages of free flaps and identifies issues that continue to be unresolved about the use of this technique. The use of free flaps for a variety of reconstructive tasks is also discussed.

Advantages

Microvascular surgery provides the capability of reestablishing blood flow to a variety of tissues transferred into the head and neck from distant sites, so that reconstruction can be completed in one operation. This is in contrast to other tissue-transferring techniques, such as regional flaps, which often require a second operation to detach the pedicle of the tissue used in reconstruction. The only regional flap that provides for immediate one-stage transfer of tissue into the defect comparable to free flap techniques are the musculocutaneous flaps. But free flaps oftentimes provide greater versatility than the regional flaps, including the musculocutaneous flaps, because the thickness of the tissue can be controlled by the selection of a particular free flap. A free flap can be thick, such as the musculocutaneous rectus abdominis free flap, or it can be quite thin, such as the fasciocutaneous radial forearm free flap. This ability to select the thickness of tissue represents a unique advantage for the free flaps.

Free flaps also provide an opportunity to transfer a variety of types of tissue into the head and neck. Depending on the selection of free flap, it is possible to transfer skin and subcutaneous tissue as a single entity, as well as muscle, fascia, bone, and even nerve–muscle combinations to achieve goals of reanimation. This flexibility to transfer a combination of different types of tissue facilitates surgical creativity to tailor precisely the reconstruction to the defect by replacing the type of tissue that has been destroyed by cancer or trauma. It therefore provides an enhanced ability to achieve the objectives of restoration of form and preservation of function that is superior to alternative reconstructive techniques.

Disadvantages

As with any technique, there are disadvantages. One of the primary disadvantages of microvascular surgery is that it continues to be a technically challenging technique that requires expertise and experience. There is no debate about this issue, and it is clear that continuing surgical experience elevates the expertise and success rate. It is doubtful that the surgeon who occasionally performs microvascular surgery can achieve the proficiency of one who regularly makes use of these techniques. There is also no question that the surgeon who regularly performs tissue transfer techniques with the regional flaps also improves proficiency and success, although this is probably less impacted by frequency of utilization with the pedicled musculocutaneous flaps than it is for microvascular surgery.

Although not totally established, many would state that free flaps add operative time compared with some of the alternative tissue-transferring techniques.[9] In addition, most free flap transfers are performed by a second operative team which is not necessary for reconstructions involving regional flaps.

Another potential disadvantage is that free flaps are often dependent on donor vessels that are within the field of treatment, whether that be surgery or radiation therapy. Both therapeutic modalities, whether performed before, during, or after the free flap transfer, have the potential to have an adverse impact on the flap's success or failure. Once again, this is in distinction to the regional flaps that are not reliant on donor vessels within the treated area. Free flaps are also limited more than the regional flaps by the patient's comorbid conditions. Any health problems that can affect the blood vessels have to be viewed as a concern and possibly a contraindication for the use of microvascular surgery. Therefore, conditions such as diabetes mellitus or atherosclerosis, or both, can become relative, or even absolute contraindications to free flap transfer. The presence of such conditions, however, is not a contraindication to the use of regional flaps.

Another potential disadvantage is the reality that the failure of a free flap oftentimes results in total loss of the tissue that has been transferred. Once again, this differs from the regional flaps where partial failure can occur which does not always result in the need for another operation to transfer tissue.

Unfortunately, many of the advantages and disadvantages cited are based on opinions from experienced reconstructive surgeons, rather than facts. As a result, there continues to be a wide array of unresolved issues regarding which reconstructive technique is most appropriate for a given situation.

Unresolved Issues

A variety of tissue transferring techniques are available for head and neck reconstruction, including skin grafts, regional skin flaps, acellular dermal graft (Alloderm, Lifecell Corporation, The Woodlands, TX),[10] musculocutaneous flaps, and free flaps. All these techniques have been published in the literature. However, a major issue remains unresolved: which reconstructive technique represents the optimal approach for a particular defect or deformity.

The critically important first step in resolving such a controversy is to agree on the goals of reconstruction. The traditional goals are restoration of form and preservation of function. However, contemporary dynamics in health care in the United States require that other goals be included. Reconstructions of defects created with ablation of advanced-stage malignancies really need to be completed at the time of the resection, rather than with a technique that requires multiple stages. The primary reason is that patients with advanced-stage lesions are now part of multimodal therapeutic protocols that require administration of adjuvant therapy within a specific time period, for optimal impact on disease erradication. Therefore, those tissue-transferring techniques that are capable of completing the reconstruction in one stage certainly are preferred.

Many issues affect the overall cost of the reconstructive procedure achieved in the most cost-effective fashion—a clear goal. The assumption is that microvascular surgery can be more costly because it adds operative time and is usually undertaken with two separate surgical teams. However, the added cost associated with these two factors could be offset by the claims of some that length of stay is shorter with free flaps because of the presumed decreased incidence of fistulization or other wound-healing problems associated with regional flaps. Although some investigators have looked into the issue of cost, comparing hospitalization costs associated with free flap reconstruction with the costs associated with regional flaps,[11,12] an accurate total cost of care for patients undergoing different reconstructive techniques remains to be calculated. The cost of rehabilitation is also an issue that can impact this consideration.

In addition to the cost of two surgical teams, when free flaps are used, it is a labor-intensive undertaking that creates a component of inefficiency of time—when one surgical team is not doing the entire procedure, this inefficiency adds indirectly to the cost of the reconstruction.

A variety of unresolved issues also remain with regard to the advantages for a variety of reconstructive approaches. Although this issue is discussed in greater detail in a subsequent section, suffice it to say that it remains to be established unequivocally whether (1) pharyngeal reconstruction using sensate free flaps actually improves swallowing function, (2) free flap mandibular reconstruction is truly something other than cosmetic surgery, or (3) reinnervated muscle free flaps translate into superior approaches to achieving the goals of reconstruction.

The literature, although it does contain some information, is somewhat compromised in resolving these issues because publications have been predominantly single-institution uncontrolled reports. Although some publications seemingly address these issues,[9,12] current study designs are still open for criticism. The "gold standard" of a prospective randomized multi-institutional trial has not been undertaken to help resolve some of these issues regarding the superior reconstructive technique for a particular reconstructive task when assessed by virtue of its ability to restore form and function in a cost-effective manner.

As experience with these techniques continues to expand, it appears that the potential for conducting well-controlled randomized trials has diminished as a result of surgeons developing a bias based on their personal experience with a particular reconstructive approach. This bias interferes with objectivity and subsequent willingness to participate in a randomized study that creates potential to use a reconstructive technique not favored by the particular surgeon.

However, it appears that the increasing trend to practice evidence-based medicine will create pressure from third-party payors to develop outcomes studies that address these issues so that payors can make rational decisions about the appropriateness of certain techniques based on fact rather than opinion. These unresolved issues exist for the full spectrum of the reconstructive tasks encountered by the otolaryngologist–head and neck surgeon.

Reconstructive Tasks

ORAL CAVITY AND OROPHARYNX

Reconstruction of soft tissue defects involving mucosa and underlying musculature within the oral cavity and oropharynx can be completed with skin grafts, acellular dermal grafts, musculocutaneous flaps, or free flaps in one stage. The literature documents the efficacy of skin grafts for these reconstructions.[13-15] Some investigators are hesitant to rely on a thin skin graft as a barrier to saliva drainage into the tissues of the neck of an incompletely healed wound. This hesitance forces the surgeon to decide between the appropriateness of the musculocutaneous flap or free flap. Both can be used effectively. There are those who claim that the bulk of the musculocutaneous flaps can be a deterrent to successful reconstruction. However, the literature has demonstrated that the oral cavity and oropharynx can be functionally restored with the musculocutaneous flaps.[16-18] There is certainly information that suggests that the transfer of sensate free flaps can potentially enhance swallowing function.[19-22] However, this matter is a classic example of an unresolved issue.

We tend to favor musculocutaneous flaps for partial oral cavity and oropharyngeal reconstructions as one-stage reconstructions that achieve the ability to restore function in a cost-effective fashion. There are certainly times when free flaps appear to be clinically advantageous. Because they are not tethered by a pedicle, free microvascular musculocutaneous flaps have a theoretical advantage in larger tongue defects in maintaining mobility. Free flaps also avoid donor site morbidity associated with musculocutaneous flaps, such as the pectoralis major flap, which may be a concern among female patients.

HYPOPHARYNX

Reconstruction of the hypopharynx introduces another variable that influences the selection of the optimal reconstructive technique because of the proximity to the larynx. Once again, the musculocutaneous or free flaps are frequently used for these reconstructions. Partial hypopharyngeal reconstructions can be effectively achieved in a one-stage fashion with either musculocutaneous flaps or free flaps that have the ability to restore function.[23-26] We usually prefer musculocutaneous flaps because of the high success rate and shorter operative time as compared with the free flaps.

PARTIAL DEFECTS OF THE LARYNGOPHARYNX

The musculocutaneous and free flaps are also effective techniques for organ function-preserving surgery in cases of partial defects of the laryngopharynx. In this example, these techniques appear to have enhanced the patient's quality of life. No longer is it necessary to perform a total laryngectomy in these patients, as reconstruction of a partial laryngopharyngeal defect is not feasible with maintenance of function. Reports in the literature support the use of both the musculocutaneous flaps[27] as well as free flaps[28,29] for this defect.

TOTAL DEFECTS OF THE HYPOPHARYNX AND CERVICAL ESOPHAGUS

Reconstruction of total defects involving the hypopharynx and cervical esophagus is an example of free flaps that have proved clearly advantageous over other approaches. Regional skin flaps can be used for total pharyngocervical esophageal defects. However, they require multiple stages to complete and are subject to compromise of the functional results as a result of a high incidence of stenoses at the distal anastomosis of the remaining esophagus to the flap. The use of musculocutaneous flaps offers the potential to complete this reconstruction in one stage. However, past experience demonstrates that the frequency of a successful reconstruction is still unsatisfactory using the musculocutaneous flaps.[23,24] Free flaps provide the opportunity for transferring a thin piece of vascularized tissue that reestablishes the continuity of the conduit and seemingly has a lower incidence of stenosis at the distal junction. This enables restoration of swallowing function and the potential for vocal rehabilitation with creation of a tracheoesophageal fistula and insertion of a voice prosthesis.

However, which free flap provides superior results remains somewhat controversial. Jejunal segment free flaps have been described in the literature as an effective reconstructive approach.[30,31] Apparent disadvantages to jejunal free flaps are their association with increased morbidity because other body cavities (i.e, the abdomen) are entered, and they require yet another surgical team to harvest the flap. Jejunal segments also do not undergo neovascularization from the surrounding tissues, and, accordingly, subsequent operations that are performed in the area of the vascular pedicle for recurrent cancer or other problems can put the total viability of the jejunal segment in jeopardy. In addition, it is unusual to achieve voicing with tracheoesophageal speech in those patients who have undergone reconstruction of the pharyngoesophagus with jejunal segment. As a result, radial forearm free flaps have emerged as a popular approach to this reconstructive task and provide a highly vascular reliable flap that appears to have a high rate of successful restoration of swallowing and speaking function.[25,32,33]

MANDIBULAR RECONSTRUCTION

Mandibular reconstruction is another area in which the free flaps provide enhanced capabilities versus alternative reconstructive techniques. A vascularized osseous, osseocutaneous, or osseomyocutaneous free flap has a distinct advantage in primary reconstruction of mandibular defects. The free flaps have a higher rate of success compared with nonvascularized bone grafts in primary reconstruction. Mandibular plate reconstruction without bone is always an option. We prefer to use plates for lateral defects. Anterior defects and larger defects are associated with a higher rate of complications, and vascularized flaps are favored in this setting.[34]

Mandibular reconstruction has been and continues to be one of the major challenges facing the otolaryngologist–head and neck surgeon. A variety of free flaps have been described for mandibular reconstruction. The most popular include transfer of portions of the scapula, iliac crest, and fibula.[35-39] Fibular free flaps have emerged as the most common technique. This technique has minimal donor site morbidity, and the bone provides the rigidity necessary to maintain soft tissue in the appropriate position. Any type of vascularized bone free flap transfer also provides the opportunity for either primary or secondary insertion of osseointegrated implants that enable denture application. There is conflicting information about whether these types of mandibular reconstruction dramatically restore chewing function of a normal mandible.[40-42] It may be that mandibular reconstruction with free flaps may provide more of a cosmetic than a functional benefit.

FACIAL REANIMATION

Facial reanimation is another reconstructive challenge where there is cautious optimism about the use of microvascular surgery for the transfer of nerve–muscle units that are neurologically connected to crossover nerve grafts with the ultimate goal of reestablishing movement in the paralyzed face. An advantage of providing viable motor end plates and a vascularized donor nerve is the restoration of facial movement in patients with longstanding paralysis. This type of work is being done for the rehabilitation of facial paralysis that cannot be resolved with the other reanimation techniques.[43,44] The results are still far from ideal.

There are those who have described using free flaps for the closure of cranial base defects.[45-47] However, we have rarely found it necessary to use free flaps for this particular reconstructive task.[48] Regional pericranial flaps coupled with calvarial bone grafts and skin grafts appear to be sufficient to seal the intracranial cavity in a one-stage procedure in the majority of instances. In specialized instances, free flaps are used when a cranial base defect is coupled with a large facial bony and soft tissue defect created by the resection of a large malignancy.

Conclusion

Over the past 25 years, free flap reconstruction using microvascular surgery has been demonstrated to be both feasible and efficacious for a variety of reconstructive challenges in head and neck surgery. In some reconstructive tasks, this approach is clearly superior, but it has potential disadvantages that sometimes can be addressed more effectively with alternative reconstructive techniques. There is a need for objective well-designed outcomes studies to help decide which reconstructive techniques best achieve the goals of restoration of form and preservation of function. Their feasibility has been clearly established. It is now time to identify more clearly the clinical settings in which a particular reconstructive approach is preferred.

REFERENCES

Schuller et al.—CHAPTER 15

1. Panje WR, Bardach J, Krause CJ. Reconstruction of the oral cavity with a free flap. *Plast Reconstr Surg* 1976;58:415–418
2. Serafin D, Rios AV, Georgiade N. Fourteen free groin flap transfers. *Plast Reconstr Surg* 1976;57:707–715
3. Zuker RM, Manktelow RT, Palmer JA, et al. Head and neck reconstruction following resection of carcinoma, using microvascular free flaps. *Surgery* 1980;88:461–466
4. Schlenker JD, Robson MC, Parsons RW. Methods and results of reconstruction with free flaps following resection of squamous cell carcinoma of the head and neck. *Ann Plast Surg* 1981;6:362–373
5. Nagahara K, Hirose A, Iwai H. Laryngeal reconstruction by free flap transfer. *Plast Reconstr Surg* 1976;57:604–610
6. Daniel RK. Mandibular reconstruction with free tissue transfers. *Ann Plast Surg* 1978;1:346–371
7. Panje WR, Krause CJ, Bardach J, et al. Reconstruction of intraoral defects with the free groin flap. *Arch Otolaryngol* 1977;103:78–83
8. Soutar DS, Scheker LR, Tanner NS, et al. The radial forearm flap: a versatile method for intra-oral reconstruction. *Br J Plast Surg* 1983;36:1–8
9. Brown MR, McCulloch TM, Funk GF, et al. Resource utilization and patient morbidity in head and neck reconstruction. *Laryngoscope* 1997;107:1028–1031
10. Rhee PH, Friedman CD, Ridge JA, et al. The use of processed allograft dermal matrix for intraoral resurfacing. *Arch Otolaryngol Head Neck Surg* 1998;124:1201–1204
11. Kroll SS, Evans GR, Goldberg D, et al. A comparison of resource costs for head and neck reconstruction with free and pectoralis major flaps. *Plast Reconstr Surg* 1997;99:1282–1286
12. Tsue TT, Desyatnikova SS, Deleyiannis FW, et al. Comparison of cost and function in reconstruction of the posterior oral cavity and oropharynx. Free vs pedicled soft tissue transfer. *Arch Otolaryngol Head Neck Surg* 1997;123:731–737
13. McConnel FM, Teichgraeber JF, Adler RK. A comparison of three methods of oral reconstruction. *Arch Otolaryngol Head Neck Surg* 1987;113:496–500
14. Schramm VL Jr, Johnson JT, Myers EN. Skin grafts and flaps in oral cavity reconstruction. *Arch Otolaryngol* 1983;109:175–177
15. Zieske LA, Johnson JT, Myers EN, et al. Composite resection reconstruction: split-thickness skin graft—a preferred option. *Otolaryngol Head Neck Surg* 1988;98:170–173
16. Stein DW, Schuller DE. Advantages of pectoralis musculocutaneous flap pharyngeal reconstruction. *Laryngoscope* 1989;99:691–696
17. Baek S, Lawson W, Biller HF. An analysis of 133 pectoralis major myocutaneous flaps. *Plast Reconstr Surg* 1982; 69:460–469

18. Krespi YP, Sisson GA. Reconstruction after total or subtotal glossectomy. *Am J Surg* 1983;146:488–492
19. Urken ML. The restoration or preservation of sensation in the oral cavity following ablative surgery. *Arch Otolaryngol Head Neck Surg* 1995;121:607–612
20. Urken ML, Biller HF. A new bilobed design for the sensate radial forearm flap to preserve tongue mobility following significant glossectomy. *Arch Otolaryngol Head Neck Surg* 1994; 120:26–31
21. Urken ML, Weinberg H, Vickery C, et al. The combined sensate radial forearm and iliac crest free flaps for reconstruction of significant glossectomy-mandibulectomy defects. *Laryngoscope* 1992;102:543–558
22. Civantos FJ Jr., Burkey B, Lu FL, et al. Lateral arm microvascular flap in head and neck reconstruction. *Arch Otolaryngol Head Neck Surg* 1997;123:830–836
23. Schuller DE. Reconstructive options for pharyngeal and/or cervical esophageal defects. *Arch Otolaryngol* 1985;111: 193–197
24. Schuller DE. Pectoralis myocutaneous flap in head and neck cancer reconstruction. *Arch Otolaryngol* 1983;109:185–189
25. Urken ML, Weinberg H, Buchbinder D, et al. Microvascular free flaps in head and neck reconstruction: report of 200 cases and review of complications. *Arch Otolaryngol Head Neck Surg* 1994;120:633–640
26. Kelly KE, Anthony JP, Singer M. Pharyngoesophageal reconstruction using the radial forearm fasciocutaneous free flap: preliminary results. *Otolaryngol Head Neck Surg* 1994; 111:16–24
27. Schuller DE, Mountain RE, Nicholson RE, et al. One-stage reconstruction of partial laryngopharyngeal defects. *Laryngoscope* 1997;107:247–253
28. Urken ML, Blackwell K, Biller HF. Reconstruction of the laryngopharynx after hemicricoid/hemithyroid cartilage resection. Preliminary functional results. *Arch Otolaryngol Head Neck Surg* 1997;123:1213–1222
29. Chantrain G, Deraemaecker R, Andry G, et al. Wide vertical hemipharyngolaryngectomy with immediate glottic and pharyngeal reconstruction using a radial forearm free flap: preliminary results. *Laryngoscope* 1991;101:869
30. Gluckman JL, McDonough J, Donegan JO, et al. The free jejunal graft in head and neck reconstruction. *Laryngoscope* 1981;91:1887–1895
31. Coleman JJ III, Searles JM Jr, Hester TR, et al. Ten years experience with free jejunal autograft. *Am J Surg* 1987; 154: 394–398
32. Harii K, Ebihara S, Ono I, et al. Pharyngoesophageal reconstruction using a fabricated forearm free flap. *Plast Reconstr Surg* 1985;75:463–476
33. Hussain A, Dolph JL, Padilla JF III, et al. Tubed, folded radial forearm free flap for pharyngeal reconstruction and voice rehabilitation. *Ann Plast Surg* 1993;30:541–544
34. Nicholson RE, Schuller DE, Forrest LA. Factors involved in long- and short-term mandibular plate exposure. *Arch Otolaryngol Head Neck Surg* 1997;123:217–222
35. Sullivan MJ, Baker SR, Crompton R, et al. Free scapular osteocutaneous flap for mandibular reconstruction. *Arch Otolaryngol Head Neck Surg* 1989;115:1334–1340
36. Urken ML, Buchbinder D, Costantino PD, et al. Oromandibular reconstruction using microvascular composite flaps: report of 210 cases. *Arch Otolaryngol Head Neck Surg* 1998;124:46–55
37. Urken ML. Composite free flaps in oromandibular reconstruction: review of the literature. *Arch Otolaryngol Head Neck Surg* 1991;117:724
38. Moscoso JF, Urken ML. The iliac crest composite flap for oromandibular reconstruction. *Otolaryngol Clin North Am* 1994;27:1097–1117
39. Hidalgo DA. Fibula free flap mandibular reconstruction. *Clin Plast Surg* 1994;21:25–35
40. Komisar A. The functional result of mandibular reconstruction. *Laryngoscope* 1990;100:364–374
41. Curtis DA, Plesh O, Miller AJ, et al. A comparison of masticatory function in patients with or without reconstruction of the mandible. *Head Neck* 1997;19:287–296
42. Urken ML, Buchbinder D, Weinberg H, et al. Functional evaluation following microvascular oromandibular reconstruction of the oral cancer patient: a comparative study of reconstructed and nonreconstructed patients. *Laryngoscope* 1991;101:935–950
43. Harii K. Microneurovascular free muscle transplantation. In: Rubin L, ed. *The Paralyzed Face*. Philadelphia: Mosby–Yearbook; 1991:178–200
44. Aviv JE, Urken ML. Management of the paralyzed face with microneurovascular free muscle transfer. *Arch Otolaryngol Head Neck Surg* 1992;118:909–912
45. Jones NF, Sekhar LN, Schramm VL. Free rectus abdominal muscle flap reconstruction of the middle and posterior cranial base. *Plast Reconstr Surg* 1986;78:471
46. Urken ML, Catalano PJ, Post K, et al. Free tissue transfer for skull base reconstruction: analysis of complications and a classification scheme for defining skull base defects. *Arch Otolaryngol Head Neck Surg* 1993;117:1318
47. Funk GF, Laurenzo JF, Valentino J, et al. Free-tissue transfer reconstruction of midfacial and cranio-orbito-facial defects. *Arch Otolaryngol Head Neck Surg* 1995;121:293–303
48. Schuller DE, Goodman JH, Miller CA. Reconstruction of the skull base. *Laryngoscope* 1984;94:1359

6

Outcomes in Sinus Surgery—Management Parameters

"Meticulous post-operative debridement and medical therapy are the best manner in which to achieve a successful objective and subjective outcome in the long-term. However, the cost-effectiveness of such a management strategy has never been demonstrated. Intuitively, avoidance of revision surgery with its associated costs and risks would seem advantageous."

David W. Kennedy

"By correcting the anatomic abnormalities and providing improved ventilation and drainage of the paranasal sinuses, the effects of mucosal edema, obstruction, and subsequent infection can be minimized. In turn, this provides for a cured or significantly improved patient."

Charles W. Gross

"Measurement demonstrates the relative burden of disease and the efficacy of therapy. By including cost as an outcome and understanding the relationship between health status and cost, economic models can be developed to demonstrate the relative value of procedures on the overall cost of chronic disease."

Richard E. Glicklich

Outcomes in Sinus Surgery—Management Parameters

CHAPTER 16

David W. Kennedy and Erin D. Wright

Since the mid-1980s, there has been an enormous improvement both in our understanding of rhinosinusitis and in our ability to manage patients with this disorder. According to the emerging theories, there is general agreement that chronic rhinosinusitis is a disorder in which there is a tendency toward hyperreactivity, whether associated with chronic infection, atopy, ASA (Salycilate) intolerance, or idiopathic. More recent hypotheses also propose a role for underlying osteitis in the perpetuation of the chronic inflammatory process. The management of these patients is multifaceted and includes medication, specific allergy treatment, and endoscopic sinus surgery. Thus, chronic rhinosinusitis can be said to be a medical disease in which surgery plays a therapeutic role. Consequently, close postoperative follow-up is an integral part of the management of this disorder. What has been repeatedly demonstrated in recent years is that there is often a discrepancy between the subjective symptoms experienced by patients and their objective endoscopic findings.[1,2] The controversy that remains is to evaluate whether the subjective or objective outcomes are more important and/or relevant from a prognostic perspective. Obviously, from the patient's point of view, and from the standpoint of third-party carriers, what may be most important is the short- to medium-term symptomatic relief. However, we have demonstrated that this does not correspond to long-term disease resolution or freedom from the potential for recurrent surgery. In a 7.8-year follow-up of surgical patients, we demonstrated that endoscopic resolution of disease by 1.5 years postoperatively correlated with subsequent avoidance of further surgical intervention.[1] Indeed, no patients whose cavity was normal or almost normal endoscopically at 1.5 years required further surgical intervention during the subsequent period.

Evaluation Scales and Staging Systems

Several evaluation scales currently exist for patients with chronic rhinosinusitis.[3] For subjective evaluation there are general health status instruments, such as the Medical Outcomes Study Short Form-36 (SF-36), as well as disease-specific instruments such as the Chronic Sinusitis Survey (CSS), the Rhinosinusitis Outcome Measure (RSOM-31)/Sinonasal Outcome Test (SNOT-20), and the Rhinosinusitis Disability Index (RSDI). A recently released comprehensive tool for the subjective evaluation of chronic rhinosinusitis is the Chronic Sinusitis TyPE Specific Questionnaire, published by the Health Outcomes Institute.

Objective staging systems for rhinosinusitis also exist. Although an ideal and widely accepted staging scale remains elusive, two staging systems have achieved reasonable acceptance and utility. Kennedy's[1] detailed analysis of a patient cohort permitted the proposal of a rational staging system that incorporated surgical findings and radiological appearance and this system has been shown to be predictive of outcome. The more recently proposed Lund–MacKay[4,5] system also uses radiologic findings as its primary determinant and was recently recommended by the Rhinosinusitis Task Force[6] for validation in large clinical studies because of its ease of use and high degree of inter- and intra-observer agreement.

Subjective Outcomes Measures

The SF-36 is a general health status instrument that permits the evaluation of a patient's overall response to treatment.[7] It provides information concerning the functional well-being of the individual and may serve to evaluate not only the response to treatment, but also the need for subsequent intervention through medical or surgical means. The limiting factor of general health status measures is that they do not provide specific evaluation of the disease in question.

Disease-specific health measurement tools are available as well. The CSS, developed at the Massachusetts Eye and Ear Infirmary, is duration-based and monitors both symptoms and need for medical therapy over an 8-week period.[8] Studies have demonstrated that the CSS is statistically reliable and is sensitive to clinical change over time. The CSS has been used as a research tool to evaluate the outcomes of sinus surgery on quality of life and seems like a reasonable candidate to use in the evaluation and management of patients with chronic rhinosinusitis.[9] This clinical use remains to be formally evaluated and the potential shortcomings for the CSS include a limited range of symptoms and psychometric data.

The RSOM-31 includes components that address health status and quality-of-life measures.[10] It permits the evaluation of both the magnitude of a symptom and its importance to the patient. In this sense, the RSOM-31 is perhaps a more sensitive instrument. The RSOM-31 has undergone modifications since its original publication and now exists in its newest incarnation as the SNOT-20. The more cumbersome RSOM-31 has been reduced by 11 items and the SNOT-20 is easier and faster to complete. With respect to the responsiveness to therapeutic intervention, the RSOM-31 has been shown to be sensitive; however, the responsiveness of the SNOT-20 remains to be determined, and this would clearly be required before its use in a clinical or research setting.

The RSDI is a unique disease-specific outcome measure in that it evaluates the self-perceived impact of chronic rhinosinusitis in a first-person descriptive format.[11] It is unclear whether this format is more helpful in gathering useful clinical or research data but this measurement tool has been tested and found reliable and valid.

Another recently released tool for outcomes assessment is the Chronic Sinusitis TyPE (Technology of Patient Experience) Specification form, which has been used in recent outcomes studies.[12] This instrument has three forms, the first of which provides an initial evaluation of the patient and previous interventions, if any. The third component is a post-treatment survey. This TyPE Specific Questionnaire is publicly available and has been recommended by the Rhinosinusitis Task Force for thorough evaluation.

In terms of clinical value in the management of patients with chronic rhinosinusitis, the CSS and TyPE (third component) appear to be simple to use and provide temporal information regarding the efficacy of treatment. The Post-Treatment Survey portion of the Chronic Sinusitis Form (TyPE Specification) is similar to the CSS in that both examine symptoms and requirement of medication over an 8-week period. After statistical and clinical validation in a controlled fashion, these forms appear to provide the best potential for usefulness as management parameters.

Objective Outcome Measures and Staging Systems

In an effort to objectify the severity of chronic rhinosinusitis and the response to medical therapy, numerous staging systems have been proposed. Theoretically, a uniform reporting scheme and a uniformly accepted staging system would improve scientific and accurate communication between otolaryngologists. Such a staging system might also permit the subsequent re-staging of patients after therapeutic intervention and thus become a management tool. To date, however, such a staging system has remained elusive.

Early attempts to devise such objective staging systems incorporated measures of disease severity (e.g., localized vs diffuse disease) combined with the presence or absence of related factors (e.g., asthma, allergy, polyposis).[13,14] Extensions and refinements of these techniques have been proposed more recently. The first significant step forward was made by Kennedy[1] in 1992 and, more recently, the Lund–MacKay staging system was endorsed by the Rhinosinusitis Task Force for future outcomes research.[3]

Kennedy's close follow-up and data collection of a patient cohort was the first to emphasize the importance of objective endoscopic follow-up after surgery. Kennedy pointed out that early recurrent disease is often detectable objectively on nasal endoscopy before the development of subjective symptoms. This provided the opportunity to treat such recurrent disease, either medically or with surgical debridement, at an early stage, when it is more manageable.

With respect to outcome measures and prognostic factors, Kennedy's study identified extent of disease as the primary predictor. Other seemingly related and important factors such as asthma, allergies, and ASA sensitivity, when severity of disease was factored in, were not independently related to outcome and prognosis. However, in stage IV disease (diffuse sinonasal polyposis), asthma did worsen the prognosis. The primary assessment of extent of disease was made using radiographic and intraoperative data, and similar evaluations were used when the initial staging system was proposed.

TABLE 16–1
Staging for Chronic Rhinosinusitis (Kennedy)

Stage	Description
I	Anatomic abnormalities All unilateral sinus disease Bilateral disease limited to ethmoid sinuses
II	Bilateral ethmoid disease with involvement of one dependent sinus
III	Bilateral ethmoid disease with involvement of two or more dependent sinuses on each side
IV	Diffuse sinonasal polyposis

SOURCE: Adapted from Kennedy DW. Prognostic factors, outcomes and staging in ethmoid sinus surgery. *Laryngoscope* 1992;102(suppl):1–18

The staging system proposed by Kennedy stratified patients into 4 categories of increasing severity (Table 16–1). Based on the preliminary study performed by Kennedy, this staging system was demonstrated to have strong prognostic and predictive value. This permits patient comparisons independent of other miscellaneous factors.

A modified Lund–MacKay staging system has been recommended by the Rhinosinusitis Task Force for use in outcomes research. This system was originally based on a numeric score derived from computed tomography (CT) scan analysis. The Task Force recommended the addition of demographic data, description of the presence of anatomic variants, as well as a surgery score, a symptom score, and the endoscopic appearance (Tables 16–2 to 16–7). The endoscopic appearance, which appears to have significant postoperative prognostic importance, is not formally included in the staging system, but its recording is recommended.

It is becoming apparent that objective evaluations incorporating relevant comorbid conditions, extent of radiologic and operative disease, and the endoscopic response to therapeutic intervention are objective measurement parameters that have prognostic value. These prognostic indicators will likely be demonstrated in the future to impact on and influence the management of chronic rhinosinusitis, including the decision for additional medical or surgical intervention.

Long-Term Outcomes—Management Issues

Until very recently, there were no long-term follow-up data regarding outcomes in endoscopic sinus surgery. Although short-term follow-up evaluation has demonstrated excellent subjective results, several studies have shown that this symptomatic

TABLE 16–2
Radiologic Staging of Chronic Rhinosinusitis (Lund–MacKay)*

Sinus	Left	Right
Maxillary		
Anterior ethmoid		
Posterior ethmoid		
Sphenoid		
Frontal		
Ostiomeatal complex		
Total for each side:		

* Scoring: Sinuses: 0 = no abnormalities; 1 = partial opacification; 2 = total opacification.
OMC: 0 = not occluded; 2 = occluded.
SOURCE: Adapted from Lund VJ, MacKay IS. Staging in rhinosinusitis. *Rhinology* 1993;107:183–184.

TABLE 16–3
Demographic Information (Rhinosinusitis Task Force)*

Last Name:	Operation:
First Name:	Date of Surgery:
Sex:	Surgeon:
Date of Birth:	Nasal Diagnosis (0-4):
Age:	Systemic Diagnosis:
Hospital Number:	Anesthetic Duration (min):
Postoperative Medications:	
Complications:	

* Nasal diagnosis: 1 = chronic rhinosinusitis; 2 = recurrent acute; 3 = nasal polyposis; 4 = miscellaneous.
SOURCE: Adapted from Lund VJ, Kennedy DW. Staging for rhinosinusitis. *Otolaryngol Head Neck Surg* 1997;117(suppl):S35–S40.

TABLE 16–4
Radiologic Grading: Anatomic Variants (Rhinosinusitis Task Force)*

Anatomic Variant	Left	Right
Absent frontal sinus		
Concha bullosa		
Paradoxic middle turbinate		
Everted uncinate process		
Haller cells		
Agger nasi cells		

* Scoring: 0 = no variant; 1 = variant present.
SOURCE: Adapted from Lund VJ, Kennedy DW. Staging for rhinosinusitis. *Otolaryngol Head Neck Surg* 1997;117(suppl):S35–S40.

TABLE 16–5
Surgery Score (Lund–Mackay/Rhinosinusitis Task Force)*

Surgical Procedure	Left	Right
Uncinectomy		
Middle meatal antrostomy		
Anterior ethmoidectomy		
Posterior ethmoidectomy		
Sphenoidectomy		
Frontal recess surgery		
Reduction of middle turbinate		
Total for each side		

* Scoring: 0 = no procedure; 1 = procedure done (range 1–14).
SOURCE: Adapted from Lund VJ, Kennedy DW. Staging for rhinosinusitis. *Otolaryngol Head Neck Surg* 1997;117(suppl):S35-S40.

TABLE 16–6
Symptom Score (Lund–MacKay/Rhinosinusitis Task Force)*

Symptom	Before Surgery	After Surgery			
		3 months	6 months	1 year	2 years
Nasal blockage/congestion					
Headache					
Facial pain					
Altered sense of smell					
Nasal discharge					
Sneezing					
Overall symptom					
Total points					

* Scoring: Visual analogic scale for each symptom (0–10): 0 = not present, 10 = most severe.
SOURCE: Adapted from Lund VJ, Kennedy DW. Staging for rhinosinusitis. *Otolaryngol Head Neck Surg* 1997;117(suppl):S35–S40.

TABLE 16–7

Endoscopic Appearance (Lund–MacKay/Rhinosinusitis Task Force)*

Characteristic	Baseline	3 months	6 months	1 year	2 years
Polyp, left					
Polyp, right					
Edema, left					
Edema, right					
Discharge, left					
Discharge, right					
Scarring, left[a]					
Scarring, right[a]					
Crusting, left[a]					
Crusting, right[a]					
Total points					

* Scoring: Polyps: 0 = absence of polyps; 1 = middle meatal polyps; 2 = beyond middle meatus. Edema/Scarring/Crusting: 0 = absent, 1 = mild, 2 = severe. Discharge: 0 = no discharge, 1 = clear, thin discharge, 2 = thick, purulent discharge.

[a] Postoperative scores to be used for outcomes assessment only.

SOURCE: Adapted from Lund VJ, Kennedy DW. Staging for rhinosinusitis. *Otolaryngol Head Neck Surg* 1997;117(suppl):S35–S40.

improvement does not necessarily correlate with objective endoscopic findings.[1,2] These findings have been corroborated by medium-term follow-up (18-month) studies.[1,14,15] The obvious extension of these conclusions is that without objective endoscopic evaluation, significant yet potentially reversible or treatable disease may not become apparent for years. Delayed detection of such recurrent disease might render it impossible to treat without revision surgery and its attendant risks.

Senior et al.[17] recently reported long-term follow-up over an average of 7.8 years and supplemented their endoscopic evaluation with CT scan data. Their aim was to determine whether patients with persistent endoscopic evidence of inflammation were more likely to have symptomatic recurrence and require surgical intervention. Overall they demonstrated that in their cohort of 72 patients who responded, 98.4% reported continued subjective improvement compared with preoperative symptoms. Consistent improvement in specific symptoms such as headache, nasal discharge, nasal congestion, recurrent infections, and asthma was noted. Medication usage was reduced, and only 18% of patients required revision surgery.

The conclusion drawn by Senior and colleagues was that excellent long-term subjective results could be obtained after endoscopic sinus surgery provided patients received appropriate postoperative care. Appropriate postoperative care was defined in this study as meticulous inspection and aggressive debridement and medical therapy. These investigators also validated the concept that patients whose cavities can be normalized on endoscopic inspection after surgery are much less likely to recur, obviating the need for revision surgery. Their data demonstrated a significant correlation between endoscopic persistence of disease at initial follow-up and the need for subsequent revision surgery.

Current Management Strategies

The results of the recent outcome studies discussed are providing increasingly compelling evidence that subjective improvement, particularly in the short to medium term (18 months), does not equate with disease resolution in chronic rhinosinusitis, hence is not predictive of a long-term successful outcome. The extension of this concept is that the most significant parameter for management of patients after sinus surgery is the objective endoscopic appearance during the healing period.

Subjective assessment of outcomes after treatment of chronic rhinosinusitis, however, has significant initial relevance. These assessments are of paramount importance to the patient. They are also important to the analysis of cost–benefit evaluations and quality-of-life issues, which are being increasingly scrutinized in modern health care. In the future, with refinements of measurement tools and with establishment of staging systems such as those seen in the CSS and the third portion of TyPE Specification (Fig. 16–1), subjective evaluations during the treatment course may assume a greater import with respect to management decisions. Subjective assessments are not as predictive or as useful, from a management perspective, as the available objective measures.

As the surgical techniques and available technology have improved over the past 15 years, there has been a trend toward mucosal preservation. It is now understood that the avoidance of mucosal stripping in the ethmoid cavity and in the frontal recess is critically important and can compromise the results of an otherwise well-performed surgery. Mucosal stripping and the resultant neo-osteogenesis and osteitis can make postoperative

Mode of Collection	
Self-Administered	1 ☐
Personal Interview	2 ☐
Telephone Interview	3 ☐
Mail	4 ☐
Other	5 ☐

OFFICE USE ONLY

DATE: MO DAY YR

PATIENT QUESTIONNAIRE

CHRONIC SINUSITIS FORM 12.3

Sanford R. Hoffman, M.D.
George W. Facer, M.D.
David W. Kennedy, M.D.
Eugene B. Kern, M.D.
Donald A. Leopold, M.D.
Dale H. Rice, M.D.
Steven D. Schaefer, M.D.

TyPE Specification
CHRONIC SINUSITIS 10/08/93-M394
©Health Outcomes Institute, 1993

CHRONIC SINUSITIS FORM 12.3

Post-Treatment Survey

1. During the past eight weelos, how often have you had: *(circle one number in each row)*

	Never	1	2	3	4	5	6	7
a. Sinus headaches, facial pain, or pressure	0	1	2	3	4	5	6	7
b. Significant postnasal drainage	0	1	2	3	4	5	6	7
c. Marked nasal congestion	0	1	2	3	4	5	6	7
d. The need to take sinus medications such as over-the-counter decongestants or antibiotics	0	1	2	3	4	5	6	7
e. Sinus infections	0	1	2	3	4	5	6	7
f. Breathing difficulties	0	1	2	3	4	5	6	7
g. Tooth pain	0	1	2	3	4	5	6	7

(Column heading: Number of times)

2. Who completed this form? *(circle one number)*

I filled it out with no help	1
I filled it out with help from family or friends	2
I filled it out with help from a health care provider	3
Family or friends	4
Health care provider	5

©Health Outcomes Institute, 10/08/93-M394
-2-

Figure 16–1 Third portion of Chronic Sinusitis Form 12.3 from TyPE Specification questionnaire. The Health Outcomes Institute has released this questionnaire for general and unrestricted use. Its primary use is for the short-term evaluation of a specific therapeutic intervention.

management more difficult and prolonged and may also result in a poor subjective and objective outcome. With newer through-cutting and powered instrumentation, mucosal preservation is now much more easily achieved and should be the goal of endoscopic sinus surgeons.

Areas in the healing sinus cavity that demonstrate polypoid swelling are often areas with persistent inflammation, frequently due to a reaction to underlying neo-osteogenesis or osteitis. Aggressive postoperative debridement of devitalized bone in such areas will frequently result in improved epithelialization of the sinus cavity. This is attributed to removal of the underlying source of the chronic inflammation. Postoperative inspection and debridement may also help avoid postobstructive fluid retention and inflammation.

Hand in hand with this aggressive postoperative debridement must come aggressive management of infection and inflammation. This most typically involves the use of prolonged antibiotic therapy and long-term topical corticosteroids, sometimes combined with a period of systemic steroids. The management decisions for the use of these medications are generally predicated on the endoscopic assessment and not upon subjective symptoms. Patients experiencing a protracted healing period with evidence of continued inflammation would remain on these medications for a longer period. Thus, each visit to the clinic will involve a nasal endoscopy that determines the treatment recommendations. The literature is accumulating to support the use of topical corticosteroids in the management of chronic rhinosinusitis. These medications form the backbone of management of this disease, both preoperatively and postoperatively.

Discharge of the patient from intensive postoperative follow-up occurs when the sinus cavity demonstrates a return to normal or near normal. A well-epithelialized cavity with patent sinus ostia and absence of mucosal edema or swelling constitutes a normal appearance. These patients will require relatively close surveillance to detect early exacerbations but, as outlined by Senior and colleagues, if they achieve a normal-appearing cavity at 18 months postintervention, they are likely to maintain their result and avoid additional surgery or significant recurrence.

When To Consider Revision Surgery

Based on the management scheme outlined, patients receive intensive follow-up after endoscopic sinus surgery for chronic rhinosinusitis. Such meticulous surveillance generally avoids significant recurrence. Patients who receive suboptimal follow-up, whether for logistical reasons or poor compliance, are more likely to develop bulky recurrence of their disease with neo-osteogenesis. This forms one group of patients who are more likely to require revision surgery. However, a significant number of such patients will be able to be managed nonsurgically with aggressive medical and debridement therapy as outlined.

A group of patients who are more likely to require revision surgery are those who have had incomplete surgery with residual bony partitions and bulky persistent or recurrent disease. Poor healing in strategic areas with attendant scarring (e.g., frontal recess, posterior ethmoid/sphenoid) or evidence of recirculation in an iatrogenic maxillary antrostomy that does not communicate with the natural ostium are other indications for revision surgery. Decisions with respect to revision surgery are again made significantly on objective grounds, having considered the radiographic and endoscopic appearance, as well as the subjective data.

Conclusion

Chronic rhinosinusitis is a complex multifactorial illness that is managed in a comprehensive fashion with the incorporation of surgical and medical therapy. Objective assessments are currently the primary factors in formulating management decisions. Instruments for subjective evaluation are available and are important with respect to outcomes research and quality-of-life issues. These instruments evaluate our success in managing this disease process but are not sensitive enough to use in the formulation of management decisions. Indeed, there is a clear dichotomy between subjective results and objective evidence of disease resolution. Disease-specific tools that incorporate temporal data and the requirement for medical therapy show promise and are worthy of further evaluation.

Short-term subjective outcomes in chronic rhinosinusitis are typically excellent. However, without meticulous and aggressive postoperative therapy based on objective endoscopic findings, these results appear doomed to failure. The best predictor of a good long-term outcome appears to be the ability to achieve a normally epithelialized sinus cavity at 18 months after surgery (medium-term). It also appears that, in order to minimize the possibility of revision surgery, intervention during the postoperative period (long-term or short-term), based on the objective endoscopic appearance, is indicated before the patient becomes symptomatic.

Future Directions

Meticulous postoperative debridement and medical therapy are the best manner in which to achieve a successful objective and subjective outcome in the long-term. However, the cost-effectiveness of such a management strategy has never been demonstrated. Intuitively, avoidance of revision surgery with its associated costs and risks would seem advantageous. However, aggressive postoperative follow-up and the use of prolonged systemic steroid therapy and antibiotics are not without risk and cost. It is our strong clinical impression that maintaining a patent cavity and minimizing inflammation and persistent/recurrent disease permit the inflammation and mucosal hyperreactivity to slowly resolve during the years after surgical intervention. Thus, these patients slowly continue to improve clinically and require fewer medications. However, this observation requires further longitudinal documentation. If not validated, it is possible that periodic revision surgery could be more cost-effective and appealing for patients with chronic rhinosinusitis. It is hoped that future studies will serve to resolve such issues.

REFERENCES

Kennedy and Wright—CHAPTER 16

1. Kennedy DW. Prognostic factors, outcomes and staging in ethmoid sinus surgery. *Laryngoscope* 1992;102(suppl):1–18
2. Vleming M, De Vries N. Endoscopic paranasal sinus surgery: results. *Am J Rhinol* 1990;4:13–17
3. Leopold D, Ferguson BJ, Piccirillo JF. Outcomes assessment. *Otolaryngol Head Neck Surg* 1997;117(suppl 3):S58–S68
4. Lund VJ, MacKay IS. Staging in rhinosinusitis. *Rhinology* 1993;107:183–184
5. Lund VJ, Kennedy DW. Quantification for staging sinusitis. In: Kennedy DW, ed. International conference on Sinus Disease: Terminology, Staging Therapy. *Ann Otorhinol Laryngol* 1995;104(suppl 167):17–21
6. Lund VJ, Kennedy DW. Staging for rhinosinusitis. *Otolaryngol Head Neck Surg* 1997;117(suppl 3):S35–S40
7. Ware JE, Sherbourne CD. The MOS 36 item short-form health survey (SF-36). I. Conceptual framework and item selection. *Med Care* 1992;30:473–483
8. Gliklich RE, Metson R. Techniques for outcomes research in chronic sinusitis. *Laryngoscope* 1995;105:387–390
9. Gliklich RE, Metson R. Effect of sinus surgery on quality of life. *Otolaryngol Head Neck Surg* 1997;117:12–17
10. Piccirillo JF, Edwards D, Haiduk A, et al. Psychometric and clinimetric validity of the 31-item rhinosinusitis outcome measure (RSOM-31). *Am J Rhinol* 1995;9:297–306
11. Benninger MS. The development of the rhinosinusitis disability index. *Arch Otolaryngol Head Neck Surg* 1997;123: 1175–1179
12. Hoffman SR, Mahoney MG, Chmiel JF, et al. Symptom relief after endoscopic sinus surgery: an outcomes-based study. *Ear Nose Throat J* 1993;72:413–414, 419–420
13. Lawson W. The intranasal ethmoidectomy: an experience with 1077 procedures. *Laryngoscope* 1991;101:367–371
14. Sogg A. Long-term results of ethmoid surgery. *Ann Otorhinol Laryngol* 1989;98:699–701
15. Rice D. Endoscopic sinus surgery: results at 2-year follow-up. *Otolaryngol Head Neck Surg* 1989;101:467–479
16. Levine H. Functional endoscopic sinus surgery: evaluation, surgery, and follow-up of 250 patients. *Laryngoscope* 1990; 100:79–84
17. Senior BA, Kennedy DW, Tanabodee J, et al. Long-term results of functional endoscopic sinus surgery. *Laryngoscope* 1998;108:151–157

Outcomes in Sinus Surgery—Management Parameters

Charles W. Gross and Scott E. Harrison

CHAPTER 17

Sinusitis affects approximately 35 million Americans. Nasal inflammation and sinus disease cause patient discomfort and loss of productivity and have a negative impact on the quality of life of those affected. The cost of treating this disease surpasses $2 billion per year.[1] Most people who experience sinus infections can be treated medically without entertaining surgical intervention. However, deciding which patients require surgical intervention can be difficult.

Most patients will respond to medical therapy. Adequate medical therapy may include the use of saline irrigation, topical and/or systemic decongestants, topical nasal steroids, systemic corticosteroids, mucolytic agents, appropriate antihistamine use, and the appropriate use of oral antibiotics for an appropriate treatment duration. The evaluation and treatment of systemic disease such as allergy (inhalant or food), immunodeficiency, cystic fibrosis, diabetes mellitus, and the evaluation of environmental factors (e.g., smoke, inhaled irritants, drug use) may increase the number of patients who will be successfully treated without surgery. It is not uncommon to treat a patient for 6 to 10 weeks before an infection resolves. Medical failures can often be traced to patient noncompliance, but if a compliant patient fails maximal therapy for 12 weeks or more, surgery should be considered.

The development and acceptance of functional endoscopic sinus surgery[2] have offered a variety of treatment options for patients who fail medical therapy and continue with debilitating sinus conditions. Functional endoscopic sinus surgery provides a method of excellent visualization that aids in the precise and meticulous eradication of paranasal sinus disease. Most patients receive surgery on an outpatient basis, have a minimal recovery time, and have excellent long-term results.[3,4]

The evaluation of a patient for sinus surgery begins with the assurance that all other treatment options have been used, and the patient continues with unrelenting disease. There are obvious cases for which sinus surgery is indicated, including unilateral nasal masses, invasive fungal disease, obstruction with nasal polyps, and complications such as subperiosteal, orbital, or intracranial extension of infection. Patients who are immunocompromised and have sinusitis should be considered eligible for surgery at a much earlier point, as they tend to respond poorly to medical management and have an increased propensity to develop orbital or intracranial complications. These patients comprise a minority of surgical candidates; the usual candidate requires a more careful evaluation. In addition, many patients undergoing sinus surgery will require ongoing treatment for underlying systemic or recalcitrant disease.

The decision to operate must be based on clear historical, clinical, and radiographic evidence. If the patient is a child, the decision becomes even more complicated. The major anatomic differences between adult and pediatric paranasal sinuses are smaller sinus size and lesser degree of pneumatization. In evaluating a child who is considered a possible candidate for sinus surgery, an immature but still developing immune system, the role of tonsils and adenoids, and other factors must be considered. Support for aggressive medical therapy before surgery has been well established;[5] however, certain conditions do benefit from surgical intervention. Most cystic fibrosis patients are within the pediatric age group and experience sinusitis. Sinusitis may progress to a life-threatening condition in this population. Sinus inflammation leads to congestion and stasis of secretions and forms a reservoir for pathogen growth. Sinus pathogens seed the lower respiratory tract and can lead to pneumonia, particularly in those who have lung transplants.[6] A decreased ability to clear secretions, the propensity to develop polyps, common colonization with *Pseudomonas* organisms, and progressive general deterioration of the patient are reasons sinus surgery is performed. Surgery is directed toward removing disease, relieving obstruction, ventilating the paranasal sinuses, and eradicating pathogenic organisms. Sinus surgery serves to mediate, not cure, the sinus disease or pulmonary involvement. The creation of widely patent middle meatus with large maxillary sinus antrostomies or "mega-antrostomies" is advocated. The "mega-antrostomy" involves opening the maxillary ostia both posteriorly and inferiorly with the removal of the posterior inferior turbinate and inferior meatus, to allow secretions to drain toward the floor of the nose and nasopharynx. Surgery often provides drastic and prolonged improvement in these patients.[7] Revision sinus surgery is not uncommon, as sinus surgery improves the general health of cystic fibrosis patients but does not cure the underlying disease. Tenacious secretions associated with cystic fibrosis are difficult to expel, and impair the function of cilia within the nasal cavity. The resultant stasis will continue to cause recurrent episodes of sinusitis, but the severity of the infection and the potential for life-threatening sequelae are most often lessened.

Ciliary dyskinesia may result from different causes. As described, cystic fibrosis causes altered secretions that commonly leads to ciliary failure. Bacterial and viral infections damage ciliated epithelium; however, most patients regain mucociliary clearance after the infection has cleared and the cilia regenerate. Cilia regeneration occurs over approximately 10 weeks. Patients with Kartagener's syndrome have congenital dysfunction of cilia. Patients with suspected primary ciliary disorders require a mucosal biopsy to establish the diagnosis. Often this will be followed by functional surgery to widen areas of constriction to improve ventilation and mucus clearance.

Any cause of ciliary dysfunction causes ineffective mucus transport, resulting in stagnation and ultimately infection.

There is a well-established relationship between sinusitis and asthma;[8] and convincing clinical evidence indicates that sinusitis may play a part in the pathogenesis of bronchial asthma.[9] Clearing disease from the paranasal sinuses with removal of offensive bacterial organisms often results in improvement of asthma.[10] Therefore, applying the principles of functional sinus surgery to medically resistant sinusitis has proved helpful in the well-being of these patients. Asthmatics are at higher risk of postoperative pulmonary complications, and this should be considered before surgery begins.

Allergic or nonallergic rhinitis has been sited as one of the most common causes of chronic or recurrent sinusitis.[11] Rhinitis is differentiated from sinusitis by the presence of sneezing, itching, and clear rhinorrhea. Surgery in itself will not cure allergic rhinitis, but allergies can lead to such severe mucosal edema and chronic inflammation that the sinus mucosa becomes permanently damaged, leading to mucosal changes and polyp formation. If such a condition exists, surgical removal of sinus obstruction and opening of sinus ostia relieves the discomfort associated with disease; improved ventilation provides access for topical steroids that further improve the patient's overall condition. Allergic rhinitis may also be due to noninvasive fungal sinusitis. Patients with allergic fungal sinusitis typically have carried the diagnosis of chronic sinusitis and have had multiple sinus surgeries before the correct diagnosis was discovered.[12] The allergic response to the fungus may initiate massive polypoid growth with significant mass effect. The diagnosis requires demonstration of allergic mucin containing fungal elements. Surgery is indicated to remove polyps and allergic mucin and restore the patency of the paranasal sinuses.

Invasive fungal sinusitis usually presents in patients who are immunocompromised. Patients who have received an organ transplant, been treated for malignancy, or have allergies or asthma should be considered at risk. The diagnosis requires a surgical biopsy with evidence of mucosal penetration that may include blood vessel or bone involvement.[13] Acute fulminate invasive fungal sinusitis (usually mucormycosis) is a medical and surgical emergency. It is characterized by rapid spread of fungus via vascular routes into the orbits or brain with the presentation of fever, headache, mental status changes, epistaxis, and a characteristic dark rust-colored or black eschar within the nasal cavity. Therapy involves aggressive surgical debridement of nonviable tissue until healthy tissue is discovered. Systemic amphotericin B is also indicated.

There are situations in which chronic or recurrent sinusitis is the result of anatomic abnormalities within the nasal cavity. Most of the structures within the nasal cavities can have deformities that lead to functional obstruction of the sinus outflow tracts, particularly the anatomically narrow osteomeatal complex. Deflection of the nasal septum (either cartilaginous, bony, or both) can result in a significant narrowing of the nasal cavity. Abnormalities of the middle turbinate including a paradoxical curvature or pneumatization (concha bullosa) can impinge on the region of the hiatus semilunaris resulting in compromise of the osteomeatal complex. An enlarged inferior turbinate can obstruct nasal airflow and sinus drainage. Anatomic variation within the ethmoid system including large agger nasi cells, hypertrophy of the anterior or posterior ethmoid air cells, infraorbital ethmoid cells (Haller's cells), or sphenoethmoid cells (Onodi's cells) can functionally impair the outflow tracts. Abnormal deflection of the uncinate process due to development or trauma can occlude the osteomeatal complex leading to obstruction. When these anatomic variations are present, even the most minor cause of inflammation can lead to obstruction, stasis of secretions, and the creation of an environment suitable for the proliferation of bacterial pathogens. The focus of functional endoscopic sinus surgery is on the restoration of ventilation and mucociliary clearance of the paranasal sinuses. Correcting the anatomic abnormalities and providing improved ventilation and drainage of the paranasal sinuses can minimize the effects of mucosal edema, obstruction, and subsequent infection. In turn, this provides for a cured or significantly improved patient.

The frontal sinus is a paranasal sinus that requires particular attention. Infection of the frontal sinus does not respond quickly to antibiotic therapy and therefore can lead to central nervous system infection. The posterior table of the frontal sinus can be traversed by infection and allow access to the frontal lobe area causing an intracranial abscess or meningitis. Frontal sinusitis requiring surgery may be approached either externally or internally. External trephination or osteoplastic flaps with frontal sinus obliteration are the more common external methods. An intranasal approach is now frequently advocated as the frontal recess can often be opened widely with the complete eradication of disease using endoscopic methods. The patency of the frontal recess can be maintained indefinitely. This prevents the patients from acquiring external signs of surgery such as unsightly scar formation. Frontal sinus trephination has historically involved a Lynch incision with access gained through the medial supraorbital frontal bone. A much smaller version or mini-trephination system is now available that allows access to the frontal sinus by making a minimal incision directly over the anterior table of the frontal sinus and provides a means of obtaining cultures and irrigation. Experience has shown that this sort of trephination and endoscopic frontal sinus surgery results in the resolution of frontal sinus disease.

Consideration of all these factors can lead to the development of a treatment algorithm. The first consideration is to ensure the patient has undergone a thorough evaluation concerning the possibility of systemic influence or other causes (environmental) and adequate medical therapy for an appropriate length of time. If the sinus condition persists for 12 weeks or more, surgical intervention may be indicated. The patient's overall medical condition must also be considered. Patients with systemic illness may be predisposed for sinusitis-related complications and surgical intervention may be warranted at an earlier point in time. The treatment protocol begins with a careful history followed by a physical examination, including nasal endoscopy. Attention to anatomic factors that could cause sinus outflow obstruction, or signs of acute or chronic infection are carefully assessed. It may be difficult to perform an adequate examination on an uncooperative child; for these cases, a computed tomography (CT) study of the sinuses is extremely helpful. Many rhinologists consider CT an essential part of the preoperative evaluation, as well as a diagnostic aid for the existence, severity, and extent of chronic inflammation. It can provide anatomic information that can direct the surgical procedure and add an element of safety in cases of difficult or unusual anatomy. Once all factors have been analyzed, appropriate counsel can be offered to the patient. Counseling patients with pre-existing medical conditions, such as cystic fibrosis, ciliary disorders, immunodeficiency, and diabetes, must be provided in order to maximize the benefit of endoscopic surgery. It is not unusual for some patients to require more than one surgical procedure; revision sinus surgery is not uncommon in these patients. Revisions are at times advised in those with chronic recurrent sinusitis in spite of previous surgery, appropriate medical therapy and CT studies that show no other sign of abnormality.[14]

Functional endoscopic sinus surgery has been established as an effective and safe method of treating patients who have chronic sinusitis and have not benefited from medical therapy. It is effective in treating adults and children as long as careful attention has been given to concomitant medical conditions and a careful anatomic evaluation has been performed.

REFERENCES

Gross and Harrison—CHAPTER 17

1. Kaliner MA, Osguthorpe JD, Fireman P, et al. Sinusitis: bench to bedside. *J Allergy Clin Immunol* 1997;99:S829–S848
2. Kennedy DW, Zinreich SJ, Rosenbaum A, et al. Functional endoscopic sinus surgery: theory and diagnosis. *Arch Otolaryngol* 1985;111:576–582
3. Senior BA, Kennedy DW, Tanabodee J, et al. Long-term results of functional endoscopic sinus surgery. *Laryngoscope* 1998;108:151–157
4. Danielson A, Olofsson J. Endoscopic endonasal sinus surgery: a long-term follow-up study. *Acta Otolaryngol* 1996;116:611–619
5. Parsons DS. Chronic sinusitis: a medical or surgical disease? *Otolaryngol Clin of North Am* 1996;29:1–9
6. Davidson TM, Murphy C, Mitchell M, et al. Management of chronic sinusitis in cystic fibrosis. *Laryngoscope* 1995;105:354–358
7. Gentile VG, Isaacson G. Patterns of sinusitis in cystic fibrosis. *Laryngoscope* 1996;106:1005–1009
8. Marney SR. Pathophysiology of reactive airway disease and sinusitis. *Ann Otol Rhinol Laryngol* 1996;105:98–100
9. Slavin RG. Complications of allergic rhinitis: implications for sinusitis and asthma. *J Allergy Clin Immunol* 1998;101: S357–S360
10. Bucca C, Rolla G, Scappaticci E, et al. Extrathoracic and intrathoracic airway responsiveness in sinusitis. *J Allergy Clin Immunol* 1995;95:52–59
11. Kaliner M. Medical management of sinusitis. *Am J Med* 1998; 316:21–28
12. deShazo RD, Swain RE. Diagnostic criteria for allergic fungal sinusitis. *J Allergy Clin Immunol* 1995;96:24–35
13. deShazo RD. Fungal sinusitis. *Am J Med Sci* 1998;316: 39–45
14. Lazar RH, Younis RT, Long TE, Gross CW. Revision endoscopic sinus surgery. *Ear Nose Throat J* 1992;71:131–133

Outcomes in Sinus Surgery—Management Parameters

CHAPTER 18

Richard E. Gliklich

Outcomes assessment refers to the measurement of health and medical results toward the goal of improving care. Although outcomes assessment in itself is not controversial, controversy arises when attempts are made to standardize methodology. There are several valid ways to approach outcomes assessment and management in sinus surgery. The best means to eliminate controversy is for the reader to understand that the relevant criteria for choosing an outcomes management system should be based on the individual needs of a particular practice or a particular study and the performance characteristics (e.g., type of measure, reliability, ease of use) of the available measures and staging systems.

Sinusitis is an increasingly common cause for patient visits to the doctor in the United States and is the prinicipal diagnosis in nearly 2% of all patient visits. Surgery for the treatment of chronic sinusitis is performed more than 200,000 times per year in the United States alone, making sinusitis both a common and, in aggregate, an expensive illness.

Sinusitis is a predominantly ambulatory disease that afflicts a working-age population. In many ways, sinusitis is a model to explain the practical steps necessary in developing outcomes management systems for chronic ambulatory diseases as well as the information that can be obtained and used from an effective program. The elements of an outcomes management system for sinus surgery include staging and stratification, process measurement, outcomes measures, and feedback.

Staging and Stratification

The challenge of developing outcomes management systems rests in adequately defining and stratifying starting points and in accurately quantifying endpoints. In sinusitis, for example, a great deal of attention has been focused on the appropriate method to stage a preoperative computed tomography (CT) scan of the paranasal sinuses. Yet, the factors that comprise a good staging system (i.e., validity, reliability, statistical distribution, comprehensiveness, and the ability to predict outcome) are rarely considered or objectively evaluated. In two studies of clinician-based staging systems,[1,2] we have found wide variations in reliability (both intra-rater and inter-rater) and the lack of substantial correlations to postoperative outcome. Nevertheless, for consistency in reporting results, it is necessary to choose a staging system. Table 18–1 describes several proposed staging systems that have been evaluated. In the comprehensive evaluation by Metson et al.,[2] which included staging systems by Kennedy,[3] Friedman et al.,[4] and May et al.,[5] the Harvard system[6] and the Lund–MacKay staging systems[7] were found to be the most reliable, whereas the Harvard system was the easiest to use. In 1996, in a report of the Rhinosinusitis Task Force Committee Meeting, Drs. Lund and Kennedy recommended the modified Lund–MacKay staging system for further outcomes research.[8] Ultimately, the best staging system will be chosen by evaluating outcomes studies to determine which factors are most predictive of the result. That will not be possible until additional data are collected.

Outcomes Measures

Assessing endpoints or outcomes is the next step in developing outcomes management systems. Although traditional endpoints such as complications and mortality rates are important, they are imprecise for nonmorbid disease processes such as sinusitis. Therefore, these measures must be supplemented by more precise and useful measurements. Unlike hearing or vision loss, patients with sinusitis suffer in ways that are less easily measured but that certainly affect their functioning and well-being. Therefore, it is clear that patient-based quality-of-life measures should be a vital element of any studies in patients with sinusitis. The recommended elements of a quality-of-life outcomes monitor for sinusitis include a general health assessment, which is a global view of the patient's well-being as well as a disease-specific assessment that focuses more narrowly on the disease entity and that is usually more sensitive to clinical change with treatment.[6,9,10]

Probably the most widely tested instrument used for general health assessment today is the SF-36 Health Survey, or some form of it.[11] This 36-item survey measures 8 domains of general health grouped into physical and mental health areas. In a study of 165 patients presenting to otolaryngologists with chronic sinusitis, patients with chronic sinusitis demonstrated significant decrements from expected normative levels of functioning when tested with this survey in such areas as physical role functioning, bodily pain, general health, vitality, and social functioning.[10] Whenever a quality-of-life measurement is reported, it is important to put it into perspective. For example, the vitality score reported in chronic sinusitis refractory to medical therapy can be thought of as indicating that one-fourth of these patients would be expected to report that they are tired most or all of the time. As a generic measure, the SF-36 also permits comparisons between diseases, to understand the relative health impact of chronic sinusitis as com-

TABLE 18–1
Examples of Computed Tomography Staging Systems*

Stage	Description	
Staging system proposed by Kennedy[a]		
0	Normal	
I	Anatomic abnormalities, all unilateral sinus disease, bilateral disease limited to ethmoidal sinuses	
II	Bilateral ethmoidal disease with involvement of one dependent sinus	
III	Bilateral ethmoidal disease with involvement of two or more dependent sinuses on each side	
IV	Diffuse sinonasal polyposis	
Staging system proposed by Gliklich and Metson (Harvard System)[b]		
0	Normal (<2 cm mucosal thickening on any sinus wall)	
I	All unilateral disease or anatomic abnormality	
II	Bilateral disease limited to ethmoidal or maxillary sinuses	
III	Bilateral disease with involvement of at least one sphenoidal or frontal sinus	
IV	Pansinus disease	
Grading of sinus systems proposed by Lund and Mackay[c]		
Sinus system	Left	Right
Maxillary		
Anterior ethmoidal		
Posterior ethmoidal		
Sphenoidal		
Frontal		
Ostiomeatal complex		
Total points for each side:		

* Scoring: For all sinus systems, except the ostiomeatal complex: 0 = no abnormalities, 1 = partial opacification, 2 = total opacification. For the ostiomeatal complex: 0 = not occluded, 2 = occluded.

SOURCE:[a] Adapted from Kennedy DW. Prognostic factors, outcomes and staging in ethmoid sinus surgery. *Laryngoscope* 1992;102(suppl 57):1–18

SOURCE:[b] Adapted from Gliklich RE, Metson, R. A comparison of sinus computed tomography (CT) staging systems for outcomes research. *Am J Rhinol* 1994;8:291–297

SOURCE:[c] Adapted from Lund VJ, Mackay IS. Staging in rhinosinusitis. *Rhinology* 1993;107:183–184

pared with other chronic illnesses. Such comparisons show that patients with chronic sinusitis have SF-36 scores in domains such as general health and vitality similar to scores of patients with other chronic illnesses, such as chronic obstructive pulmonary disease. Using generic health measures in this way gives us a better understanding of the relative public health impact of one illness versus another.

In order to obtain the measurement precision necessary to accomplish effective outcomes management systems, it is helpful to include condition-specific measures as part of the health status assessment. Although recommendations have been made in the literature over which particular instrument should be declared the "standard," there are significant hazards to this approach. Outcomes measures are classified according to purpose. Diagnostic tests are judged by their correlation with a clinical diagnosis. Prognostic measures predict a trait or a result. Discriminative indices classify patients as with or without the disease or characteristic. Evaluative measures track change over time. It is therefore the purpose of the study that determines which instrument is most suitable.[12] One size does not fit all. In general, for therapeutic interventions such as surgery, evaluative measures are usually most appropriate.

TABLE 18–2
Outcomes Measures Used in Chronic (Rhino) Sinusitis

Measure	Year Reported	Reliability Reported	No. of Published Studies[a]
Chronic Sinusitis TyPe Specification	1993	No	2
Chronic Sinusitis Survey (Nasal Outcome Survey)	1995	Yes	10+
Rhinosinusitis Outcomes Measure-36 or the Sinonasal Outcomes Test-20	1995	Yes	<5
Rhinosinusitis Disability Index	1997	Yes	1

*SOURCE:[a] Based on Medline search through 1998.

Available Measures

Table 18–2 presents several available instruments and the number of published studies identified in a Medline search through 1998. I do not recommend any one particular instrument. For different purposes, different instruments will be most suitable. For example, the rhinosinusitis outcome measure (RSOM-31,)[13] and its derivative, the Sinonasal Outcomes Test (SNOT-20), was developed in primary care practices in order to better ascertain which symptoms are best correlated with the diagnosis of sinusitis. As such, it has potential to be used as a discriminative test to help differentiate patients who have sinusitis from those who do not.

The Chronic Sinusitis Survey (CSS), (also known as the Nasal Outcome Survey),[6] was developed as a brief, highly sensitive evaluative instrument designed to measure change with therapy. This makes it particularly useful for clinical trials or for following patients who are undergoing surgery. Of all the reliable sinusitis instruments, it is the least burdensome to administer and the most widely used to date. In addition to patient symptom information, it generates data on medication usage and cost.

The Rhinosinusitis Disability Index (RSDI)[14] is another instrument that has been tested for validity and reliability. The RSDI includes more questions on general health effects, potentially making it useful as a stand-alone instrument without a general health assessment.

The Rhinoconjunctivitis Quality-of-Life Questionnaire[15] is a reliable measure that was developed primarily for allergy symptoms, although it has been used in a few sinusitis studies.

Applications

The largest body of published outcomes information in chronic rhinosinusitis is based on the CSS (10+ published studies), in combination with the SF-36. Several interesting findings demonstrate the range of information that can be collected using appropriate outcomes measures. Figures 18–1 and 18–2 demonstrate the application of our outcomes management system to two different patients undergoing surgery. When this type of management system is applied to an entire population of patients, we are able to derive meaningful information.

In a study of 100 patients with chronic sinusitis undergoing sinus surgery, this outcomes measurement system was applied to understand the effect of sinus surgery on patient quality of life.[16] In this study, patients demonstrated significant improvements on all items of the CSS. The mean symptom score improved by 95%, mean medication-based score by 36%, and the total score by 58%. In using quality-of-life measures to report results of interventions, it is necessary to root such measures to clinically significant change. For sinusitis, an 8-point change in the CSS total score requires a 50% change in duration of symptom or medication usage, making this a clinically meaningful improvement. On the basis of this definition, at 12 months after surgery, 82% of patients were improved, 7% unchanged, and 11% worse.

Using the general health measure, the SF-36, patients demonstrate significant improvements in all domains of the SF-36. In fact, the mean normative level is reached for all domains except role-functioning physical scores, which relate to a person's ability to work.

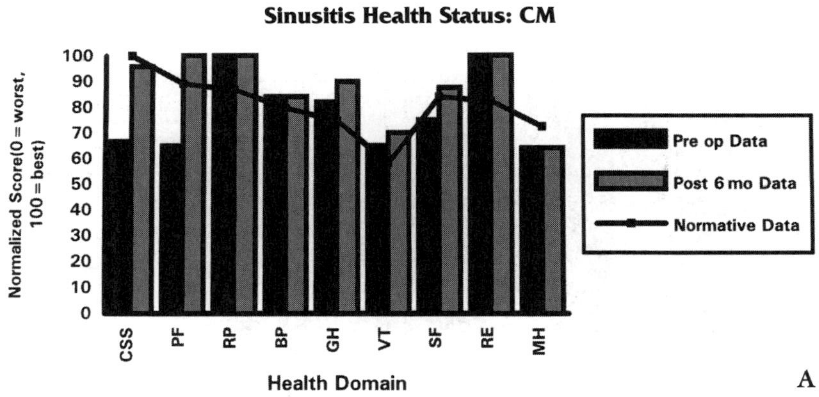

A

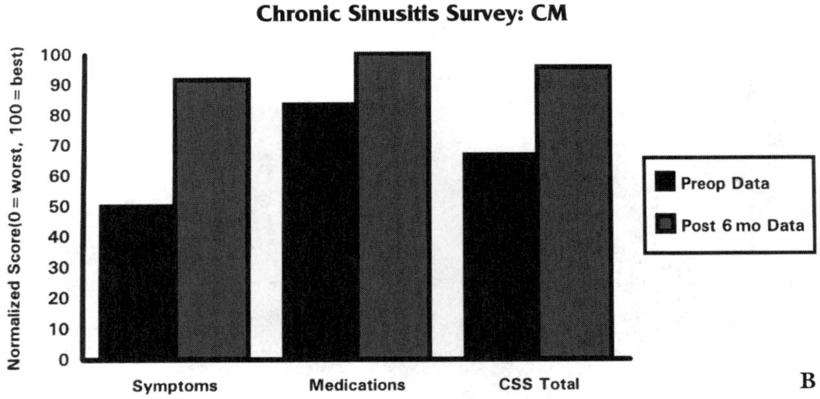

B

Figure 18–1 (**A**) Preoperative and postoperative scores are shown versus normative data for patients with sinusitis, CM (black line) 0. 0 is the worst possible score and 100 the best. The first column shows the Chronic Sinusitis Survey (CSS) total score; the remaining 8 pairs of columns are the domain scores for the SF-36. At 1 year after surgery, this patient has demonstrated significant improvement in the total CSS score and the physical functioning score of the SF-36. (**B**) Preoperative and postoperative CSS score results for this patient. Note that the CSS allows us to track an overall score and both symptom and medication usage scores. This patient has had significant improvement in symptoms and less of an improvement in medication usage (off all medications at 1 year indicated by CSS = 100).

Outcomes measures can also be used to construct economic models. In one study, 100 consecutive patients undergoing primary endoscopic sinus surgery were prospectively followed using the CSS and the SF-36 and by recording actual payor reimbursements for surgery and medication costs and usage. Data for work disability, hospital expenditures, and physician visit rates were derived from the health status measures.[17]

Mean surgical cost was taken as the sum of the actual reimbursements for the hospital, the surgeon, and the anesthesiologist and totaled $6490. Medication costs preoperatively and postoperatively were based on actual reported usage rates for over-the-counter medications, nasal sprays, and antibiotics. Preoperatively, costs averaged $1220 per patient per year for medications; postoperatively, they averaged $629 per patient per year, a difference of $591, or 48%. In addition, indirect cost-savings of $645 per patient per year were achieved after surgery because of a significant reduction in projected work-related disability due to sickness.

Conclusion

Outcomes management in sinus surgery provides a model for outcomes measurement and management of many ambulatory conditions. Measurement demonstrates the relative burden of disease and the efficacy of therapy. By including cost as an outcome and understanding the relationship between health status and cost, economic models can be developed to demonstrate the relative value of procedures on the overall cost of chronic disease. The single most important cause of current controversy surrounding outcomes measures for sinus disease and surgery stems from attempts to force standardization, rather than evaluating each measurement system or staging system on its relative value for a particular purpose. An improved understanding of outcomes measures will enable clinicians and researchers to choose the approach that best suits their needs.

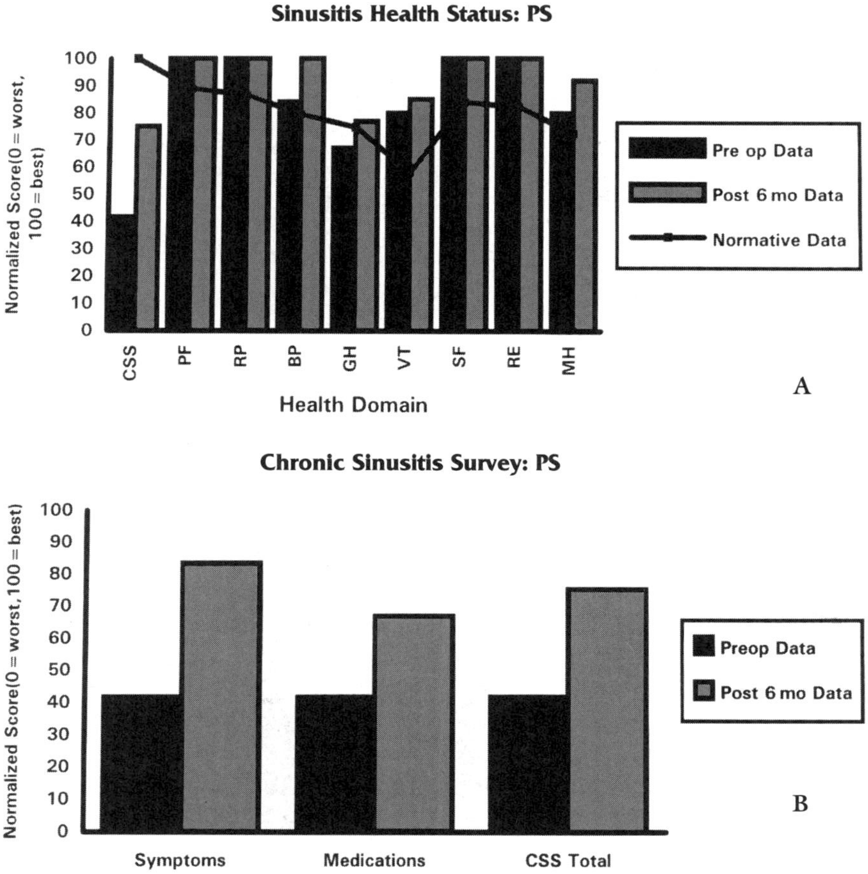

Figure 18–2 **(A)** Sinusitis Health Status results including the Chronic Sinusitis Survey (CSS) and the SF-36 Health Survey demonstrate that patients can have near-normal SF-36 scores while still demonstrating significant decrements in sinus-specific health. After surgery, this symptomatic patient with pansinus disease and nasal polyps reaches the normative level for general health (GH) and maintains that level for all other subscales of the SF-36. This patient shows significant improvement in the total CSS score but does not reach normative levels. **(B)** A closer look at the breakdown of the CSS scores demonstrates significant improvement in the CSS total score, which is mostly due to the improvement in the CSS symptom score. Improvements in medication usage score are more modest in this patient, who has continued to use nasal steroid sprays and antihistamines.

REFERENCES

1. Gliklich RE, Metson R. A comparison of sinus computed tomography (CT) staging systems for outcomes research. *Am J Rhinol* 1994;8:291–297
2. Metson R, Gliklich RE, Stankiewicz JA, et al. Comparison of sinus computed tomograpy staging systems. *Otol Head Neck Surg* 1997;117:372–379
3. Kennedy DW. Prognostic factors, outcomes and staging in ethmoid sinus surgery. *Laryngoscope* 1992;102(suppl 57):1–18
4. Friedman WH, Katsantonis GP, Sivore M, et al. Computed tomography staging of the paranasal sinuses in chronic hyperplastic rhinosinusitis. *Laryngoscope* 1990;100:1161–1165
5. May M, Levine HL, Schaitkin B, et al. Results of surgery. In: Levine H, May M, eds. *Rhinology and Sinusology.* New York: Thieme Medical Publishers; 1993:176–192
6. Gliklich RE, Metson R. Techniques for outcomes research in chronic sinusitis. *Laryngoscope* 1995;105:387–390

7. Lund VJ, Mackay IS. Staging in rhinosinusitis. *Rhinology* 1993;107:183–184
8. Lund VJ, Kennedy DW. Staging for rhinosinusitis. *Otolaryngol Head Neck Surg* 1997;117:S35–S40
9. Gliklich RE, Hilinsky J. Longitudinal sensitivity of generic and specific health measures in chronic sinusitis. *Qual Life Res* 1995;4:27–32
10. Gliklich RE, Metson R. The health impact of chronic sinusitis in patients seeking otolaryngologic care. *Otol Head Neck Surg* 1995;113:104–109
11. Ware JE Jr, Snow KK, Kosinski M, et al. *SF-36 Health Survey: Manual and Interpretation Guide*. Boston: The Health Institute; 1993
12. Gliklich RE. Outcomes measures. In: Gliklich RE, Isenberg S, eds. *Profiting from Quality: Outcomes Strategies for Medical Practice*. San Francisco: Jossey-Bass; 1999:75–82
13. Piccirillo JF, Edwards D, Haiduk A, et al. Psychometric and clinimetric validity of the 31-item rhinosinusitis outcome measure (RSOM-31). *Am J Rhinol* 1995;9:297–306
14. Benninger MS. The development of the rhinosinusitis disability index. *Arch Otolaryngol Head Neck Surg* 1997;123: 1175–1179
15. Juniper EF, Guyatt GH. Development and testing of a new measure of health status for clinical trials in rhinoconjunctivitis. *Clin Exp Allergy* 1991;21:77–83
16. Gliklich RE, Metson R. The effect of sinus surgery on quality of life. *Otolaryngol Head Neck Surg* 1997;117:12–16
17. Gliklich RE, Metson R. Economic implications of chronic sinusitis. *Otolaryngol Head Neck Surg* 1998;118:344

7

Quality-of-Life Issues in Head and Neck Cancer Management

"Quality of life and quality of death are opposite sides of the same coin and both are presumably optimized when the likelihood of locoregional cancer recurrence is minimized."

Sharon L. Collins

"It is however vital for oncologists to appreciate the only way that meaningful therapeutic decisions regarding our patient's well-being can be made is to incorporate these QOL instruments into our decision-making algorithm."

Jack L. Gluckman

"The great physicians never stop learning, and recognize the roles our patients play as teachers. It is our responsibility to occasionally pause and reflect on what we know works, what doesn't, and what new avenues might be explored."

Nancy L. Snyderman

Quality-of-Life Issues in Head and Neck Cancer Management

CHAPTER 19

Sharon L. Collins

As we go beyond the year 2000, health care professionals, regardless of their area of practice, will be required (like it or not) to participate in evolving areas of medical practice that have not been part of the traditional medicine of earlier decades: outcomes assessment, patient quality-of-life (QOL) issues, statistical methods such as decision analysis and meta-analysis, and new areas of patient interest such as alternative medicine, to name a few.[1] A voluminous literature already exists concerning QOL assessment in head and neck cancer (HNC) patients, but it is too embryonic to have fostered distinct controversies at this point. This chapter presents a brief overview of where we have been, where we are, and where we are going on issues related to QOL in HNC patients. The goals of this presentation are to make health care professionals aware of (1) new issues that must be dealt with; (2) how espousing, rather than resisting, these new trends can optimize relationships with patients and foster compliance with any desired treatment regimen; (3) current deficiencies in the existing literature toward the goal of correcting them expeditiously; and (4) what can be done now in daily practice to enhance the QOL of HNC patients.

What Is QOL and Why Should We Study It?

QOL refers to a spectrum of factors that, in aggregate, comprise "well-being," a concept that is currently being defined.[2-13] Global well-being includes physical, functional, emotional, and social domains as influenced by a person's beliefs, expectations, and perceptions, and as influenced by the patient's education and knowledge about expected outcomes of therapy. Such perceptions may change during the course of therapy and in conjunction with the patient's disease/health status, cancer-free or not. The person under discussion is the patient—not the health care professional. An individual's past experience, personality, and ethnic background lead to different expectations regarding health and varying ability to cope with limitations and disability. Two people with the same health status may have different QOL related to different perceptions of health and satisfaction with life. QOL outcomes are often impacted by functional factors involved in cancer treatment. For example, two patients who are "cured" of larynx cancer may experience disparate levels of satisfaction if one has a persistent tracheotomy and/or feeding tube, and the other does not. But QOL is a multidimensional construct in which functional ability is only one component. Outcomes assessment has shown that the severity of physiologic or functional measures often correlates minimally with global QOL, which correlates more accurately with patient satisfaction and is manifested as increased compliance with treatment regimens.

Interestingly, traditional cancer outcome measures (e.g., response rates, sites of failure, disease control, overall survival, cause of death, treatment toxicities) do not always correlate with patient benefit, especially in advanced cancer patients, which makes assessing QOL essential. The ultimate goal of adding such assessments is that the combination of symptoms, function, QOL, cost, and cancer treatment endpoints will lead to better definition of treatment efficacy to facilitate the choice of treatment.[9] Interestingly, in a completion of the circle, there is evidence that optimizing global QOL may be a significant predictor of survival time and that improving the QOL of cancer patients may result not only in better quality-adjusted survival, but in longer survival as well.[14]

QOL issues differ when considering curative intent versus palliation. In the former approach, aggressive attempts to control locoregional cancer may be justified despite attendant toxicities that negatively impact on QOL. In the latter situation (incurable metastatic disease), such an aggressive stance is less appropriate and symptom control—especially pain control—becomes paramount. QOL is also important in the context of adjuvant treatment, which, by definition, is given in patients without symptoms and without objectively evident cancer in whom the main criteria of effectiveness are relapse-free survival and long-term survival.

Except for the inclusion of constitutional B symptoms in lymphoma staging, cancer staging systems have included only factors related to the tumor, and not to the patient. The complexity of the tumor–host interaction in HNC patients has been reemphasized in the recent literature[15] and the effect of having left out the patient half of the equation in the past may well negate the putative incremental improvements in cancer control claimed with some of the newer treatment strategies. For example, two recent articles demonstrate that the variable of alcohol consumption (none versus heavy) is associated with a 40 to 50% difference in survival,[16,17] which is much more than the less than 10% differences that can currently be related to variations in cancer treatment for HNC, and that reversing alcoholism correlates with improved survival over time.[16] Certainly, in view of these results, this usually neglected factor, often considered impossible to assess accurately in unreliable HNC patients, deserves renewed attention.

The most important goal of QOL assessment is to have a cured and intact patient who can assume as near-normal function as possible for the duration of his or her lifetime. An important practical application of studying QOL is identifying patients and/or families who will have, or are having, problems adapting to their illness and its treatment. The identification of these problems at their onset can lead to expeditious implementation of psychosocial treatment, behavior modification, and instruction in coping mechanisms so that both patient and spouse/family can make a more rapid transition to psychological stability.

One gets the feeling from the existing HNC QOL literature that there should be no morbidity associated with any type of treatment for advanced HNC. In fact, by its very nature, HNC is a mutilating disease. Treatment of any type intrudes on an individual's physical, emotional, and social well-being, in contradistinction to the age-old perception that the morbidity of HNC treatment relates largely to the surgical component. The achievement of complete normalcy in the treated HNC patient is an unrealistic expectation. Persistent pain, dysphagia, altered voice, and the need for tracheotomy and/or feeding tubes can accompany initial treatment with chemo- and radiotherapy or altered fractionation radiation or traditional radiation with curative intent, as well as with surgical regimens. Among the QOL studies emerging from the University of Chicago, one showed that the 40% of patients who had pain before aggressive chemo- and radiotherapy also continued to experience pain after treatment,[18] demonstrating that an objective tumor response does not always correlate with freedom from distress. Another study showed that in a group of patients free of disease at 1 year after organ preservation treatment (although biased toward a favorable result due to selecting cancer-free survivors), that the most important performance impairment was the inability to eat a normal, solid food diet, with 50% of the patients able to eat only soft foods or liquids.[19] Obviously, when cancer affects the complex and compact anatomy of the head and neck, the important functions of speech, swallowing, breathing, and appearance will inevitably be affected. It is unrealistic to use the patient's premorbid condition as the baseline for comparison of functional and QOL results. It is more realistic to focus on the degree of compromise of structure, function, and ensuing psychosocial morbidity to be expected with HNC of various stages and sites, and currently such information is not available. A large standardized sample study including oncologic, functional, and QOL outcomes in the HNC population would help establish such norms.

QOL issues relate not only to patients with recurrent/persistent cancer, but also to cancer survivors. "Successful" cancer treatment (often prematurely defined) has resulted in a class of "walking worried,"[20-23] such as treated prostate cancer patients who regularly focus on their prostate-specific antigen (PSA) levels or breast cancer survivors who participate in ongoing hormone or chemotherapy trials. Ongoing anxiety over maintenance of the cancer-free status can become an important health problem. Patients may look and feel physically well, but they are not well emotionally. Survivorship issues for HNC patients relate to long-term use of Salagen[24] or participation in chemoprevention trials, with daily medications being an ongoing reminder of potential disease and treatment, as well as ongoing monitoring for second primary tumors. Many studies now assess the cost/benefit of follow-up regimens for treated cancer patients, and an important emerging issue is whether the omnipresent reminders of such surveillance outweigh the potential benefit to well-being of less rigorous follow-up. Such questions raise obvious ethical concerns but are inherent in the modern era of cost containment in medical practice. This leads to an additional reason for health care providers to get involved in QOL and other types of outcomes research. Many other groups (medical consortia, HMOs, federal agencies, insurers) are engaged in synthesizing outcome and economic data toward the development of clinical practice guidelines. Some of the tools of modern medical practice include the development of evidence-based medicine (the 10 to 15% of the medical literature that is considered scientifically valid, based on a randomized, controlled, prospective format), cost-containment research, and outcomes research. It is inevitable that in the not too distant future, health care providers may have to justify their treatment plan to health care payors based on outcomes data and patient satisfaction responses. The "sciences" of practice guideline development and implementation are both in their infancy and too embryonic to serve as a basis for treatment decisions in the individual patient, but there is also no question that investigating health care and documenting health care outcomes is now an industry in its own right in the United States. This fact cannot be ignored. A new class of entrepreneurs has emerged—private companies who are vendors of outcomes instruments. Many flashy systems are available, but the descriptive data collected often have limited usefulness. The push for further development in QOL and related areas now appears to come largely from third-party payors. Unless the medical community actively participates in research that will lead to valid information based on deep medical expertise, outcomes analysts will soon be dictating what success is based on more superficial analysis. In particular, a specialist should not sacrifice involvement in the post-treatment aspects of patient management in an era when surveillance of treated cancer patients is being directed away from them and toward family physicians. Currently, about 40 articles in the QOL literature (often published in journals such as *Medical Decision Making*, *Quality of Life Research Journal*, and *Journal of the Medical Information Association*) document the cost-effectiveness and importance of ongoing specialist intervention.

QOL Assessment Instruments

QOL issues, heretofore considered too soft and subjective for specialists to deal with are, in fact, objectively quantifiable and do not merely represent the absence of disease. QOL is generally measured by structured questionnaires that can be scored and quantified to generate hard data. Most widely used QOL assessments include measures of physical, psychosocial, economic, and global well-being. There is an explosion in the QOL literature, with more than 30 generic tools available (to assess global QOL and health considerations) and more than 300 disease-specific tools available, including 35 to 45 for cancer patients. The otolaryngologist–head and neck surgeon who ventures into the QOL literature published in journals of psychology, epidemiology, health science, psychosomatic medicine, and sociology may well be confused by the statistical methodology and jargon encountered, such as, "Construct validity was examined in this study through factor analysis using principal components and orthogonal rotation, which revealed that the average scores were function and network properties which did load onto three factors."[25]

Different methodologies assess different health outcomes. For example, QOL scales (self-assessment questionnaires) measure the patient's perceived quality of health retrospectively, whereas utility scales measure projected health state. An example of the latter is the time/trade-off method that identifies the number of years of perfect health the interviewee (often not a patient) is willing to exchange for 5 to 10 years in each health state. Products of outcomes research often apply linear analogue scoring or category rating not only to physical status, but also to psychological and social well-being by assessing variables such as pain, mobility, capacity for sexual relationships, and symptom-free days. Additional complexity arises when cost-effectiveness of treatment alternatives is included.

In general, articles in the QOL literature show that whatever instrument is under evaluation, is reliable (yields consistent values), valid (targets what it claims to measure), responsive (detects changes over time), sensitive (reflects true changes in individual patients), and practical to administer. Instruments that fail to document these parameters probably do not get published, although it would be interesting to see some scales that have not fulfilled these criteria; possibly much could be learned from them. Often lacking are articles that demonstrate the reproducibility of a given instrument; there appears to be more interest among authors in generating a slightly different instrument that is better than any of the others rather than in validating someone else's. All instruments vary slightly in methodology (e.g., self-response vs proxy, telephone vs mail vs interview) and psychometrically in what is included in the questionnaire. Outcomes research has demonstrated that patients generally like to fill out questionnaires (satisfied patients generally respond more than dissatisfied ones who manifest their dissatisfaction in other ways), but there is concern over how the information gathered will be used; to discriminate against patients in a punitive way? There is also significant concern on the part of providers who are often reluctant to participate in such studies; will patient satisfaction results be used to punish (or reward) providers ("report cards")? The theoretical desire to include all relevant outcomes and costs is daunting, and there are already too many tools to choose from. It is more realistic to select a QOL product that meets most of the needs of the patient population under consideration and to use it in a prospective, longitudinal manner in large numbers of patients.

QOL studies must be performed prospectively and longitudinally over time, as a cancer patient's perception of health often changes, and if QOL is assessed at only one point or over a short interval, a distorted picture will emerge. Recall bias is a well-known factor, and responses often differ when they are asked near to or far after an event. An individual's satisfaction with QOL early after treatment often differs significantly from that perceived years later, especially if side effects become more troublesome or if the cancer recurs. One example from the prostate cancer literature shows that with longer follow-up, persistent incontinence may dampen early enthusiasm over having had a successful operation.[26] An analogy in the area of HNC might be that patients who require delayed or have long-term tracheotomies and difficulty swallowing may become depressed, whereas they were initially happy to have their larynx preserved. These conditions may not develop for years after nonsurgical organ preservation treatments, as a result of progressive soft tissue fibrosis in the head and neck, and may not be recognized if cancer follow-up terminates at 5 years, the traditional cure endpoint. Additional surveillance of HNC patients for second primaries should continue indefinitely with yearly chest radiographs that can detect early, operable second primary lung cancers.

Thus, measurement of QOL is dynamic, rather than static, and requires periodic reassessment. Short-term results cannot be extrapolated to reflect long-term outcome. It is likely that prospective, long-term, longitudinal studies, which are lacking in the HNC literature, may better elucidate the patient's true experience in the future. Similarly, isolated observations in long-term survivors are biased if they are meant to represent the population at large, because patients who have had less favorable cancer-control results and outcomes have already expired or otherwise been selected out.[27]

How often QOL outcomes should be measured depends on the condition and the treatment given. Assessment before treatment and after each component of multimodality treatment, if clearly definable, as well as longer-term assessment, might be reasonable for the HNC population. For example, in patients who undergo surgery followed by radiation or chemoradiotherapy, assessment before treatment, after surgery/before radiotherapy, after radiotherapy, 6 months after the end of treatment, and 1, 3, and 5 years after treatment seems logical. Even longer assessment, at 10 years, for example, is probably indicated to assess functional changes over time caused by progressive tissue fibrosis.

The fact that outcomes and QOL research are not yet exact sciences is demonstrated by highlighting some of the problems in the existing literature. Table 19–1 lists some general problems with questionnaire studies. For example, depending on how questions are phrased, it is easy to get the desired response; a fact that pollsters are well aware of. If identical probabilities are proposed to subjects but are asked in two different ways (chance of survival vs chance of death), subjects usually make different decisions, even though the probabilities are identical.[28,29] Table 19–2 lists areas of apparent consensus in the QOL literature.

HNC QOL Perspective: Where Have We Been and Where Are We Now?

Before about 1985, the major focus of solid tumor surgical oncology was to cure the patient and/or increase the length of survival. Any degree of organ resection with its accompanying physical and functional "mutilation" was acceptable, as the alternative was death. Treatment planning was based on

TABLE 19–1
Problems with the Existing QOL Literature

1.	Potential for bias: How the questions are phrased Who administers the questionnaire (biased when data are interpreted by interested parties with an agenda favoring a particular treatment) Reporting long-term results including only survivors or cancer-free patients (eliminating patients with recurrent/persistent cancer or unfavorable outcomes)
2.	Lack of prospective, long-term data reporting that includes all relevant inputs
3.	Failure to report oncologic, functional, and QOL outcomes in the same publication, which would highlight the overall value of a given treatment strategy
4.	Lack of assessing impact of differences related to ethnicity and culture
5.	QOL studies include too few patients who have undergone comparable therapies for HNC arising in similar anatomic locations
6.	Significance of anti-intuitive and conflicting literature results
7.	Using group-mean QOL data to predict an individual patient's QOL status/concerns; studies emphasizing the results of groups of patients, rather than individuals, may obscure important individual differences

QOL, quality of life, HNC, head and neck cancer.

TABLE 19–2
Current Consensus in QOL Issues

1.	The severity of physiologic measures often correlates minimally with QOL. QOL correlates with patient satisfaction. Patient satisfaction influences treatment compliance.
2.	QOL studies must be formatted as prospective and long-term.
3.	QOL considerations respect the patient's wishes; patients who are empowered to participate in their treatment planning and rehabilitation generally manifest higher QOL.
4.	Any type of treatment for HNC is associated with negative QOL impact. Functional and QOL compromise is not exclusively associated with surgical regimens, but also accompanies nonsurgical treatments (radical radiotherapy, chemoradiotherapy).
5.	QOL considerations include many more aspects than functional status alone.
6.	Negative functional consequences are more common in patient-reported outcome surveys than are reported in the medical literature.
7.	Because the population at large of patients with HNSCC have both cancer-related and general health/comorbidity issues, QOL outcomes should be assessed with both general health measures and HNC-specific measures.
8.	Patients with cancer are often unwilling to sacrifice any length of life for a shorter life of putatively better quality. Therefore, the relevance of time/trade-off methods of QOL analysis using surrogate models needs reevaluation.
9.	There is lack of correlation between physician and patient ratings of QOL and emotional well-being. Physicians do not accurately predict what is important to patients in the physical, functional, emotional, and QOL realms. Many articles show both that physicians consider many treatment defects more mutilating than patients do and that patients consider many long-term sequelae of treatment more negative on QOL than physicians do.[a]
10.	The elitist assumption of health care professionals that patients cannot evaluate and assess the QOL impact of their cancer treatments seems incorrect.

QOL, quality of life; HNC, head and neck cancer; HNSCC, head and neck squamous cell carcinoma.

[a]Dirksen SR. Theoretical modeling to predict subjective well-being. *West J Nurs Res* 1990;12:629.

tumor-related factors. The patient's nonphysical status was not a priority. The literature largely consisted of retrospective cancer treatment reports of oncologic results. During the 1960s, some articles appeared on rehabilitating surgically imposed deficits, and attention focused on certain postoperative conditions, such as the "oral cripple." The literature on QOL for HNC patients was largely nonexistent, with the exception of one contribution, which was subsequently widely misquoted.[30] A holistic approach to the patient was considered the domain of general medical practitioners. For the most part, this approach failed to enter the realm of specialty training, where the focus is on technical advances. Topics such as communicating with patients,[31] psychosocial considerations in patient management, and disease prevention/behavior modification,[32] were largely absent from medical school curricula.

Starting in the 1980s, changes in the focus of surgical oncology were motivated by patient demands for less mutilating treatment options (e.g., lumpectomy vs radical mastectomy). Over time, this led to a function-preserving emphasis (in selected patients) such as sphincter-preserving operations for gastrointestinal and genitourinary cancers, limb-preserving sarcoma operations, and nerve-sparing prostatectomy. This functional approach to solid tumors has led to a minimally invasive strategy in general surgical oncology, as exemplified by the increased use of laparoscopic techniques for cancer resection. However, such a modus operandi has largely failed to penetrate HNC surgery, with the exception of more widespread use of selective neck dissection and transoral laser excision of laryngeal tumors by some practitioners. In HNC surgical oncology, the popularity of free-flap reconstruction during the 1990s led to the philosophy that there is no longer a need to "scrimp and save" because large organ territories can be resected and adequately reconstructed. The functional validity of these reconstructive techniques has largely been assumed, rather than documented in the literature, however. Although an organ preservation strategy has not developed in the area of HNC surgical oncology for advanced tumors, this is the focus of strategies using various combinations of chemo- and radiotherapy as the initial treatment in patients with advanced (and now less advanced) HNC, in an effort to avoid initial surgery altogether—presumably a response to widespread aversion to the traditional radical, mutilating operations for advanced HNC. The organ preservation strategies of the past 10 to 15 years, synonymous with using nonsurgical combinations of chemo- and radiotherapy in the initial treatment of HNC patients, have become (surprisingly, based on the lack of evidence-based support in their favor), a community standard of care in many parts of the United States.[33] The multimodality management of HNC remains controversial in many aspects, which are beyond the scope of this chapter, but which have been reviewed in the recent literature.[15] For patients who present with advanced cancer that is difficult to cure, maintaining QOL assumes greater importance.

Consistent with this new emphasis in head and neck oncology, QOL studies are now appearing in addition to the omnipresent retrospective cancer treatment reports in the HNC literature. The "state of the art" of HNC QOL is currently to report functional outcomes related to various treatments (only a small component of global QOL/well-being), as well as validating a variety of QOL instruments that assess the general health as well as the disease-specific status of these patients.

There appears to be competition between academic institutions in generating better QOL instruments for HNC patients, and there are a plethora of these.[18,19,34-38,67] Concomitantly, there appears to be little interest in verifying the validity of someone else's instrument. Most published reports are still retrospective in nature, resulting in a large number of studies on small numbers of patients, further complicated by the many stages and natural histories of HNC in different sites. However, there now appears to be a realization that the proper format for QOL data collection is prospective. There is a need to select one good instrument and to apply it uniformly to the HNC population in the form of national prospective studies, in order to produce the type of data that are necessary to generate valid practice guidelines.

In the context of documenting function and relating it to various treatments, the tendency is to generate very sophisticated technical and multivariate analysis such as objective measures of vocal function and to use these data to demonstrate the advantage of one treatment over another. By now, the reader of this chapter should be able to deduce that such high-tech quantitative assessments of function may have relatively little relationship to a patient's perceived QOL, although these measures may have intrinsic interest from a research viewpoint.

A question that arises from recent publications is what to do with anti-intuitive or contradictory results. For example, one study from the University of Chicago[19] found that dry mouth, the most frequent and severe residual effect of the chemoradiotherapy strategy under study, was not associated with the outcome of diet, depression, or QOL. Certainly most treatment managers would expect dry mouth, as well as ongoing pain and fatigue, to be major factors affecting QOL in irradiated HNC patients. Would, or should, such a contradictory result from a single study reverse the impression of years of unsolicited patient testimonials to the contrary? Such anachronistic results highlight the recognized fact that patients under stress have internal adaptive processes that often maintain their QOL at an acceptable level in ways that defy measurement by external criteria and that tend to even out QOL comparisons between apparently very divergent treatments. Despite the adverse effects of therapy, patients often express overall satisfaction with their outcomes, although there are wide variations in individual responses. For some patients, QOL scores may actually increase after treatment because QOL has been compromised by the presence of cancer before treatment. Most patients can accommodate to virtually any treatment-related deficit if it is not too divergent from what they were led to expect, highlighting the importance of generating realistic expectations through patient and family education. If the same anachronistic result is demonstrated repeatedly in the literature, its credibility will increase, leading to change in the perception of the significance of a particular QOL parameter and to refocusing on other areas which have not been considered as important theretofore.

For example, in the HNC QOL literature, the primacy of voice quality has been the major parameter assessed because doctors have considered it most important. Preservation of the larynx has been a primary QOL endpoint to the virtual exclusion of other considerations until recently, although the importance of this factor and the negative impact of surgery in the initial treatment plan have largely been assumed, rather than documented in the literature. For example, functional voice results from the VA study were not published until 7 years[39] after the landmark 1991 study conducted by the Veterans Affairs Laryngeal Cancer Study Group,[40] which launched the nonsurgical organ preservation strategy for patients with advanced HNC. During the interim, a number of articles have documented the fact that an individual HNC patient's overall QOL is not dependent on a particular therapeutic strategy. Treatments as diverse as total laryngectomy, hemilaryngectomy, and radiotherapy for larynx cancer may not differ significantly when QOL assessment is performed,[37] although such findings are undoubtedly counterintuitive to many treatment managers who typically think of surgery as the treatment for HNC most associated with mutilating consequences. It has been widely assumed that postradiation voices are normal, although clinical and experimental evidence now suggests that many patients experience a decrease in voice quality and overall QOL after radiotherapy.[34,41] Such results have also been found in other areas of solid tumor surgical oncology; for example, some sarcoma studies have failed to prove that QOL is higher in patients who have had limb salvage than in those who undergo amputation.[22,42,43]

The fact that such findings are unexpected may relate to the influence of a seminal study published in 1981[30] (that has been widely misinterpreted) in demonstrating the preference of HNC patients for radiotherapy rather than surgery for laryngeal cancer. That study was a utility analysis (time/trade-off technique) in which 37 healthy volunteers (12 firefighters and 25 executives) were asked to choose treatment options based on perceived changes in QOL after treatment with a laryngectomy. The investigators estimated that 20% of subjects would choose a treatment to preserve their larynx, even if it meant potentially shorter survival, related to the perceived decrement in QOL pursuant to laryngectomy. The use of surrogates to respond to questionnaires concerning cancer treatment impact, which they themselves have not experienced, is not considered appropriate by many, and cannot be used as the basis for formulating QOL outcome statements, which by definition concern patient satisfaction.[34,41] Stewart et al.[28] argued, "The decisions on health status and QOL made by healthy volunteers should not be assumed to coincide with the values and decision of patients with laryngeal cancer, who usually have decreased functional status and QOL at the time of decision making." In a pilot study of patients with HNC from New Zealand, a surprisingly high proportion of patients indicated that they would not sacrifice 1 day of their present existence in exchange for a better QOL.[44] According to Morton,[45] "Many patients treated may have disability or dysfunction which a clinician regards as unacceptable, but which may be quite acceptable to the patient who is grateful to be alive and participating."

Two points have now been substantiated by replication in multiple HNC QOL studies (Table 19–2): (1) health care professionals have little ability to predict what is important to patients undergoing various treatments, and (2) the patient's perception of factors affecting QOL often differs significantly from the physician's perspective. In one retrospective study comparing the relative importance of various QOL dimensions as ranked by patients undergoing laryngectomy and by health care professionals, ranking differed significantly between the two groups. Health care professionals ranked impaired communication, self-image, and self-esteem as the most important, whereas patients ranked physical consequences and interference with social activities as the two most important QOL dimensions. To patients, communication was only third and self-image/self-esteem were seventh.[46] These differences may relate to physicians projecting their own values onto patients and responding to QOL questionnaires based on what they consider important. Voice is, admittedly, essential to psychological identity, and having a normal voice is very important to a practicing physician. However, many HNC patients, both male and female, especially in the rural population, tend to be verbally circumspect. To such patients, the loss of a voice that they normally do not use much anyway may not be very significant. In fact, there is considerable evidence that patients who have undergone a total laryngectomy are more bothered by the presence of a stoma with draining secretions than by the loss of voice, which can usually be adequately rehabilitated.[46-48] One study of postlaryngectomy patients using a tracheoesophageal prosthesis (TEP) reported an improvement in speech intelligibility over the preoperative voice.[49]

A recent report[28] demonstrated that the health status of 80 veterans who had undergone treatment for laryngeal cancer (surveyed in 1996), was affected by factors other than voice handicap. Unexpectedly, many patients who had TEP after laryngectomy showed less voice handicap than did patients treated with radiotherapy. Patients who had undergone a laryngectomy actually reported better overall health on a single-item scale than did patients treated with radiotherapy. Pretreatment prediction by experienced speech pathologists was a poor predictor of eventual voice outcome. Additional evidence showed that the "perception of changes in functional status and QOL by health professionals is a poor predictor of the changes reported by patients with laryngeal cancer themselves." These investigators concluded that their data "refute the common perception that sparing the larynx during treatment will result in improvements in verbal communication," noting that "much of the difference in QOL was caused by other [unmeasured] factors." They cited swallowing and airway protection as other relevant issues when considering outcomes after larynx-sparing treatment. Similarly, a long-term single assessment study[27] from the VA trial[40] showed similar speech scores in the group of patients who received chemo- and radiotherapy as those who received total laryngectomy. The former group had better QOL scores, but this was related more to freedom from pain, better emotional well-being, and lower levels of depression than to the preservation of the speech function. Such a single-point, long-term study may be biased because it assesses only long-term survivors who respond to questionnaires, a selected subgroup of patients who have had considerable time to adjust to any treatment-imposed deficits. Such a study would be more useful had comparison points at earlier stages in the treatment sequence been available, and if sequential data had been accumulated in a prospective, longitudinal format.

Some have commented that it is invalid to compare voice handicap and QOL outcomes after different treatments because (1) many studies are retrospective, (2) there is a lack of female patients from Veteran's Administration hospitals, and (3) treatment and voice rehabilitation methods are almost never assigned in a randomized manner, so the possibility for selection bias exists. These objections again emphasize the need for prospective QOL studies. Interestingly, in one QOL study of patients who had total laryngectomy, a preoperative counseling visit by a laryngectomee was the only significant factor determining later QOL/satisfaction.[48] It has been pointed out that identifying the coping strategies of patients who have been through the experience and incorporating them in pretreatment counseling might be useful, especially for patients with poor coping skills.[45]

The importance of factors other than voice, such as problems with diet/swallowing and residual pain,[50] have emerged as significant QOL factors in multivariate HNC QOL studies. A study from the University of Chicago showed that pain relief correlates with better physical functioning, mood, and sense of well-being. In that study, 23% of patients were depressed, and this was associated with past problems related to alcohol abuse.[19] In other QOL studies, about 22% of patient populations screen positive for major depression when tested[51-53]

HNC QOL Perspective: Where Are We Going?

The number of articles addressing QOL in the HNC literature should heighten the awareness of practitioners as to the importance of such considerations, although the current focus is largely still on the rather basic and incomplete aspect of functional status accompanying various cancer treatments. The mind–body–spirit connection is being addressed in the QOL literature at large, although such factors are still largely absent in the HNC literature. Several examples are included in this discussion to illustrate these considerations and how they may be addressed in daily practice. It is easy to anticipate resistance to addressing issues such as religion and spirituality in medicine. Some or many physicians may believe that such considerations are unimportant (except regarding blood transfusions in Jehovah's Witnesses) because they mean little to them personally. However, there is increasing evidence that attention to such concerns is important[54] in the areas of prevention, coping, and recovery.[55]

Although it is unrealistic to expect office time-challenged otolaryngologists–head and neck surgeons who have previously used only closed-ended questioning with patients (i.e., questions that can be answered with a "yes" or "no") to facilitate brief encounters, to suddenly start asking patients whether they are happy, depressed, and alcoholic, and how they feel about their cancer treatment, it is necessary to be aware of the domains encompassed in "well-being" and to be aware of issues relating to patient empowerment. Failure of medical practitioners to concern themselves with such issues is a factor in the burgeoning industry of alternative medicine into which patients are currently pouring billions of dollars and more practitioner visits than to family doctors.[56]

Well-being remains to be clearly defined in patients with altered states of health. It is tentatively defined as a person's perception of life quality, a personal experience that is influenced by both the individual's past experiences and current expectations. This emphasizes the importance of imparting realistic expectations in cancer treatment planning to the patient before treatment is administered. One article illustrates the types of domains that are taken into consideration in attempting such definitions.[25] This study is described in some detail to indicate the complex and sophisticated level to which QOL research has developed, and to illustrate the types of factors currently thought to be relevant and that are probably not typically taken into consideration by many HNC treatment managers. Well-being under a stressful life circumstance such as illness may be mediated by three factors: (1) the extent to which people see themselves as being in control of their environment; (2) the access to, and use of, family, friends, and associates; and (3) judgments one makes concerning self-worth. In formulating a theoretical model to predict subjective well-being, these three factors—presumably related to well-being in individuals diagnosed with cancer—were examined:[32] influence of locus of control, social support, and self-esteem.

It is believed that psychosocial morbidity, of which many clinicians are unaware, is reduced when people have the ability to exercise choice and to retain a sense of self-sufficiency (locus of control), strengthened by support from a social matrix, and the maintenance of self-esteem and integrity. According to Rotter's 1954 social learning theory, an individual's behavioral response to a specific event is contingent on one's locus of control (LOC), which may be internal or external. External LOC relates to luck, to chance, and to "powerful others." Medical personnel are typically conceptualized as the "powerful others," but in Dirksen's study,[25] 25% of subjects express a personal belief that God was in control of the cancer. Therefore, a "powerful other" may also be a religious figure. The importance of LOC is that persons who believe that chance governs an unordered environment will behave differently from those who believe that "powerful others" are in control. Depending on which LOC the patient favors, feeling that "powerful others" are in control of the cancer can either add to or subtract from a sense of well-being. Those who are comfortable with others being in control might find a traditional health care model comforting, in which physicians assume a paternalistic role in the doctor/patient relationship. Those who do not would presumably have enhanced well-being if empowered to make some of their own decisions. The "chance" LOC is often associated with helplessness; a lack of perceived control over life events can result in depression and anxiety, a decreased perception of well-being, and feelings of low self-esteem.

Social support has been hypothesized to play a major role in alleviating stress when illness occurs and is thought to be a good predictor of subsequent well-being.[57] Self-esteem is defined as positive judgment of self-worth and indicates the degree to which a person feels capable, significant, successful, and worthy. Self-worth is based on the ability to influence and control events and the attention received from others. Satisfaction with self-esteem has been identified in some studies as a strong predictor of an individual's perceived well-being. In persons with chronic illness, low self-esteem may have more of an impact on perceived well-being than the disability or the disease itself.

Dirksen's study used several instruments to assess these apparently important aspects of well-being: the cancer health locus of control scale (18 items with 6 in each of 3 locus of control subscales), the Norbeck Social Support Questionnaire and Personal Resource Questionnaire (used to measure the multiple dimensions of social support), and the Self-Esteem Inventory and Index of Well-Being (to measure the cognitive dimensions of subjective well-being, which rates present satisfaction with life on a 7-point continuum). The time required to complete all the questionnaires was approximately 1 hour. It was found that upon finishing, subjects would frequently want to discuss how their life had been affected by the cancer experience. Obviously, such evaluations can be complex and lengthy, and their interpretation is probably not totally within the purview of the cancer clinician. The importance of such factors suggests the need to have someone qualified and interested in psychosocial morbidity (a "psychosocialist") who will listen and be able to interpret as a new team member for the HNC patient.

The mind–body connection is under investigation in many areas of cancer. One hypothesized example is that hormonal and other somatic aspects of depression (including hypercortisolemia) might exert some influence on tumor growth, and molecular mechanisms have been proposed whereby hormone levels can influence the expression of cancer oncogenes in humans related to depression, by analogy with the finding in animals that overactivation of the adrenocorticotropic hormone (ACTH)-cortisol system can lead to more rapid tumor progression.[58] Other postulated mechanisms include the immunosuppressive effects of glucocorticoids. The impact of stress-induced or alcohol-induced immunosuppression in cancer surveillance is also complex, possibly relevant, and deserving of more study.[59] Some studies have shown no association between psychological distress and rate of relapse or mortality from cancer, although it is intuitively logical that suppression of distress, active coping strategies, and psychosocial intervention would be beneficial.

Measuring distress is complex and multifaceted.[58] This subject is not straightforward because patients who try to suppress affect are often, if anything, more anxious and depressed than those who are less defensive. Measures of stress scales may reflect a genuine absence of anxiety, depression, and other symptoms or lack of awareness of such problems or breakthrough of symptoms despite genuine efforts to repress them. The theory holds that people with substantial distress, despite efforts to avoid coming to terms with that distress, are at most risk of stress-induced somatic symptoms. Conversely, some studies have shown that coping styles predict medical outcome, with an attitude characterized as "fighting spirit" associated with longer survival among some cancer patients. There are few answers in this area, but the need to study the effects of psychological intervention on disease progression has been recognized. Clearly, there is a growing interest in the interaction between psychological and medical variables in cancer as well as other diseases. There is a need for better definition of psychological constructs and controlled intervention trials. "It is not simply mind over matter, but instead... in future research, it may be possible to determine how mind does matter."[59]

Patient Empowerment

Outcomes assessment includes an important component relating patient satisfaction to medical care, and there is considerable evidence that patients are more satisfied (Table 19–3) if they have some sense of empowerment; the ability to participate in their own treatment decision making. Patient empowerment is widely considered to have far-reaching beneficial psychological effects in giving the patient a sense of some control over his or

TABLE 19–3
Some Patient Concerns That Influence Satisfaction/Dissatisfaction

Family/spouse relationships
Faith in God
Health/health care
Long life
Sex life
Stress/worry
Unemployment/employability/insurability/financial independence
Government influence
Length of treatment
Financial burden of treatment
Disfigurement
Dysfunction
Substance abuse
Concerns about the future
Inability to do things
Fear, anxiety, depression, anger, loneliness
Survivorship issues

SOURCE: Arrzouman JM, Dudiss S, Farance CE, et al. Quality of life of patients with sarcoma post-chemotherapy. *Oncol Nurs Forum* 1991;18:889–894.

her destiny. There is increasing need to recognize that treatment decisions are not up to the physician; rather, they are the patient's decision. Treatment managers often lose sight of this. A rapidly expanding new literature suggests that patient satisfaction may directly relate to the degree to which the patient is allowed to become involved in decision making concerning the treatment process, and that the more empowered patients are, the more satisfied (and less litigious) they are with the treatment outcome, although the outcome may be what a doctor would consider unfavorable (e.g., cancer recurrence). Again, it is important to be aware that physician and patient opinions on what constitutes an unfavorable treatment outcome may differ significantly. For example, physicians typically consider cancer persistence/recurrence the ultimate unfavorable outcome and fear litigation for failure to control cancer with treatment but this may not occur to a patient who is "satisfied" by having been allowed to participate in treatment decision making, if a choice of treatments exists. Patient satisfaction can also be optimized if treatment managers indicate "up front" that cancer cure cannot be guaranteed—which patients readily understand, in my experience—and also do not make premature statements that the treatment has cured the patient based on initial tumor "response," such as at the conclusion of initial treatment.

The "patient empowerment" trend is in direct contrast to the decades-old paternalistic attitude of doctors who often made treatment decisions without discussing options with the patients or their families, or even indicating that there were treatment options. The classic example is that the patient with cancer was often not told of the diagnosis, although members of the family might have been. There may also be a particular tendency to dehumanize the "typical" HNC patient who has often been somewhat stigmatized by the presumed risk factors associated with the disease. A history of alcoholism, lack of gainful employment, lack of family and social support, poor educational level, etc., may contribute to the impression that patients are not qualified to participate in their own treatment planning, with physicians often assuming that the patient has neither the requisite intelligence, interest, nor reliability. This is documented to some extent by studies that have shown that physicians perceive the need for surrogate studies concerning QOL issues in HNC patients rather than questioning the patients themselves.[60]

During the past decade or two, this attitude has been corrected somewhat by a more concerted attempt to present the patient with available multidisciplinary treatment options by having patients talk to each subspecialist involved. However, the presentation is often heavily biased and may actually represent form more than substance. Physicians may feel that empowering the patient might be construed as a sign of weakness on their part, assuming that patients want a strong authority figure managing their medical care who is always in control and knows exactly what to do (a "powerful other"). It is important that physicians begin to realize that facilitating patient empowerment does not imply weakness on the part of the physician. Physicians can provide an environment of patient empowerment by giving the patient a sense of control; by exhibiting care, concern, and reassurance; and by respecting the patients and their identity in allowing them to participate in the decision-making process. Such factors rank high on patient satisfaction surveys, more so than the impact of technology, as patients can more easily evaluate their interpersonal relationship with their doctor than they can technical expertise.

Another aspect of patient empowerment by physicians is encouraging patients to live a healthy lifestyle, to change their diet, to engage in physical activity, and to eliminate habits that constitute risk factors, as this type of activity can also provide a sense of personal contribution to health and improve well-being. Issues relating to QOL and "well-being" are much more complex and global than assessing the impact of treatment on a particular function (swallowing, airway, voice, appearance) and QOL outcome depends largely on factors relating to the patient (e.g., "will to live," personality, support systems) of which the doctor may have little awareness based on a brief acquaintance with the patient and family.

Another area of oversight on the part of physicians that is being increasingly recognized[54,55] is the impact of religion and spirituality in medicine. In 1910, William Osler wrote about "the faith that heals." Spirituality and research on religious factors in health has become as sophisticated as any other growth area within epidemiology. Recent surveys reveal that nearly 80% of Americans believe in the power of God or prayer to improve the course of illness. Nearly 70% of physicians report religious inquiries for counseling on terminal illness, but only 10% of physicians ever inquire about the patient's religious beliefs or practices. "This oversight is a result of the focus on the etiology of disease and effect of therapies, at the expense of fostering caring and humane concern for patients."[54] Increasingly, medical education is introducing humanistic concepts through curricular innovations in didactic clinical and postgraduate training. Considerable data document that religious commitment may play a positive role in promoting physical and mental health. Religious commitment may help prevent many clinical problems, including depression, substance abuse, physical illness, and early mortality. The impact of religious belief may have significant relevance in the areas of prevention, coping, and recovery of cancer patients. Some researchers have recommended that physicians consider the religious orientations of their patients when designing or implementing a clinical treatment plan. In a recent survey, more than 75% of patients surveyed thought that their physician should address spiritual issues as part of their medical care.[55] Religious considerations may be of new or increased importance to a patient who has received a diagnosis of cancer. Nevertheless, the dichotomy between religion and science has pervaded Western intellectual endeavor for 400 years, and the two will not be amalgamated overnight.

Many currently practicing physicians have not been trained in ways to address such nonscientific patient concerns, but terminology used in Matthews's article[55] can be modified to address a number of such issues. It was suggested that clinicians might ask "is your religion (or faith) helpful to you in handling your illness?" If the answer is yes, they might follow with "what can I do to support your faith or religious commitment?" This might be a "politically correct" way to inoffensively derive information on a variety of sensitive issues. If physicians were to ask these questions more routinely in medical care, they would presumably gain access to potentially valuable information on how to integrate such factors into the care plans of particular patients, especially those suffering from chronic or severe illnesses. An adoption of any of these practices is likely to lead to enhanced quality of care and patient satisfaction. Physicians can also refer patients to clergy or chaplains as an adjunct to standard medical care. The involvement of clergy might be especially important in support of patients who have little social support from family members.

One example of how physicians could more frequently empower HNC patients in participating in their own treatment decisions relates to the controversial management of the N0 neck. The impact of widefield (non-parotid-sparing) radiotherapy even in elective doses (which have progressively increased over the years) is multifactorial (dry mouth, difficulty retaining and gagging on dentures and other intraoral appliances, profound, often long-term fatigue, and appetite disturbances) and presumably has impact on the patient's QOL. This leads to the hypothesis that the QOL of many patients would be enhanced if there were equally effective alternatives to widefield radiotherapy. Admittedly, in some treatment regimens (initial chemoradiotherapy) there is little option to decrease the radiation portals and, even if surgery is the initial treatment, postoperative radiotherapy may need to be widefield in order to provide adequate coverage of the primary resection bed. However, a plan that spares the contralateral parotid could be considered for many lateralized primary tumors with a low incidence of cancer spread to the contralateral neck. The patient could participate in the decision as to whether the opposite neck is operated electively (END), irradiated electively (ENI), or observed expectantly. Although physicians are treatment oriented and generally feel more comfortable with some type of treatment rather than observation, when the evidence-based (scientifically valid) data are examined, it is clear that the issue is still controversial and that any of the three options is acceptable and does not deviate from the "standard of care."[61]

The patient could be presented with numbers relating to the likelihood of cancer recurrence for each of these options, the likelihood of negative consequences (shoulder syndrome with END, xerostomia associated with ENI), as well as the salvageability of recurrent cancer in a neck that has been treated or observed. If one contrasts a likely contralateral incidence of occult lymph node metastases of 15 to 20% on average (which might be controlled by the host immune response), the virtual 100% guarantee of negative consequences related to xerostomia with widefield non-parotid-sparing radiotherapy, the impact of the treatment decision becomes clear. Salvageability of recurrent cancer is often optimized in the "observed" neck, as surgery and postoperative radiotherapy are still available. In one study, recurrent neck cancer was half as common after END as ENI and three times as salvageable in observed as in treated N0 necks.[62] Obviously, allowing patients to talk with others who have had such treatment is also recommended. The patient's choice (treatment vs observation) is likely to relate to their personality and risk-taking tendencies. Some patients may be uncomfortable with the potential for cancer growth and would like to feel that everything possible is being done to prevent it, thus choosing treatment, whereas others may prefer to enjoy the enhanced QOL that presumably accompanies the absence of xerostomia. Such considerations are discussed in more detail in the recent literature.[61]

Conclusion

What can we do to improve QOL in HNC patients now, while we are waiting for documented guidelines to emerge from patient-derived, evidence-based studies (Table 19–4)? The following suggestions seem reasonable based on the current HNC QOL literature:

TABLE 19–4
Recommendations to Enhance QOL of HNC Patients

Attention to the following issues before instituting cancer treatment:

- Set up meeting between prospective patient and other patient(s) who have undergone similar treatment.
- Add a professional counselor to the team managing HNC patients who can address detected problematic areas in more depth than can the busy oncologist.
- Screen for major depression and personality disorders in a psychosocial questionnaire.
- Recognize alcoholism and develop a treatment plan for it before, and subsequent to, institution of cancer treatment.
- Make treatment modifications that presumably optimize QOL (e.g., parotid-sparing postoperative radiotherapy[61]; choice of operation for tongue base cancer[64]).
- Give the patient realistic expectations. Patients can adjust to amazing deficits if prepared. Honesty in describing the likely effects of treatment solidifies the doctor/patient relationship as credibility accrues.

Broaden the scope of post-treatment educational and support group meetings to include common issues of interest to patients with all sites of HNC.

QOL, quality of life; HNC, head and neck cancer.

1. Participate in the acquisition of valid information. Nationwide data collection in the form of simple surveys that amalgamate oncologic, functional, and QOL results (possibly under the auspices of the American Head and Neck Society) could help clarify both optimal cancer treatment and QOL maneuvers relatively quickly. Standardized, prospective, uniform, longitudinal data collection is necessary to accumulate the HNC patient numbers from which conclusions can be drawn, rather than continuing to report institutional experiences using a variety of instruments that vary slightly but not substantially in content.

   By analogy with other ongoing nationwide studies/surveys, such questionnaires could be widely disseminated rapidly using PC software. It is necessary to formulate an appropriate instrument quickly so that uniform outcome data can be collected and collated, before treatment guidelines are dictated by health care agencies that lack the deep expertise of health care professionals.

   Generate an appropriate QOL instrument from the research realm, tailored into a repeatable format that is simple, expeditious, valid, and comprehensible to clinicians (a major challenge). Many of the existing instruments are based on the assumption that physicians know what are the most critical elements in the oncological, functional and QOL outcomes relating to HNC patients. Perhaps it would not be unreasonable to take a short step backward and have patients respond to open-ended, general, unguided questions such as "name five differences between your life before and after cancer treatment" or "five ways in which your life has changed for the better or worse since your cancer treatment." This could be applied to patients who have had the spectrum of contemporary treatments, in order to get an idea as to whether the types of currently measured factors are, in fact, important to HNC patients, rather than just to the doctors who manage them. There is evidence in the literature,[28] reflected in correlation coefficients of <0.5—that there is a large amount of unexplained variance representing unmeasured factors in the existing HNC QOL literature.

   It would be appropriate at this juncture to include new parameters in the staging system for HNC whose importance has been realized in recent years, such as the impact of positive retropharyngeal nodes and the patient's alcohol consumption status,[16, 17] both of which can impact on survival outcomes to a much greater extent than variations in current treatment.

   Ideally, future contributions to the HNC literature should include oncological, functional and eventually QOL data in the same rather than separate manuscripts to provide a more easily accessible overview of the multiple factors which are relevant to the patient's outcome. Adding cost-related factors will add to the complexity.
2. Use the most oncologically effective treatment first in this population. Quality of life and quality of death are opposite sides of the same coin. Presumably both are optimized when the likelihood of locoregional cancer recurrence is minimized. Although many people now perceive that standard treatment for advanced HNC is no longer surgery followed by radiotherapy, but rather initial treatment with some combination of chemotherapy and radiation, Forastiere[63] maintains that a change in the standard of care requires:
   - A high rate of organ preservation to justify the expense, morbidity of chemotherapy, and delay of definitive treatment for the whole population
   - A low requirement for salvage surgery
   - Locoregional failures to be salvageable

   None of these points has been convincingly documented, as extensively discussed in the recent literature.[15]
3. If a spectrum of equivalent options exists within the chosen treatment modality (often difficult to define from the retrospective HNC literature), consider choosing the option that presumably optimizes QOL. For example, in patients with base of tongue tumors, the "organ preservation" operation most discussed in the literature has been total glossectomy with preservation of the larynx. This, however, leaves most patients severely impaired from the viewpoint of verbal communication, unable to taste, and often gastrostomy-dependent. In contradistinction, an operation that carefully mobilizes and preserves one or both hypoglossal nerves, can allow the anterior mobile tongue to be preserved and the base of tongue tumor to be removed in the manner of an "extended total laryngectomy," although sacrificing the larynx. The consequences of the latter operation are likely to be less severe from a QOL viewpoint in most patients who would traditionally be facing a total glossectomy. A patient who has had a total laryngectomy extended to include the base of tongue can take food by mouth, taste the food, and have speech capabilities rehabilitated with a tracheoesophageal puncture if a mobile anterior tongue is preserved. (Many patients with base of tongue tumors can have operations that preserve functional organ territories in both the remaining tongue and the larynx.[64] The validity of a strategy of organ preservation surgery for advanced HNC in several poor prognosis sites has been presented in the recent literature[15]). Similarly, the QOL consequences of the options for managing the N0 neck differ and afford an opportunity for patient choice.
4. Facilitate patient empowerment. It is quite possible that QOL is optimized by allowing patients to participate in their own treatment planning more than by differences in the actual cancer treatments currently available. Truly involving the patient in treatment planning is much more than simply discussing multidisciplinary treatment options with them. The role of the physician can change from paternalistic dictator to one of facilitator and remain just as powerful, if not more so.
5. Physicians should try to avoid projecting their own needs on the patient. An example would be to use toxic treatment plans "off protocol," especially in the palliative setting, due to a perceived "need to do something" that may often relate more to the doctor's needs than to the patient's. One must remember that QOL, by definition, involves the patient's reactions to treatment, not the doctor's.

6. Learn to talk to patients in a manner that will elicit useful information. A strategy as simple as switching from closed-ended to open-ended questions is recommended.[31] A strategy at the initial encounter that includes the sentence, "tell me about yourself and your family," may be all that is necessary to stimulate a lengthy and appropriate response from the patient. Avoid letting family members answer this question for the patient, although you may later specifically direct similar questions to them.
7. Increase attention to the multifactorial consequences of smoking[32] and alcoholism in the HNC patient population.[65,66] This factor has been poorly quantified in the existing retrospective HNC cancer treatment literature. However, new evidence of the seminal importance of the patient's alcohol status on cancer survival[16,17] (a 40 to 50% difference—much larger than any we can currently attribute to variations in cancer treatment), and the fact that reversing a patient's alcoholism can have a positive impact on survival, should furnish compelling reasons to reemphasize the importance of this factor. This impact on survival may relate to optimized nutrition with its beneficial impact on the immune response, to more cohesive family support with less alienation, and to related factors. Alcohol consumption status should possibly be included in the HNC staging system, by analogy with constitutional B symptoms in lymphoma staging.

   Alcohol counseling should be instituted from the outset in HNC patients who need it. Depression in HNC patients prominently relates to alcoholism and has a major impact on compliance with treatment recommendations. Addressing alcoholic patient's rehabilitation from the outset would be expected to have benefits not only with regard to cancer survivorship, but also in improving social interactions with family and engaging the positive processes attendant to rehabilitating such relationships. Therefore, normalizing this aspect of the patient's life appears to be exceedingly important. An interested counselor or other professional who can competently address psychosocial issues in both the alcoholic and nonalcoholic HNC population should be included as a new HNC team member. This team member can also assess and address the spouse's and family's level of psychosocial stress. Family members may have a different assessment of the patient's QOL than that of the patient. Their needs in this regard need to be addressed for their own benefit as well as the patient's.

   Although busy HNC treatment managers will wonder how a pre-treatment consultation with a psychologist can be worked in, a precedent certainly exists, as HNC patients often require pre-treatment evaluation by several team members (e.g., dental, speech/swallowing).
8. Expand support groups to include all HNC patients, in the manner of the "voice clubs" now common for patients who have had total laryngectomy. There is evidence that patients and their spouses who participate in short-term psychosocial and educational group programs report less depression, anxiety, and social isolation (feel they have better control over their lives) and deal more effectively with the illness and with treatment-related problems.[25] Participation in educational seminars, post-treatment resource programs, and support groups may be important variables that influence both QOL and survival. A support group for alcoholics is often neglected but particularly important. Generalized HNC cancer patient support group meetings could address topics of interest regardless of the site of cancer and one could even consider a pre-treatment "support group" meeting to assist in treatment planning that presents options for local and systemic therapy and contact with patients that have had various treatments. Post-treatment support groups could deal with coping mechanisms related to the tracheotomy and G-tube appliances often required, regardless of treatment, and helping patients to adjust to living with the uncertainty of being a cancer patient, as well as to the side effects of the common forms of treatment.
9. Increase attention to QOL assessment before cancer treatment is instituted. Because outcomes reflect inputs, it is intuitively logical that attention to QOL issues should be increased before cancer treatment is decided and instituted, since accurate assessment and patient empowerment in decision making cannot be retroactively instituted. The "garbage in, garbage out" adage is especially relevant here. Giving more attention to assessing the individual patient and his or her family, support mechanisms, personality, educational background, and religious preferences, is indicated as a prerequisite for optimal treatment planning. HNC patients have generally had their condition and symptoms for many months and, in the absence of airway obstruction, there is no need to institute cancer treatment on an emergent basis. Time can be taken to perform the necessary pre-treatment assessments. This involves more than simply preoperative education concerning a given treatment to be instituted (e.g., how to manage a tracheotomy).

Taking additional time before treatment is instituted is not only beneficial from the viewpoint of assessing QOL issues, but also humane. People require time to adjust to the cancer diagnosis and to absorb the treatment options presented. Rapid institution of a treatment protocol may not foster patient well-being. For many years I have used the basic guideline that once I know a patient needs an operation, I like to perform it within 2 weeks. However, I generally do not make any attempt to rush the patient to the operating room, all other things being equal. A 2-week interval allows time for multiple appointments with team members and ensures that information imparted will be remembered by the patient. Such a time interval can help with consideration of patient factors as well as tumor factors. If definitive treatment is begun within 1 week of the initial encounter, there is little opportunity for the treatment managers to familiarize themselves with the patient's personality, family, situation, or personal desires. Such factors have generally not been considered important and have taken a back seat to more traditional aspects of cancer treatment planning. The literature suggests, however, that such factors may be at least as important as the tumor factors typically assessed in planning treatment and heightening awareness of these considerations is, in my opinion, a major contribution of the current emphasis on QOL in the HNC literature. Thus, as appropriate outcome measures for HNC cancer treatment and QOL are being generated, probably the best we can do for our patients right now is to take additional time and effort pretreatment to assess what QOL issues are relevant to the individual patient (based on their input) and facilitate encounters between the new patient and other patients who have had similar treatment.

Although other traditional pretreatment assessments relative to tumor staging will inevitably be considered more important by physicians, the major purpose of this chapter is to direct attention to the fact that other issues may, in fact, be at least as important, if not more so.

REFERENCES

Collins—CHAPTER 19

1. Reinertsen JL. Physicians as leaders in the improvement of healthcare systems. *Ann Intern Med* 1998;128:833–838
2. Cella DF, Cherin EA. Quality of life during and after treatment. *Compr Ther* 1988;14:69–75
3. Cella DF, Tulsky DS, Gray G, et al. Functional assessment of cancer therapy scale: development and validation of the general measure. *J Clin Oncol* 1993;11:570–579
4. Cella DF, Tulsky DS. Quality of life in cancer: definition, purpose, and method of measurement. *Cancer Invest* 1993;11: 327–336
5. Chaturvedi SK, Shenoy A, Prasad KM, et al. Concerns, coping and quality of life in head and neck cancer patients. *Supp Care Cancer* 1996;4:186–190
6. Fletcher AE. Measurement of quality of life in clinical trials of therapy. *Recent Results Cancer Res* 1988;111:216–249
7. Kunkel EJ, Rodgers C, Field HL, et al. Treating the patient who is disfigured by head and neck cancer. *Gen Hosp Psychiatry* 1995;17:444–450
8. McHorney CA. Generic health measurement: past accomplishments and a measurement paradigm for the 21st century. *Ann Intern Med* 1997;127:743–750
9. McQuellon RP, Hurt GJ. The psychosocial impact of the diagnosis and treatment of laryngeal cancer. *Otol Clin North Am* 1997;30:231–241
10. Pfister DG, Ruchlin HS. Outcome and economic issues in head and neck cancer. In: Thawley SE et al., eds. *Comprehensive Management of Head and Neck Tumors.* Vol 1. 2nd ed. Philadelphia: WB Saunders; 1999:296–309
11. Rapoport Y, Kreitler S, Chaitchik S, et al. Psychosocial problems in head-and-neck cancer patients and their change with time since diagnosis. *Ann Oncol* 1993;4:69–73
12. Shapiro CL. Relevance of quality of life assessment to the evaluation of combined-modality therapy. *Semin Surg Oncol* 1993; 9:65–69
13. Welch-McCaffrey D. Cancer, anxiety, and quality of life. *Cancer Nurs* 1985;8:151–158
14. Stockler M, Osaba D, Goodwin P, et al. Validation of the PROSQOLI: a pragmatic outcome measure for clinical trials in advanced prostate cancer. *Proc Am Soc Clin Oncol* 1995;14:244
15. Collins SL. Controversies in multimodality therapy for head and neck cancer: clinical and biologic perspectives. In: Thawley SE, et al., eds. *Comprehensive Management of Head and Neck Tumors.* Vol 1. 2nd ed. Philadelphia: WB Saunders; 1999:157–282
16. Deleyiannis FW-B, Thomas DB, Vaughn TL, Davis S. Alcoholism: independent predictor of survival in patients with head and neck cancer. *J Natl Cancer Inst* 1996;88:542–549
17. Vokes EE, Kies M, Haraf DJ, et al. Induction chemotherapy followed by concomitant chemoradiotherapy for advanced head and neck cancer: impact on the natural history of the disease. *J Clin Oncol* 1995;13:876–883
18. List M, Haraf D, Ciston A, et al. A longitudinal study of quality of life and performance in head and neck cancer patients on a concomitant chemoradiotherapy protocol. Abstract 248. In: *Proceedings of the Fourth International Conference on Head and Neck Cancer*, Toronto. July 1996:120
19. List MA, Mumby P, Haraf D, et al. Performance and quality of life outcome in patients completing concomitant chemoradiotherapy protocols for head and neck cancer. *Qual Life Res* 1997;6:274–284
20. Andersen BL. Surviving cancer. *Cancer* 1994;74(suppl 4): 1484–1495
21. Anderson B, Lutgendof S. Quality of life in gynecologic cancer survivors. *Cancer CA* 1997;47:218–225
22. Arrzouman JM, Dudiss S, Farance CE, et al. Quality of life of patients with sarcoma post-chemotherapy. *Oncol Nurs Form* 1991;18:889–894
23. DeCosse JJ, Cennerazzo WJ. Quality-of-life management of patients with colorectal cancer. *Cancer CA* 1997;47: 198–206
24. Lieke JW, Haferman MD, Johnson JT. Oral pilocarpine for radiation-induced xerostomia: integrated efficacy and safety

results from two prospective randomized clinical trials. *Int J Radiat Oncol Biol Phys* 1995;31:661–669
25. Dirksen SR. Theoretical modeling to predict subjective well-being. *West J Nurs Res* 1990;12:629–643
26. Herr HW. Quality of life in prostate cancer patients. *Cancer CA* 1997;47:207–217
27. Terrell JE, Fisher SG, Wolf GT, et al. Long-term quality of life after treatment of laryngeal cancer. *Arch Otolaryngol Head Neck Surg* 1998;124:964–974
28. Stewart MG, Chen AY, Stach CB. Outcomes analysis of voice and quality of life in patients with laryngeal cancer. *Arch Otolaryngol Head Neck Surg* 1998;124:143–148
29. Tversky A, Kahneman D. The framing of decisions and the psychology of choice. *Science* 1981;211:453–458
30. McNeil BJ, Weichselbaum R, Pauker SG. Speech and survival: tradeoffs between quality and quantity of life in laryngeal cancer. *N Engl J Med* 1981;305:982–987
31. King M, Novik L, Citrenbaum C. *Irresistible Communication: Creative Skills for the Health Professional.* Philadelphia: WB Saunders; 1983
32. Collins SL. Smoking cessation and prevention of head and neck cancer. In: Thawley SE et al., eds. *Comprehensive Management of Head and Neck Tumors.* Vol 1. 2nd ed. Philadelphia: WB Saunders; 1999:346–360
33. Harari PM. Why has induction chemotherapy for advanced head and neck cancer become a U.S. community standard of practice? *J Clin Oncol* 1997;15:2050
34. Bjordal K, Ahlner-Elmquist M, Tollesson E, et al. Development of a European Organization for Research and Treatment of Cancer (EORTC) questionnaire model to be used in quality of life assessments in head and neck cancer patients. *Acta Oncol* 1994;33:879–885
35. Browman GP, Levine MN, Hodson I, et al. The head and neck questionnaire: a morbidity/quality-of-life instrument for clinical trials of radiation therapy in locally advanced head and neck cancer. *J Clin Oncol* 1993;11:863–872
36. Hassan SJ, Weymuller EA Jr. Assessment of quality of life in head and cancer patients. *Head Neck* 1993;15:485–496
37. List MA, Ritter-Sterr CA, Baker TM, et al. Longitudinal assessment of quality of life in laryngeal cancer patients. *Head Neck* 1996;18:1–10
38. Weymuller EA Jr, Ahmad K, Casiano R, et al. Surgical reporting instrument designed to improve outcome data in head and neck cancer trials. *Ann Otol Rhinol Laryngol* 1994;103: 499-509
39. Hillman RE, Walsh MJ, Wolf GT, et al. Functional outcomes following treatment for advanced laryngeal cancer. *Ann Otol Rhinol Laryngol* 1998;172:1–27. Review
40. Veterans Affairs Laryngeal Cancer Study Group. Induction chemotherapy plus radiation compared with surgery plus radiation in patients with advanced laryngeal cancer. *N Engl J Med* 1991;324:1685
41. Bjordal K, Kaasa S. Psychological distress in head and neck cancer patients 7–11 years after curative treatment. *Br J Cancer* 1995;71:592–597
42. Sugarbaker PH, Barossky I, Rosenberg SA, et al. Quality of life assessment of patients and extremity sarcoma clinical trials. *Surgery* 1982;91:17–23
43. Weddington WW Jr, Segraves KB, Simon MA. Psychological outcome of extremity sarcoma survivors undergoing amputation or limb salvage. *J Clin Oncol* 1985;3:1393–1399
44. Morton RP. Quality of life: current status and future directions. In: *Proceedings of the Fourth International Conference on Head and Neck Cancer*, Toronto. July 1996
45. Morton RP. Laryngeal cancer: quality-of-life and cost-effectiveness. *Head Neck* 1997;19:243
46. Mohide EA, Archibald SD, Tew M, et al. Post-laryngectomy quality-of-life dimensions identified by patients and healthcare professionals. *Am J Surg* 1992;164:619–622
47. DeSanto LW, Olsen KD, Perry WC, et al. Quality of life after surgical treatment of cancer of the larynx. *Ann Otol Rhinol Laryngol* 1995;104:763–769
48. Stam HJ, Koopmans JP, Mathieson CM. The psychosocial impact of a laryngectomy: a comprehensive assessment. *J Psychosoc Oncol* 1991;9:37
49. Blom ED, Singer MI, Hamaker HL. A prospective study of tracheoesophageal speech. *Arch Otolaryngol Head Neck Surg* 1986;112:440–447
50. Clinical Practice Guideline. *Management of Cancer Pain: Adults.* AHCTR Publication Number 94-0593. Washington, DC: US Department of Health and Human Services, Agency for Healthcare Policy and Research; 1994
51. Beck A, Beamasderfer A. Assessment of depression: the depression inventory. *Mod Probl Pharmacol Psychiatry* 1974; 7:151–169
52. D'Antonio LL, Long SA, Zimmerman GJ, et al. Relationship between quality of life and depression in patients with head and neck cancer. *Laryngoscope* 1998;108:806–811
53. Henderson JM, Ord RA. Suicide in head and neck cancer patients. *J Oral Maxillofac Surg* 1997;55:1217–1222
54. Levin JS, Larson DB, Puchalski CM. Religion and spirituality in medicine: research and education. *JAMA* 1997;278: 792–793
55. Matthews DA, McCullough ME, Larson DB, et al. Religious commitment and health status. *Arch Fam Med* 1998;7: 118–124
56. Weil A. *Health and Healing.* New York: Houghton Mifflin; 1995
57. Mathieson CM, Logan-Smith LL, Phillips J, et al. Caring for head and neck oncology patients. Does social support lead to better quality of life? *Can Fam Physician* 1996;42: 1712–1720
58. Spiegel D. Psychological distress and disease course for women with breast cancer: one answer, many questions. *J Natl Cancer Inst* 1996;88:629

59. Spiegel D. Psychosocial intervention in cancer. *J Natl Cancer Inst* 1993;85:1198
60. MacKillop WJ, Palmer MJ, O'Sullivan B, et al. The expert surrogate system. In: Williams OJ, ed. *Introducing New Treatments for Cancer: Practical, Ethical and Legal Problems.* New York: John Wiley & Sons; 1992:459
61. Collins SL. Controversies in management of cancer in the neck. In: Thawley SE et al., eds. *Comprehensive Management of Head and Neck Tumors.* Vol 2. 2nd ed. Philadelphia: WB Saunders; 1999:1479–1564
62. Muzaffar K, Collins SL. New perspectives on controversies in the management of the N0 neck. *Br J Cancer* 1998;77:24
63. Forastiere AA. Another look at chemotherapy for organ-preservation in patients with head and neck cancer. *J Natl Cancer Inst* 1996;88:855
64. Collins SL. "Narrow margin" surgery for cancer of the base of tongue: organ preservation, oncological and functional results. Abstract 61. In: *Annual meeting of the Society of Head and Neck Surgeons, Cancun, Mexico.* April 1997:141
65. Fabian MC, Irish JC, Brown DH, et al. Tobacco, alcohol, and oral cancer—the patient's perspective. *J Otolaryngol* 1996;25:88–93
66. U.S. Department of Health and Human Services; National Institutes of Health, National Institute on Alcohol Abuse and Alcoholism. *The Physician's Guide to Helping Patients with Alcohol Problems.* Bethesda, MD: National Institutes of Health; 1995
67. Terrell JE, Nanavati KA, Esclamado RM, et al. Head and neck cancer-specific quality of life. Instrument validation. *Arch Otolaryngol Head Neck Surg* 1997;123:1125–1132

Quality-of-Life Issues in Head and Neck Cancer Management

CHAPTER 20

Jack L. Gluckman and Tapan A. Padhya

Advanced squamous cell cancer of the head and neck presents an enormous challenge to the oncologist. This devastating disease is associated with pain, disfigurement, loss of essential bodily functions, and a tremendous sense of loss of self-image and self-esteem. These events, occurring in patients who usually already suffer from significant comorbidity by virtue of their longstanding self-abuse from excess alcohol and tobacco usage, result in an enormously fragile human being in desperate need of kind and compassionate care from the health care provider.

How best to treat these patients without further adding to their problems and misery is a great source of anguish to the head and neck oncologist and for which there remains no clear-cut solution. There are essentially three options available for treating these patients:

1. An aggressive attempt at cure, understanding clearly the reality that in spite of our best efforts, only a small percentage of these patients can be expected to survive long term—Radical surgery is usually the cornerstone of this approach with adjunct radiation or chemotherapy, or both, usually added. Although most believe that this approach offers the best chance at cure, there is a price to pay, including mutilation and further impairment in quality of life. The question that haunts the surgeon is whether one is doing more harm than good.
2. Purely palliative care—This treatment may be limited to protection of the airway, nutritional support, and pain management. However, occasionally it may consist of radiation or palliative resection (debulking), or both, to improve function and decrease pain. This ultraconservative approach would be used in those cases in which it is believed that although heroic radical surgery is possible, the chances of cure are so slight that it is just not worth the effort or in the patient's best interest to pursue this. Examples may include stomal recurrence after laryngectomy or recurrent nasopharyngeal cancer. Although theoretically this approach can be intellectualized in principle, in practice this philosophy is difficult to implement, as it consists essentially of "giving up" on the patient from the outset and thereby condemning him or her to certain death. This "playing God" is in general an anathema to most contemporary physicians, especially in the absence of any clear-cut indicators that would determine which patients should fall into this category.
3. A compromise "organ-sparing" approach consisting of less aggressive therapy geared to preservation of the vital organs affected by the malignancy, minimizing the cosmetic and functional sequelae—This approach usually consists of using nonsurgical modalities (e.g., chemotherapy and radiation in various combinations) but may use innovative surgical techniques that are modifications or extensions of traditional conservation surgery (e.g., partial laryngectomy procedures). The basic premise of this approach is that the cure rates are equal to the more aggressive approach, but function, cosmesis, and a more meaningful quality of life (QOL) can be preserved.[1-17] Unfortunately, it remains unclear that this is an accurate assumption. Survival rates may be compromised and the promise of improved QOL may not be realized. This approach remains a work in progress, and it may be many years before the answer to this question is available.

While we await clarification of this debate, the question of what to offer our patients remains. The oncologist clearly wishes to do the right thing, that is, to optimize the chances of cure without causing the patient unnecessary harm. Unfortunately, no body of scientific evidence clearly supports one approach over another, and the "experts" remain divided in their approach. Likewise, no prognostic indicators (biomarkers) are yet available that can accurately predict tumor behavior sufficiently to convincingly dictate one approach over another. The oncologist is therefore compelled to rely on experience and instinct in managing these patients, together with the patient's physical and emotional state, as well the characteristics of the tumor—hardly the most scientific of approaches in making these life-altering decisions.

Evaluation of Therapy in Advanced Head and Neck Cancer

As we ponder which of the approaches to advocate for our patients, it is important to have clear in our mind what ultimately determines success. Survival has always been the gold standard by which a particular therapy has been judged. However, in these advanced cancers there is no clear-cut evidence that any one approach offers a better chance at survival. In fact, as stated by Weymuller in 1994,[18] "using the therapeutic end points of survival and loco-regional control, it is true that no multi-institutional study that has utilized surgery as a form of treatment has demonstrated a significant separation between the control and distant arms." Yet it remains the impression of most surgical oncologists that this is incorrect and that in most situations those who undergo radical surgery have a better chance at survival and better palliation but without real scientific data to support this.

If survival cannot be used as an endpoint, the morbidity associated with these approaches needs to be compared. Radical surgery is certainly associated with significant functional deficits, as is radical radiation with or without chemotherapy. Comparing the deficits after the different approaches would be useful, but this can be quite difficult given the myriad of surgical and reconstructive procedures available and the different organ preservation approaches used.

The increased sophistication of the reconstructive techniques employed following radical ablative surgery has certainly leveled the playing field in comparing the radical and organ preservation approaches resulting in improvement of not only cosmesis but function as well (e.g., pharynx, esophagus, mandible, and skin defects of the head and neck).[19] Some structures (e.g., tongue and larynx) defy meaningful reconstruction, and it is cancer of these structures that creates the greatest therapeutic dilemma. Using function and form after radical ablation with reconstruction and organ preservation approaches may be impossible as often the organ saved may be dysfunctional.

In the final analysis, it appears that the ultimate goal sought after treating these patients with advanced cancer is a meaningful QOL for their remaining days. What exactly constitutes this quality and whether we best achieve it by radical surgery, organ preservation approaches, or merely palliating the symptoms remain elusive issues; however, real efforts are now being made to clarify this.

Quality of Life

What exactly constitutes QOL? It is not equivalent to functional status, rather, it is a complex sense of well-being related to expectations, perception, experience, religion, and community and is dependent on actual outcome, duration of survival, support systems, and the patient's relationship with the physician. Cella[20] describes QOL as "representing the gap between one's actual functional level and one's ideal standard." He regards QOL as having two basic components: subjectivity and multidimensionality. Subjectivity relates to the patient's cognitive processing of basic concepts like perception of one's illness, perception of treatment options, expectations from self and the estimation of morbidity and mortality.

Multidimensionality encompasses four areas: (1) physical well-being, which includes disease symptoms, treatment toxicity, and the patient's sense of well-being; (2) functional well-being, which relates to the patient's ability to accomplish personal needs, ambitions and family integration; (3) emotional well-being, defined as a bipolar entity (i.e., reflecting a positive affect versus negative affect or distress); and (4) social well-being, a constellation of measures that are hard to quantify, including social support, family dynamics, financial status, and sexual intimacy.

Once one understands the concepts of QOL, the next step is to appreciate that it is now possible to measure QOL with reasonable accuracy. Numerous QOL instruments (questionnaires) have been developed both for general health and for specific disease.[21-37] By necessity, these instruments have been designed to be consistent across socioeconomic class and cultural differences.[35] In administering these tests, it is important to appreciate that the health care provider's and the patient's perception of QOL are significantly different. Disease recurrence and survival tend to be the focus of the provider, whereas the patient feels that functional status and self-image are paramount. Therefore, the best QOL measures are evaluated not by the provider but rather by patient self-reporting, by either an interview or questionnaire format. In general, the patient self-administered questionnaire has proved the best and least time-consuming. Ideally, QOL should be measured (1) at pretreatment, (2) at the midpoint of treatment, (3) immediately posttreatment, and (4) at varying intervals in follow-up management. In head and neck cancer patients, the optimal intervals are not yet clarified.

A large body of work has documented the psychosocial issues, functional capabilities, and communicative skills of the patient with head and neck cancer.[38-51] In addition, over the past 10 years, multiple QOL instruments have been developed specifically designed for patients with head and neck cancer. The most significant of these include the EORTC QLQ-30 for head and neck, FACT-H&N, University of Washington QOL, and PSS-H&N.[22,28,33,34] These instruments look at swallowing, communication, local discomfort, and pain. In spite of scientific validation of these general and disease-specific instruments, the medical community, and particularly surgeons, have been slow to accept the results of these studies or to incorporate them in their practices. The reasons include a lack of familiarity with these studies, the fact that they are time-consuming to administer, and a reluctance to accept that the patient's perception of outcome is as important as the physician's.

It is vital for oncologists to appreciate that the only way that meaningful therapeutic decisions regarding the patient's well-being can be made is to incorporate these QOL instruments into our decision-making algorithm. These instruments will go a long way toward eliminating personal and specialty bias and enable us to do "the right thing" for our patients. It is only after this has been done that we can remotely hope to address the more formidable societal issue of the cost-effectiveness of these therapies.

REFERENCES

Gluckman and Padhya—CHAPTER 20

1. Lavertu P, Adelstein DJ, Saxton JP, et al. Aggressive concurrent chemoradiotherapy for Squamous cell head and neck cancer. *Arch Otolarynogol Head Neck Surg* 1999;125:142–148
2. Corvo, R, Sanguineti G, Benasso M. Biological and clinical implications for multimodality treatment in patients affected by squamous cell carcinoma of the head and neck. *Tumori* 1998;84:217–222
3. Harrison LB, Lee HJ, Pfister DG, et al. Long term results of primary radiotherapy with/without neck dissection for squamous cell cancer of the base of tongue. *Head Neck* 1998;20:668–673
4. Lefebvre JL. Larynx preservation—the discussion is not closed. *Otolaryngol Head Neck Surg* 1998;118:389–393
5. Vokes EE. Enhancing the therapeutic index of concomitant chemoradiotherapy for head and neck cancer. *Ann Oncol* 1998;9:471–473
6. Kies MS, Haraf DJ, Athanasidis I, et al. Induction chemotherapy followed by concurrent chemoradiation for advanced head and neck cancer—improved disease control and survival. *J Clin Oncol* 1998;16:2715–2721
7. Brizel DM, Albers ME, Fisher SR, et al. Hyperfractionated irradiation with or without concurrent chemotherapy for locally advanced head and neck cancer. *N Engl J Med* 1998;338:1798–1804
8. Lefebvre JL, Chevalier D, Luboinski B, et al. Larynx preservation in Pyriform sinus cancer—preliminary results of a European Organization for Research and Treatment of Cancer Phase III trial. *J Natl Cancer Inst* 1996;88:890–899
9. Vokes EE, Haraf DJ, Mick R, et al. Induction chemotherapy followed by concomitant chemoradiotherapy for advanced head and neck cancer—impact on the natural history of the disease. *J Clin Oncol* 1995;13:876–883
10. Shirinian MH, Weber RS, Lippmann SM, et al. Laryngeal preservation by induction chemotherapy plus radiotherapy in locally advanced head and neck cancer—the M.D. Anderson Cancer Center experience. *Head Neck* 1994;16:39–44
11. Wolf GT, Hong WK, Fisher SG, et al. Induction chemotherapy plus radiation compared with surgery plus radiation in patients with advance laryngeal cancer. *N Engl J Med* 1991;324:1685–1690
12. Karp DD, Vaughan CW, Carter R, et al. Larynx preservation using induction chemotherapy plus radiation therapy as an alternative to laryngectomy in advanced head and neck cancer—long term followup report. *Am J Clin Oncol* 1991;14;273–279
13. Demard F, Chauvel P, Santini J, et al. Response to chemotherapy as justification for modification of the therapeutic strategy for pharyngolaryngeal carcinomas. *Head Neck* 1990;12: 225–231
14. Adelstein DJ, Sharan VM, Earle AS, et al. Long term results after chemoradiotherapy for locally confined squamous cell head and neck cancer. *Am J Clin Oncol* 1990;13:440–447
15. Chang TM. Induction chemotherapy for advanced head and neck cancers—a literature review. *Head Neck* 1988;10:150–159
16. Clavel M, Cognetti F, Dodion P, et al. Combination chemotherapy with methotrexate, bleomycin, and vincristine with or without cisplatin in advanced squamous cell carcinoma of the head and neck. *Cancer* 1987;60:1173–1177
17. Al-Sarraf M, Pajal TF, Marcial VA, et al. Concurrent radiotherapy and chemotherapy with cisplatin in inoperable squamous cell carcinoma of the head and neck—an RTOG study. *Cancer* 1987;59:259–265
18. Weymuller EA Jr. Moratorium on multi-institutional head and neck cancer trials. *Head Neck* 1994;16:529–530
19. Urken ML, Buchbinder D, Weinberg H, et al. Functional evaluation following microvascular oromandibular reconstruction of the oral cancer patient—a comparative study of reconstructed and nonreconstructed patients. *Laryngoscope* 1991;101:935–950
20. Cella DF. Quality of life—concepts and definition. *J Pain Symp Mgmt* 1994;9:186–192
21. Clements KS, Rassekh CH, Seikaly H, et al. Communication after laryngectomy—an assessment of patient satisfaction. *Arch Otolaryngol Head Neck Surg* 1997;123:493–496
22. Aaronson NK, Ahmedzai S, Bergman B, et al. The European Organization for Research and Treatment of Cancer QLQ-C30: a quality of life instrument for use in international clinical trials in oncology. *J Natl Cancer Inst* 1993;85:365–375
23. Cella DF, Tulsky DS, Gray G, et al. The functional assessment of cancer therapy scale: development and validation of the general measure. *J Clin Oncol* 1993;11:570–579
24. Terrell JE, Fisher SG, Wolf GT, et al. Long-term quality of life after treatment of laryngeal cancer. *Arch Otolaryngol Head Neck Surg* 1998;124:964–971
25. Terrell JE, Nanavati KA, Esclamado RM, et al. Head and neck cancer—specific quality of life (instrument validation). *Arch Otolaryngol Head Neck Surg* 1997;123:1125–1132
26. Ruhl CM, Gleich LL, Gluckman JL. Survival, function, and quality of life after total glossectomy. *Laryngoscope* 1997;107: 1316–1321
27. Long ST, D'Antonia LL, Robinson EB, et al. Factors related to quality of life and functional status in 50 patients with head and neck cancer. *Laryngoscope* 1996;106:1084–1088
28. List MA, D'Antonio LL, Cella DF, et al. The performance status scale for head and neck cancer patients and the functional assessment of cancer therapy—head and neck scale. *Cancer* 1996;77:2294–2301

29. List MA, Ritter-Sterr CA, Baker TM, et al. Longitudinal assessment of quality of life in laryngeal cancer patients. *Head Neck* 1996;18:1–10
30. D'Antonia LL, Zimmerman GH, Cella DF, et al. Quality of life and functional status measures in patients with head and neck cancer. *Arch Otolaryngol Head Neck Surg* 1996;122:482–487
31. DeSanto LW, Olsen KD, Rohe DE, et al. Quality of life after surgical treatment of cancer of the larynx. *Ann Otol Rhinol Laryngol* 1996;104:763–769
32. Bjordal K, Kassa S, Mastekassa A. Quality of life in patients treated for head and neck cancer—a followup study 7 to 11 years after radiotherapy. *Int J Radiat Oncol Biol Phys* 1994;28:847–856
33. Hassan SJ, Weymuller EA: Assessment of quality of life in head and neck cancer patients. *Head Neck* 1993;15:485–496
34. Bjordal K, Kaasa S. Psychometric validation of EORTC core quality of life questionnaire, 30-item version and a diagnosis-specific module for head and neck cancer patients. *Acta Oncol* 1992;31:311–321
35. Aaronson NK, Meyerowitz BE, Bard M, et al. Quality of life research in oncology—past achievements and future priorities. *Cancer* 1991;67:839–843
36. Mohide EA, Archibald SD, Tew M, et al. Postlaryngectomy quality of life dimensions identified by patients and health care professionals. *Am J Surg* 1992;164:619–622
37. Dropkin MJ, Malgady RG, Scott DW, et al. Scaling of disfigurement and dysfunction in postoperative head and neck patients. *Head Neck* 1983;6:559–570
38. Schuller DE, Bier CM, Sharma PK, et al. Tissue conserving surgery for prognosis, treatment and function preservation. *Laryngoscope* 1998;108:1599–1604
39. Morton RP. Laryngeal cancer—quality of life and cost effectiveness. *Head Neck* 1997;19:243–250
40. Acherstaff AH, Hilgers FJM, Aaronson NK, et al. Communication, functional disorders and lifestyle changes after total laryngectomy. *Clin Otolaryngol* 1994;19:295–300
41. Devins GM, Stam HJ, Koopmans JP. Psychosocial impact of laryngectomy mediated by perceived stigma and illness intrusiveness. *Can J Psychiatry* 1994;39:608–616
42. Jones E, Lund VJ, Howard DJ, et al. Quality of life of patients treated surgically for head and neck cancer. *J Laryngol Otol* 1992;106:238–242
43. Maas A. A model for quality of life after laryngectomy. *Soc Sci Med* 1991;33:1373–1377
44. Koster META, Bergsma J. Problems and coping behaviour of facial cancer patients. *Soc Sci Med* 1990;30:569–578
45. Mathieson CM, Henderikus JS, Scott JP. Psychosocial adjustment after laryngectomy—a review of the literature. *J Otolaryngol* 1990;19:331–336
46. Breitbart W, Holland J. Psychosocial aspects of head and neck cancer. *Semin Oncol* 1988;15:61–69
47. Pruyn JF, de Jong PC, Bosman LJ, et al. Psychosocial aspects of head and neck cancer—a review of the literature. *Clin Otolarygol* 1986;11:469–474
48. Morton RP, Davies ADM, Baker J, et al. Quality of life in treated head and neck cancer patients. *Clin Otolaryngol* 1984;9:181–185
49. Stevens MH, Gardner JW, Parkin JL, et al. Head and neck cancer survival and life-style change. *Arch Otolaryngol* 1983;109:746–749
50. Harwood AR, Rawlinson E. The quality of life of patients following treatment for laryngeal cancer. *Int J Radiat Oncol Biol Phys* 1983;9:335–338
51. Gates GA, Ryan W, Cooper JC, et al. Current status of laryngectomee rehabilitation—results of therapy. *Am J Otolaryngol* 1982;3:1–7

Quality-of-Life Issues in Head and Neck Cancer Management

CHAPTER 21

Nancy L. Snyderman

I have vivid memories as a little girl of taking my father's otolaryngology textbooks from the shelf and looking for hours at the faces staring back at me. There were the black-and-white photos of people missing chins, cheekbones, and eyes. I saw pictures of forearms sewn to foreheads and great tubes of skin bridging a shoulder to a cheek. "Andy Gumps" shared their profiles, and patients with tracheostomes and pharyngostomes posed for the camera. Each description was more poetic than the other. The text referred to how tumors were resected, how long a forearm would stay in this less than natural position, and when the staged flap would be completed.

The procedures were heralded, with technical wonders and cures spoken of interchangeably. How to take things apart and put them back together again was the focus. Cure was the goal. I was comforted in knowing that the people on these pages were being treated by the best surgeons in the field. These steps were necessary in saving their lives. But at that tender age, the curiosity was one of peering in someone else's window. I never asked the obvious questions. Did they go outside looking like this? Did they stay in the hospital away from family and friends? Did they know other people who looked just like they did? Did they ever get depressed and wonder whether it was all worth it?

This was an era in which the patient was not invited to be part of the decision-making process, and issues of quality of life took a back seat to getting the patient and tumor separated. I found the pictures fascinating in a macabre way and did not understand in my youth how those pictures would later affect my life as a head and neck surgeon.

Twenty years later, I began my career as most young, aggressive head and neck surgeons do. I considered the whole "world preop" and a personal failure if I could not find a protocol for each of my patients to fit into. I quite easily divorced the physical from the spiritual. After all, I could always call in the social worker or psychiatrist if a patient was having trouble coping or getting the blues. Rarely did we talk about the bigger psychosocial issues before scheduling a patient for surgery. There was this unspoken assumption that if the tumor could be resected, the patient would manage without his larynx or the ability to swallow the steak that had been a part of Friday night ritual for most of his adult life.

It is true that we celebrate our successes but we learn from our failures. One of my most striking failures came early in my career and smacked me in the face with the overriding issues of quality of life when taking care of the patient with a head and neck malignancy.

As a young staff surgeon, I performed a routine composite resection on a farmer with a squamous cell cancer of the retromolar trigone. The operation went without a hitch, and he segued into postoperative life, able to swallow and talk. I considered him an early success. I thought I was listening, he seemed to trust me, and yet I slid into what I now call a doctor/patient disconnect. I lost the ability to really hear.

He started complaining of pain that radiated from the surgical site over his occiput. I scanned him, and scoped him, and assured him that there was no sign of tumor. I gave him one of my "buck up Bucky" pep talks and sent him on his way. The following Saturday night I got a call from the emergency room that my patient had just been brought in. He had put a shotgun in his mouth and blown his head off. He had been depressed, in pain, and very ashamed of the way he looked. I never got it. What I considered a cure, he considered a huge stone wall. I offered him a skilled surgical team and missed the mark.

Today, the issues are not particularly different. We must consider cure and try to figure out a way to achieve it, but no longer at the cost of everything else. Quality of life refers to quality of our patients' lives—not ours. It means putting patients back in the middle where they belong and encouraging them to be a vocal part of the team. It means really listening and knowing when to stop treatment. It means putting the entire body back together again and treating the patient as a whole—the physical, emotional, and spiritual parts that should never have been dismembered in the first place.

In many ways the public has driven the discussion of death and dying and quality of life issues and has forced us to come along with them. Best-selling books such as *How We Die* and *The Final Exit* have urged patients to take control of the decision making in the final days of life, just as they would for other everyday matters. Although the physician has not always been comfortable with such topics, the public discourse has not gone away, nor will it. In fact, it has taken on new extremes with very in-your-face spectacles of Dr. Jack Kevorkian and television shows like *60 Minutes* showing a physician-assisted suicide (some would say murder). The length of life has taken a back seat to the quality of life. States are putting referenda on the ballots that would allow doctors to assist their patients in their deaths. It is not uncommon for the average person to have a health care proxy or someone designated as a power of attorney for health care decisions. Why? It all comes back to the quality of one's life. How you and I define it may be quite different. But it doesn't take long to figure out what you would allow to have done to you in the name of a cure and what you would be willing to walk away from.

In treating the patient with head and neck cancer, the results of treatment are usually there for everyone to see. That makes our task as the patient advocate all the more important. Everyday, all of us do three things we take for granted. We speak, breathe, and swallow. Unfortunately, with many of the modalities we use in treating a patient with a head and neck tumor, one or all of those things will be altered, many times forever. A 32-year-old district attorney with a cancer of the tongue begs you to get rid of the cancer but to return her to the courtroom. A vintner with a lesion of the nasopharynx pleads with you to treat the tumor but to preserve his sense of smell. A ballerina with a cancer of the larynx implores you to save her airway so she can continue to dance. No case comes with promises. But the failure of the physician not to listen to the underlying concerns of the patient means that we fail in the doctor–patient relationship. And when we fail there, the cure becomes secondary.

So what is our role? I believe it is multifaceted. First and foremost, we are the patient's advocate. The patient's concerns and well-being come before anything else. The patient comes to us for direction and wants to know what we would do. In that regard, I imagine the patient as my brother or sister. Would I urge a family member to have the same operation I am considering for this patient, or is this a time to assess the problem and offer nonoperative treatment?

The second role is to be a good listener. The importance of listening to the patient has not changed since the days of Osler. Listen to the patient and he will tell you not only what is wrong, but the concerns he has about treatment and the quality of his life.

The third role of the physician is to be honest. We have a responsibility not to delude. We know the fine line between being a cheerleader and keeping someone's hopes alive and lying about what the outcome may be. The tact and forthrightness of the conversation will change with the psychiatric makeup of each patient and with the timeline of the course of treatment. But the underlying responsibility is not to the protocol, or the patient's family, or to your whim. It is to the patient who entrusts you with guiding him through complicated surgery and the psychological repercussions that can follow.

Along the way, don't forget the power of touch. After the drains are out and the dressing is off, take a moment. A minute sitting on the patient's bed will seem like a half-hour to her. Touching a hand or shoulder connects the healer to the patient in a way that an examination never can.

We tend to minimize such simple acts, but they lay the groundwork for the quality of our treatment and have a profound psychological impact on how the patient perceives his role as patient and yours as the physician. The quality of life issues don't start 3 weeks after a patient is discharged from the hospital. They start in your examining room and are bridged by your attitudes and by nonverbal communication during hospitalization and long after. The challenge is to recognize these moments and use them.

The great physicians never stop learning, and recognize the roles our patients play as teachers. It is our responsibility to pause occasionally and reflect on what we know works, what doesn't, and what new avenues might be explored. It is our role to help balance the quality of our patients' lives. Their struggle should be our primary concern. To miss the opportunities to guide, to listen, to heal, and to learn, with the quality of life always in the forefront, is to miss one of the richest rewards of being a doctor.

SUGGESTED READINGS

Snyderman—CHAPTER 21

Bronheim H, Strain JJ, Biller HF. Psychiatric aspects of head and neck cancer. Part 1. New surgical techniques and psychiatric consequences. *Gen Hosp Psychiatry* 1991;13:165

Conley J. Rights of the dying patient. *Arch Otolaryngol* 1969; 90:405

DeSanto LW, Olsen KD, Perry WC, Rohe DE, Keith RL. Quality of life after surgical treatment of cancer of the larynx. *Ann Otol Rhinol Laryngol* 1995;104:763–769

Kubler-Ross E. *On Death and Dying*. New York: Macmillan; 1969

Lucente FE. Thanatology: a study of 100 deaths. *Trans Am Acad Ophthalmol Otolaryngol* 1972;76:334–339

Lucente FE. Psychiatric problems in otolaryngology. *Ann Otolaryngol* 1973;82:340–346

Lucente FE. Psychological problems in otolaryngology. *Laryngoscope* 1973;83:1684–1689

Lucente FE. Psychological impact of ENT disorders. *Med Times* 1978;106(9):87–94

Lucente FE. Treatment of head and neck carcinoma with noncurative intent. *Am J Otolaryngol* 1994;15:99–102

Lucente FE, Fleck S. A study of hospital anxiety in 408 medical and surgical patients. *Psychosom Med* 1972;34:304–312

Lucente FE, Strain JJ. Psychological implications of laryngeal disease and laryngectomy. In: Fried M, ed. *The Larynx: A Multidisciplinary Approach*. Boston: Little, Brown; 1988: 615–623

Lucente FE, Strain JJ. Wyatt D. Psychological problems in the head and neck tumor patient. In: Thawley SE, Panje WR, eds. *Comprehensive Management of Head and Neck Tumors*. Philadelphia: WB Saunders; 1987:69–79

Lucente FE, Joseph EM, Weiner ED. Psychiatric and ethical issues in patients with head and neck cancer. In: *Comprehensive Management of Head and Neck Tumors*. vol 1. 1999:310–320

Terrell JE, Fisher SG, Wolf GT. Long-term quality of life after treatment of laryngeal cancer. *Arch Otolaryngol* 1998;124:964–971

8

Static versus Dynamic Management of the Paralyzed Face

"In our practice Gore-Tex suspension has become the primary modality for management of facial paralysis against which other techniques must show significant superiority before being recommended to patients."

Kevin A. Shumrick

"When assessing which procedure(s) to perform, one should not simply look at the problem as dynamic vs. static reanimation of the entire face. Rather, it is best to approach the analysis by dividing the regions of the face to be reanimated into upper third, middle third, and lower lip, then determine the functional deficits, cosmetic deformity in each region, and the patient's desires."

Maisie L. Shindo

"There is a role for muscle transfer even in the setting of expected nerve recovery, and there is a role for static procedures even in patients who are a good anesthesia risk, who have isolated functional complaints relative to their facial palsy."

Mack L. Cheney

Static versus Dynamic Management of the Paralyzed Face

CHAPTER 22

Kevin A. Shumrick

The facial muscles are the only muscles of the human body that have direct connections to the overlying integument. Using these connections, the facial muscles are able to perform a variety of functions of both physiologic and sociologic importance. Physiologically, the facial muscles provide sphincters for the eye and mouth that are crucial for eye protection, eating, drinking, and speaking. The facial muscles also function to modify the diameter of the nostrils, affecting breathing through the nose. Although these functional considerations are important, they are perhaps overshadowed by the role played by the human face in social interactions. The human face is unique across the animal kingdom because of its ability to express a wide range of emotions and intents. In lower animals, facial expressions are used primarily to express anger or aggression. The human face is capable of clearly signaling to other humans the four major emotions—fear, anger, happiness, and sadness—as well as more subtle nuances—sympathy, disgust, amusement, disbelief, and surprise. Facial expressions have clearly evolved to aid in the social interaction of humans. Paralysis of the face significantly compromises an individual's ability to function effectively in society. Patients with a facial paralysis have a distinctly abnormal appearance, which makes others uncomfortable. Human societies have always tended to marginilize those who are considered "different." In addition, there may be the unspoken fear that whatever is affecting the face is contagious and, as a result, routine physical contact, such as handshaking, is avoided. The appearance of a paralyzed face is often interpreted as one of anger or disapproval, which can be intimidating to others, especially children. Patients with a facial paralysis typically avoid having photos taken and eventually drop out of a family's photographic record. Also, patients with a facial paralysis begin to avoid social functions and family gatherings. Social isolation may be compounded at the workplace, where job advancement, and even hiring, may be adversely affected.

Goals of Rehabilitating the Paralyzed Face

Facial paralysis has two major consequences: loss of volitional facial muscle motion and loss of baseline muscle tone. The loss of muscle motion leads to the functional debilities noted with facial paralysis, such as the inability to blink, to purse the lips, and to flare the nostrils. The loss of baseline facial muscle tone is responsible for many of the changes in facial appearance associated with facial paralysis, such as drooping of the ipsilateral face and deviation of the nose to the contralateral side. The ultimate goal of rehabilitating the paralyzed face would be to restore normal facial tone and function. However, it must be recognized by both physician and patient that no single technique (or combination of techniques) will restore normal facial tone and motion. It is the responsibility of the treating physician to be knowledgeable with regard to the various treatment options and to present these options to the patient in such a fashion that an informed decision may be made by the patient. For example, an 80-year-old individual with facial paralysis and multiple medical problems may be very satisfied with simple restoration of eyelid closure alone, whereas a 25-year-old individual may strive to have every nuance of facial motion restored. It remains for the surgeon to weigh the therapeutic options available against what is appropriate for each patient.

Management of the Paralyzed Eye

Most of the changes associated with facial paralysis are not life-, or even health-, threatening and are primarily quality-of-life issues. However, the ability to blink and lubricate the eye is crucial to providing a stable and comfortable eye. Toward this end, upper lid loading with gold weights and lower lid tightening have supplanted older techniques, such as slings and springs. Therefore, management of the paralytic eye is not discussed further in this section.

Methods of Rehabilitating the Paralyzed Face

The closer one is to restoring the facial nerve to its native state, the closer to a normal-appearing and functioning face will be the result. The best results are obtained on patients with facial paralysis who have an intact nerve with mild neuropraxia; the worst results occur in cases in which the integrity of the facial nerve is completely lost. There is no question that if the nerve is transected, but the proximal and distal ends are available, either a primary anastamosis or interposition nerve graft is preferable. However, if the continuity of the nerve cannot be reestablished then there are three possible conventional solutions: hypoglossal to facial nerve crossover, temporalis muscle transposition, and static facial suspension. Free muscle transfer with cross-facial nerve grafting has been mentioned in the literature, but the numbers are low and results sporadic. Although free muscle transfer may be a mainstream choice in the future, it is probably best reserved for young patients with no other options.[1-4]

Hypoglossal to Facial Nerve Transfer

The hypoglossal to facial nerve transfer has been a popular choice for facial reanimation because it reestablishes neuronal impulses to the facial muscles and supplies a base line resting tone. However, simply regaining tone and some facial motion does not ensure a satisfactory outcome. With hypoglossal to facial transfer, it is very rare for a patient to regain any movement that could be considered spontaneous or emotive. In fact, it is rare for patients to achieve voluntary movement of discrete regions of the face; instead, they have mass motion of all ipsilateral facial muscles. Those few patients likely to regain control of individual regions of the face are highly motivated, undergo extensive training, and, most importantly, have the crossover performed early (within 2 years) after injury to the facial nerve.[5,6] A review of several large series of patients with hypoglossal to facial nerve transfers shows that patients obtain "excellent" results only approximately 40 to 50% of the time.[7-9] The major reasons for a less-than-excellent result with hypoglossal to facial nerve transfers are synkinesis, facial movement on eating or talking, hypertonicity with excessive resting tone, and exaggerated movement with attempts at volitional movement. The hypertonicity and synkinesis can be so severe and the appearance of the face so grotesque (particularly with eating, where the face moves in concert with the motions of the tongue) that it becomes a deformity rivaling the original facial paralysis in terms of disability. In addition, when the entire hypoglossal nerve is sacrificed, there is a certain degree of morbidity due to the resultant hemitongue flaccidity, and eventual tongue atrophy, which may cause difficulty with speaking, eating, and swallowing. The actual incidence of significant postoperative morbidity varies from series to series, but it may be as high as 74% of patients.[9] The hypoglossal facial nerve jump graft, in which a cable graft is sewn to a partially transected hypoglossal nerve and distal end of the facial nerve, described by May et al.[10] would theoretically alleviate many of the shortcomings of the hypoglossal facial crossover by intentionally limiting the strength of the hypoglossal neuronal input and preserving most of the hypoglossal connections to the tongue. However, other surgeons are reporting difficulty obtaining significant facial movement with this technique (G.B. Hughes, personal communication, 1996).

Temporalis Muscle Transposition

Contiguous muscle transposition for restoration of facial tone and movement has been a popular alternative to hypoglossal facial crossover, particularly when the distal nerve is not available or the patient is being treated on a delayed basis. The masseter muscle has been mentioned as a possible donor site, but most current investigators consider this muscle a poor choice because of its short length and suboptimal direction of pull. Temporalis muscle transposition has traditionally been the procedure of choice for facial reanimation if a hypoglossal to facial nerve crossover was not an option. Use of the temporalis muscle for facial reanimation is relatively straightforward and, despite a number of possible complications, they are usually minor. However, there are several shortcomings of temporalis muscle transposition for management of facial paralysis: (1) a temporal depression is left from transfer of the muscle; (2) the bulk of the muscle over the zygoma is usually quite apparent, even with thinning of the underlying zygoma; (3) the muscle does not always provide a sufficiently strong contraction to bring about significant facial movement; (4) contraction of the temporalis is not an emotive response and requires training to achieve a semblance of a smile; (5) in order to achieve significant elevation of the upper lip and oral commissure substantial overcorrection is required, which can produce an unsightly appearance, reminiscent of a snarl; (6) the procedure usually requires a general anesthesia with 2 to 3 hours of operating time.

Static Suspension for Facial Rehabilitation

Although there is no question that the ideal to strive for in the management of patients with facial paralysis is restoration of voluntary facial motion, with good resting tone, this is not always achievable. There are many reasons why facial motion may not be restored, but the most common is lack of a usable distal facial nerve to hook up a hypoglossal to facial nerve jump graft or crossover graft. Degeneration or loss of facial muscles may also preclude the use of a reinnervation procedure. Denervation or loss of the temporalis muscle (common in extensive skull base procedures) may prevent the use of a temporalis transposition for facial reanimation. Finally, patients who have incurred a facial paralysis as a result of a rather involved skull base procedure are generally reluctant to pursue further surgery, which they perceive (rightly or wrongly) as extensive. They choose instead to live with their facial paralysis.

For patients in whom facial reanimation is not an option, or who have an intact nerve with expected recovery on a prolonged basis, a reasonable second choice is to provide the illusion of facial tone with a static suspension. In fact, a static suspension, well done, may go a long way toward ameliorating much of the morbidity and deformity of facial paralysis without imparting any particular morbidity of its own. The major goal of a static suspension has been to elevate the corner of the mouth and to change the expression from one of severe anger or sorrow to one of neutral emotion, or even happiness. An additional benefit of a static suspension is that it can help control drooling of food and liquids, as well as keeping the cheek against the teeth so that food does not become trapped in the buccal space. A static suspension will also improve speech by keeping the cheek against the teeth and not allowing it to blow outward when saying words with "p" in them. Although most of the static suspensions we have performed have been directed at suspension of the lower face, we have been performing suspensions of the forehead with increasing frequency. Initially, we performed forehead suspension only on patients with severe brow ptosis causing visual-field deficits or entropions; however, we have been employing brow suspension for aesthetic improvement with increasing frequency. The value of a brow suspension becomes obvious once the lower face has been elevated and the ptotic brow now stands out in stark contrast to the elevated lower face.

In the past, static suspensions for facial paralysis were performed primarily with fascia lata as the suspending material. However, fascia lata requires a donor site, with considerable morbidity, and the fascia tends to stretch out over time, with loss of facial suspension. To compensate for this loss of tone, the initial suspension had to be overcorrected significantly producing an unnaturally tight appearance during the immediate postoperative period; later, after some loosening, the face returned to the flaccid state associated with facial paralysis. An additional difficulty with performing the traditional fascia lata suspension was that there was no easy way to attach the fascia lata to the zygoma, often requiring suturing around the zygoma, which was cumbersome.

Currently, our material of choice for facial suspension is Gore-Tex strips (1 mm or 2 mm thick) for several reasons[11,12]: (1) with Gore-Tex, there is no donor site morbidity, (2) Gore-Tex is easy to work with and comes in a variety of lengths and thickness, (3) Gore-Tex appears to have excellent tensile strength with little stretching over time, and (4) Gore-Tex is well tolerated with extensive applications elsewhere on the body. We now attach the Gore-Tex to the zygoma, with titanium screws replacing the clumsy suturing techniques used in the past.

Recently, we have begun to employ static suspension of the lower face for patients with facial paralysis after skull base surgery (typically acoustic neuroma) who are known to have an intact facial nerve and are expected to regain some degree of facial function. Typically, recovery of facial nerve function due to an injury at the skull base takes 12 to 18 months. During this recovery time, patients must endure all the sequelae of facial paralysis, often a source of considerable distress, particularly for those with high-profile jobs. We have found that suspension of the lower face improves speech, eating and drinking, and cosmesis and improves self-confidence during the recovery period. Once the nerve recovers, and the face begins to move, it has not been necessary to remove the Gore-Tex implants and, in fact, there is often residual benefit from the suspension, even after nerve recovery, presumably because the nerve does not recover fully.

Over the past 6 years, we have come to see several benefits of Gore-Tex suspension for rehabilitation of the paralyzed face: (1) it is easily performed with local anesthesia on an outpatient basis, (2) there is immediate improvement of appearance and function, (3) no donor site morbidity occurs, and (4) it can be easily revised and, if necessary, reversed. The disadvantages of Gore-Tex suspension are the fact that facial motion is not restored and there is a possibility of implant extrusion.

Technique of Gore-Tex Suspension

Gore-Tex is obtained in sheets of 1- or 2-mm thickness and cut into strips 3 to 4 mm wide and 7 to 8 cm long. Incisions are planned at the lateral border of the obicularis oris muscle, which closely corresponds to the melolabial crease, and over the body of the zygoma at the junction of the cheek skin and lower eyelid skin. The zygoma is exposed superiorly and a deep subcutaneous tunnel connecting the two incisions is created and a strip of 2 mm Gore-Tex is passed. The inferior end of the strip is then sutured to the obicularis muscle with 4-0 or 5-0 permanent sutures (Mersilene, Ethobond, nylon, or Gore-Tex suture). The superior end of the strip is then placed on tension and the corner of the mouth elevated to the desired position. Some overcorrection should be included in the original positioning, but much less than the amount needed for fascia lata or temporalis muscle. The Gore-Tex strip is then secured to the zygoma with one or two 1.5-mm titanium screws passed through the Gore-Tex and into the underlying bone using the screw head to secure the Gore-Tex. This is facilitated by the use of self-tapping and self-drilling screws. For forehead suspension, a horizontal inferior incision is marked in a suprabrow crease approximately 5 to 10 mm above the brow just lateral to the midbrow point. The inferior incision is carried into the subcutaneous tissue and dissection directed inferiorly until the edge of the orbicularis oculi muscle is identified. Superiorly, a vertical incision is marked in the hairline (if available). The superior incision is carried through the galea aponeurosis and a supraperiosteal dissection performed until the inferior incision is reached. A strip of 1-mm-thick Gore-Tex is then passed and the inferior end sutured to the orbicularis with any of the previously mentioned suture material. The superior end is then placed on traction and, when the brow has been elevated to its desired height, it is tacked to the underlying skull with a 1.5-mm-diameter and 4-mm-long titanium screw. The scalp incision is closed with staples and the skin incisions closed with fast-absorbing chromic.

Pros and Cons of Gore-Tex Suspension of the Paralyzed Face

When compared with the two most popular alternative procedures (hypoglossal to facial nerve crossover and temporalis muscle transposition) for facial rehabilitation (Table 22–1), Gore-Tex suspension has several advantages. It is a straightforward procedure, performed under conscious sedation on an outpatient basis. The results are immediate with no lag time before the nerve regenerates or the muscle starts to move. There is no donor site morbidity, such as ipsilateral tongue weakness or temporal depression, and it is easily reversible by explanting the Gore-Tex strip. It is also the only procedure that can ameliorate the symptoms of facial paralysis while an intact nerve with neuropraxia is regenerating.

TABLE 22–1
Comparison of Modalities for Rehabilitation of the Paralyzed Face

Modality	Advantages	Disadvantages	Summary
Hypoglossal to facial nerve transfer	Restores neuronal input to facial muscles, with resulting strong resting facial tone	Significant synkinesis; movement of face with eating and speaking; excessive resting tone; hemitongue paralysis; requires fairly involved surgery; forehead rarely improved	Good choice for young motivated patients who can accept donor site morbidity and synkinesis
Temporalis muscle transfer	Uses contiguous muscle, not nerve; low donor site morbidity; provides elevation of the oral commissure; and allows some conscious (but not spontaneous) movement of the corner of the mouth	Temporal depression; bulk of muscle overlying the zygoma may be apparent; movement of corner of mouth is not spontaneous and may not be very strong; surgery requires general anesthesia and 2–3 hours operating time; forehead not improved	May be a reasonable choice for patients who want some movement of oral commissure, but should be reserved for young motivated patients; amount of successful movement obtained is variable
Gore-Tex suspension	No donor site morbidity; simple procedure with local anesthesia on an outpatient basis; can improve both oral commissure and brow; improves facial symmetry, function, and appearance at rest	No movement of face possible; possibility of implant extrusion; possibility of loosening of suspension	Nice alternative to other procedures with few down sides; when combined with upper eyelid gold weights, a very acceptable rehabilitation of the paralyzed face may be achieved

The disadvantages of Gore-Tex suspension are the fact that it is a static procedure with no chance of facial movement. There is the additional disadvantage of potential loosening of the suspension and extrusion of the Gore-Tex implant, both of which have been very uncommon in our experience.

Conclusion

Static suspension of the face with Gore-Tex strips for rehabilitation of the paralyzed face has provided our patients a reasonable alternative to more invasive procedures such as hypoglossal to facial nerve crossover or temporalis muscle transposition. When combined with upper lid loading, using gold weights, Gore-Tex suspension significantly improves many of the sequelae of facial paralysis in a simple, one-step procedure that is reversible and that is associated with no donor site morbidity. A major application of Gore-Tex suspension is in the management of patients with intact facial nerves but with paralysis after skull base surgery. While awaiting regeneration of the nerve, Gore-Tex suspension ameliorates many of the sequelae of facial paralysis and continues to add support after the nerve has begun to function. Other strong candidates for Gore-Tex suspension are patients with loss of the ipsilateral temporalis muscle or distal facial nerve, or both (as in lateral face or skull base malignancies) in whom there are no good alternatives. To date the vast majority of Gore-Tex implants we have used have been well tolerated with good maintenance of suspension and only one extrusion.

In our practice, Gore-Tex suspension has become the primary modality for management of facial paralysis against which other techniques must show significant superiority before being recommended to patients.

REFERENCES

Shumrick—CHAPTER 22

1. Ueda K, Harii K, Yamada A. Free vascularized double muscle transplantation for the treatment of facial paralysis. *Plast Reconstr Surg* 1995;95:1288–1296
2. Rubin LR. Discussion of free vascularized double muscle transplantation for the treatment of facial paralysis by Ueda et al. *Plast Reconstr Surg* 1995;95:1297–1298
3. McO'Brien B, Kumar PAV. Cross-face nerve grafting with free vascularized muscle grafts. In: Rubin LR, ed. *The Paralyzed Face.* 2nd ed. St. Louis: Mosby–Year Book; 1991:201–212
4. Harii K. Microneurovascular free muscle transplantation. In: Rubin LR, ed. *The Paralyzed Face.* 2nd ed. St. Louis: Mosby–Year Book; 1991:178–200
5. Sobol SM, May M. Hypoglossal-facial anastomosis: its role in contemporary facial reanimation. In: Rubin LR, ed. *The Paralyzed Face.* 1st ed. St. Louis: Mosby–Year Book; 1991:137–143
6. Conley J, Baker D. Hypoglossal-facial nerve anastomosis for reinnervation of the paralyzed face. *Plast Reconstr Surg* 1979; 63:63–72
7. Pitty LF, Tator CH. Hypoglossal-facial nerve anastomosis for facial nerve palsy following surgery for cerebellopontine angle tumors. *J Neurosurg* 1992;77:724–731
8. Kunihiro T, Kanzaki J, O-Uchi T. Hypoglossal-facial nerve anastomosis. *Acta Otolaryngol (Stockh)* 1991;487:80–84
9. Pensak ML, Jackson CG, Glasscock ME, Gulya AJ. Facial reanimation with the VII-XII anastomosis: analysis of the functional and psychologic results. *Otolaryngol Head Neck Surg* 1986;94:305–310
10. May M, Sobol SM, Mester SJ. Hypoglossal-facial nerve interpositional-jump graft for facial reanimation without tongue atrophy. *Otolaryngol Head Neck Surg* 1991;104:818–825
11. Konoir RJ. Facial paralysis reconstruction with Gore-Tex soft tissue patch. *Arch Otolaryngol Head Neck Surg* 1992;118:1188–1194
12. Petroff MA, Goode RL, Levet Y. Gore-Tex implants: applications in facial paralysis rehabilitation and soft-tissue augmentation. *Laryngoscope* 1992;102:1185–1189

Static versus Dynamic Management of the Paralyzed Face

Maisie L. Shindo

CHAPTER 23

Facial paralysis can lead to a variety of troubling symptoms for the patient, including ocular problems, speech difficulties, drooling, and nasal obstruction (Table 23–1). Facial paralysis can be devastating for patients because of the emotional impact from the facial disfigurement as well as difficulties with communication, eating, and drinking in a social setting. Numerous options are available for rehabilitation of prolonged facial paralysis (Table 23–2). The rehabilitation procedures can be divided into dynamic and nondynamic reanimation procedures; the latter include static slings, ocular protective procedures, and adjunctive cosmetic procedures. When assessing which procedure(s) to perform, one should not simply look at the problem as dynamic versus static reanimation of the entire face. Rather, it is best to approach the analysis by dividing the regions of the face to be reanimated into upper third, middle third, and lower lip and then to determine the functional deficits, cosmetic deformity in each region, and the patient's desires. Furthermore, one must determine the feasibility of performing the procedures for achieving the desired goals.

Three basic questions need to be answered in the decision tree:

1. What are the patient's functional and aesthetic needs?
2. What is the potential for spontaneous recovery?
3. Is the patient medically fit to undergo a long operative procedure?

TABLE 23–1
Problems Frequently Experienced by Patients with Facial Paralysis*

Problems	Reasons
Eye irritation	Inadequate eye closure and corneal protection
Epiphora	Inability to effectively "pump" tears into the lacrimal drainage system
Visual-field defect	Ptosis of brow and soft tissues of the forehead
Speech difficulties	Lip incompetence, resulting in diffi culty pronouncing consonents such as P and B
Drooling and difficulties eating/drinking	Lip incompetence and frequent biting on buccal mucosa, which protrudes into the oral cavity
Nasal obstruction	Collapse of nasal alar rim from flattened nasolabial fold

* In addition to lack of facial motion.

Figure 23–1 presents a suggested algorithm based on the answer to these questions. This logical and rational approach to facial analysis for rehabilitation of the paralyzed face takes into consideration the aesthetic units that need to be restored, specific functional deficits and patient's desires, duration of paralysis, patient's medical condition, and the status of the distal facial nerve fibers and motor end plates.

Rehabilitation of the Upper Third of the Face

The main problems to be addressed in this region are improvement of eye closure and correction of laxity of the lower eyelid. Although dynamic muscle procedures have been described to restore eyelid function, most surgeons today rehabilitate the eye with static procedures because they are simple and effective. Inadequate eye closure can be improved by placement of a gold weight in the upper eyelid or insertion of an eyelid spring. Most surgeons prefer gold weight insertion over springs because the procedure is simple and easier to perform. The disadvantage of gold weight is that it requires gravity on the weight of the gold to pull the eyelid down and thus does not work effectively when the patient is supine. The advantage of a spring over gold weight is that its function is not dependent on gravity; therefore, it automatically protects the cornea during sleep. However, it is much more complicated and difficult to place a spring, and the potential for complications is greater. Paralytic ectropion of the lower lid can be corrected by performing wedge excision of the lateral lower eyelid and lateral canthopexy. Severe paralytic ectropion may also require medial canthopexy. The second, and often overlooked, problem in the upper third of the face is ptosis of the eyebrow, which aside from the obvious asymmetry may result in obstruction of peripheral vision due to lateral hooding. Brow ptosis is corrected with a forehead and brow lift, which can be performed through a forehead incision if the patient has a prominent wrinkle; otherwise, it can be performed endoscopically or through a coronal incision.

Rehabilitation of the Middle Third of the Face

Management options for correction of the mid-face disfigurement are much more varied, as shown in Figure 23–1. They range from simple procedures to restore symmetry at rest, such as a static sling or face lift, to complex dynamic rehabilitation with microneurovascular free flaps. Selection of procedure(s)

TABLE 23–2

Procedures for Rehabilitation of Prolonged Facial Paralysis after Parotidectomy

Dynamic Reanimation	Static Reanimation and Cosmetic Procedures
Interposition nerve grafts	Eyelid procedure
Crossover reinnervation procedures	Goldweight
Hypoglossal	Spring
Ansa hypoglossi	Lower lid tightening
Cross-facial	Brow and forehead lift
Regional muscle transfer	Correction of midfacial deformity
Temporalis	Slings
Masseter	Fascia lata
Digastric	Alloplastic sheets
Microneurovascular free flap	Malar augmentation
Gracilis	Facelift
Latissimus dorsi	Lower lip wedge resection
Rectus abdominis	Botulinum toxin
Serratus anterior	
Pectoralis minor	
Abductor hallucis	
Extensor digitorum brevis	

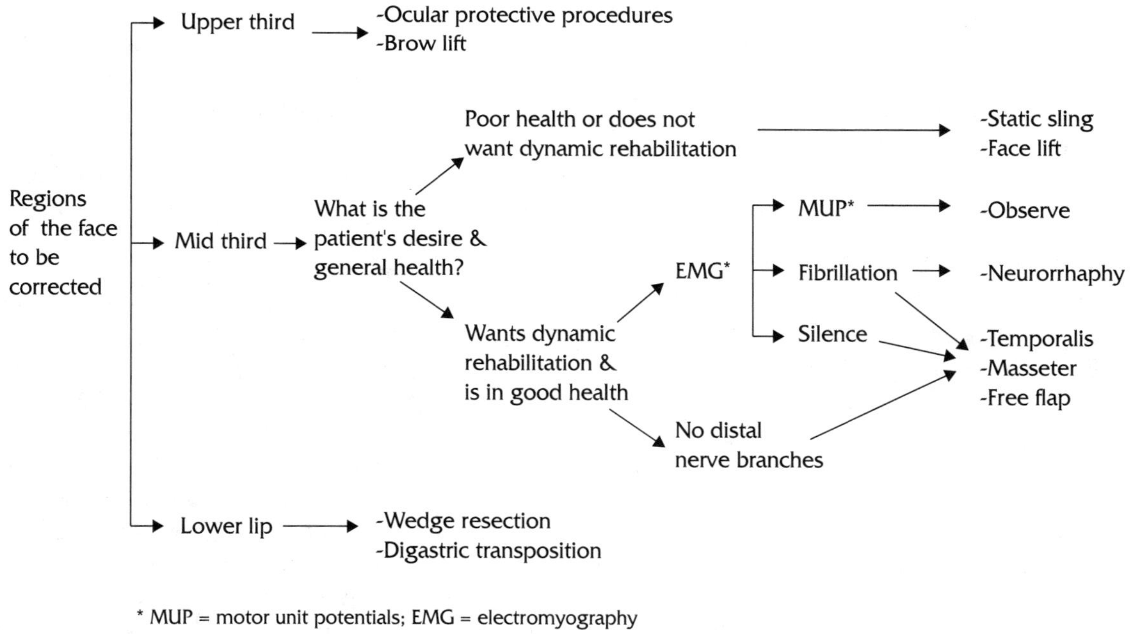

Figure 23–1 Rehabilitation of chronic facial paralysis.

for this region depends on both the patient's desires and underlying medical condition as well as the potential for spontaneous recovery.

When the facial paralysis is deemed permanent, such as when the facial nerve was not grafted at the time of resection (i.e., radical parotidectomy, acoustic neuroma surgery), any of the static or dynamic procedures listed in Table 23–2 can be offered to the patient at any time. By contrast, if the facial paralysis is thought to be a result of contusion such as after temporal bone fracture, or of surgery such as mastoidectomy, acoustic neuroma surgery, or parotidectomy, where the surgeon is confident that the nerve was left intact, reinnervation procedures should be delayed. The patient should be allowed to recover for approximately 1 year; reanimation procedures for the mid-face can then be considered if the patient does not demonstrate any clinical evidence of reinnervation. Selection of the rehabilitation procedure depends on the availability of the distal nerve fibers, associated soft tissue defect, the patient's desires, and the operative risks. The algorithm in Figure 23–1 outlines a proposed decision tree based on these factors. The next step in deciding what to offer the patient is to determine the patient's goals or wishes and to assess the patient's underlying medical problems. If the patient simply wants to restore facial symmetry at rest to improve speech and mastication functions, or is a very high operative risk, static procedures such as an alloplastic sling or face lift under local anesthesia would be most appropriate. By contrast, if the patient is in fairly good health and would also like to restore facial motion, dynamic reanimation procedures should be offered. The choice of the dynamic procedure depends on the status of the distal facial nerve fibers and motor endplates. If distal facial nerve fibers are available for neurorrhaphy, reinnervation can be achieved with neurorrhaphy procedures such as interposition grafts or crossover reinnervation. Before performing these neural reanastomosis procedures, the status of the motor endplates should be evaluated with electromyography (EMG) of the facial musculature. Spontaneous recovery is expected if the EMG demonstrates polyphasic motor unit potentials; neurorrhaphy procedures should not be performed. Fibrillation potentials on EMG indicate persistent denervation, in which case neurorrhaphy procedures are appropriate. Lack of electrical activity on EMG implies that the motor endplates are no longer viable due to longstanding denervation, indicating that neurorrhaphy procedures are not likely to be successful. If the distal nerve fibers are not available for neurorrhaphy, or EMG shows electrical silence, innervated muscle flaps such as temporalis transposition, masseter transposition, or gracilis free flap are required for dynamic rehabilitation.

Neural Reinnervation Procedures

These procedures are generally performed if the duration of paralysis has been longer than 1 year and EMG demonstrates primarily denervation potentials. Two types of neural anastomosis procedures can be used to reinnervated the paralyzed face. The first method is direct reanastomosis or interposition nerve grafting, which can be attempted if the proximal and distal ends of the facial nerve can be isolated. Mastoidectomy may be required to expose the intratemporal portion of the facial nerve to attain a healthy proximal stump for anastomosis. Nerve anastomosis is best performed under magnification with loops or a microscope using fine, atraumatic interrupted sutures, usually 9-0 or 10-0 nylon. Repair of the extratemporal facial nerve can be accomplished by placing the sutures through the epineurium, the perineurium, or each fascicle. The theoretical advantage of the perineural or fascicular repair is that the fascicles can be topographically matched to achieve reinnervation with minimal synkinesis. There is no convincing evidence for the superiority of one particular technique over another. Epineural repair is the easiest to perform and is most commonly used. The number of epineural sutures needed for repair depends on the diameter of the nerve. The goal should be to place the fewest number of sutures that will tightly coapt the nerve ends and prevent axon escape, which can result in neuroma formation and prevent successful regeneration. In general, six to seven sutures are required to repair the proximal stump and three to four for distal branches. It is extremely important to achieve a tension-free anastomosis. An anastomosis performed under tension can result in scar formation, which impedes axonal regeneration beyond the anastomotic site. If tension-free repair cannot be achieved, the proximal stump can be mobilized to gain some length, or an interposition nerve graft should be used. Successful axonal regeneration and reinnervation are highly dependent on good anastomotic techniques. In general, direct end-to-end anastomosis yields superior results over interposition grafts.[1] However, a tension-free anastomosis is essential in order to achieve good results with primary repair; thus, it is better to use a cable graft if the repair is under significant tension.

The second neural anastomosis method is crossover reinnervation, where the distal stump of the facial nerve is anastomosed to a nerve other than the ipsilateral proximal facial nerve (i.e., another donor nerve). The motor function of the facial musculature is then driven by that donor nerve. Certainly, if the proximal facial nerve is available, it is better to perform interposition nerve grafting between the two stumps rather than crossover reinnervation so that the patient has a chance of restoring spontaneous emotional facial expressions, which is controlled by neural input from the proximal facial nerve. Thus, crossover reinnervation procedures are generally indicated when the distal facial nerve stump is available, but the ipsilateral proximal facial nerve stump is not, such as following acoustic neuroma surgery or temporal bone resection. The major disadvantages of crossover reinnervation over primary reinnervation are potential morbidity associated with sacrifice of a donor nerve, and lack of spontaneous emotional expression, as the motor input to the facial musculature is not being driven by the appropriate motor cortex. The most commonly used donor nerve is the hypoglossal nerve. Potential problems that can result from hypoglossal-facial (XII to VII) crossover reinnervation are speech and swallowing difficulties from hemitongue paralysis, and hyperkinesis and synkinesis after reinnervation. Modifications of the XII to VII procedure have been described to avoid these potential problems. One option is to split the hypoglossal fibers and use only approximately half to preserve normal tongue function. May et al.[2] also described the use of an interposition ("jump") graft, usually the great auricular nerve, between the hypoglossal and the distal facial nerve(s). With this technique, approximately half of the diameter of XII is transected, and an end-to-side anastomosis is performed between the partially cut XII and the interposition nerve graft. Another potential donor nerve for crossover reinnervation is a buccal branch of the contralateral facial nerve. This technique is known as cross-facial nerve (VII to VII) grafting and is a two-stage procedure. In the first procedure, a sural nerve graft is anastomosed to one of the normal contralateral buccal nerve branches and tunneled across the upper lip to the buccal region on the paralyzed side. The axons are allowed to generate across the graft for approximately 1 year, at which time the distal stump of the graft is exposed and anastomosed to the distal stump of the paralytic facial nerve. Axonal regeneration in the sural nerve can be monitored clinically by eliciting a Tinel's sign, where the patient experiences paresthesia when the nerve is tapped at the site of regenerated axons. The results with the procedure have generally been inconsistent and less than favorable. The disadvantages of cross-facial nerve grafting are potential paralysis of the contralateral mid-face, and a lower success rate of reinnervation.

With successful axonal regeneration, the patient can be expected to have facial tone (e.g., restoration of melolabial fold) in approximately 6 months, and progressive restoration of motion one to three months thereafter. If the site of nerve repair involves the main trunk, the best functional result that can most likely be achieved is a grade III by House-Brackmann scale, as synkinesis is generally expected with reinnervation.[3-5]

Muscle Transposition

TEMPORALIS TRANSPOSITION

The principle of the temporalis transposition procedure is to transpose an innervated, vascularized strip of temporalis muscle for immediate restoration of facial symmetry at rest and potentially to restore facial motion. The muscle is innervated by a motor branch of the trigeminal nerve and derives its blood supply primarily from the deep temporal branch of the internal maxillary artery, which enters the muscle on its deep surface. Through a hemicoronal incision, a 2-cm strip of the muscle is elevated, rotated over the zygomatic arch, and sutured to the lateral edge of the orbicularis oris muscle to achieve the desired upward pull and restore symmetry at rest. The distal end of the muscle is split and sutured around the commissure. Overcorrection of the upward pull is essential. The patient then learns to smile by activating the innervated temporalis flap through motions such as biting or clenching teeth. Indications for temporalis muscle transposition include (1) absence of distal facial nerve fibers, (2) motor endplates not likely to be viable, (3) associated soft tissue defect in the cheek, and (4) alternative to or failed neural anastomosis procedures. The advantages of temporalis muscle transfer are ease of performance, immediate restoration of midfacial symmetry, and potential for restoring movement. Its disadvantages are (1) the restored facial motion is not spontaneous and has to be learned by activating the temporalis muscle, (2) chronic temporal mandibular joint pain from loss of temporalis function, (3) bulkiness over the zygomatic arch, and (4) temporal depression, which can be minimized by reconstructing the temporal fossa. If the defect is not very deep, a temporoparietal fascial flap (TPFF) may be sufficient to prevent postoperative temporal fossa hollowing. The temporoparietal fascia is a thin fascial layer between the subcutaneous fat and the superficial layer of the temporalis fascia supplied by the superficial temporal artery. The TPFF is elevated and set aside prior to elevation of the temporalis muscle and can later be rotated into the temporal defect. If additional augmentation is required, an alloplastic implant, such as a Silastic block, Gore-Tex (W.L. Gore & Associates, Flagstaff, AZ), AlloDerm (Life Cell Corp., Woodlands, Tx) or hydroxyapatite cement (Bone-Source, Leibinger, Carrollton, TX) can be placed in the temporal fossa and covered with the TPFF.

MASSETER TRANSPOSITION

Masseter transposition has limited applications in rehabilitation of facial paralysis because of the limited upward pull, its potential long term effects on mastication, and availability of many other better options. One useful application of the masseter flap is in reconstruction of a buccal defect associated with sacrifice of the lower division(s) of the facial nerve. In such a situation, through a transoral approach, the anterior portion of the masseter muscle can be detached from the lower border of mandible and transposed into the buccal defect. The distal end of the rotated muscle is then sutured to the orbicularis oris muscle fibers of the lower lip to reanimate the paralytic lip. If there is an associated buccal mucosal defect, a skin or mucosal graft can be placed on the masseter muscle and sutured to the edges of the mucosal defect.

Microneurovascular Free Tissue Transfer

The most ideal circumstance for using an innervated, vascularized muscle free flap for facial reanimation is a defect created by radical parotidectomy, where the flap is used for dynamic reanimation of the paralytic face and to reconstruct the soft tissue deficit at the same time. It is also indicated when the paralysis has been present for years, especially if facial atrophy is present; an innervated microvascular free muscle flap will allow not only dynamic facial reanimation, but also some soft tissue augmentation. Although temporalis transfer is a good alternative to free flaps, free flaps have distinct advantages over the temporalis flap. Most importantly, free flaps can be reinnervated with motor input from the proximal stump of the facial nerve, which would then allow potential restoration of spontaneous emotional expression. If the proximal stump is not available, such as after resection of a cerebropontine angle tumor, a sural nerve graft can be interposed between the nerve of the free muscle flap and a buccal branch of the contralateral facial nerve to achieve the desired results. The second advantage is that muscle free flaps yield superior aesthetic results over the temporalis flap when there is an associated large soft tissue defect because a large volume of muscle can be harvested, with a cutaneous paddle if necessary, and "custom fitted" into the defect. The most commonly used free flap for facial reanimation is the gracilis muscle flap. For facial paralysis associated with a large parotidectomy and soft tisssue defect, an inferior rectus abdominis muscle flap is ideal.

Excellent functional and cosmetic results have been reported with muscle free flaps for facial reanimation.[6] This chapter will briefly describe the flap design and insetting methods for the gracilis and rectus flaps.

GRACILIS FLAP

The gracilis muscle is a long, thin muscle arising from the anterior margins of the symphysis pubis and the ramus of the ischium, and inserts into the medial surface of the tibia. Removal of this muscle does not result in any significant functional disability. The muscle derives its predominant blood supply from a muscular branch of the profunda femoris artery, and venous drainage is via two paired venae commitantes that accompany the artery. The anterior branch of the obturator nerve, the motor nerve to the muscle, is also harvested with the flap. The gracilis muscle is divided superiorly near its origin and then inferiorly at a pre-measured length that matches the appropriate length on the face that achieves the desired correction of the midfacial ptosis. The inferior edge of the muscle is split and sutured around the oral commissure described for the temporalis muscle transfer. The superior edge is trimmed to achieve the desired pull and anchored to the zygomatic arch. As in the temporalis muscle transfer, overcorrection is essential. The anterior obturator nerve is anastomosed to the proximal stump of the facial nerve. In some instances, the inferior vertical segment of the mastoid portion of the nerve may need to be exposed to attain an adequate segment for anastomosis. If a previously implanted cross-facial sural nerve graft is to be used as the recipient motor nerve, it is exposed in the buccal region and anastomosed to the motor nerve of the gracilis. Other potential recipient nerves are the ansa hypoglossi and the motor branch of the masseter muscle. The ansa is much easier to isolate, is a better size match to the anterior obturator nerve, and does not result in any morbidity for the patient. Certainly, if the facial nerve is not used for neural input, the patient must learn to activate facial motion by clenching the teeth or swallowing, depending on which nerve is used as a donor nerve. After the neural anastomosis, the arterial and venous anastomoses are performed. The superficial temporal or the facial are usually used as recipient vessels.

RECTUS ABDOMINIS FLAP

The rectus abdominis muscle arises from the pubic crest and symphysis pubis and inserts into the fifth, sixth, and seventh ribs. The muscle has a dual blood supply from the superior and inferior epigastric arteries; the latter is most commonly used for free tissue transfer. The motor innervation to the muscle is from multiple segmental intercostal nerves. The flap can be harvested with or without a skin paddle, depending on the nature of the defect. After making the proper skin incisions, the superior border of the muscle is transected, and the flap is elevated off of the posterior rectus sheath with one of its motor nerves from cephalad to caudad direction. The vascular pedicle is readily identified on the posterior surface of the muscle and dissected down to its origin at the external iliac vessels. After isolating the pedicle, the muscle is then transected inferiorly off of the symphysis pubis. The vascular pedicle is then transected and the flap is transferred to the face. The muscle insetting and neurovascular anastomosis are performed as described for the gracilis flap. The transverse tendinous inscriptions of the rectus muscle help hold the sutures that are placed through the muscle for anchoring. When reconstructing large skin and soft tissue defects over the parotid region, an ipsilateral rectus myocutaneous flap with the skin paddle placed in an oblique orientation is ideal. This flap design allows the rectus muscle to be suspended between the zygomatic arch and the lip for facial reanimation, and the bulky obliquely oriented skin paddle then provides both skin coverage and soft tissue augmentation over the parotid region.

Static Rehabilitation Procedures

A static sling procedure is generally indicated when the patient does not desire restoration of facial motion or is not medically fit to undergo a more extensive procedure under general anesthesia. Although static sling procedures do not restore facial motion, they do improve facial aesthetics for the patient by providing facial symmetry at rest and often will improve oral incompetence. Traditionally, a fascial graft, such as fascia lata from the thigh, is harvested and anchored from the zygomatic arch to the orbicularis oris, using the same techniques described for muscle transfer. In recent years, availability of highly biocompatible alloplastic implants has obviated the need for harvesting autologous fascia, which eliminates donor site scar and morbidity as well minimize operative time. The most commonly used alloplastic material for midfacial suspension is Gore-Tex,[7] although Alloderm is also currently being used. The procedure is simple and easy to perform. A sheet of the implant, either Gore-Tex or AlloDerm is trimmed to an estimated appropriate size, and a vertical slit is made in the lower part of the implant. Small incisions are made in the melolabial crease and preauricularly over the root of the zygoma. A subcutaneous tunnel is dissected connecting the two incisions. The implant is placed in the subcutaneous pocket and brought out through both incisions. The inferior edge of the implant is sutured to the orbicularis oris muscle as described previously. The other end of the implant is pulled superiorly to achieve the desired elevation of the cheek and upper lip and then anchored to the zygomatic arch with permanent sutures. Some overcorrection is necessary, although not as much as the muscle flaps.

Face lift, performed either alone or in conjuction with a static sling, is also very helpful in reanimation of the paralyzed midface. A deep plane face lift generally yields superior results over the standard superficial lift by SMAS suspension or plication for rehabilitation of the paralyzed face.

Rehabilitation of the Lower Lip

With paralysis of the marginal mandibular nerve, the lower lip may drift in a downward and/or medial direction, which can result in oral incompetence, drooling, and difficulties with annunciation. These functional difficulties usually occur when the paralytic lip drifts down and medially. Correction of this deformity requires static suspension with a sling from the lateral lip to the zygomatic arch and/or a deep plane face lift to pull the corner of the lower lip up. If a midfacial paralytic deformity is being corrected at the same time, the muscle flap or alloplastic sling can be sutured to the lateral lower lip to correct this deformity. For an isolated marginal mandibular nerve paralysis that results in a medial and downward drift of the lower lip, a static sling can be performed. The sling should be tunneled superficially along the cheek to prevent injury to the intact buccal and zygomatic branches. If the lip is only deviated medially, it is primarily a cosmetic problem and can generally be corrected with a lateral lower lip wedge excision.[8] However, wedge resection alone will not correct a medial and downward deviation. As previously mentioned, this type of deformity requires a combination of static suspension, such as a sling or deep plane face lift, and wedge resection. Coneley[9] also described cheiloplasty for this deformity, where a wedge resection is performed in conjunction with transposition of a viable portion of the contralateral lip to create a smaller mouth opening and establish a dynamic sphincteric lip.

Management of Synkinesis and Hyperkinesis

Injection of botulinum toxin can be quite helpful for patients who develop hyperkinesis following reinnervation (e.g., after XII to VII cross-innervation). It may also be helpful for patients who have severe synkinesis that results in excessive facial twitches. The toxin is injected into the orbicularis oculi muscle for eyelid spasms and into the zygomaticus major muscle for midfacial spasms. EMG may be helpful in localizing the muscle for injection. An initial dose of 5 to 10 U can be injected into the orbicularis oculi and 10 to 20 U into the zygomaticus and then repeated if necessary to achieve the desired results. The duration of effect lasts approximately 3 months, and patients will require repeated injection.

Conclusion

Facial paralysis is a devastating problem that significantly alters the quality of life for patients. Patients can be helped by a variety of static and dynamic procedures. The best outcome can only be achieved by systematically evaluating the patient and selecting the appropriate procedure(s) that are likely to work, that suit the needs of the patient, and that will not cause additional morbidity.

REFERENCES

1. Spector JG, Lee P, Peterein J, et al. Facial nerve regeneration through autologous nerve grafts. A clinical and experimental Study. *Laryngoscope* 1991;101:537–554
2. May M, Sobol SM, Mester SJ. Hypoglossal-facial nerve interpositional-jump graft for facial reanimation without tongue atrophy. *Otolaryngol Head Neck Surg* 1991;104:818–825
3. Green JD, Shelton C, Brackmann DE. Surgical management of iatrogenic facial nerve injuries. *Otolaryng Head Neck Surg* 1994;111:606–610
4. May M, Sobol SM, Mester SJ. Management of segmented facial nerve injuries by surgical repair. *Laryngoscope* 1990; 100:1062–1067
5. Stephanian E, Sekhar LN, Janecka IP, et al. Facial nerve repair by interposition nerve graft. Results in 22 patients. *Neurosurgery* 1992;31:73–76
6. O'Brien BM, Pederson WC, Khazanchi RK, et al. Results of management of facial palsy with microvascular free-muscle transfer. *Plast Reconstr Surg* 1990;86:12–22
7. Biel MA. Gore-Tex graft midfacial suspension and upper eyelid gold-weight implantation in rehabilitation of the paralyzed face. *Laryngoscope* 1995;105:876–879
8. Glenn M, Goode R. Surgical treatment of the marginal mandibular nerve deformity. *Otolaryngol Head Neck Surg* 1987;97:462–468
9. Coneley J. Cheiloplasty in the treatment of facial paralysis. *Laryngoscope* 1986;96:140–145

Static versus Dynamic Management of the Paralyzed Face

CHAPTER 24

Tessa A. Hadlock and Mack L. Cheney

The management of longstanding facial paralysis presents a unique surgical challenge. It has been established that during the first several years after facial nerve sacrifice or injury, techniques that reestablish neural input to the native facial musculature yield the most satisfactory clinical results.[1] In the case of primary or cable graft repair of the facial nerve, the restoration of neural input from the facial motor nucleus directly to existing facial musculature offers the only chance for return of natural, emotive expression. In cases in which the proximal facial nerve is not available for grafting, reinnervation techniques with alternative proximal neural sources provide direct innervation of facial muscles. This type of repair may yield satisfactory resting tone and function during voluntary smiling, but lacks spontaneous emotive function.

Perhaps the most challenging clinical situation is one in which reinnervation of the facial muscles themselves is not possible. This occurs when the distal facial nerve stump is either absent or severely fibrotic or when the facial musculature is atrophic beyond contractile capability. Efforts to restore facial symmetry and tone then involve static and dynamic tissue transfer techniques. These methods routinely provide less satisfactory functional and aesthetic results, and controversy surrounds which procedures are best employed in different clinical situations. There are numerous static and dynamic approaches to facial reanimation, and various techniques have proved to be well matched to particular clinical situations.

Background

Whereas the entity of facial paralysis was described and linked to damage of the facial nerve almost two centuries ago, efforts to perform corrective procedures evolved very slowly. Until 30 years ago, the problem was thought of by most as a permanent deformity. However, increasing interest in correction of the problem was generated during the 1960s. Electrophysiologic techniques for measurement of neural function, classification schemes for the measurement of recovery, and surgical techniques for correction were developed.

In this contemporary era, the first-line approach to reanimation of the atrophic paralyzed face has been to perform a regional muscle transfer to provide dynamic facial movement.[2,3] Both masseter and temporalis muscles have been used; currently, the temporalis muscle is favored. The middle third of the muscle is brought down to the oral commissure, and the donor site defect filled with an ipsilateral temporoparietal fascia flap (TPFF).[4] An accompanying eye procedure, such as gold weight implantation, is usually executed for eyelid closure. Drawbacks to the temporalis muscle transfer include a persistent soft tissue defect in the donor site despite partial fill-in with the TPFF and the fact that the resulting oral commisure movement is not physiologic. Physical therapy helps train individuals to elicit a smile by biting down; however, emotive expression is never restored.

Techniques for the transfer of free muscle grafts for dynamic facial reanimation have also been developed over the past two decades.[5] Gracilis, pectoralis minor, latissimus dorsi, and serratus anterior muscle slips have all been used. Microneurovascular transfer is carried out in conjunction with a cross-facial jump graft for innervation. Results from these free muscle transfers vary substantially. Drawbacks include nasolabial distortion, excessive cheek fullness, and flap failure. For these reasons, they tend to be reserved for congenital facial palsy patients (i.e., Mobius syndrome).

Static reanimation techniques have traditionally been employed in clinical situations in which more lengthy muscle transfer techniques are not a viable option. This would include the management of patients in whom the longer anesthesia time presents too high an operative risk or in patients whose overall prognosis is poor. It is recognized that the goals of surgery do not include dynamic function of the afflicted side. The procedures simply help restore symmetry at rest and improve functional oral competence.

The restoration of resting facial symmetry can be achieved with a wide variety of surgical techniques, depending on the anatomy of the individual and the precise functional deficits. Among the most common static procedures are superficial musculoaponeurotic system (SMAS) plication, brow-lifting procedures, and oral commissure Z-plasties designed to ameliorate speech slurring and drooling.[1] Additional procedures, including judicious lower lip resections and nasolabial fold resections, have been designed to achieve more precise facial symmetry. The nasal valve collapse that sometimes accompanies facial paralysis can be managed with standard nasal valve widening procedures, and the paralyzed eye can be managed with tarsorrhaphy, medial canthoplasty, and/or spring or gold weight implantation.

Discussion

Selecting an appropriate approach to the chronically deinnervated paralyzed face is complex. The present-day paradigm, employing dynamic muscle reanimation as a first-line approach, with static methods as a fallback, is an oversimplified algorithm that requires refinement. Specific clinical scenarios arise in which a deviation from this strategy is called for in order to achieve the desired outcome. Acknowledging that, in general, dynamic muscle transfer offers superior results in complete, longstanding paralysis (House–Brackmann grade V–VI recovery), we highlight special clinical situations in which static methods may provide comparable or superior outcomes. In addition, clinical situations exist in which early dynamic muscle transfer provides an adjunct to reinnervation of the transiently completely paralyzed face. Figure 24–1 shows a schematic illustrating one possible facial paralysis management strategy, which includes these particular scenarios.

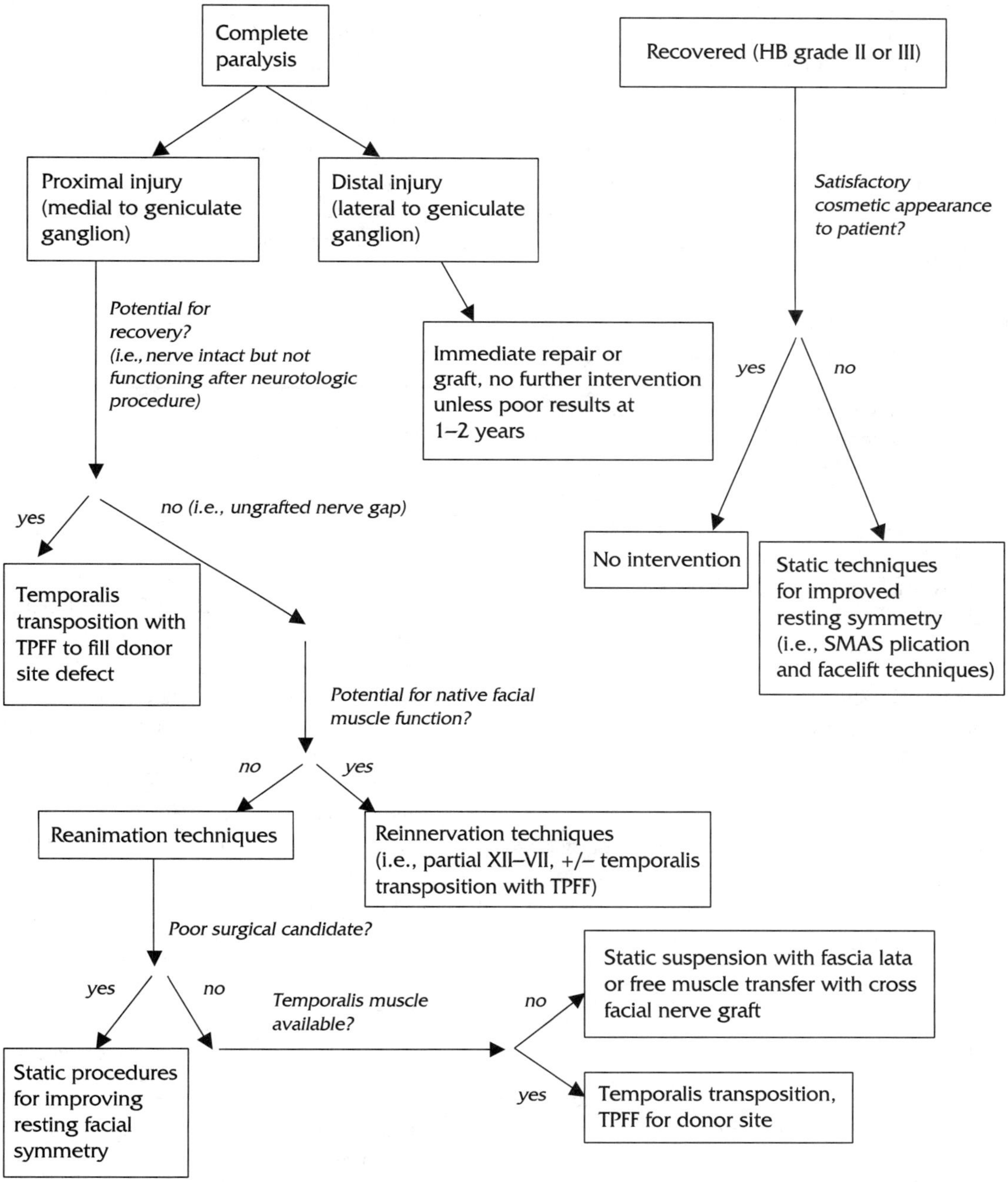

Figure 24–1 Schematic illustrating management strategy for facial paralysis. HB, House–Brackmann; SMAS, superficial musculoaponeurotic system; TPFF, temporoparietal fascia flap.

STATIC PROCEDURES FOR THE RECOVERED FACIAL PALSY PATIENT

Patients with partially recovered facial palsy present an interesting problem. Often after a severe but transient facial nerve insult, such as Bell's palsy, recurrent facial paralysis from Melkerson-Rosenthal syndrome, or iatrogenic neuropraxia, patients recover to a House–Brackmann grade II or III level. They have better function than could be expected with grafting procedures but still have complaints relative to facial asymmetry. In these patients, muscle transfer would play no role at all, as they maintain a fair amount of mimetic function. In order to improve resting facial symmetry, a limited, "mini" facelift technique can provide increased resting support to the affected side, without jeopardizing residual dynamic function. If the affected side has developed a contracture so that the normal side appears flacid in comparison, the unaffected side can be operated on in order to match the contractured side. This is done through standard anterior rhytidectomy incisions. Subdermal flaps are elevated, and the SMAS is simply plicated to an appropriate degree according to the resting position of the opposite side. This asymmetric facelift technique allows the resting position of the two sides of the face to match more closely.

STATIC PROCEDURES FOR THE PATIENT WITH CONTRAINDICATIONS TO TEMPORALIS FLAP USE

There is a group of patients in whom temporalis muscle transposition would be the procedure of choice, but in whom the temporalis muscle is unavailable for use. This group includes patients in whom the muscle is absent (from previous use) or is involved in a disease process (skull base processes involving both cranial nerves V and VII). In these patients, it is often preferable to use static methods, such as fascia lata slings, rather than to employ free muscle grafts.

DYNAMIC MUSCLE TRANSPOSITION AS AN EARLY INTERVENTION IN THE PATIENT EXPECTED TO RECOVER FACIAL FUNCTION

A topic of controversy has been how to manage the face of the patient in whom facial nerve recovery is expected to occur over a prolonged time course. This can arise after acoustic neuroma resection, severe Ramsay-Hunt syndrome, certain temporal bone fractures, and a variety of other facial nerve insults. In these patients, it is critical not to jeopardize regeneration through either an anatomically intact facial nerve or one that has been primarily repaired or grafted at the brainstem or intratemporally. However, the addition of a dynamic reanimation procedure during the early postoperative period dramatically improves resting facial tone, significantly reducing the cosmetic deformity.

We have established a role for early temporalis muscle transposition in the treatment of this subgroup of patients, with excellent results.[4] The surgical technique has been refined to deal effectively with both donor site defect problems and hypertrophic scarring at the oral commisure. Using this dynamic muscle transfer as an adjunct procedure permits efficient restoration of facial tone, symmetry, and purposeful facial movement in a patient population that previously waited up to 3 years after paralysis for any reanimation procedure. Not only is early function restored, but the natural regeneration of facial nerve fibers is not interfered with, so that ultimate restoration of innervation to the muscles of facial expression may still occur.

Although this early intervention is still not in widespread use, we believe it improves short-term postoperative outcome significantly and will be more frequently employed as its benefits become more widely recognized.

Conclusion

Surgical planning for reanimation of the chronically paralyzed face continues to be a challenge. This is related to the fact that even the most advanced reanimation techniques in the best hands often yield disappointing cosmetic or functional results.

We have outlined our specific approach as it has evolved over the past decade (Fig. 24–1) and have defined clinical scenarios that deviate from the dogma that reinnervation techniques come first, followed by dynamic muscle transfer, leaving static techniques as a last resort. These procedures are not mutually exclusive; specific clinical goals must dictate therapy. For example, there is a role for muscle transfer even in the setting of expected nerve recovery, and there is a role for static procedures even in patients who are a good anesthesia risk, who have isolated functional complaints relative to their facial palsy.

As more techniques for both static and dynamic reanimation of the paralyzed face are developed, a growing number of tools will be at our disposal for the treatment of what continues to be a suboptimally managed problem.

REFERENCES

Hadlock and Cheney—CHAPTER 24

1. Cheney M, ed. *Facial Surgery, Plastic and Reconstructive.* Baltimore: Williams & Wilkins; 1997:665–684
2. Baker D, Conley J. Regional muscle transposition of rehabilitation of the paralyzed face. *Clin Plast Surg* 1979;6:317–331
3. May M. Muscle transposition for facial reanimation: indications and results. *Otolaryngol Head Neck Surg* 1984;92:85–87
4. Cheney M, McKenna M, Megerian C, Ojemann R. Early temporalis transposition for the management of facial paralysis. *Laryngoscope* 1995;105:993–1000
5. O'Brien B, Franklin J, Morrison W. Cross-facial nerve grafts and microneurovascular free muscle transfer for long established facial palsy. *Br J Plast Surg* 1980;33:202–215

9

SMAS Surgery versus Deep-Plane Rhytidectomy

"Today the debate seems to be whether one operation gives a superior result to the other, which is missing the real crux of the controversy. The debate should be focused on the total clinical presentation of the patient and the patient's goals of what the surgery will achieve."

Douglas D. Dedo

"It is difficult, if not impossible, to compare these techniques objectively because of the subjective nature of the results and the lack of an endpoint to determine the length of time the results 'last.'"

Frank M. Kamer

"Elevation of this 'musculofascial' plane is a key component of the biplane facelift described in this chapter. In my opinion, no other operation provides the elegant upper facial rejuvenation that is characteristic of this operation. This is especially true when there is an indication to correct a downward slope of the lateral canthal region."

Howard A. Tobin

SMAS Surgery versus Deep-Plane Rhytidectomy

Douglas D. Dedo

CHAPTER 25

The evolution of the facelift during the twentieth century was dependent on technologic breakthroughs and the understanding of the anatomy responsible for the vagaries of aging. With better lighting and the development of low-reacting suture materials that self-absorbed over weeks and months, surgeons were able to see, manipulate, and secure tissue planes that were previously impossible to work with. During the early 1900s, simple skin excision with minimal if any undermining was the standard.[1] With fiberoptic lighting, dissection could be extended farther and farther under the skin with improved results. As late as the 1960s and 1970s, the need to do little more than lift the skin remained controversial. With Mitz and Peyronie's[2] landmark anatomic work on the subcutaneous musculoaponeurotic system (SMAS), the innovators were stimulated to plicate, imbricate, excise, and manipulate this layer in a variety of ways. Depending on the approach used by a specific surgeon, varying degrees of success and longevity could be added to the standard skin-flap facelift. It was not until Hamra[3] fully mobilized the SMAS layer in continuity with the obicularis oculi muscle to release the zygomatic ligament that the deep-plane facelift came into practice. The old controversy of the need to even operate on the subcutaneous layers now had added an extra caveat: Does the deep-plane lift improve the mid-face laxity and the overall results of a SMAS-manipulated facelift, to justify the increased risk and morbidity to the patient?

Background

Aufricht[4] defined the SMAS layer in his article reviewing 15 years of SMAS surgery as "the area overlying the parotid and underlying the skin of the face and cheek. This sheet, present in the embryo, is made of fibrous tissue and of some muscular fibers; superiorly, it is related to the obicularis and frontal muscles and inferiorly by the platysma. Lying between the muscles of facial expression and the skin, it arches over the zygoma and stretches from the tragus to the nasolabial fold, fanning into labial musculature" (Fig. 25–1). Aufricht[4] was among the first to advocate plication of this fibrous layer in an effort to enhance the postoperative result and achieve a longer lasting result. Skoog[5] also popularized the manipulation of this layer to improve the results.

IMBRICATION

Webster et al.[6] performed a series of operations in 1982 in which they attempted to show that imbrication, the undermining and advancement of the SMAS, failed to increase the amount of posterior displacement of aesthetically important landmarks as compared with simple plication of this layer. Despite these results and an ongoing debate in the literature concerning the efficacy of SMAS surgery, the standard approach to the SMAS is extensive freeing of the skin in the cheek area to the cheek–lip fold. In the neck, the skin is undermined across the midline in most patients. When imbricating, the SMAS is incised horizontally 1 cm below the zygomatic arch. The vertical limb runs inferiorly in front of the ear to connect with the platysma along the anterior border of the sternocleidomastoid muscle. The dissection of this SMAS flap extends to the anterior border of the parotid gland, avoiding any injury to the facial nerves. As the SMAS runs in continuity with the playsma, the extent of the subplatysmal dissection can vary from 1 to 2 cm, to meet in the midline, negating the need for a submental incision.[7] This SMAS flap is then advanced posteriorly and superiorly. The excess is excised above the zygomatic arch and in front of the ear with subsequent reapproximation of the cut edges. The posterior flap is sutured to the sternocleidomastoid fascia. Present-day PDS sutures permit ample time for fibrosis and healing before being absorbed 6 months later.

PLICATION

Plication of the SMAS layer involves the same amount of skin undermining as for imbrication, but this layer is not incised. Approximately 3 cm below the zygomatic arch, the SMAS is grasped with a pair of forceps and pulled posteriorly and superiorly while the effect on the skin flap, ptotic jowl fat, and labial commissure is observed. The goal is to advance and elevate the SMAS layer and the contiguous structures as much as possible. Once this point is found, double-looped sutures of 3/0 PDS are placed through it to fix and tighten this pseudofascial layer.

The deep-plane facelift described by Hamra[3] was an extension of the sub-SMAS facelift, with the dissection extending beyond the anterior border of the parotid, superiorly over the malar eminence, and anteriorly into the nasolabial fold. Inferiorly, it stops at the jawline. The skin is undermined only 2 to 3 cm before creating a composite musculocutaneous flap that stays above the zygomaticus muscles to release the zygomatic

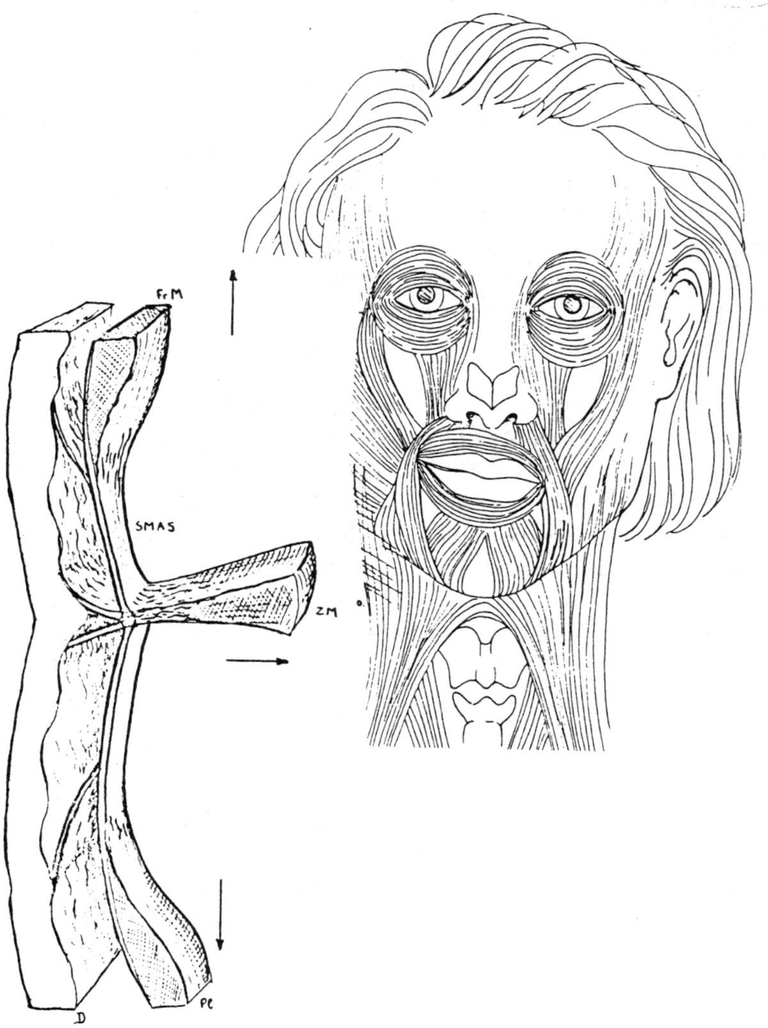

Figure 25–1 The SMAS is a fibrous layer that extends over the cheek from the tragus to the nasolabial fold. Superiorly, it is contiguous with the temporalis fascia with fusion to the zygomatic arch. Inferiorly, it is part of the fascia surrounding the platysma muscle.

ligaments. When the SMAS is released, the skin, subcutaneous fat, and fascial layers are all elevated and advanced superoposteriorly. The dermis of the flap is secured with absorbable sutures to the temporal fascia.

Discussion

The search for perfection and the multitude of articles published annually attest to the fact that the ultimate universal facelift has yet to be discovered. I might add that it will never be—the aesthetics, surgical ability, patient's anatomy, and desires offer too great a variability to be defined by one operation. What is enlightening is the multitude of facelift procedures being used to correct the vagaries of the aging process. During the early 1980s, I formulated a classification of the neck.[9] The goal was to identify specific pathologic conditions in order to tailor the facelift surgery to the patient's needs. Today the debate seems to be whether one operation gives a superior result to the other. This misses the real crux of the controversy. The debate should be focused on the total clinical presentation of the patient and on the patient's goals of what the surgery will achieve. SMAS surgery in and of itself offers a quantum leap in the postoperative result as compared with simple skin advancement. Although Webster showed that there was no significant difference in the width of skin excised between SMAS plication and imbrication, there is a postoperative difference in the submandibular and submental contouring. In some patients in whom the SMAS is plicated, a bulge of fat/muscle is visible in the submental triangle. For years, I followed Webster's dictum about the efficacy of plication. I too believed that SMAS plication, which is faster and virtually eliminates any possibility of salivary leaks, produced the same long-term result achieved with imbrication. This conclusion was based on the case of a patient who had a superficial parotidectomy on the right side with a SMAS flap facelift. Three months later, a simple SMAS plication facelift was performed on the left side. One year later, there is no difference between the two sides and the cheek–lip folds are identical.

A problem that sometimes arose with the simple SMAS plication was the submental bulge. When the SMAS is created into flaps and is advanced posterosuperiorly, the surgeon has more control on the vectors of the SMAS–platysma flap. Instead of directing the pull superiorly, the inferior portion of the flap at the angle of the mandible can be directed more posteriorly, eliminating the postoperative bulge. Does this mean that simple plication is obsolete and useless? I don't think so. Today safety is as important as quality and longevity. The patient who has zero tolerance for any complication and who presents with a pure class III neck is a candidate for SMAS plication.

The decision between a sub-SMAS or deep-plane facelift should be made on the basis of the particular pathology to be corrected and the patient's clinical picture. Age, social history, patient tolerance, primary or multiple lifts, malar and cheek fat composition, oral commissure slope, chin ptosis, jowl fat, and neck classification are factors that need to be considered.

The age of the patient is extremely important in the preoperative planning of the surgical procedure. Younger patients in their late 30s or early 40s with a class II neck do not need extensive neck and facial surgery. In the absence of jowls and deep cheek–lip folds, a simple SMAS plication facelift will suffice. With the fifth and sixth decades, more extensive facial work is required as the jowls droop and the platysma sags.

The social history of smoking is one of the few absolute indications for the deep-plane facelift procedure. Before Hamra's work, patients were instructed to stop smoking both 4 weeks before and 4 weeks after surgery to protect the flaps from the vasoconstrictive effects of nicotine. Rees et al.[9] demonstrated a 12-fold higher incidence of skin slough in smokers over nonsmokers. Subsequently, most cosmetic surgeons refused to operate on any patient who failed to stop smoking. The thick musculocutaneous flaps preserve the vasculature to the skin in the deep-plane approach, reducing the need for cessation of smoking.

Patient tolerance and expectations for the recovery time affect the choice of the surgical procedure. After a SMAS facelift (barring any complications), the patient is presentable in a minimum of 2 weeks after surgery. With the deep-plane lift, the patient should be prepared for a minimum of 4 weeks up to 6 months to recover, as disruption of the mid-face causes prolonged edema and healing. Furthermore, on animation, the insertion of the zygomatic muscle in the cheek is accentuated and can produce a dimple that resembles a marionette line. Obviously, the improvement in the mid-face and nasolabial folds should negate the presence of this dimple.

A significant problem with secondary facelifts is distortion of the labial commissure. A pulled, windtunnel, or widemouth frog look is a dead give-away of multiple facelifts. This effect, combined with the fibrosis and scarring of the first lift or two, makes the deep-plane lift a good alternative to any other approach. After the deep-plane facial flap is elevated and its rotation is adjusted, the oral commissure can be elevated without pulling it laterally and distorting it. Furthermore, the sub-SMAS dissection is in a virgin plane deep to the fibrotic layer of the previous lifts, greatly facilitating the surgery.

The position and composition of the malar and cheek fat present the surgeon with multiple challenges. When the malar fat atrophies and/or descends from its normal position over the malar eminence, two alternatives are available to rejuvenate this area. The sublabial insertion of cheek and malar implants is a fast and safe way to augment the aging face. Not only do these implants augment the skeleton; they also soften the cheek–lip fold groove as the skin is elevated. Furthermore, they have withstood the test of time. Extended dissection into, and suspension of, the fat through the deep-plane facelift is another approach popularized by Owsley.[10] The hollow cheek or gaunt look of facial atrophy has limited options for improvement. Whereas fat injections have immediate and dramatic results, their permanence is limited with respect to absorption and present-day grafting techniques.

The oral commissure succumbs to the effects of gravity, and patients will complain of looking sad when the corners of their mouths droop. Direct excision to elevate the oral commissures is an operation that can be staged with a facelift or done as a separate procedure. Another alternative is the deep-plane facelift. Because the fibromuscular layer of the facial muscles (including the orbicularis oris) is mobilized, it is very easy to direct the pull superiorly, thus reversing the droop of the corner of the mouth.

Chin ptosis may be corrected through a submental incision. After elevating the skin and fat from the deep mental muscle, the muscle is incised above the mental crease and undermined laterally, as is done with a chin implant. The cut muscle is sutured down over the mental crease, tightening this area. Chin implants and sliding genioplasty are two other alternatives to this problem. By increasing the skeletal support, the chin pad is elevated and the cervical skin stretched with an implant. Although a sliding genioplasty does achieve the same result, it is at the expense of a more involved procedure.

Ptotic jowl fat is one of the pathognomonic signs of aging, as it interrupts the distinct separation of the face and neck. Both the SMAS and deep plane operations address this problem. The older and heavier the patient, the more difficult it is to maintain the suspension and postoperative result. Recurrent jowling occurs as fat accumulates and tissues stretch and sag.

Management of the neck should be based on the particular pathology. In Hamra's original description of the deep-plane surgery, he describes a midline excision and suturing of the anterior platysma borders to extend below the thyroid cartilage. Thus, he pulls the muscle complex anteriorly, while leaving the posterior border untouched. If the patient is not a class IV with anterior platysma muscle laxity, there is little to be gained from this maneuver. If there is only fat (class III), liposuction is indicated. Personally, I believe the posterior edge of the platysma muscle should be mobilized and advanced posteriorly over the sternocleidomastoid muscle to create a sling in the neck and maintain the support for the underlying structures (submaxillary glands).

The last consideration for choosing a particular operation is the potential for complications. In our litigious society, in which a perfect result is expected every time, we must weigh the potential risks versus the benefits to be achieved as we put our careers and reputations on the line for our patients. Simple SMAS plication shortens the operating time and does not introduce any significant sequelae. However, when the SMAS is undermined, the risk of parotid fistulas can become an issue. The latter problem is caused by exposure and trauma to the parotid gland. Fortunately, expectant waiting solves the problem much as it does after fistulas that develop after superficial parotidectomy.

When the deep support of the cervical area has been reestablished, patients will complain of difficulty swallowing as well as a choking sensation. Again, this tight sensation gradually loosens over several weeks; the longer the patient complains of tightness, the longer the postoperative result.

Fortunately, hematomas that develop postoperatively in the deep planes of the face do not compromise the vasculature of the skin. However, they take many months to resolve and require hours of patient reassurance.

Facial nerve injury is heightened as the dissection extends beyond the parotid gland. When the deep-plane operation is done correctly, one is literally dissecting between branches of the facial nerve. Weakness in the buccal branch is most commonly seen. Here is when one begins to question the advantage of one operation over the other. Most of the time there is gradual return of function.

Conclusion

This year, the controversy is the SMAS layer and the extent of its dissection. Next year it could well be the subperiosteal facelift. Regardless of the controversy and new developments in facelift surgery, certain basic principles must guide surgeons as they consider adding new techniques to their armamentarium. First is patient safety. What are the complications and potential sequelae to the patient? Do the benefits outweigh the potential risks of the procedure? Second, are the results described by the originator of the technique capable of being consistently reproduced by others? Third, what is the learning curve of the operation? Familiarity with basic surgical skills and anatomy allows the average surgeon to learn and stay abreast of the new procedures. However, a 1-month fellowship to learn a new technique might cause one to pause before attempting the procedure. Last, what is the cost to the surgeon and to the patient? New instrumentation, as seen with endoscopic or laser surgery, prompts serious consideration of the capital investment before it is incorporated into the practice. In addition, is there a charge that has to be passed along to the patient for each procedure? When we look at these guiding principles as they relate to this chapter, we see that there is a definite learning curve in doing a deep-plane facelift. Cadaver dissection to refamiliarize oneself with the anatomy is mandatory. In specific instances (e.g., smoking, secondary or revision facelifts), the deep-plane operation is the surgery of choice. As a parameter of the efficacy of the deep-plane operation, Kamer[11] used the frequency of doing a tuck-up procedure. He found that 11.4% of SMAS patients required a tuck, whereas only 3.3% of the deep-plane lifts required the tuck-up procedure. Based on this statistic, Kamer concluded that the deep-plane technique was more effective. However, when one considers all the factors of morbidity, complications, and other factors, I believe that the SMAS operation is probably the procedure of choice in most cases.

REFERENCES

Dedo—CHAPTER 25

1. Passot R. II. La correction chirurgicale des rides du visage. *Bull Acad Natl Med* 1919;82:112
2. Mitz V, Peyronie M. The superficial musculoaponeurotic system (SMAS) in the parotid and cheek area. *Plast Reconstr Surg* 1976;58:80–86
3. Hamra ST. The deep-plane rhytidectomy. *Plastic Reconstr Surg* 1990;86:53–61
4. Aufricht G. Surgery for excessive skin of the face. *Transactions of the Second International Congress of Plastic Surgery*. Livingstone, Edinburgh. 1960:495
5. Skoog T. *Plastic Surgery: New Methods and Refinements*. Stockholm: Almqvist & Wiksells; 1974
6. Webster RC, Smith RC, Papsidero MJ, Karolow WW, Smith KF. Comparison of SMAS plication with SMAS imbrication in face lifting. *Laryngoscope* 1982;92:901–912
7. Owsley JQ. The sub-SMAS facelift. *Plast Surg Clin North Am*
8. Dedo DD. A preoperative classification of the neck for cervicofacial rhytidectomy, *Trans Am Assoc Cosm Surg* 1981;1:47
9. Rees TD, Liverett DM, Guy CL. Smoking in the facelift patient. *Plast Reconstr Surg* 1984;73:911
10. Owsley JQ. The extended facelift. *Plast Reconstr Surg* 1998
11. Kamer F. SMAS rhytidectomy versus deep plane rhytidectomy: an objective comparison. *Plast Reconst Plast Surg* 1998;102:878–881

SMAS Surgery versus Deep-Plane Rhytidectomy

CHAPTER 26

Frank M. Kamer and Andrew S. Frankel

Techniques for facelift surgery have advanced rapidly over recent years in order to provide for optimal aesthetic results, minimal postsurgical recovery time, and few complications. As patients have become more sophisticated and demanding, increased competition has fueled the already ongoing pursuit for the ideal surgery, further stimulating the development of improved methods of rhytidectomy. Despite a multitude of techniques for facelifting, each can be effective in the right hands, and there is no single best method that is universally applicable. The specific technique or techniques employed by a surgeon depend largely on his or her background, training, and experience. As with any other surgical procedure, the rhytidectomy technique should be based on sound scientific and surgical principles. It should also yield reliable time-tested results, with complications occurring at a rate comparable to that of the existing gold standard. Ultimately, the success of a facelift technique is based on patient acceptance and satisfaction, the basis for a fulfilling surgical practice.

Although there are several different ways to perform a facelift, an ongoing debate continues regarding the subcutaneous musculoaponeurotic system (SMAS) and deep-plane rhytidectomy techniques. This may be because the SMAS lift has been the most widely used technique for an entire generation of surgeons, and the deep-plane technique is closely related, differing in only a few important technical points. Unlike the subperiosteal or endoscopic lifts, which require advanced instrumentation and novel concepts regarding tissue rearrangement, healing, and aesthetics, the deep-plane operation may seem somewhat familiar to those surgeons who routinely perform the SMAS lift, and thus more worthy of consideration. In fact, it may be the close similarity between these two techniques that has stimulated their differentiation and comparison among the surgical community. Those surgeons who routinely perform SMAS lifts believe the differences in outcome are not worth making the change. They also argue that there is an increased risk of nerve damage with the deep-plane technique and that this outweighs any perceived aesthetic benefit one might obtain.[1,2] Advocates of the deep-plane technique consider the results extremely beneficial, with few complications, and contend that performing a less effective lift would be doing a disservice to their patients.[3,4]

It is difficult, if not impossible, to compare these techniques objectively because of the subjective nature of the results and the lack of an endpoint to determine the length of time the results last. Therefore, rather than attempt to provide a purely objective analysis, this discussion is based on reports from the literature as well as the experience of the senior author, who was for many years an innovator and leading proponent of the SMAS lift until making the transition to the deep-plane rhytidectomy. The background of these procedures, as well as their technical details, is described, with specific controversial issues addressed. It is hoped that the reader will be stimulated to consider alternative options when performing facelifts in the future.

Background

Historically, rhytidectomy began during the early twentieth century as a very limited procedure involving minimal subcutaneous undermining and excision of redundant skin.[5] The modern concept of facelift surgery began in 1974, when Skoog[6] described a subplatysmal technique in a deeper anatomic plane of the face that he believed was useful for facelift surgery. The research conducted by Mitz and Peyronie,[7] which identified and clarified the relationship and dynamics of the superficial musculoaponeurotic system (SMAS) and the platysma, fostered a generation of surgeons, the senior author included, who advocated the aesthetic benefits of the SMAS lift. The 1980s generated a number of variations of the SMAS technique, most having to do with vectors of pull and management of the midline platysma fibers. The senior author in 1981, and Owsley in 1983, each described a sub-SMAS and subplatysmal dissection with superoposterior suspension of the lower face and neck combined with subcutaneous undermining and lateral traction of the mid- and upper cheek to produce a "bidirectional" rhytidectomy.[8,9] During this same period, a few practitioners of the Skoog technique modified and advanced the subplatysmal concepts that culminated in the refinements described by Lemmon and Hamra. In 1980, Lemmon and Hamra[10] published a variation of the Skoog technique involving a series of 577 patients. Lemmon and Hamra reported fewer contour irregularities in the face and a longer-lasting result in the neck with no increase in complications. After improving on his initial operation, Hamra[11] originally described the deep-plane rhytidectomy in 1990. Since that time there has been increased acceptance and use of the deep-plane technique, which is used by the authors and described in this chapter.

The senior author's experience with the SMAS technique began during the mid-1970s and involved approximately 2500 facelift operations over the next 15 to 20 years. The results were found to be aesthetically superior, more predictable, and longer lasting than had been obtained with the previous, less extensive, dissection techniques. Nevertheless, some inadequacies and small problems associated with the SMAS technique ultimately served as the incentive to search for an improved facelift technique. In 1996 the results of Kamer's[12] first 100 consecutive deep-plane facelifts were analyzed and reported, demonstrating the benefits of this technique and the lack of associated complications. Since that report, the senior author has performed the deep-plane operation predominantly, and the results have been under continual assessment.

Technique

The sub-SMAS (deep-plane) facelift is based on sound surgical principles of tissue mobilization, advancement, and repair. It is important to remember, when repositioning tissue, that the structures influenced by undermining are usually from the point of incision to the most distal point of dissection, but not beyond. The surgical incisions for the two operations are identical.

Platysmal plication is performed when there is notable laxity to the anterior platysmal fibers. The technique for this portion of the operation is also identical for both the SMAS and deep-plane operations.

A subcutaneous dissection is begun in the pretragal area and is extended approximately 3 to 4 cm toward the cheek. It continues inferiorly into the neck, below the body of the mandible. This preplatysmal plane is widely undermined toward the midline, joining the subcutaneous submental dissection overlying the previously plicated anterior platysmal bands.

In the scalp, the temporoparietal fascia and galea are separated from the deep temporal fascia in an areolar plane, with care taken to avoid injury to the temporal branch of the facial nerve as the dissection proceeds anteriorly toward the lateral brow.

Entrance to the sub-SMAS deep plane in the face is facilitated by retracting the skin and subcutaneous tissues, tenting up the SMAS and the platysma. An incision is outlined (leaving approximately a 1-cm "tongue" of SMAS attached to the skin) from the malar region, extending inferiorly toward the posterior border of the platysma, just beneath the angle of the mandible. Traction is maintained as the SMAS is dissected from the deeper parotidomasseteric fascia. Dense fibrous attachments between the superficial and deep fascias exist along the zygomatic arch, overlying the parotid gland, and along the anterior border of the masseter muscle. A less adherent areolar plane exists between the superficial and deep fascias in the cheek, directly overlying the masseter muscle, and beneath the platysma. Dissection is facilitated by vertically spreading the scissors directly along the underside of the platysma, peeling the fat and loose areolar tissue off this structure. Sharp dissection is required to transect the parotidocutaneous, masseteric cutaneous, and zygomatic osteocutaneous ligaments. The sub-SMAS plane is suprisingly avascular, but for a perforating branch of the transverse facial artery, which is relatively constant in the cheek.

The extent of anterior dissection is dependent on the amount of mobilization necessary to attain the required aesthetic result. To influence the malar bags, dissection must proceed beneath the inferior border of the orbicularis, transecting the thick osteocutaneous ligaments of the malar pad (MacGregor's patch). The nasolabial fold is approached by undermining the fascial-fatty layer of the cheek overlying the major and minor zygomatic muscles. Blunt finger dissection easily separates this plane overlying the mimetic muscles and continues anteriorly toward the nose and upper lip. As the facial nerve innervates these muscles from their deep surfaces, it is important for the surgeon to remain in a plane superficial to the zygomatic muscles. If this area is approached from the inferior subplatysmal dissection, the nerve can become subject to injury, as the SMAS envelops these muscles, and there is danger of dissecting beneath them into this deeper plane. The dissection of the prezygomatic area can be connected with the subplatysmal undermining as the dissection proceeds inferiorly. Fibrous attachments between the two planes are severed, but the confluence of mimetic muscles at the corner of the mouth (modiolus) is not disturbed.

The jowl area is undermined. An areolar plane exists overlying the masseter muscle, allowing the SMAS to be rapidly elevated by means of a blunt technique from the anterior border of the parotid gland as far forward as the anterior border of the masseter, where the fibrous septae of the masseteric-cutaneous ligaments are encountered. These are severed, and the dissection in the subplatysmal plane is continued anteriorly over the masseter muscle border and inferiorly to the border of the mandible, extending anteriorly to where the facial artery crosses. As long as the underlying parotidomasseteric fascia is not violated during this dissection, injury to the marginal mandibular nerve and vessels is highly unlikely. Further subplatysmal dissection inferior to the mandible is unnecessary. A subcutaneous plane in the neck has already been created.

Once the flap is adequately mobilized, hemostasis is ensured and the resultant widely undermined multiplane, musculocutaneous flap can be advanced to attain the desired aesthetic effect. The temporal brow area is elevated by superior advancement of this flap. Excess tissue is excised beginning at the most anterior extent of the wound. Inappropriate tension to elevate the eyebrow should be avoided. As closure proceeds inferiorly in the area of the superior pinna, the sideburn is brought more posterior rather than elevated, to prevent the temporal tuft from being overlifted. Before closure of the cheek flap, redundant preauricular subcutaneous tissue is excised to better define the tragus from the preauricular area. To facilitate advancement, the SMAS and the platysma are freed from the overlying skin for about 1 to 2 cm, creating a small strip of SMAS that can be used for suturing. The cheek flap is closed by suturing this SMAS tongue to the firm preauricular tissues with 4-0 polyglycolic acid sutures. These sutures, tied under some tension, determine the direction of the vector forces on the mobilized flaps and take tension off of the skin before closure. The superior suture advances the cheek in a posterosuperior direction. Three intermediate sutures anchor the flap posteriorly just anterior to the tragus, softening the melolabial fold and jowl while substantially obliterating the subcutaneous preauricular dead space. The inferior suture's vector is almost directly posterior, anchoring the platysmal flap to the dense fascia of the retrolobular area. This helps to restore the lower jowl and to delineate the jawline and the upper part of the neck. The excess SMAS flap and any irregular fascial-fatty tissues are trimmed and smoothed with scissors. Any areas of dog-ears or puckering can be dealt with by judicious subcutaneous undermining; however, to retain the compound flap, more extensive undermining between skin and SMAS should be avoided.

After the flaps have been adequately mobilized and advanced, the skin is trimmed and sutured. Excision proceeds in a sequential fashion. To better delineate the tragus, the small flap of skin advanced over it is judiciously defatted and closed without tension with interrupted fine nylon sutures. Cervical skin is likewise excised and sutured without tension, making sure that hairline disruptions or step deformities do not interrupt the normal individual anatomical configuration of the postauricular and occipital area. Subcuticular 5-0 plain catgut is used to close the postauricular wound, and stainless steel staples are used for the hair-bearing incisions.

Drains are used routinely. They emerge from a separate occipital stab incision and are connected to a negative-pressure reservoir. The drain and dressings are removed the day after surgery, and the incisions are examined. A looser protective dressing is applied for another 2 days, after which the patient can shower and wash his or her hair daily. The sutures and staples are removed after 1 week.

The traditional SMAS technique differs from the above deep-plane technique primarily in that the skin is undermined widely and it is separated completely from the underlying SMAS layer. This requires that a long skin flap be created which is at some risk of ischemia at the edges. In the SMAS technique the SMAS is incised parallel and 1 cm below the zygomatic arch from the pretragal area anteriorly for approximately 4 to 5 cm and undermined and raised in continuity with the posterior border of the platysma. The platysmal flap is begun by continuing the incision of the SMAS flap downward along the midportion of the sternocleidomastoid muscle. At the posterior border of the platysma muscle the flap is elevated anteriorly approximately 7 cm or as far as the anterior platysmal border if necessary. The superior limit of this undermining is a line running 2 cm below the border of the mandible in order to prevent injury to the marginal mandibular nerve. Next the flaps are separately positioned with the SMAS advanced posterosuperiorly, the platysma posteriorly, and the skin usually in a slightly different vector than that of the SMAS flap, to prevent a "pulled look."

The operating time should be similar for the two procedures if not less for the deep-plane technique because it requires that only one flap be elevated, rather than two, and there is usually less bleeding in the sub-SMAS dissection plane than in the subdermal dissection plane.

Discussion

When debating the value of these two facelift techniques, the first question that arises is usually: Which technique offers better aesthetic results? Attempts have been made to answer this in the literature but no solid conclusions can be made. Ivy et al.[13] found no significant difference in the results obtained from SMAS, extended SMAS, or deep-plane (composite) lifts. By contrast, Hamra and others,[14-16] have presented data suggesting superiority of the deep-plane technique over SMAS techniques. In several anecdotal reports, the investigators render opinions and make claims as to the advantages of one technique over the other without any objective data whatsoever.[2] We believe that this question of which technique offers better aesthetic results is rather general and is best handled by analyzing specific elements that make up the aging face. Deep nasolabial folds benefit more from the deep-plane technique because, in addition to initial undermining in the sub-SMAS plane, as is done in the traditional SMAS procedure, the fascial-fatty tissues and skin of the nasolabial fold anterior to the zygomatic muscles are separated from the underlying SMAS and musculature to the upper lip. Therefore, traction on the compound flap not only advances the SMAS, but also allows for redistribution of the skin over the nasolabial groove resulting in softening of the nasolabial fold. This finding is supported by the anatomic studies of Yousif et al. which demonstrated that traction on the SMAS lateral to the nasolabial fold may actually deepen the fold while traction on the fascial-fatty tissue and skin restores the ptotic elements and provides for an improved appearance in the nasolabial fold.[17,18] Jowls and the mandibular line should theoretically be improved equally well with either of these rhytidectomy techniques. However, the deep-plane procedure allows for more extensive dissection and greater tissue mobilization, which ultimately results in a tighter lift. Although incisions routinely heal well after any type of facelift, there is a definite advantage in being able to minimize tension on the closure. In the SMAS lift the skin incision is closed without any deep supporting sutures. This is in contrast to the deep-plane lift where the preauricular incision is relieved of any tension by the underlying SMAS sutures. In the routine case, this may not make any difference, but in any patients with a prior history of hypertrophic scarring, smoking, diabetes, or any other condition in which there may be vascular compromise, the decreased tension may result in better incisional healing. One other aesthetic feature that deserves mention is the long-term outcome. Critical analysis of patients who previously underwent a SMAS rhytidectomy occasionally reveals misdirected rhytides extending from the oral commissure in a sweeping pattern up to the earlobe. We believe that this deformity is a result of improper orientation of separate tissue layers during the closure of SMAS lifts. This has also been noted by Stuzin et al.,[19] who postulated that this deformity resulted from use of the skin flap as the vehicle to suspend facial fat. This stigma of prior facelift surgery is only associated with techniques involving subcutaneous undermining and is not possible after a deep-plane lift because the tissues are all mobilized and suspended together.

The question of which technique provides for longer-lasting results is difficult to assess because of the lack of a definitive endpoint to determine when the benefits of surgery have worn off. However, a recent objective study comparing the tuck rate after the SMAS and deep-plane rhytidectomy techniques revealed significantly fewer tucks being performed after the deep-plane technique.[20] In this retrospective study of 634 facelifts, the overall tuck rate was 7.5%, whereas the tuck rate after SMAS lifts was 11.4% and that after deep-plane lifts was 3.3%. Therefore, tucks were necessary 71% less frequently after deep-plane rhytidectomies than after SMAS rhytidectomies, implying that the deep-plane lift is more effective than the SMAS lift (Table 26–1). One explanation for these results is that there is more extensive undermining in the deep-plane operation, severing the facial retaining ligaments and allowing for greater mobilization of the flaps. In further support of this is the fact that a similar trend was noted in a 1981 report that demonstrated a higher tuck rate for patients undergoing a minimal lift with SMAS imbrication as compared to those undergoing sub-SMAS dissection and mobilization of a SMAS/platysma flap.[8] It may also be that keeping the skin in continuity with the underlying SMAS provides for better cutaneous support and prevents it from sagging.

Most reluctance to begin performing deep-plane facial surgery has to do with the perception of an increased chance for complications, most notably nerve injury. In his original report in 1990, Hamra[11] noted 4 transient weaknesses after 403 deep-plane lifts. More recently, the senior author cited no nerve injuries, temporary or permanent.[12] These statistics are well within the range considered acceptable for SMAS surgery or facelifts in general. The deep-plane procedure, as described earlier, is based on identifiable anatomical landmarks, and if the operation is performed correctly there exists no more risk of nerve injury than there is when performing the SMAS procedure. Indeed, the SMAS operation is performed in exactly the same deep tissue plane.

Hematomas are still reported at a rate of up to 3.9% of SMAS procedures.[21] The senior author's hematoma rate for deep-plane lifts was 6% during the first 100 performed. The hematoma rate has since been 2.1%. This is comparable to the overall rate reported for facelifts. It is important to note that all these occurred in the neck. Hamra[14] reported that he has never seen a hematoma under the facial flap, and he attributes this to the thickness of the flap coupled with the applied tension and absence of subcutaneous dissection. Although a hematoma in the neck is always possible with the deep-plane technique, the inability for it to extend into the face dissection facilitates evacuation through the retroauricular incision and minimizes any visible scarring. The lack of dead space achieved with the composite flap also eliminates the chance for subcutaneous collections to occur in the cheeks as occasionally happens with the SMAS patients. These small collections present only minor problems for the patients, but they can result in permanent scars or irregularities in the skin leading to dissatisfaction with the procedure overall.

Descriptions of facelift techniques have documented a lower incidence of skin slough with sub-SMAS techniques than with subcutaneous techniques; 3.6% of 4806 subcutaneous lifts resulted in skin slough, whereas only 0.4% of 3733 SMAS lifts exhibited skin slough.[21] Despite this, Whetzel and Mathes[22] recently performed an anatomic study that concluded that the SMAS layer does not provide increased vascularity to the lateral facial skin. Rather it is the perforating vessels and their relationship to a large subdermal arterial structure that is the most important factor. The deep-plane technique with its composite flap ensures excellent vascularity; not by including the SMAS layer, but by protecting this subdermal plexus, which could be injured during a routine SMAS lift when the skin is elevated from the SMAS. A study by Schuster et al.[23] further supports that there is improved vascularity to a composite facelift flap than to an extended skin flap and that there is no significant blood supply carried by the SMAS layer itself. Increased heartiness of the facial flap with the deep-plane dissection is of particular benefit in smokers or other persons with compromised vascularity, and may also provide for more rapid and improved healing when concomitant laser procedures are being performed.[24,25] Although there is little chance of having skin slough in the preauricular area after a deep-plane operation the postauricular area is still at some risk, and this is no different than with the SMAS technique.

TABLE 26–1
Comparison of Tuck Rates for Various Techniques

	1975 Skin Only	1997 SMAS Flap	1997 Deep-Plane
Tuck rate	21.7%	11.4%	3.3%
	(56/258)	(32/279)	(12/355)

SOURCE: From Kamer FM, Frankel AS. SMAS rhytidectomy vs deep-plane rhytidectomy: an objective comparison. *Plast Reconstr Surg* 1998;102:880.

Postoperative healing is slightly different for the two facelift techniques. The deep-plane lift is associated with more swelling in the preauricular area, but there is less swelling and bruising in the cheek as compared to the SMAS lift. Also, after a deep-plane rhytidectomy there are occasionally pleats in the preauricular skin from the deep sutures that can persist for 2 to 3 weeks, but these resolve as edema dissipates. Healing takes longer after the deep-plane surgery because of increased edema. Although most patients return to their normal lifestyle within 2 to 3 weeks, they do not reach their optimal appearance for nearly 3 months.

Indications and Contraindications

The deep-plane technique can be considered for most cases of primary rhytidectomy, except in the unusual situation, when simple skin redundancy is the only concern. It is particularly effective for advanced jowls and heavy nasolabial folds and for patients who smoke or have some other condition that predisposes them to compromised vascularity or infection. Patients with extremely thin skin in whom minor subcutaneous irregularities would be more evident are also better suited for the deep-plane rhytidectomy, as are those who are suceptible to hypertrophic scarring.

Revision of a primary rhytidectomy that involved dissection in the sub-SMAS plane could conceivably increase the risk of facial nerve injury due to distortion of surgical landmarks by scar tissue. This will not be determined until more of these patients present for revision. Other contraindications are not specific to the deep plane technique and include patients with improper motivation for surgery, persistently unrealistic expectations as to possible results, certain psychiatric disorders, serious medical conditions, and prior life-threatening anesthetic complications.

Since becoming acclimated with the deep-plane technique more than 5 years ago, the senior author has not performed any SMAS–platysma operations. Despite an enormous variety in the types of patients presenting for surgery, there has not seemed to be any indication to perform a SMAS lift over a deep-plane lift. The deep-plane lift seems to satisfy all the requirements for performing safe, effective treatment of the aging face.

Conclusion

Numerous techniques are available to the facelift surgeon performing a rhytidectomy. The SMAS lift has been the most widely used for more than two decades and has yielded consistently good results. The deep-plane lift is based on similar principles but represents an evolution in technique in order to provide for improved aesthetic results that are longer lasting. The main difference between techniques is the establishment of a well-vascularized compound flap of facial skin, fat, and muscle that allows for more extensive dissection, greater tissue mobilization, and skin closure under less tension. There is no objective proof as to the aesthetic superiority of one facelift technique over another, and there probably never will be. Therefore, it is left to individual surgeons to determine which technique works best in their hands for their particular patients.

REFERENCES

Kamer and Frankel—CHAPTER 26

1. Baker DC. Deep dissection rhytidectomy: a plea for caution. *Plast Reconstr Surg* 1994;93:1498–1499
2. Lassus C. Cervicofacial rhytidectomy: the superficial plane. *Aesth Plast Surg* 1997;21:25–31
3. Hamra ST. Letter to the editor; reply. *Plast Reconstr Surg* 1998;101:550–551
4. Pina DP. Aesthetic and safety considerations in composite rhytidectomy: a review of 145 patients over a 3-year period. *Plast Reconstr Surg* 1997;99:670–678
5. Passot R. La chirurgie esthetige des rides du visage. *Presse Med* 1919;27:258
6. Skoog T. The aging face. In: *Plastic Surgery: New Methods and Refinements.* Philadelphia: WB Saunders; 1974:300–330
7. Mitz V, Peyronie M. The superficial musculoaponeurotic system (SMAS) in the parotid and cheek area. *Plast Reconstr Surg* 1976;58:80–88
8. Kamer FM, Halsey W. The two layer rhytidectomy. *Arch Otolaryngol* 1981;107:450–453
9. Owsley JQ SMAS–platysma face-lift. *Clin Plast Surg* 1983;10: 429–440
10. Lemmon ML, Hamra ST. Skoog rhytidectomy: a five-year experience with 577 patients. *Plast Reconstr Surg* 1980;63:283–297
11. Hamra ST. The deep-plane rhytidectomy. *Plast Reconstr Surg* 1990;86:53–61
12. Kamer FM. One hundred consecutive deep-plane face-lifts. *Arch Otolaryngol Head Neck Surg* 1996;122:17–22
13. Ivy EJ, Lorenc ZP, Aston SJ. Is there a difference? A prospective study comparing lateral and standard SMAS face lifts with extended SMAS and composite rhytidectomies. *Plast Reconstr Surg* 1996;98:1135
14. Hamra ST. Composite rhytidectomy and the nasolabial fold. *Clin Plast Surg* 1995;22:313–323

15. Hamra ST. Composite rhytidectomy: finesse and refinements in technique. *Clin Plast Surg* 1997;24:337
16. Furnas DW. The deep-plane rhytidectomy (discussion). *Plast Reconstr Surg* 1990;86:62–63
17. Yousif NJ, Gosain A, Matloub HS, Sanger JR, Madiedo G, Larson DL. The nasolabial fold: an anatomic and histological reappraisal. *Plast Reconstr Surg* 1994;93:60–69
18. Yousif NJ, Gosain A, Sanger JR, Larson DL, Matloub HS. The nasolabial fold: a photogrammetric analysis. *Plast Reconstr Surg* 1994;93:70–77
19. Stuzin JM, Baker TJ, Gordon HL, et al. Extended SMAS dissection as an approach to midface rejuvenation. *Clin Plast Surg* 1995;22:295–311
20. Kamer FM, Frankel AS. SMAS rhytidectomy vs. deep-plane rhytidectomy: an objective comparison. *Plast Reconstr Surg* 1998;102:878–881
21. Duffy MJ, Friedland JA. The superficial-plane rhytidectomy revisited. *Plast Reconstr Surg* 1994;93:1392–1401
22. Whetzel TP, Mathes SJ. The arterial supply of the face lift flap. *Plast Reconstr Surg* 1997;100:480–486
23. Schuster RH, Gamble WB, Hamra ST, et al. A comparison of flap vascular anatomy in three rhytidectomy techniques. *Plast Reconstr Surg* 1995;95:683–690
24. Ramirez OM, Pozner JN. Subperiosteal minimally invasive laser endoscopic rhytidectomy: the SMILE facelift. *Aesth Plast Surg* 1996;20:463–470
25. Guyuron B, Michelow B, Schmelzer R, Thomas T, Ellison MA. Delayed healing of rhytidectomy flap resurfaced with CO_2 laser. *Plast Reconstr Surg* 1998;101:816–819

SMAS Surgery versus Deep-Plane Rhytidectomy

CHAPTER 27

Howard A. Tobin and Angelo Cuzalina

Facelifting dates back to the early 1900s. A few surgeons in Europe and in the United States were experimenting with the removal of small skin strips from in front of and behind the ears.[1] Dr. Jacques Joseph,[2] in 1921, and Dr. Bettman,[3] in 1920, were the first surgeons to publish before-and-after photographs of their facelift results. During the first 60 years of facelift surgery, dissection was limited to the subcutaneous plane. It was not until the 1950s in the United States that the "classic" wide skin undermining facelift became the norm. This technique was not significantly challenged until Skoog[4] in 1974.

Facelift surgery in the first half of the twentieth century was considered to be an act of extreme vanity. Surgeons who performed such "risky and unnecessary" operations were looked down upon by society and the medical community. Increased public demand and affluence have led to a dramatic rise in facelifting. Consequently, the number of facelift techniques has also markedly increased.

Successful manipulation of facial tissues other than skin for facelifting began during the early 1970s due to a better understanding of facial anatomy as well as surgical anesthesia improvements. In 1974 Skoog first described his "deep-plane" facelift, which emphasized the presence of an interconnected "skin-fat-musculofacial unit" that, if elevated together, improved facelift results. Owsley[5] further described use of the platysmal muscle for lifting in 1977. Other surgeons quickly began reporting additional techniques involving the platysma.[6,7]

Innovations over the past 20 years have led to the development of the "composite,[8,9] deep-plane,[10] subperiosteal,[11-13] laser, and endoscopic[14] facelifts. Skoog's elevation of the platysma muscle in his advancement flap sparked the interest in the musculofascial plane or superficial musculoaponeurotic system (SMAS), initially described in 1976 by Mitz and Peyronie.[15] The SMAS was more accurately detailed in 1984, when Jost and Levet's publication challenged the previous SMAS concept.[16] There continues to be a great deal of disagreement, as well as confusion, regarding the best plane of dissection, not to mention the definition of surgery. The manipulation of a musculofascial plane to achieve improved and longer-lasting results has become common practice for many cosmetic surgeons. Elevation of this musculofascial plane is a key component of the biplane facelift described in this chapter.

General Approach to Facelift Surgery

In the senior author's practice, which spans a career in facelifting of 25 years, the biplane facelift has become the workhorse operation and is used for most patients. Newer innovations, including the use of laser dissection and the skin-sparing technique described later in this chapter, basically have not altered the approach that has been in use for more than 15 years. In patients who are seeking additional upper facial rejuvenation, the biplane facelift can easily be combined with either a direct or endoscopic coronal lift. However, for patients who are concerned primarily about upper facial rejuvenation, the extended subperiosteal coronal lift is still the operation of choice.

In the senior author's opinion, no other operation provides the elegant upper facial rejuvenation that is characteristic of this operation. This is especially true when there is an indication to correct a downward slope of the lateral canthal region. Although the technique of the extended subperiosteal coronal lift is beyond the scope of this chapter, it is important to understand that, when this operation is selected, lower facelifting must be sharply modified.

The plane of dissection for the subperiosteal lift extends down to the mandible, making it essential to avoid additional mid-face dissection when carrying out lower lifting. For this reason, when lower facelifting is combined with a subperiosteal lift, a biplane neck dissection is performed, but very little subcutaneous undermining is carried out in the face. A subperiosteal lift effectively lifts not only the upper face but also the midface; subcutaneous dissection in the cheek area is only necessary to remove redundant skin.

Regardless of the facelift technique used, there will always be some secondary relaxation. We suggest to all our lower facelift patients that they consider a secondary tuck (a mini-facelift) 12 to 24 months after the original surgery. When this secondary procedure is carried out, it is done under local anesthesia and involves reopening the incision around the ear, both anteriorly and posteriorly. Very limited undermining is carried out, and the skin is slightly advanced and excised.

The wound is subsequently closed in two layers, using 4-0 Monocryl and a running 6-0 plain gut. No dressings are applied, and patients are able to return to essentially normal activity the day after surgery. In spite of the limited undermining and advancement, it is remarkable how this procedure enhances the effect of the original operation.

Over the course of many years, we have had a considerable number of patients who have returned every few years for a secondary tuck, effectively eliminating the need for a second facelift. Because of the limited morbidity and risk associated with the procedure, we believe this technique deserves more widespread emphasis. Because of the network of subcutaneous scar tissue that has developed through the subcutaneous dissection of the facelift, this secondary tuck seems to provide a very strong and lasting lift that far exceeds what one would anticipate from so minor a procedure.

Since its introduction by Hamra,[17] the term *deep-plane facelift* has been widely used. The term can be confusing because not every surgeon is following the technique as originally described by Hamra, but the term has generally come to be accepted as a type of facelift that is carried out in a plane deeper than the subcutaneous plane.

The term *sub-SMAS* is commonly used for this type of dissection, but we prefer to avoid use of the term *SMAS*, again because there is often confusion on the part of surgeons as to the precise meaning of this term. As one approaches the anterior border of the parotid, the SMAS becomes so thin as to become an almost microscopic layer. For that reason, we prefer to use the term *musculofascial layer* as described by Jost and Levet.[16]

When carrying out a deep-plane dissection, it is essentially the same as simply using the deeper plane of the biplane lift (see below). Although the deep-plane lift sacrifices some of the versatility of the biplane lift, it does offer an advantage of safety, as the subcutaneous flap is very limited and, in fact, after the excess skin is trimmed, it becomes nonexistent. For this reason, we tend to favor the deep-plane approach in patients who are smokers and diabetics, and increasingly for patients who are undergoing combined laser resurfacing with facelift. Because the biplane facelift is our workhorse operation, the technique is described in some detail.

Introduction to the Opportunistic Biplane Facelift

The biplane facelift described in this chapter is based on principles that increase aesthetics and longevity with limited morbidity. Facial aging is most pronounced from changes occurring in the deeper musculofascial plane that result in ptosis of the malar fat pad, jowl region, nasolabial folds, and neck. Precise elevation and rotation of this plane is accomplished using this biplane facelift technique. We call the operation "opportunistic," because there is no set anatomic limit to the deep-plane dissection. Rather, it is based on the concept of elevating tissue to the point where the flap can be easily advanced with the effect of providing adequate lift in the mid- and lower midface regions. Generally, this point is quite obvious. A rather sharp release is effected when sufficient elevation is accomplished, and the surgeon observes a marked lifting effect around the anterior cheek and the corner of the mouth.

Lifting the musculofascial flap anteriorly until adequate release is obtained allows the surgeon to obtain an improved lift with better control of the multivector pull necessary in this deeper plane of musculofascial tissue. We have not had any incidence of periauricular wound margin necrosis since adopting this technique. A natural appearance is achieved as a result of the deep multivector lift, with minimal skin tension after redraping.

The term *opportunistic* also applies to the concept of recognizing that, in some patients, the musculofascial layer becomes so attenuated as the dissection proceeds anteriorly that the resulting biplane flap would lack sufficient strength to provide adequate pull. In these cases, the surgeon wisely retreats and depends on plication for deeper support.

Tumescent anesthesia and fine cannula lipodissection, combined with electrocautery and laser dissection, all help minimize operative time (which averages $1\frac{1}{2}$ hours) and postoperative morbidity. Because the primary lift is in the deeper plane, we have essentially eliminated skin excision in the temple and occipital regions. Skin bunching in the mastoid area subsides after a few weeks, resulting in a completely hidden scar within the hair and a decreased incidence of skin injury behind the ear. We depend entirely on the deeper pull for the effectiveness of the lift. Skin excision in front of the ear is very conservative. This has produced much better healing and finer scars because of the total absence of pull on the skin.

We have long abandoned postoperative drains or extensive head wraps and have seen no increase in postoperative hematomas. Our incidence of hematoma requiring surgical drainage was 2% (4 out of the past 200 cases) after biplanar facelifts without the use of drains or dressings, compared with a prior incidence of 4% when dressings had been routinely used. Part of the difference is attributable to the ability to recognize early small hematomas during recovery that can be treated conservatively by milking the flap, thus avoiding large hematomas when dressings are removed 24 hours after surgery. In addition, it appeared to us that hematomas would sometimes occur on removal of the drain and may have actually been caused by abrasion of the drain removal. Avoidance of dressings promotes patient comfort and may help avoid the swelling that can result from the tourniquet effect of compressive dressings.

Submusculofascial dissection has been reported to increase the risk of facial nerve injury; arguments have been made that plicating the SMAS is safer and as effective as the deeper plane techniques. In our experience, no permanent facial nerve injuries have occurred. There is no question that expert knowledge of the facial anatomic planes and neurovascular distribution is a requirement to avoid this complication with any facelifting techniques. Furthermore, our use of operating loops and laser dissection minimizes the risk of facial nerve injury. We expect to see the buccal nerve fibers during the course of dissection overlying the masseter muscle and, in fact, feel more comfortable when they are in view. Frequently, portions of the ramus mandibularis are seen as we begin dissection of the posterior platysma.

SMAS plication facelifts can improve facial aesthetics,[18, 19] but limited improvement is often seen in the malar and mandibular border due to the inability of this technique to free the restraining fibers (zygomatic and mandibular ligaments) in these regions. The biplane lift breaks these adhesions during the submusculofascial dissection. As mentioned, the "opportunistic" description given to this lift is based on the concept of only dissecting far enough anteriorly to release the flap. Should poor flap quality (thickness or continuity) exist, the procedure can easily be converted to a simple SMAS plication procedure.

Biplane Facelift Technique

PREOPERATIVE MARKING

Initial marking is confined to outlining the incisions in the temple and in the mastoid region (Fig. 27–1). We begin by determining the proposed lift vector. A line is then drawn perpendicular to that vector, constituting the temporal and occipital ends of the facelift incision. These lines are marked with the patient sitting and before induction of anesthesia. The remaining incisions can easily be marked in the operating room.

PREPARATION AND ANESTHESIA

Nearly all our surgery is carried out under endotracheal anesthesia, although it can be carried out using analeptic technique. The incisions in the scalp are prepared by shaving hair conservatively around the incision site.

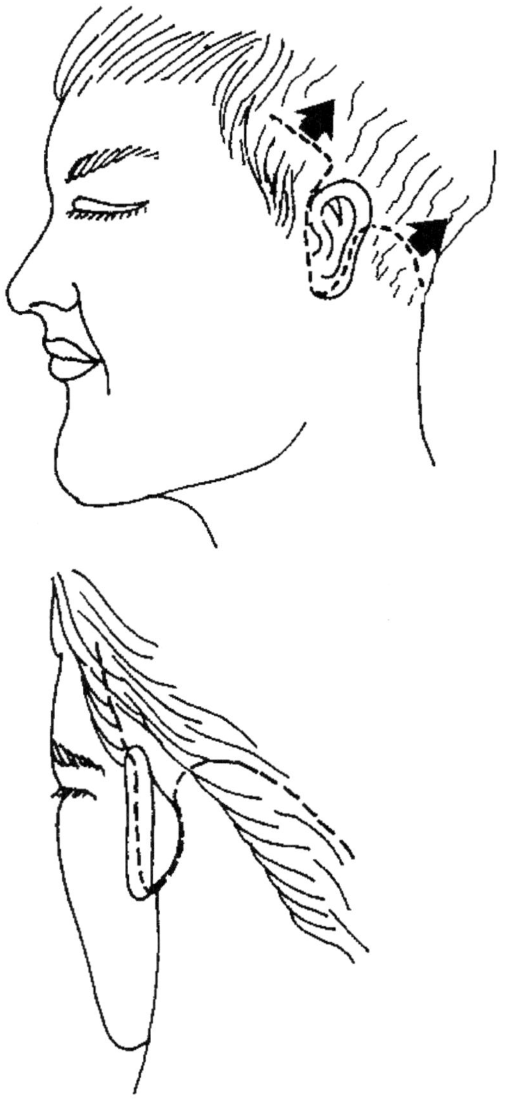

Figure 27–1 Location of incisions.

After the initial preparation, a modified tumescent infiltration is accomplished. We use a solution containing 250 ml of saline, 50 ml of 2% lidocaine, and 1 ml of 1:1000 epinephrine. The infiltration is facilitated by using a self-filling syringe in line with the tumescent solution. Infiltration is begun with the deep dermis of the temporal and occipital incision sites and then subcutaneously over the entire face and neck, with care taken to limit the injection to the subcutaneous plane in these areas. The layer between the temporoparietal and temporalis fascia is flooded to facilitate later blunt dissection in that area.

It is important to avoid infiltrating beneath the platysma. The reason for this is related to the fact that we use "lipodissection." Lipodissection involves the use of fine liposuction cannulas without associated suction. This creates a honeycombing in the subcutaneous plane that will greatly facilitate the subsequent sharp dissection. If the tumescent infiltration is carried out in the subplatysmal plane, it is possible that the lipodissection will be too deep and may damage our platysmal flap.

With injection in the subcutaneous plane, we find that a fair amount of the fluid still diffuses into the deeper tissue layers providing significant hemostasis and facilitating later elevation of the platysmal flap. It is especially important to get a tumescent infiltration in the area just below and behind the earlobe, as the dissection planes in this area are quite thin. After infiltration, the patient is again prepared and draped.

LIPODISSECTION

Before making incisions, flap elevation with lipodissection is accomplished. The term is derived from the use of liposuction cannulas used for dissection rather than suction. In fact, very little liposuction is even completed. We have found from past experience that the technique of aggressive facial liposuction, although often providing good initial results, often led to later changes that were undesirable as patients aged. Patients who were followed for long periods have an excessive loss of subcutaneous tissue from aggressive liposuction surgery in the face, neck, and jowls. We now limit suctioning to areas in which there is truly a fatty tissue excess. This will generally be in the jowl and submental areas. Suctioning along the anterior jowl with microcannulas can be very useful but, again, fat removal should be conservative. In the submental area, there is often excess fat. In this case, we will do liposuction but we avoid removing all the fat between the anterior bands of the platysma muscle to avoid producing a hollowing effect in this area, sometimes referred to as a "cobra neck deformity."

The lipodissection is accomplished by using small cannulas of diameter varying from 1.5 to 2 mm. Approaches are made through punctures just in front of the upper attachment of the helix of the ear, below the lobule, in the mastoid area and in the submentum. A small trochar is used to puncture the skin, lipodissection is carried out using a very gentle movement. The small cannulas should easily identify the subcutaneous plane above the deeper musculofascial layers.

In all cases, the cannula opening is down, facing platysma, and not toward the undersurface of the skin to prevent injury to the dermis which could cause skin dimpling. The extent of lipodissection extends from beneath the zygomatic arch anteriorly beyond the extent of the parotid gland, partially overlying the masseter muscle. Along the angle of the mandible, suction is carried out toward the chin. While approaching the chin, it is critical to remain in a superficial plane since the mandibular branch of the facial nerve is quite superficial in this area and is not covered by muscle. It is very important to carry the lipodissection far forward toward the chin to facilitate release of mandibulocutaneous attachments in that region. Adequate rehabilitation of the jowl is dependent on this release. In the neck, dissection is carried down to the hyoid and posteriorly to the sternocleidomastoid muscle.

Overlying and posterior to the sternocleidomastoid muscle, there are often thick attachments between the skin and the deeper structures of the neck and it may not be possible to develop a superficial plane with the cannula. If there is resistance in this area, we desist and depend on later sharp dissection. This is also true in the posterior triangle of the neck. It is important to avoid going too deep in the posterior triangle as the spinal accessory nerve may be at risk. We avoid all lipodissection beneath the hair bearing skin in the occipital scalp to avoid damage to hair follicles, which can easily result in permanent alopecia.

MANAGEMENT OF THE ANTERIOR PLATYSMA

The "opportunistic" biplane facelift depends primarily on posterior pull of a platysmal flap for neck rehabilitation. Even anterior cervical laxity is well corrected by this procedure. However, if the patient has significant anterior platysmal banding, we do carry out an anterior platysmaplasty. If there is distinct banding, posterior platysmal pull is usually not sufficient, and it is helpful to secure the platysma in the midline. This occurs in approximately 20% of our cases.

Before surgery, we mark the platysmal bands. We make a 2- to 3-cm transverse incision in the submentum, attempting to use a natural crease. The skin is then elevated off the underlying anterior platysma muscle which is usually quite easy to identify as a result of the lipodissection. An Aufricht or small right-angle retractor is inserted into the wound for visualization. Any residual excess fat is clamped and trimmed with scissors. Silk sutures (3-0) are then placed between the platysmal bands and are secured across the midline from the chin to within 1 or 2 cm of the hyoid bone. This is rather easily done through a small incision when the surgeon is using a headlight and loops. Inspection will confirm that adequate approximation has been carried out. Wide undermining of the skin of the neck is important to allow proper draping at the end of the procedure.

INCISIONS

The skin incisions are then made using a scalpel or an electrosurgical unit. For electrosurgical incision, we use a pure cutting current and a Colorado needle tip. Long-term experience has shown that the scars are indistinguishable between the two techniques. We prefer to use a blade on younger patients and electrosurgery on older patients who have more lax skin, which tends to make it more difficult to get an even cut with the blade.

We begin with an oblique temporal incision that is perpendicular to the desired direction of temple lifting. This incision need only be long enough to allow introduction of a finger. The incision is made just through the dermis. The posterior extent of that incision joins an incision inferior along the upper anterior helix, going along the edge of the tragus, then sweeping around the earlobe in the crease behind the ear and up on the occiput. Although many investigators have advocated making the postauricular incision on the conchal cartilage because of subsequent migration of the scar, we find this unnecessary, as our technique avoids any pull on the skin and thus eliminates scar migration.

TEMPLE DISSECTION

The dissection begins in the temple, lifting and separating the skin edges with double-prong hooks, dissection is carried through the temporoparietal fascia to the temporalis fascia. Branches of the superficial temporal artery or vein may be encountered here. These vessels should be controlled; it is helpful to try to identify them before cutting. Blunt dissection is used to elevate over the temporalis fascia, working as far forward as the temporal crest and inferiorly to just above the zygomatic arch. Both superiorly and posteriorly, the dissection is also carried out so that a flap is mobilized which can later be elevated and secured to the temporalis fascia. The fibrous attachments of the temporal crest are broken to allow better mobilization of the temple flap. This permits better elevation of the lateral brow area. After completion of the lower dissection, this flap will be firmly advanced, and the temporoparietal fascia will be secure to the deep temporal fascia.

LOWER FACIAL DISSECTION

The plane of dissection for the midface is entirely separate from the temporal dissection. As stated, the temporalis dissection is beneath the temporoparietal fascia. As dissection is carried inferior to the zygomatic arch the plane abruptly switches to the subcutaneous level. Subcutaneous dissection is carried forward sharply in the midface until visualizing the honeycomb perforations that were created during the lipodissection. As dissection proceeds inferiorly around the ear toward the mastoid area, very careful, sharp dissection is required. If the plane is too superficial, the flap may be compromised. If dissection goes too deeply, there will be bleeding from the muscle and possible injury to the great auricular nerve.

The incision extending posteriorly from the post auricular crease is made deeply and extends through the underlying fascia. When the mastoid and occipital regions are dissected, care must again be taken to keep the plane of dissection deep in the upper part of the flap. This is essential because the flap will later be advanced by securing it to the superior occipital fascia with deep permanent sutures. As dissection continues inferiorly in the occipital region, the plane become more superficial but still must remain beneath the hair follicles to avoid producing alopecia. As a general rule, if you see hair follicles, they probably are damaged. Flap elevation is carried out from behind, working toward the sternocleidomastoid muscle. In this area, sharp dissection will be required. We prefer to use the electrosurgical unit, but dissection can be carried out with a blade or scissors.

A very important part of the dissection is the upward dissection in the occipital scalp, the dissection extends just above the fascia, for a distance of 3 or 4 cm. The scalp is released superiorly to allow for later advancement of the lower occipital flap during closure. While this flap is firmly advanced, little or no skin will be excised. Rather, the skin will be allowed to loosely lie and often creates a small "sausage" roll that will slowly flatten over a period of weeks. This loose skin allows a very nice realignment of the posterior hair line, as there is really no tension of the skin edge.

As the dissection proceeds inferiorly and forward to the sternocleidomastoid muscle, we are careful to avoid injury to the external jugular vein and great auricular nerve. Once in front of the sternocleidomastoid muscle, we will again see the perforations produced by lipodissection. Now the remainder of the subcutaneous dissection is usually quite simple. We typically complete the dissection by simply sweeping our finger across the residual fine bands of connective tissue. If necessary, we use open scissors, which we advance for a rapid elevation.

The general anterior extent of the subcutaneous dissection is to a line drawn from the corner of the eye to the mental foramen. This varies and, in keeping with our "opportunistic" approach, we will be more conservative if the dissection is more difficult, or if there is more than minimal bleeding. In the neck, superficial dissection is generally carried out completely across the midline. Because of the tumescent infiltration, the dissection is almost always bloodless, but meticulous hemostasis is accomplished with electrocoagulation.

DEEP-PLANE DISSECTION

We keep referring to this as an "opportunistic technique" since the extent of the dissection of the deep flap is not based on anatomic landmarks, but rather on determining what is required to give the elevation necessary for the patient. Dissection of the deep-plane usually begins in the neck.

The first step is to identify the posterior border of the platysma. If this structure is not clearly evident, we use a technique of open liposuction to remove the fatty tissue off the posterior extent of the muscle. A No. 6 spatula type liposuction cannula is attached to standard wall suction and, using an open technique, the fatty tissue is suctioned off of the muscle. Once the posterior border of the platysma is evident, a flap is started. It is developed by incising along its posterior border from the lower edge of the parotid inferiorly to the level of the upper thyroid cartilage. This incision can be made with a knife or electrosurgically, but we prefer the laser because of its precision and hemostasis. Once the incision is complete, scissors are used to undermine the posterior platysma for about 4 or 5 cm. A lower transverse incision is then made across the platysma to create a flap that can be advanced posteriorly. The anatomic development of the platysma muscle varies considerably from individual to individual. In some patients, the platysma can be clearly identified, extending upward into the face, whereas in other individuals it attenuates at the level of the mandible. Even in cases where it attenuates, a fibrous remnant usually persists.

The posterior incision in the platysma is continued upward into the face following the posterior border of the muscle to the angle of the jaw. From there, it continues upward in the midface, about 2 cm in front of the helix.

Flap elevation is then carried out using the laser. The deep-plane of the dissection is either the thin areolar tissue overlying the parotid gland, or, if that layer is not apparent, the parotid gland itself. The upper level of the incision is slightly below the zygomatic arch. At this point, the incision curves forward, proceeding anteriorly toward the true zygoma.

In this fashion, a deep flap is elevated that is continuous with the lower platysmal flap. Superiorly, the anterior dissection extends into the fibro-fatty tissue of the cheek. Further inferiorly, a discrete plane is clearly apparent. Ideally, this plane is within the loose areolar tissue immediately overlying the parotid gland.

Anterior dissection is carried forward with the laser to and beyond the anterior border of the parotid gland. As the dissection proceeds forward, beyond the anterior limit of the gland, the masseter muscle is apparent, and one usually sees fibers of the facial nerve resting on that muscle within a thin layer of areolar tissue.

Here again, the use of magnification facilitates the dissection. As mentioned before, we are more comfortable when we actually see the nerve fibers. Similarly, we can also sometimes see Stenson's duct with an associated buccal branch.

The nerve fiber that is probably most at risk is the marginal mandibular. Although we do occasionally see this nerve, it is usually not apparent. Careful meticulous laser dissection is carried out, and flap elevation is most conservative over the angle of the mandible.

The important decision to make is just how far we need to elevate this flap. Again, the answer depends on the individual patient. As we proceed with the dissection, we are constantly pulling on the flap to see whether we get the desired lift. Once we reach a point where there is a general freeing of the flap, we can usually see the desired pull on the cheek, nasolabial fold and the corner of the mouth. In simple terms, when we get the pull that we need, the dissection is complete.

Most commonly, we find that it is the malar portion of the flap that binds us down the most. This is the most difficult area of the dissection, because we are working within the bulk of the malar fat pad and not in a true anatomic plane. We like to make the flap fairly deep in this area because we feel that by staying deep, we actually lift up the malar fat pad itself. This gives a natural form of malar augmentation.

Once the flap is elevated and hemostasis maintained the flap can be secured. Using a strong permanent suture (3-0 braided silk), the upper part of the flap is attached to the temporalis fascia, exerting a strong pull. Next, the platysma muscle is pulled back, attaching it to the mastoid fascia. Immediately, we can see a marked tightening of the face and neck. These are the two primary anchoring sutures. We continue to suture the posterior border of the platysma to the fascia overlying the sternocleidomastoid muscle using interrupted 3-0 silk suture. The pull is actually in a posterior superior direction, such that the platysmal flap actually forms a sling that supports the ear lobe and tends to prevent subsequent inferior migration of the ear, which can result in the deformity commonly called "pixie ear." In the facial region, the flap is attached to the parotid fascia in the preauricular area. A firm pull is applied, as this forms the primary support of the facelift.

SKIN EXCISION AND CLOSURE

Once this flap is secured, a re-draping of the skin and removal of excess tissue in front of the ear is accomplished. Before excising skin, we gently pull our skin flaps upward and backward to mark the new location of the inferior portion of the lobule. A slit is then made on the skin so that there will be no downward tension in this area. Avoiding traction on the earlobe is essential to prevent a pixie ear, elfin deformity. The hammock effect of the posteriorly placed platysmal flap also assists in preventing this deformity. Once this point is marked, the subcutaneous tissue is inset to the subcutaneous tissue beneath the lobule, ensuring a relaxed closure.

Next the temple tissues are elevated. No skin is removed, but a strong permanent suture to the underlying dermis and temporoparietal fascia of the inferior temporal flap is placed and advanced posteriorly and superiorly, securing it to the temporalis fascia. By avoiding any skin excision, the scar will be thin, with little chance of hair loss. Still, this strong deep suture provides effective elevation of the temple area without a stretched look.

Elevation of the neck is then carried out in the mastoid area using a similar technique of attaching the subcutaneous tissue to the occipital fascia. Having previously undermined the superior flap in this area allows significant advancement. When there is significant laxity in the neck, it may be necessary to trim a small amount of occipital hair bearing skin, but the excision is kept to a minimum, allowing a closure with no tension. The skin is then advanced superiorly in the postauricular area, securing the closure with deep sutures (3-0 or 4-0 Monocryl). This smoothes out any pleating that might occur near the lobule of the ear.

Excess skin in front of the ear is trimmed with minimal tension after excision, and the skin immediately in front of the tragus is defatted, using either the laser or scissors. A subcutaneous closure with 4-0 Monocryl is carried out in this region that results in approximation of the skin edges. We do not want any pull on the skin from the skin sutures.

Skin closure in the hair bearing skin is with staples, but the preauricular area is closed with a simple running 6-0 plain gut suture. Because the subcutaneous closure actually provides the strength of the skin approximation, this very fine skin closure is quite adequate and virtually never leaves stitch marks. The suture usually dissolves in 1 week. The postauricular crease is simply closed with 4-0 Monocryl. Skin sutures are not used here to allow for drainage and evacuation of small hematomas should they occur in the immediate postoperative period. Again, as there is no tension on this closure, the subcutaneous closure is quite adequate.

POSTOPERATIVE CARE

Drains and dressings have not been used at our center for about 8 years. Dressings are more likely to hide problems than to prevent them. Long experience with suction drains indicated that they did not reduce the chance of hematoma. By leaving the surgical site open, small hematomas can promptly be identified in the recovery room where they can often be treated by simply expressing them. When larger hematomas are present, we can identify them much more quickly, allowing for an early definitive correction. A normal blood pressure is maintained in the recovery room, as postoperative hypertension is one of the primary causes of hematoma after facelift. Medication is promptly given if the patient shows signs of nausea or hypertension. Preoperative dimenhydrinate (Dramamine) and postoperative oxygen are used in the recovery room to help allay nausea.

Patients are instructed to keep their heads elevated for the first few days after surgery. They are permitted to wash their hair and face the day after surgery. They are to apply a thin layer of antibiotic ointment to the incisions and to cleanse the suture lines with peroxide as needed. Surgical staples are removed from the hair 1 week to 10 days after surgery. The sutures in the skin dissolve and do not require removal.

COMBINED FACELIFTING AND LASER RESURFACING

Regardless of the surgical technique used for facelifting, some sort of surface modification is needed to improve fine and deep lines etched in the skin. In our practice, CO_2 laser resurfacing has entirely replaced deep chemical peeling. When we first began to use the laser, we followed the old accepted principles of only doing regional resurfacing of the perioral region in association with the lift. Full face resurfacing was staged.

Based on the experience of two well-known Texas cosmetic surgeons, Bill Miles of Fort Worth and John Pate of El Paso (personal communication), we have come to modify our approach. Both of these surgeons, the former using chemical peel and the latter working with laser, have shown that resurfacing can safely be combined with surgery. About 4 years ago, we began combining laser resurfacing with selected patients undergoing facelift surgery. Our initial approach was to combine the resurfacing with our traditional biplane approach. Because we were concerned about the possibility of injury to the flaps, we would diminish the laser intensity toward the periphery of the face.

We have now modified our technique, and currently we favor a deep-plane approach when we combine surgery with resurfacing. Our deep-plane approach is essentially the same as our biplane approach except for the skin undermining in the cheek area. In the neck, the approach is identical. In the face, subcutaneous undermining only goes far enough forward to allow for skin excision (usually about 3 to 6 cm). Dissection is then carried down to the parotid after elevation of the lower platysmal flap. The same opportunistic advancement in the deep-plane is accomplished until adequate release of the flap is evident. Because we don't undermine the skin, we do lose a little of the cutaneous tightening. This does, however, allow us to apply full laser energy to the entire face. Essentially, we believe that, in selected cases, we gain more from the laser than we lose from the added biplane facial undermining.

LASER TECHNIQUE

Although beyond the primary scope of this chapter, it is worthwhile to briefly discuss our laser technique when combined with deep-plane facelifting. We classify our laser technique as moderately aggressive. Because settings vary from instrument to instrument, it is important to realize that wise surgeons will always start at low intensities until they are familiar with the effects of their unit. We use a Luxar CO_2 laser. Before surgery, we mark the deepest lines of the patient. After prepping, and before surgery, we etch the deepest lines with several passes using a superpulse setting of 6 to 8 W. The char is wiped off and we then proceed with the facelift.

After the facelift is complete, using a computerized scanner, we treat the entire face with a single pass using 9 W of energy with the scanner set at maximum density. We feather into the neck to avoid a demarcated line. We do not wipe the char, but rather apply a layer of Catrix, which the patient is instructed to reapply frequently during recovery. Complete healing of the wound is expected in 8 to 10 days.

There is no question that patient satisfaction seems higher in our patients undergoing combined treatment compared with facelift alone. We expect that this practice will become much more accepted in the future.

SECONDARY FACELIFTING

Although nearly all our patients undergoing primary facelift are treated with either a biplane or deep-plane approach, our attitude toward secondary facelift is much more conservative. As previously discussed, we are strong advocates of the secondary tuck 1 or 2 years after the primary lift. About 25% of our patients elect this program. For patients who come back several years later, we offer an intermediate procedure that we call a "secondary lift."

Conclusion

The argument over the ideal facelift will not be solved in the near future. There are far too many variables to permit a totally scientific approach to this issue. It remains to be proved that deep-plane techniques actually add longevity to the results of facelifting. Those of us who advocate these procedures do so because we have an impression that they produce better and longer-lasting results, but this has not been proved and is disputed by many surgeons.

This technique has been used by the senior author (H.T.) for more than 14 years in several hundred cases, with excellent results. Complications have been few, limited to relatively minor problems, including unsatisfactory posterior scars, delayed recovery related to hematoma, and relatively minor but unacceptable elevation of the temporal hair tuft in a few cases. One case of excessive preauricular scarring occurred in a patient who sustained pulmonary compromise after surgery that resulted in a period of significant hypoxia related to a pulmonary embolus. Fortunately, the patient recovered and had a satisfactory result after scar revision. We have had no cases of motor nerve injury in spite of the extensive dissection.

Not every patient can undergo the complete biplane dissection. Each patient's treatment plan is individualized. Occasionally, a decision is made preoperatively to limit the dissection to the superficial plane.

Patients who return for second facelifts often maintain a layer of scar tissue that appears to offer more holding power even if the surgery was performed several years earlier. Most of these patients do not need the effects of the deeper lift, if the dissection of their first lift was substantial. In fact, aggressive secondary lifting can occasionally elevate tissue too much, leading to an unnatural look.

The decision to carry out a biplane approach may be modified during the actual surgery if more than average bleeding occurs or if a thin musculofascial layer prevents adequate deep-plane flap elevation.

Over the past 12 years, most of our patients have undergone the biplane facelift. The technique is safe and effective and one that can be modified to suit the needs of the individual patient.

REFERENCES

Tobin and Cuzalina—CHAPTER 27

1. Holländer E. XVII. Die kosmetische Chirurgie. In: Joseph M, ed. *Handbuch der Kosmetik.* Leipzig: Verlag von Veit; 1912:688
2. Joseph J. Hängewangenplastik (Melomioplastik). *Dtsch Med Wochenschr* 1921;47:287
3. Bettman AG. Plastic and cosmetic surgery of the face. *Northwest Med* 1920;19:205
4. Skoog T. *New Methods and Refinements: Plastic Surgery.* Philadelphia: WB Saunders; 1974
5. Owsley JQ. Platysma-fascial rhytidectomy. A preliminary report. *Plast Reconstr Surg* 1977;59:12:843–850
6. Connell BF. Cervical lift: surgical correction of fat contour problems combined with full width platysma muscle flap. *Aesth Plast Surg* 1978;1:355
7. Gurerro-Santols J. The role of the platysma muscle in rhytidoplasty. *Clin Plast Surg* 1978;5:29
8. Hamra ST. *Composite Rhytidectomy: Concepts and Elements of Composite Rhytidectomy.* St Louis, MO: Quality Medical Publishing; 1993:1–25
9. Hamra ST. Composite rhytidectomy, finesse and refinements in technique. *Clin in Plast Surg* 1997;24:337–346
10. Tessier P. Facelifting and frontal rhytidectomy. In: Ely JF, ed. *Transactions of the Seventh International Congress of Plastic and Reconstructive Surg.* Rio de Janeiro. 1980:393
11. Tobin HA. The extended subperiosteal coronal lift. *Am J of Cosmet Surg* 1993;10:47–57
12. Ramirez OM. The subperiosteal rhytidectomy: the third-generation facelift. *Ann Plast Surg* 1992;28:218–234
13. Ramirez O, Maillard G Musolas A. The extended subperiosteal face lift: a definitive soft-tissue remodeling for facial rejuvenation. *Plast Reconstr Surg* 1991;88:227–238
14. Ramirez OM. Endoscopic full face lift. *Aesthetic Plast Surg* 1994;18:363
15. Mitz V, Peyronie M. The superficial musculo-aponeurotic system (SMAS) in the parotid and cheek area. *Plast Reconstr Surg* 1976;58:80–88
16. Jost G, Levet Y. Parotid fascia and face lifting: a critical evaluation of the SMAS concept. *Plast Reconstr Surg* 1984;74:42–51
17. Hamra ST. Composite rhytidectomy. *Plast Reconstr Surg* 1978;86:53
18. Webster R, Davidson TM, White MF, Bush JE, Smith RC. Conservative facelift surgery. *Arch Laryngol* 1976;102:657–682
19. Webster R, Smith R, Smith K. Facelift. IV. Use of superficial musculoaponeurotic system suspending sutures. *Head Neck Surg* 1984;6:780–791

10

Skin Resurfacing—Laser or Peel

"Structure and surface should be analyzed separately and then melded into a therapeutic plan for the individual facing you across the consultation room."

Leonard J. Singer

"Since the mid 1990s, laser-assisted skin resurfacing has rapidly replaced chemical peels and physical dermabrasion as the most common means of skin exfoliation. Remarkably this has taken place with alarming rapidity and despite the lack of comparative trials. Evidence-based medicine has taught us the value of comparative trials. Without these we must ask ourselves the fundamental questions, how and why has this happened and is it justified?"

Milton Waner

"The contemporary use of these agents began in the 1960s, and their use has flourished since that time. Well-documented research has shown the beneficial clinical and histologic changes present after the application of various chemical peeling agents."

Devinder S. Mangat

Skin Resurfacing—Laser or Peel

CHAPTER 28

Leonard J. Singer

During the past 5 years, two new industries have made a substantial mark on the cosmetic surgery world: the therapeutic skin care market, and the cosmetic laser market. As with most advances in this field, these new products and services have undergone a baptism by fire of talk-show promotion, infotainment exposé, and faddish mood swings in popularity. At this juncture, it would be useful to review a framework of knowledge and opinion that may help the practicing cosmetic surgeon organize and make sense of these new products and services.

Patients consulting with the cosmetic surgeon for improvement of the appearance of their face represent the broadest range of expression of any presenting problem in the specialty. They range from the preteen struggling with scarring from self-evacuation of acne pustules to the leathery alligatorlike skin of the working outdoorsman; from the society matron who shuns photos of her profile to the 30-year-old manager who simply wants to improve and maintain her skin. An organized, logical approach to these problems will encourage problem-oriented solutions, which should in turn result in improved outcomes and greater patient satisfaction.

When the patient is first seen, it is helpful for the surgeon to determine where the patient's concerns and priorities lie. Is the patient most concerned about problems of structure, i.e., sagging of skin around the brows, nasolabial folds, jaw line, and neck, or is the concern directed more toward skin color and tone, and surface wrinkles or acne scars? The analogy I frequently use in explaining this concept to the patient is that of the old, neglected house being considered for rehabilitation. Clearly, placing a bid without first determining the quality of the supporting structure and the need for structural repair would be foolish. Equally important is the assessment of the surface, such as paint, roof, and landscape. Structure and surface should be analyzed separately and then melded into a therapeutic plan for the individual facing you across the consultation room.

The purpose of this chapter is to address the repair of surface abnormalities specifically by laser resurfacing, but it is important to place the procedure within the context of a logical plan. Only the amateur cosmetic surgeon will address all facial concerns with one modality.

Background

It has long been observed that select patients who had sustained relatively superficial burns to the face frequently noted improvement of the texture and pigmentation of their face after the burn had healed—sometimes with a dramatic decrease in superficial wrinkling. This has been seen in flash burn injuries from gas stoves and mine gas explosions. For a number of years, attempts have been made to replicate these results in a reliable and safe way. Given that therapeutic measures affecting only the epidermis did not effectively address the stubborn problems of superficial wrinkling and acne scarring, it was recognized early on that this would require the development of a means of applying heat in a very specific fashion so as to maximize the therapeutic effect with penetration of the papillary, and even the superficial reticular, dermis. At the same time, in order to avoid the risks of pigmentary changes and scarring, it was necessary to minimize damage to the skin microcirculation, the adnexal organs, dermal melanin granules and melanocytes, and the deeper reticular dermis. This was a tall order. Direct sources of heat energy are terribly nonspecific, indiscriminately damaging anything in their paths.

With the development in the mid-1960s of a unique light source with unusual characteristics called the light amplification by stimulated emission of radiation (laser), it was immediately evident that this device held promise of being the selective source of heat which could accomplish safe and effective resurfacing. This is because the physics of lasers enabled the release of energy in a form of light that could theoretically penetrate a specific structure before changing into another form of energy: heat. Because light absorption is specific in pigmented structures and the organic world is full of pigmented structures, one could then select a laser that emits a particular "color" of light that would be maximally absorbed by a particular "colored" material in the skin (technically "wavelength" is more accurate than "color," as color refers only to the visible wavelengths). If the heat could be applied very selectively, the laser would enable specific cellular damage, permitting safe and effective resurfacing.

The first task was to choose the correct laser wavelength. For the sake of simplicity, one can assume that there are three light-absorbing structures or chromophores in the skin: melanin, hemoglobin, and water. Clearly, resurfacing attempts to apply energy superficially, avoiding melanin and hemoglobin. Since tissue water is abundant in the skin, laser wavelengths that are absorbed maximally in water are potentially those that may be useful in resurfacing. The three wavelengths that are maximally absorbed in water are CO_2, erbium-YAG, and excimer. The first two are infrared (IR); the latter ultraviolet (UV). UV light, with its propensity for breaking bonds in DNA molecules, is contraindicated in rapidly dividing skin, whereas it is very useful in the relatively acellular hydrophilic environment of the cornea.

Of the remaining two wavelengths, the erbium-YAG has a greater affinity for water; therefore, its effect is more superficial than that of the CO_2. In addition, less heat is generated with the erbium, which is advantageous in that it produces less post-inflammatory erythema, but disadvantageous in that it does not produce sufficient heat to stimulate neocollagen formation and reversal of elastosis, as occurs with the CO_2 laser. Each laser has found a different role in the resurfacing armamentarium, but the CO_2 laser remains the gold standard for the treatment of surface wrinkles and, many believe, acne scarring.

The continuous-wave CO_2 laser was one of the first available in medicine. When resurfacing was first attempted with this laser, results were decidedly mixed. The problem was that the continuous wave inevitably pumped excessive heat into the skin. Therefore, the complications of scar formation and pigmentary changes were common, and the procedure was considered too risky for adoption.

The next major advance in the field of resurfacing was the recognition that the skin model was able to divest itself of excess heat if the energy was applied very rapidly and in large amounts. The observed value for the threshold at which heat was no longer efficiently divested, and instead was conducted to adjacent tissue (leading to dermal scarring), is known as the thermal relaxation time; in human skin it is less than 1 ms in duration. CO_2 lasers capable of delivering the heat in a duration of less than 1 ms were found to be effective and safe to use for resurfacing. The laser manufacturers chose one of two methods to achieve this: one was to use collimated pulsed devices that put out discrete packets of light, each high in energy and less than 1 ms in duration. This type of laser is epitomized by the Coherent UltraPulse laser (Coherent Medical Group, Santa Clara, CA). The other method was to use a scanning device attached to a continuous-wave laser, which moved the beam very rapidly so that any one unit area of skin never received energy for more than the thermal relaxation time. The Sharplans devices (ESC/Sharplan Medical Systems, Needham, MA) took this path. Both devices are quite capable of producing excellent and safe resurfacing, but it is the author's personal opinion that the collimated, pulsed devices are inherently more user-friendly and safer. Other improvements in these devices involve ease and rapidity of use. The actual delivery of dose is a mature engineering task and has not changed dramatically during the past 5 years.

During the past 5 years, there has been a trend toward the erbium lasers and away from CO_2. This preference has been shaped by a number of factors. First, there is no doubt that the postoperative course is easier on the erbium laser patient (and surgeon) than the CO_2 laser patient. Patients treated with the erbium laser heal faster (4 to 7 days vs 8 to 10 days) and have significantly less erythema afterward. However, in my opinion, erbium laser treatment is simply unable to deliver the level of improvement seen with the CO_2 laser. This is probably because the erbium laser does not generate the 55 to 70°C necessary to stimulate neocollagen formation. Although some laser manufacturers claim that they can replicate CO_2 treatment with their erbium laser by repeated overtreatment, the reality is that the CO_2 remains the most effective treatment for deep wrinkles, acne scarring and muscle action lines. Having said that, if you wish to treat the neck or dorsal hand, it is far safer to do so with the erbium laser than the CO_2 laser.

More recently, newer devices claim to combine the two wavelengths to take advantage of both. Generally these are low-power lasers (usually on the CO_2 side). No credible published data confirm these sales claims. Likewise, the efficacy of the 1380-nm Nd-YAG laser, which purports to treat the collagen of the dermis without in any way damaging the epidermis, awaits clinical evidence.

Intraoperative Safety Considerations

EYE SAFETY

All medical lasers are considered potentially harmful to the eye in less time than it takes to blink. The Food and Drug Administration (FDA) has mandated the use of appropriate eyewear when performing resurfacing. There is a major misconception among physicians that any protective eyewear is adequate. Although the CO_2 wavelength is relatively easy to filter, that is not the case for the erbium-YAG, nor for any vascular, tattoo, or hair-removal laser. When working around the patient's eye, the use of metal scleral protectors is required.

PLUME HAZARD

Aside from the foul odor produced by resurfacing, there are concerns about both the smoke and the particles released by this procedure. The smoke contains a number of toxic gases, which over the long term may have health ramifications for the surgeon and staff. Of greater concern, however, is the fact that a number of different viable viral particles have been recovered from laser plume. The use of a high-volume smoke evacuator is a requirement.

FIRE HAZARD

The CO_2 wavelength will readily ignite drapes, gauze, clothing, curtains, and endotracheal tubes in the presence of more than 35% oxygen, especially if any concentration of nitrous oxide is also present. As most of these procedures are done under intravenous (IV) sedation, the endotracheal tube is usually not of concern. However, these patients are usually kept under deep sedation. If oxygen is administered by nasal canulla, it should be very clear whose responsibility it is to turn off the oxygen when the laser is in the ready mode. A number of large settlements have been awarded as a result of third-degree intranasal burns and resulting synechiae and contractions. Because of the high water absorbance by these wavelengths, wet towels and gauzes are protective against this hazard.

INADVERTENT SKIN DAMAGE

Inadvertent skin damage is entirely avoidable with the judicious use of wet towels and drapes. One should avoid riding the foot pedal when not lasing. It is also helpful to designate a nurse as safety officer, to ensure that the laser is in standby mode when not lasing.

Preoperative Considerations

There are four major issues with regard to the patient.

PATIENT'S SKIN TYPE

Most clinicians use the modified Fitzpatrick scale (types I–VI Table 30–1). This is based on response to UV radiation. It is generally felt that type III and above (usually tan, sometimes burn) should be pretreated b.i.d. (twice a day) with hydroquinone plus glycolic acid or Retin-A with or without topical steroids for 6 to 8 weeks before the resurfacing and beginning again after reepithelialization for several months to avoid postinflammatory hyperpigmentation. Of equal importance is absolute avoidance of UV exposure until the erythema is completely resolved. Patients with Fitzpatrick types V or VI have the additional potential problem of postoperative hypopigmentation. This is directly related to the depth of the treatment, and a conservative approach in stages is highly recommended.

HISTORY OF SEVERE HERPETIC INFECTION

Dermal ablation is believed to unroof nerve endings in which inactive herpes type I resides. Together with the warm, bacteria-free, serum-rich environment of the treated skin, this is a setup for an overwhelming herpetic infection. All full-face resurfacing patients as well as those undergoing perioral resurfacing, should have prophylaxis with Zovirax, Femvir, or Valtrex for 2 days preoperatively and 8 days postoperatively. Patients presenting with serious herpetic infection postoperatively should be admitted for IV antiviral agents.

PATIENT'S WILLINGNESS TO COOPERATE WITH THE FIRST POSTOPERATION WEEK REGIMEN

Classically, patients who present to the emergency department with facial burns are treated with an open exposure, using an occlusive ointment. The patient must cleanse the area repeatedly to avoid bacterial infection and resultant scarring. The same regimen may be used after resurfacing, but inevitably the patient becomes sleep deprived and anxious as a result of this rigorous regimen. Because the resurfacing wound is rendered sterile by the heat of the laser, it is considered safe to use one of several types of occlusive membranes to cover the area, maintaining a sterile, moist environment for rapid reepithelialization. In most cases, this membrane is changed on day 3 or 4 postoperatively. Some patients insist on switching to the open exposure method at that point. There is no good evidence that there is any clinical difference in the results with either method.

PATIENT'S WILLINGNESS TO COOPERATE WITH SUN AVOIDANCE

During the phase of postinflammatory erythema (the red phase), it is critical that the patient avoid sun exposure, as this will inevitably result in unsatisfactory hyperpigmentation for an extended period. The red phase persists for 3 to 4 months. If the patient clearly will not cooperate with intense sun avoidance, resurfacing is not recommended.

Mechanism of Action

ABLATION

Both the erbium-YAG and the CO_2 lasers will flatten elevations by purely physical ablation. The erbium laser is not hemostatic, whereas the excess heat of the CO_2 laser is hemostatic for small vessels.

COLLAGEN CONTRACTION VERSUS COMPACTION

After the epidermis is ablated, the first pass into the dermis usually produces obvious contraction. It is unclear whether this is attributable to shortening of the collagen bundles or of compaction of ground substance.

NEOCOLLAGEN FORMATION

It is postulated that the excess heat produced by the CO_2 laser stimulates fibroblast activity to produce new collagen. At the histologic level, over time this produces a shift from a thin collagen and excess elastin (solar elastosis) to the appearance of undamaged dermis (thick, parallel collagen bundles).

Comparison With Other Surface Modalities

With the proliferation of a- and b-hydoxy acids, various retinoids, numerous antioxidants, microdermabrasion, and numerous peels, it would be the height of arrogance to describe my particular regimen. Every practitioner in the field will find his or her favorites. I would, however, propose a simple "Resurfacing Ladder" which may help place these methods in a useful context for both practitioners and patients.

At the base of the "Resurfacing Ladder" are methods described as Level I. This level refers to modalities that affect only the epidermis. Included here, in my opinion, would be glycolic acid home treatments as well as micropeels, retinoids and other topicals, microdermabrasion, and superficial erbium-YAG resurfacing.

Level II methods may include trichloroacetic acid (TCA) and certain other peels, as well as deep erbium-YAG resurfacing. These methods penetrate into the superficial papillary dermis, have limited recovery downtime and post-inflammatory erythema, and are generally felt to be most useful in treating dyspigmentation.

Level III methods include CO_2 resurfacing, phenol peels, and dermabrasion. Because of deeper penetration to or beyond the papillary-reticular junction, these manifest longer recovery and post-inflammatory erythema, as well as increased risk of scarring or pigmentary changes. They also produce the most significant improvement with regard to superficial rhytids, acne scars, and solar elastosis. I believe that CO_2 resurfacing has effectively replaced the other two modalities in this level, but whether or not you agree, this algorithm may be useful in your consultation room. This simple approach permits every practitioner the ability to adapt it to his or her own preferences and needs.

SUGGESTED READINGS

Adrian RM. Pulsed carbon dioxide and erbium-YAG laser resurfacing: a comparative clinical and histologic study. *J Cutan Laser Ther* 1999;1:29–35

Anderson RR, Parish JA. Selected photothermolysis: precise microsurgery by selective absorption of pulsed irradiation. *Science* 1983;220:524–527

Baker TJ, Stuzin JM, Baker TM. *Facial skin resurfacing.* St. Louis: Quality Medical Publishing; 1998

Green HA, Burd E, Nishioka NS, Bruggemann U, Compton CC. Middermal wound healing: a comparison between dermatomal excision and pulsed carbon dioxide laser ablation. *Arch Dermatol* 1992;128:639–645

Fitzpatrick RE, Tope WD, Goldman MP, Satur NM. Pulsed carbon dioxide laser, trichloroacetic acid, Baker-Gordon phenol, and dermabrasion: a comparative clinical and histologic study of cutaneous resurfacing in a porcine model. *Arch Dermatol* 1996;132:469–471

Skin Resurfacing—Laser or Peel

Milton Waner

CHAPTER 29

Since the mid-1990s, laser-assisted skin resurfacing has rapidly replaced chemical peels and physical dermabrasion as the most common means of skin exfoliation. Remarkably, this has taken place with alarming rapidity and despite the lack of comparative trials. Evidence-based medicine has taught us the value of comparative trials. Without these we must ask ourselves the fundamental questions, how and why has this happened and is it justified?

The first of these questions must be answered against the backdrop of the state of the art at that time (i.e., when laser-assisted skin resurfacing first emerged). Chemical skin exfoliation (chemical peels) developed almost in parallel with mechanical skin exfoliation and both became established modalities during the mid- to late 1960s.[1-5] Chemical peeling is a process whereby a chemical cauterant is applied to the skin to induce exfoliation. A variety of agents can be used that produce a variety of effects, ranging from a light peel, in which the stratum corneum is affected, to a deep peel, in which necrosis can extend all the way to the reticular dermis. These include salicylic acid, trichloroacetic acid (TCA), the α-hydroxy group of acids, Jessner's solution (i.e., salicylic acid, resorcinol, lactic acid, and ethanol), and phenol.[6-10] By contrast mechanical skin exfoliation refers to dermabrasion usually accomplished with a power-driven rotary dermabrader. A direct comparison of these two modalities revealed consistent changes.[11] In general, the papillary dermis enlarged and the depth of the injury correlated well with the benefit derived from treatment to a point. Hayes et al.[12] showed that the upper reticular dermis heals by regeneration from residual adnexial structures, whereas the deeper reticular dermis heals with scar tissue formation. An injury extending down to the reticular dermis is therefore likely to leave irreversible scarring. A more superficial injury is likely to heal by regeneration. This is the fundamental basis of aesthetic and therapeutic skin exfoliation. Kligman et al.[10] studied the long-term histologic changes associated with chemical peels and noted a newly formed wide band of thin compact collagen bundles, parallel to the overlying skin. They also noted elastin fibers within the neocollagen and, once again, parallel to the surface of the overlying skin. The clinical correlation was apparent as a smoothing of the skin. Obliteration and subsequent regeneration of the epidermis from residual adnexiae resulted in elimination of dyschromias, keratoses, and the reestablishment of the normal vertical polarity of skin. The benefits of limited skin exfoliation were thus obvious.

Despite some excellent results, several limitations and some devastating complications became evident.[13] The major limitations related to a lack of precision. With regard to chemical peeling, it became evident that there was variability in the success rate among patients and that this was probably due to an inherent lack in the control of the depth of exfoliation. So many variables determined the depth of exfoliation that any classification of peeling agents was virtually meaningless.[14] For example, the application of 25% TCA with a cotton-tipped swab to the face of a patient with thick oily skin that has not been primed before treatment will result in superficial intradermal sloughing of the skin. If a piece of gauze, saturated with the same concentration of TCA (25%), is rubbed repeatedly on the face of a thin-skinned woman whose skin was primed before treatment with 0.1% retinoic acid, the extent of injury will be much deeper and will probably extend to the midpapillary dermis. The variables that determine the depth of the peel appear to be related to the type of agent used and to the technique with which it is applied:

- Peeling agent and its concentration
- Number of coats applied
- Technique used to apply the agent
- Method of skin cleansing prior to the application
- Whether the skin was pretreated in the weeks just before the peel
- Skin type
- Anatomic location of the peel
- Duration of contact with skin

Not only were there complications relating to the actual peel, such as scarring, hypopigmentation, and hyperpigmentation, but complications resulting from an adverse effect of the specific agent used became evident. Resorcinol and salicylic acid can cause systemic toxicity, and even death in rare instances, several of the other agents can provoke an allergic reaction.[13,15,16]

As with chemical peeling, during dermabrasion, an appreciation of the depth of the treatment at any point in time is difficult and only comes with experience. Once again, this lack of precision led to variability in results.[4,17] Profuse bleeding not only obscures the endpoint, but aerosolization of blood and tissue by the high-speed burrs, with the attendant risks of airborne infection, should discourage against using this technique.

This lack of precision, variability in results, and the relatively high risk of side effects kept these techniques from widespread popularity. One needed considerable experience to master these techniques and approach the safety standards demanded of cosmetic surgeons. An additional factor to consider was the changing climate of medical practice. The diminishing reimbursement rates paid out by third-party carriers and the rapid rise of managed care left many physicians disenchanted with traditional medical practice. By contrast, cosmetic procedures were strictly fee for service and were also very lucrative. Patients usually paid in advance of the service, obviating the need to generate the seemingly endless reams of paperwork demanded by the third-party carriers. Laser-assisted skin resurfacing could hardly have come at a more opportune time. The vacuum created by the problems of dermabrasion and chemical peels, together with the disaffection many physicians felt with the general trends in medicine, led to the enormous popularity of laser-assisted skin resurfacing. The next and most fundamental question is: is this justified?

The fundamental principle of laser-assisted skin resurfacing (skin resurfacing) is the limitation of thermal damage. The following sequence of events takes place during tissue vaporization:

1. ***Optical penetration***: The light emitted by the laser will penetrate to a given depth. This is a wavelength-dependent phenomenon. Infrared light is strongly absorbed by water and will thus only penetrate to a limited depth. In skin, this is generally around 60 to 80 μm.
2. ***Vaporization***: The light absorbed by water will raise the temperature of the intra- and extracellular water to the point of vaporization (100°C), at which point a layer of desiccated dead tissue will be left behind. If this dead tissue is again vaporized, it will heat to about 300°C and carbonize. It should therefore always be wiped away before any further vaporization takes place.
3. ***Thermal transmission***. Once the tissue has vaporized, the thermal energy is transmitted to surrounding tissue. In the case of skin resurfacing, this is not desirable and should be prevented.

Thermal transmission can be limited by turning off the laser just after the tissue has vaporized and before the start of thermal transmission. This span of time (i.e., the time the laser is left on to allow only optical penetration and thermal transmission) is roughly equivalent to what is known as the *thermal relaxation time*. The thermal relaxation time of epidermis is about 1000 μs. Therefore, if the patient's skin is exposed to ≤ 1000 μs one is able to vaporize to a specific depth with very little thermal damage beyond that.[18] With CO_2 lasers, the depth of vaporization will vary from 50 to 1000 μm depending on the power setting selected.[19,20] The depth of thermal damage approximates an additional 30 to 50 μm. With the Er:YAG laser, the depth of vaporization is 4 μm/joule (J) of energy used.[20,21] Therefore, at 5 J/cm^2, the depth of vaporization is 20 μm. The depth of thermal damage with this laser is only 5 μ. Therefore regardless of who is operating the laser, at a particular fluence, one pass with a CO_2 laser will reliably vaporize to a depth of 50 μm with 30 μm of thermal damage. An Er:YAG laser operated at 5 J/cm^2 will reliably vaporize to a depth of 20 μm and effectively heat a further 5 μm of tissue. This meant that one could vaporize skin with a degree of precision not seen with chemical peeling and dermabrasion. Furthermore, the same degree of precision was attainable regardless of the experience of the operator. The learning curve was much shorter, and the results were readily reproducible. Needless to say, there was still a learning curve, requiring a fundamental understanding of wound healing and light–tissue interaction. Provided one remained within the well-defined parameters, complications were few. Although no prospective comparison with chemical peeling or dermabrasion has been done, the precision, reliability, and reproducibility of laser-assisted skin resurfacing should yield a lower complication rate.[22,23]

With the passage of just a few years, advances in technology have not only given us greater precision in laser-assisted skin resurfacing, we have more versatility in what we are able to do. We now have three generations of skin-resurfacing lasers and, with each successive generation, our versatility has increased.

The first-generation lasers were the CO_2 skin-resurfacing lasers. With these we are able to vaporize skin to the desired depth both accurately and precisely. The limited thermal transmission beyond the zone of vaporization was found to be advantageous in that a degree of thermally induced collagen denaturation took place within this zone and resulted in immediate shrinkage. This appeared to persist, and its effect was advantageous. This laser was found to be most useful for patients with class 2 and class 3 rhytids.[19,20,23]

The second-generation lasers were the Er:YAG lasers. With these lasers, we are able to vaporize skin with even more precision but with significantly less thermal damage.[20,21] The resultant collagen shrinkage is present, but to a much lesser degree. It is generally accepted that this device is preferred for patients with class 1 and for some with class 2 rhytides. The main advantage is a quicker healing time and less postoperative erythema.[20]

The third-generation devices combine the above two effects and with an alteration of parameters one can obtain anywhere from a "light" predominantly Er:YAG effect, to a "deeper" peel with more thermal damage, as with a CO_2 laser. With these devices, one is more versatile and can thus tailor the treatment to suit the patient. For example, in a patient with more pronounced rhytides on her upper lip and much less obvious changes over the rest of her face, one is able to "lightly" peel the entire face with a more pronounced effect, using more thermal damage over the patient's upper lip. This added versatility meant that these devices could replace the first- and second-generation devices and that any physician purchasing a laser for the first time need only buy a third-generation device.

One of the major criticisms leveled against lasers concerns their cost. This is especially true when one compares it with the cost of a small volume of lactic acid or any other of the exfoliants. Although it is true that some skilled individuals can obtain excellent results with chemical peels, as stated previously, the learning curve is long and the risk of complications appears to be much greater. Furthermore, their lack of precision and the variability of results clearly justify the added cost of lasers. Because the standards for cosmetic surgery have become so high, the added safety afforded with a laser, as well as their greater versatility, further justifies their continued use. Lastly, given the long learning curve for the use of chemical peels, any recently trained physician is much more likely to be comfortable using a laser than with the techniques of chemical peeling. It is therefore likely that with the passage of time, fewer and fewer physicians will use chemical peeling techniques.

REFERENCES

1. Baker TJ. Chemical face peeling. *Plast Reconstr Surg* 1962;29:199
2. Baker TJ, Gordon HL. Chemical face peeling and dermabrasion. *Surg Clin North Am* 1971;51:387–401
3. Kurtin A. Corrective surgical planing of the skin. *Arch Dermatol* 1953;68(suppl):389
4. Yarborough J. Dermabrasive surgery. *Clin Dermatol* 1987;5:75
5. Spira M, Freeman R, Arfai P, Gero FJ, Hardy SB. Clinical comparison of chemical peeling, dermabrasion, and 5-FU for senile keratosis. *Plast Reconstr Surg* 1970;46:61–66
6. Rubin M. Trichloroacetic acid and other non–phenol peels. *Clin Plast Surg* 1992;19:525–536
7. Stegman S, Tromovitch TA. *Cosmetic Dermatologic Surgery.* Chicago: Year Book; 1984:27–46
8. Kligman A. Results of a pilot study evaluation the compatability of topical tertinoin in combination with glycolic acid. *Cosmet Dermatol* 1993;6:10:28–32
9. Resknik SS, Lewis LA, Cohen BH. Trichloroacetic acid peeling. *Cutis* 1976;17:127–129
10. Kligman AM, Baker TJ, Gordon HC. Long-term histologic follow-up of phenol face peels. *Plast Reconstr Surg* 1985;75:652–659
11. Stegman SJ. A comparative histologic study of the effects of three peeling agents and dermabrasion on normal and sun damaged skin. *Aesth Plast Surg* 1982;6:123
12. Hayes DK, Berkland ME, Stambaugh KI. Dermal healing after local skin flaps and chemical peel. *Arch Otolaryngol Head Neck Surg* 1990;116:794
13. Spira M, Gerow FJ, Hardy SB. Complications of chemical face peeling. *Plast Reconstr Surg* 1974;54:397–403
14. Brodland DG, Cullimore KC, Roenighk RK, et al. Depths of chemexfoliation induced by various concentrations and application techniques of trichloroacetic acid in a porcine model. *J Dermatol Surg Oncol* 1989;15:967–971
15. Pascher F. Systemic reactions to topically applied drugs. *Bull NY Acad Med* 1973:49:613–617
16. Stagnone G, Orgel M, Stagnone J. Cardiovascular effects of topical 50% trichloroacetic acid and Baker's phenol solution. *J Dermatol Surg Oncol* 1987;13:999–1002
17. Rubin M. *Manual of Chemical Peels: Superficial and Medium Depth.* Philadelphia: Lippincott-Raven; 1995
18. Fitzpatrick E, Goldman MP. CO_2 laser surgery. In: Goldman MP, Fitzpatrick RE, eds. *Cutaneous Laser Surgery.* St Louis: CV Mosby; 1994;198–258
19. Hohenleutner U, Hohenleutner S, Baumler W, Landthaler M. Fast and effective tissue ablation rates and thermal damage zones. *Laser Surg Med* 1997;20:242–247
20. Adrian RM. Pulsed carbon dioxide and erbium YAG laser resurfacing: a comparative clinical and histological study. *J Cutan Laser Ther* 1999;1:29–35
21. Kaufman R, Hibst R. Pulsed erbium YAG laser ablation in cutaneous surgery. *Lasers Surg Med* 1996;19:324–330
22. Weinstine C, Ramirez OM, Pozner JN. Postoperative care following carbon dioxide laser resurfacing: avoiding pitfalls. *Plast Reconstr Surg* 1997:100:1855–1866
23. Fitzpatrick RE, Goldman MP, Satur NM, et al. Pulsed carbon dioxide laser resurfacing for photoaged facial skin. *Arch Dermatol* 1996:132:395–402

Skin Resurfacing—Laser or Peel

CHAPTER 30

Devinder S. Mangat and Jon E. Mendelsohn

The demand for facial skin rejuvenation has seen unprecedented growth in recent times. The explosion of interest in facial skin resurfacing by the public has paralleled that on the part of the cosmetic surgeon. As newer technologies have become available, the cosmetic surgeon's armamentarium for treating aged and actinically damaged facial skin has blossomed. While the media continue to bombard the public with the latest therapies, and as we address better informed, Internet-saavy patients, facial plastic surgeons have a responsibility to be knowledgeable and to understand the advantages and disadvantages of the various types of facial skin resurfacing techniques.

Many options are available to physicians who treat patients interested in facial skin rejuvenation. The latest advances in technology have allowed physicians to treat many facial skin conditions with laser therapy. As laser technology continues to develop, many different types of lasers are becoming available. The recent debate, however, is whether the laser will supplant more traditional chemical peeling procedures. Chemical peeling agents have been used for many centuries. The contemporary use of these agents began during the 1960s, and their use has flourished. Well-documented research has shown the beneficial clinical and histologic changes present after the application of various chemical peeling agents. Similar findings have recently been shown after laser facial skin resurfacing.

Regardless of the modality used, success with these agents is based on many variables. Along with a thorough understanding of the chemical agent or laser, and its proper use by the operator, patient selection remains a crucial factor in determining a successful outcome. No single therapy can be used successfully for all patients or all skin conditions. Currently, we use both modalities in our practice and continue to do so for a variety of different problems to help our patients achieve optimal rejuvenation of their skin.

Background

Chemical peeling of the face has been performed for centuries. The ancient Egyptians used particles of alabaster mixed with milk and honey to abrade the skin in an attempt to tighten the facial skin. Substances including acids, minerals, sulfur, mustard, fire, sandpaperlike products, limestone, and plant substances have been used in an attempt to reduce facial rhytids and to reverse changes associated with photoaging.

During the early twentieth century, interest in skin revitalization again flourished as MacKee, a dermatologist, reported the use of phenol for the treatment of acne scars. Shortly after this discovery, in 1905, surgical planing, today known as dermabrasion, was pioneered by Kromayer. He is reported to have used rotating wheels and rasps for the treatment of keratoses, acne scars, and hyperpigmentation disorders. Kromayer observed that healing after skin resurfacing was related to the depth of injury created by surgical planing. He believed that when injury to the skin was restricted to the upper dermal layer, above the adnexal structures, subsequent healing would occur without scarring.

Interest in surgical planning grew after World War II as many attempts were made to improve traumatic tatoo injuries sustained during the war. Throughout the 1940s and 1950s, the medical literature became replete with descriptions related to the uses of dermabrasion. During this period, chemical peeling did not receive the same attention from the medical community because it was not applicable to the treatment of war-related injuries. However, the lay public was extremely interested in chemical peeling, as the media reported that the "fountain of youth" had been discovered.

Most operators performing chemical peels were not physicians. It was not until the late 1950s and early 1960s that plastic surgeons and dermatologists undertook scientific investigations of phenol and trichloroacetic (TCA) acids peels for their use in facial skin resurfacing. It was not until 1972, when Baker demonstrated to a group of plastic surgeons the beneficial results he had achieved using phenol, that facial skin resurfacing became widely accepted in the medical community.

Histologic Effects of Photoaging and Skin Resurfacing

Most patients seeking evaluation for skin rejuvenation have a history of significant sun exposure. Clinical signs of actinic damage include the development of coarse rhytids, rougher skin texture, pigmentary mottling, and the development of solar lentigines and actinic keratoses. Histologically, changes in the epidermis and dermis of patients with sun-damaged skin develop as well. Epidermal dysplasia occurs, indicated by thickened epidermis and the appearance of dysplastic cells. Clinically, this finding corresponds to the development of actinic keratoses and may lead to the development of basal or squamous cell carcinomas. In addition, epidermal hyperplasia and epidermal atrophy are observed in combination with irregular pigment distribution and solar lentigines. In the dermis, dermoelastosis, the degeneration of collagen and elastic fibers, is the main diagnostic feature in sun-damaged skin. Intrinsically aged skin shows similar clinical and histologic changes, except that, in actinically damaged skin, these processes are accelerated.

Chemical peeling and laser resurfacing techniques reverse the damage created in the skin as a result of photoaging. The obliteration of many of the clinical and histologic changes varies depending on the depth of the wounding agent. Knowledge of histologic changes and the histologic effects of various peeling agents must be understood in order to obtain optimal results and prevent complications.

Patient Selection

INDICATIONS

As in all facial aesthetic procedures, proper patient selection with individualization of treatment is key to a successful outcome. Technical skill must be combined with proper selection of the right patient, to avoid devastating results. Chemical peeling and laser resurfacing have well-defined indications. These treatment modalities are not appropriate for all patients or all skin conditions. In general, patients with facial wrinkles and blotchy pigmentation are candidates for either type of procedure. Patients with actinic keratoses also benefit from resurfacing techniques, as the epidermal and dermal damage is reversed. It is our experience that patients with traumatic or acne scars are more likely to respond to CO_2 laser resurfacing than to treatment with chemical peeling agents. Deeper scars may respond poorly to either of these skin resurfacing techniques.

Most patients seeking consultation for facial aging mistakenly believe that a facelift will repair their sun-damaged skin. When gravitational forces are part of the problem, surgical procedures are recommended. However, patients should understand that superficial or deep facial rhytids, pigmentary changes, and acne scarring are better treated with skin resurfacing. It is important to explore the patient's goals and expectations regarding the procedures desired.

Patient assessment begins with the evaluation of skin type and complexion, skin texture and thickness, the degree of photoaging and severity of facial rhytids, and age-related gravitational changes. Skin type and complexion are the primary factors that help determine whether laser or chemical peeling agents should be considered to yield the best outcome. Other considerations include patient lifestyle and patient expectations. The morbidity associated with early sun exposure must be weighed against the desires and goals of the patient. We use the Fitzpatrick classification as a guide for evaluating skin types (Table 30–1). Skin types under this classification scheme correlate with the patient's skin color and reaction to sun exposure. White skin that always burns is classified as Fitzpatrick type I, whereas black skin that never burns is classified as Fitzpatrick type VI. Another classification system, developed by Glogau, is more objective, but it is also very useful to help classify photoaged skin (Table 30–2).

The Fitzpatrick skin classification system is a simple guide that helps dictate which patients require pretreatment. Both patient and physician must realize that pretreatment with the use of α-hydroxy acids, retinoic acid, topical steroids, sunscreens, and bleaching agents may be a part of the pretreatment regimen. The patient's skin thickness and texture also must be factored into the plan. As opposed to patients with thin, dry, atrophic skin, those with thicker, oily, sebaceous skin may require a more aggressive pretreatment regimen, including Retin-A and glycolic acids. These patients may also require multiple applications with the peeling agent, or multiple passes with the CO_2 laser, to achieve a satisfactory result. Finally, the degree of pathology and the desire for improvement must be assessed. Superficial lentigines and fine rhytids may be treated satisfactorily with either medium-depth chemical peels or conservative CO_2 or erbium laser resurfacing. Deeper, coarse, facial rhytids require phenol chemical peeling to achieve the optimal result.

TABLE 30–1
Fitzpatrick Classification System

Type	Skin Color	Skin Characteristics
I	White	Always burns, never tans
II	White	Usually burns, tans less than average
III	White	Sometimes mild burn, tans about average
IV	White	Rarely burns, tans more than average
V	Brown	Rarely burns, tans profusely
VI	Black	Never burns, deeply pigmented

Chemical Peels

Chemical peeling involves the application of chemical agents that act to accelerate the normal process of exfoliation. A variety of chemical agents are used to produce varying effects to the skin. Sloughing of the stratum corneum, produced by superficial chemical peeling, improves skin texture by stimulating the growth of a thicker epidermal layer. These peels are also effective for the treatment of superficial skin lesions. Medium-depth peeling agents produce injury to the papillary and upper reticular dermal layers by their chemical cauterant effect. This helps reverse the effects of photoaging, including the treatment of mild to moderate facial rhytids and pigmentary dyschromias. They are also performed for the removal of actinic keratoses. Deeper escharotic peeling agents act by destroying specific layers of skin, creating necrosis and inflammation in the epidermis, papillary dermis, and reticular dermis. The deeper peeling agents are indicated for the treatment of patients with significantly photoaged skin. Some chemicals may be used as superficial, medium, or deep peeling agents. A number of factors, including the concentration, the number of layers applied to the skin, and the duration of contact of the peeling agent with the skin, may affect the depth of the peel. Understanding the properties of these chemical agents is key to their successful use (Table 30–3).

TABLE 30–2
Glogau Classification

Damage	Description	Characteristics
Type I (mild)	No wrinkles	Early photoaging Mild pigmentary changes No keratoses Minimal wrinkles Patient age: 20s or 30s Minimal or no makeup Minimal acne scarring
Type II (moderate)	Wrinkles in motion	Early to moderate photoaging Early senile lentigines visible Keratoses palpable but not visible Parallel smile lines beginning to appear Patient age: late 30s or 40s Some foundation usually worn Mild acne scarring
Type III (advanced)	Wrinkles at rest	Advanced photoaging Obvious dyschromia, telangiectasias Visible keratoses Wrinkles present even when not moving Patient age: 50s or older Heavier foundation always worn Acne scarring present—makeup does not cover
Type IV (severe)	Only wrinkles	Severe photoaging Yellow-gray skin color Prior skin malignancies Wrinkles throughout, no normal skin Patient age: 60s or 70s Makeup cannot be worn—it cakes and cracks Severe acne scarring

TABLE 30–3
Classification of Peeling Agents

Depth	Agent
Superficial	Glycolicacid 50 to 70% applied for 5 to 15 min Jessner's solution applied in 5 to 10 coats Resorcinol 50% applied for 30 to 60 min TCA 10 to 35%
Medium depth	Glycolic acid 70% applied 5 to 30 min TCA 35 to 50% applied alone or augmented with glycolic acid or Jessner's solution
Deep	Phenol 88% Baker–Gordon phenol formula

TRICHLOROACETIC ACID PEELS

TCA is perhaps the best single agent for skin resurfacing. It exhibits unique properties that afford the cosmetic surgeon tremendous flexibility and versatility in treating a variety of clinical conditions. When properly used, TCA has an overall decreased morbidity as compared with other agents. It allows patients to achieve a predictable result with the benefit of disrupting their lives to a lesser degree.

Indications

Although TCA is the most popular and most widely used chemical peeling agent, proper usage is imperative to a successful outcome. Ideal candidates for TCA peeling include patients with pigmentation disorders and those who exhibit early facial rhytids. Patients with severe actinic damage and those with coarse facial rhytids are better served by other methods.

Pretreatment

To achieve the most consistent and reliable results, pretreatment of facial skin is mandatory. This improves the ability of TCA to penetrate beyond the stratum corneum and deep to the epidermal–dermal junction in a more predictable manner. We feel that almost all patients should undergo prepeel treatment with a combination of 8% hydroquinone, 1% hydrocortisone, and 0.05% retinoic acid. This bleaching formula is prepared for us by a pharmacist. Hydroquinone affects melanocytic metabolism by increasing the degradation of melanin, while decreasing melanin formation. It acts specifically by inhibition of tyrosinase, a hormone responsible for increasing the proliferation of melanocytes. Retin-A acts synergistically by increasing the penetration of hydroquinone. An absolute indication for pretreatment is any patient with Fitzpatrick type III skin or greater. After this pretreatment regimen, TCA peeling is more predictable. This combination helps ensure a peel of consistent penetration with a lower risk of postinflammatory hyperpigmentation. Our patients use these products once daily for at least 4 weeks before undergoing their peel. Other cosmetic surgeons recommend treatment for a 6-week period. Alternative pretreatment regimens include the use of glycolic acid products ranging within 10 to 14% concentration. Glycolic acid acts to thin the stratum corneum and enhance TCA penetration. When glycolic acids are used for pretreating the skin, they are frequently used in combination with hydroquinones.

Technique

As with all chemical peeling, the skin should be degreased with an acetone-soaked sponge. The mechanical abrasion helps remove the stratum corneum, helping produce uniform penetration of the peeling agent. TCA may be applied as a 10 to 50% concentration, depending on the desired depth of penetration. We strongly discourage the use of TCA in concentrations higher than 35% because of a significantly higher risk of undesirable side effects such as scarring and hypopigmentation. We routinely use a 35% TCA concentration after the application of Jessner's solution. Jessner's solution is a keratolytic agent that acts by removing the stratum corneum to permit deeper penetration of the TCA. Unlike other peeling agents, the penetration of the TCA peel is affected by the number of layers applied. The goal is to achieve uniform frosting of the treated skin. Generally, the whiter the frost, the deeper the TCA has penetrated. It is important to note that a change in the color of the frost, from white to gray, represents penetration deep into the reticular layer and may result in hypertrophic scarring. Jessner's solution and 30% TCA can be used to treat actinic damage in the neck area.

Postpeel Care

Postpeel care may vary depending on the depth of the TCA peel. Patients undergoing superficial TCA peels are treated with occlusive agents such as bacitracin ointment, Eucerin cream, or Elta. These are applied 4 to 5 times per day by the patient for 3 to 5 days until reepithelialization has occurred. At this point, the patient may resume wearing makeup and is instructed to use a skin moisturizer. Patients undergoing deeper TCA peels are instructed to follow the same directions but should expect reepithelialization to occur several days later, usually between 5 and 7 days. It is imperative that patients be instructed to avoid sun exposure for 6 weeks after their peel.

Complications

Hyperpigmentation The most common complication of TCA peeling is postinflammatory hyperpigmentation, which is generally the result of early sun exposure. It must be stressed that during the early stages of healing, sun exposure is prohibited. In most patients in whom this complication develops, failure to comply with this instruction is the most common cause. Patients may also exhibit this complication if pretreatment was inadequate. Birth control pill intake should also cease during this peripeel period, as their use can produce pigmentary changes.

Hyperpigmentation is usually easy to treat and will respond to 0.05% Retin-A cream in combination with 8% hydroquinone. We prefer to use our bleaching formula as described previously. This is usually applied once or twice daily for about 3 weeks, but it may be used longer if necessary. Some patients may experience moderate erythema secondary to Retin-A use. This problem is less common in those who were treated with Retin-A during the prepeel period. However, should this be of concern, topical hydrocortisone may be used for several weeks as required. These patients are also instructed to use a sunscreen with a sun protection factor (SPF) of 20 or greater.

Hypertrophic Scarring The risk of producing hypertrophic scarring from medium-depth TCA peels is rare. When it does occur, it appears most commonly along the mandibular border and in the perioral region. Thin-skinned patients are at greatest risk, as the TCA is more likely to penetrate deep into the reticular dermis. We consider the use of isotretinoin during the prior 12 months a contraindication to TCA peeling, as it has been shown that its use can lead to scarring. Most practitioners recommend waiting 18 to 24 months after the use of Accutane has been stopped before performing any skin resurfacing procedure. Clinically, it is probably safe to perform a peel on patients after they begin to produce normal oil in their skin. Patients who develop hypertrophic scarring are treated most successfully with injectable steroids, although some may require surgical revision after scar maturation.

Herpes Simplex Infection Herpes simplex infection may develop in any patient after undergoing any peel or laser procedure. Patients with or without a positive history are treated prophylactically with systemic antiviral agents daily, starting 2 days before the peel and continuing for a total of 7 days. Those patients who develop postpeel herpes infection are treated more aggressively with acyclovir or valacyclovir, 800 mg 4 times per day. Treatment is usually successful, and scarring does not result.

Summary

TCA peels represent the most common chemical peel performed. In our opinion, they are the most versatile agents available and may be used to treat a variety of dermatologic conditions. They are applicable to a diverse population and most commonly used to treat sun-damaged skin that shows pigmentary changes with mild to moderate rhytids. As with all skin resurfacing techniques, the key to successful TCA peeling is appropriate patient selection and the proper pretreatment regimen.

PHENOL PEELS

Phenol represents the most common deep chemical peeling agent. It leads to dramatic results by producing a controlled chemical burn to the level of the upper reticular dermis. As healing occurs, new stratified collagen is laid down, resulting in younger-appearing skin. Phenol is an extremely effective agent for reversing facial wrinkling and irregular pigmentary changes related to sun exposure and the natural aging process.

The most commonly used phenol preparation is the Baker-Gordon formula, which contains 3 mL USP liquid phenol, 2 mL tap water, 8 drops liquid soap, and 3 drops groton oil. Although this formula remains popular, other buffered phenol solutions exist that are reported to cause less postpeel hypopigmentation. By varying the concentration of phenol, the depth of the peel will change. The lower the phenol concentration, the more deeply it penetrates. In addition, the use of croton oil appears to be especially important in enhancing or limiting phenol penetration. When the solution contains lower concentrations of croton oil, less phenol penetration is observed, limiting postpeel hypopigmentation. Although the risk of hypopigmentation decreases when the formula is varied (i.e., 88% phenol solution), the improvement of coarse facial rhytids and the degree of neocollagen formation may also be reduced. For this reason, patients who are at greater risk of developing postpeel hypopigmentation, those with Fitzpatrick type III–VI skin, should consider other skin resurfacing modalities, such as laser resurfacing.

Indications

Phenol is extremely successful in eradicating coarse wrinkles and pigmentary changes caused by chronic solar exposure, birth control pills, or pregnancy. Because of its effectiveness, the best candidates for phenol chemical peeling are those with Fitzpatrick type I skin and those with little prior sun exposure. In these patients, regional peeling can be performed more successfully because an obvious line of demarcation will not result. In Fitzpatrick type II or greater skin types, and in those patients with significant actinic damage, results are improved if the entire face is peeled. Phenol peeling is not the best option for Fitzpatrick type IV, V, or VI skin types. They may exhibit blotchy hyper- and hypopigmentary changes.

The best candidates for phenol peeling are those patients who demonstrate moderate to severe facial rhytids and those with moderate to significant pigmentary changes. Coarse facial rhytids in the perioral and periorbital regions are treated extremely well with this agent. However, unlike the medium-depth peels, additional morbidity is associated with phenol peeling. The potential toxicity of the agent itself, extended healing times, and increased postoperative sequelae mandate that the treating physician fully understand the nature of phenol peeling.

Mechanism of Action

Unlike other agents, phenol is a keratocoagulant that creates an all-or-none response. As stated above, varying the concentration of the phenol agent inversely varies the depth of the peel. This means that a more effective peel is not obtained by increasing the concentration. By contrast, a lower concentration of phenol yields a deeper peel because keratocoagulation is slowed, allowing the phenol to penetrate more deeply. A higher concentration will only increase the chances of systemic toxicity.

A potential side effect of phenol peeling is the toxicity of the agent itself. Phenol is absorbed through the facial skin and then carried through the bloodstream to the liver, where it is detoxified. The metabolic products are then excreted through the kidney. Therefore, a toxic dose of phenol that is absorbed systemically can injure both the liver and kidney. Phenol may also depress the respiratory system and the myocardium. The risk of producing cardiac dysrhythmias is lessened when phenol is applied systematically, to smaller regions of the face over time. When doing a full face peel, if it is applied sequentially over the various aesthetic units over a 1- to 2-h period, the risk of myocardial irritability and electrocardiographic (ECG) changes is rare. However, because the potential risk exists even when following these guidelines, patients undergoing phenol chemical peeling should be monitored electrocardiographically and should have an intravenous (IV) line placed. Adequate IV hydration before and during the peeling process will lower the risk of cardiotoxicity.

Preparation

Phenol is used as an 88% concentration. We use the standard Baker-Gordon formula in most cases. This consists of 3 mL USP liquid phenol (88% concentration), 2 mL water, 8 drops surgical soap (Septisol), and 3 drops of croton oil. The soap is used to help saponify the mixture. Although we use Septisol, any liquid soap should be effective. Croton oil, extracted from the seeds of *Croton tiglium*, serves as a vesicant. Croton oil enhances the mixture's keratolytic action and therefore permits deeper penetration of the solution. This formula is prepared fresh for each patient. When using this formula, it must be mixed well just before its application because chemically it does not readily combine.

Technique

Before entering the operating room, patients are instructed to wash their face well with an astringent, which helps remove the stratum corneum. Upon entering the operating room, the patient is first placed in a sitting position, and the submandibular region is marked to delineate the limit of the peel in this region. If the patient is marked while supine, the gravitational effects will not be accounted for, and peeling will not be carried into the shadow beneath the mandibular border. Failure to peel into this region will result in an obvious line of demarcation. The patient is then placed supine, as IV sedation or general anesthesia is administered by an anesthesiologist. When IV sedation is used, additional subcutaneous local infiltration of a mixture of 2% lidocaine without epinephrine and 0.5% marcaine without epinephrine in equal amounts is also used. The rate of intravenous D_5LR or NS are increased at this time so that patients receive at least 1000 to 1500 mL of fluid during the peripeel period. Epinephrine must never be used in the infilteration of local anesthetic because it can deepen the penetration of the peel solution and lead to scarring.

An acetone-soaked 4 x 4-in. gauze sponge is used to thoroughly cleanse oils from the patient's face. The mechanical action of vigorous cleansing also helps remove other debris and desquamated epithelium to allow deeper and more consistent penetration of the peeling solution. At this time, the patient's head is placed at an approximately 35-degree angle, where it remains until the procedure is completed. By using the broken end of a cotton-tipped applicator, individual rhytids are first treated with the phenol solution. Coarse rhytids extending into the vermilion are similarly treated by this method. Next, the facial subunits are treated sequentially, using a dampened cotton-tipped applicator. The aesthetic subunits include the forehead and glabella, perioral, nasal, cheek, and periorbital regions. When full face peeling is performed, we begin with the application of the peeling solution to the forehead. As the formula is applied, the skin begins to turn a frosty gray-white. As phenol does not affect hair follicles, the peeling agent may be feathered into the frontal and temporal hairline. After the application of the phenol solution to each aesthetic subunit, 20 min is permitted before applying the solution to the next subunit. Using this method, we have never had a cardiac dysrhythmia that required treatment. When treating subsequent subunits, erythema will be observed at the border of the previously treated region. The area of reactive erythema will require the application of the solution, as it is not an area that was adequately treated by the previous application.

Postpeel Care

All patients are monitored with an ECG for at least 2 h postpeel. After the peel is complete and the frost has disappeared, a wet dressing is applied over all the peeled areas. Eucerin cream is our current choice of an emollient and is applied approximately 1 h after the peel. Other agents that can be used include A&D ointment, Crisco, Elta, or other antibiotic ointments. We avoid ointments containing neomycin, as this may pose additional risk to patients who develop a dermatologic reaction to this agent. Other occlusive techniques, including taping the face, have been used in the past but have been abandoned by most. Although both techniques work well, we believe that our technique affords greater patient comfort and allows us to evaluate the peeled areas more easily. Despite giving a parenteral dose of steroids (Decadron 8 mg) before the peel, moderate to severe facial edema often occurs during the postpeel period. Patients are instructed to reapply Eucerin cream every 3 to 4 h for approximately 5 days. They are also instructed to shower twice daily during this time. During postoperative days 5 to 8, an antibiotic ointment is substituted for the Eucerin cream. Patients should be instructed not to pick or remove any eschar, as this may result in unwanted scarring. Generally, reepithelialization will occur 10 days after the peel. At this time, patients begin using Eucerin lotion liberally, and a 2.5% hydrocortisone cream two to three times daily. Patients are also allowed to begin wearing makeup to camouflage the peeled areas that now appear pink. As with all skin resurfacing techniques, patients should avoid exposure to the sun for at least 6 weeks postpeel. Patients should also be instructed to always wear a sunscreen of SPF 30 or higher when outdoors.

Complications

Toxicity Phenol has the potential to cause cardiac, renal, and pulmonary toxicity. The best management of these complications is to avoid them. If the phenol solution is applied to facial subunits sequentially, as suggested, the risk of developing any of these problems is minimal. Patients should be monitored carefully and appropriate treatment instituted should these complications develop. The use of phenol warrants extreme caution in the periorbital region, to avoid burning the eye. Extreme care must be employed when peeling these areas. An assistant should always have a clean, dry, cotton-tipped applicator in her hand. It should be used to absorb tears that may drip down onto the face or into the temporal area, which would otherwise cause deeper, unwanted penetration of the solution.

Milia Milia are tiny superficial epidermal inclusion cysts that often appear during the first few weeks of recovery. They present in small numbers or may be present diffusely all over the treated areas. Milia often resolve spontaneously with normal cleansing of the face, although at times it is necessary to uncap the persistent milia with an 18-gauge needle tip. Although annoying when present, milia are never a permanent problem.

Erythema The erythema present after phenol peeling is not a complication, but an expected result. Camouflage makeup can be worn as needed starting at approximately 10 days. Slight erythema may persist for 10 to 12 weeks but gradually subsides. Although a topical steroid cream (2.5% hydrocortisone) is used routinely, it may not diminish the erythema rapidly. At times the erythema can be severe, lasting up to 6 to 9 months. Occasionally, it may be necessary to use a short course of systemic steroids to counteract severe postpeel inflammatory response.

Hyperpigmentation Postinflammatory hyperpigmentation is a very common postoperative complication, especially in Fitzpatrick type III–VI skin types. It also occurs commonly in those who receive sun exposure too early. When it appears, a bleaching formula (described previously) is used with great success. Retin-A, glycolic acid products, lighter TCA peels, and other hydroquinone preparations may be necessary to alleviate persistent hyperpigmentation.

Undesirable Alteration of Skin Texture Several changes may occur in the skin of some patients after a Baker–Gordon peel. Although there is no scientific evidence to explain this, some patients may complain that their skin pores appear to be enlarged. Patients with telangiectias may notice a worsening of them after phenol peeling. These are easily treated with one of the vascular lasers. Nevi may appear darker after the peel. The skin may acquire a fine reticular pattern in some areas that does not represent a scar and in cases in which epithelialization occurred within a normal period of time. These patients can be treated with a fairly potent nonfluorinated topical steroid such as Elocon 0.1%, for 2 to 3 weeks with good resolution.

Infection In spite of prophylactic use of antiviral agents, patients may develop an outbreak of herpes simplex infection. This can be treated with acyclovir 800 mg 4 times per day, along with careful treatment of ulcers with emollients. Our patients are routinely placed on a prophylactic dose of Famvir or Valtrex 2 days preoperatively and are maintained for 5 days postoperatively. Although a herpes outbreak during the peripeel stage may be disconcerting, it responds rapidly to treatment and rarely causes residual scarring. A herpetic outbreak may delay complete epithelialization and cause prolonged erythema at the herpetic sites.

Scleral Show or Ectropion of the Lower Eyelid Older patients with senile lid laxity, patients who have undergone a prior transcutaneous lower blepharoplasty, and patients with extremely thin skin are predisposed to this complication after a Baker–Gordon phenol peel. When ectropion does occur, the first line of treatment is conservative care, such as massaging of lower lid skin, taping of the eyelid, especially at night, and adequate protection of the globe using Natural Tears and Lacrilube. In most cases, this is a self-limiting process that corrects spontaneously or with conservative care. Intralesional steroids or surgical repair are only considered for rare persistent cases with severe ectropion.

Skin Depigmentation Clinically and histologically, patients undergoing phenol chemical peeling may exhibit a bleaching effect. After phenol peeling, melanocytes reorganize themselves along the basement membrane. Although still present, these melanocytes lose their ability to produce melanin. Clinically, this results in a bleached appearance. This may be desired and beneficial for those patients seeking treatment of certain pigmentary problems. However, in patients undergoing regional facial peeling, this bleaching effect may become noticeable and problematic. It is often most noticeable in the jaw–neck region, where untreated skin in the neck appears more obvious as it abuts the newly rejuvenated cheek or periorbital skin.

Scarring Although rare, scarring from phenol peeling may be very disturbing to both the patient and the surgeon. The perioral area, specifically the upper lip, and the region over the mandible are the most common areas in which scars develop. Scarring may occur as a result of poor postpeel wound care. For this reason, our patients are evaluated every 2 weeks for the first 2 months to avoid preventable complications. Infections and self-inflicted wounds that result in excoriated areas should be addressed immediately to prevent scarring. Scarring may also result from poor patient selection, particularly those patients with microvascular disease resulting from underlying diabetes or as a result of smoking. Scars may also develop when the peeling agent has penetrated too deeply. When it does occur, scarring is best managed with the use of intralesional steroids. We routinely use a 20% Kenalog solution injected into the scar every 2 to 3 weeks as needed. If the surgeon is overzealous with the use of intralesional steroids, however, dermal atrophy and telangiectasia will develop. Phenol peeling in the neck is not recommended, as it can produce severe scarring.

Summary

Phenol chemical peeling produces a dramatic improvement in the treatment of coarse facial rhytids. The longevity of its results have been established. We continue to use phenol as the agent of choice for deep chemical peeling. However, we also recognize that potential pigmentary disturbances may occur; therefore, proper patient selection, proper technique, and proper postoperative care are critical to a successful outcome. For Fitzpatrick III–V skin types, we prefer phenol 88% rather than the Baker–Gordon formula. This has proved successful for the treatment of deep facial rhytids in these patients, while minimizing pigmentary disturbances. In the future, phenol may be supplanted by laser resurfacing or by newer resurfacing techniques as they are developed. For the present, phenol remains the most effective deep skin resurfacing tool.

Laser Resurfacing

Although laser physics was first described by Albert Einstein in 1917, laser technology did not appear until the 1960s. Only in recent times have the CO_2 and erbium lasers found their way into the cosmetic surgeon's armamentarium as skin resurfacing tools. These high-energy lasers have revolutionized the treatment of photoaged skin. In contrast to other forms of skin resurfacing, laser resurfacing has captured the attention of many people worldwide. When referring to laser resurfacing, the media conjure up the image of someone using a magical wand to transform a severely photoaged face into a youthful-appearing one. This fictional belief has led patients who were once fearful of undergoing chemical peeling to flock to the cosmetic surgeon's office for laser skin resurfacing. These patients have been mistakenly told that recovery from laser resurfacing will be markedly reduced and that complications are less likely. As these beliefs are not true, patients must be better informed as to the true advantages and disadvantages of laser resurfacing. The main advantage to laser resurfacing is the ability to treat certain patients who might not otherwise be candidates for other methods of skin resurfacing. This is particularly true for patients with Fitzpatrick type IV–VI skin types, who may be at greater risk of developing pigmentary problems after deep phenol chemical peeling.

HISTOLOGIC CHANGES

The histologic changes observed after treatment with high-energy pulsed CO_2 lasers are similar to those found in patients undergoing resurfacing with phenol chemical peeling. Lasers produce a controlled thermal injury that extends to the upper reticular dermis. As the wound heals, angiogenesis and fibroplasia are stimulated as new collagen is laid down. Improvement in epidermal morphology, including the reversal of epidermal atypia and a return of cellular maturation and vertical polarity, are consistent features found after laser resurfacing. Epidermal healing is usually complete by 2 weeks after the procedure, whereas dermal healing continued for 4 to 6 months. Histologically, the major difference between laser resurfacing and phenol resurfacing is the impact to the melanocyte. After phenol chemical peeling, epidermal melanocytes lose their ability to synthesize melanin. By contrast, after treatment with the CO_2 laser, melanocytes retain their ability to produce melanin. This has been demonstrated in the biopsies from black skin, in which melanocytic activity returned 3 months after laser resurfacing. For this reason, patients with darker skin types who are otherwise poor candidates for phenol peeling, may be successfully treated by CO_2 laser resurfacing. Although the laser is less detrimental to melanocyte function, there is still a risk of hypopigmentation as the depth of penetration increases. This is true of all skin resurfacing agents and should not be overlooked.

Indications

CO_2 laser resurfacing may be used for many types of clinical problems; however, we find it most useful in patients seeking treatment for dermatologic conditions affecting the reticular dermis. We have found that patients with acne scarring benefit more from CO_2 laser resurfacing than from any type of chemical peeling. In our practice, it has supplanted dermabrasion as the procedure of choice for the treatment of acne scarring. For patients with deep ice-pick type scars, the best treatment is punch excision and grafting, followed by laser resurfacing. This has produced improved results.

Laser skin resurfacing may also be used for patients seeking improvement of both fine and coarse facial rhytids. Overall, rejuvenation of photoaged skin is produced by the regeneration of elastic fibers and dermal collagen. Improvement in skin tightening and overall skin texture is comparable to results obtained with other chemical peeling agents. For the treatment of fine facial rhytids, we prefer TCA chemical peeling, as it is safer, faster, and less costly. Patients seeking treatment for epidermal dysplasias, including those with actinic keratoses, may also benefit from laser skin resurfacing. The laser's high energy results in the thermal ablation of these dysplasias. The epidermis regenerates with normal healing and, as it does, significantly improves the quality of the skin's appearance. Laser resurfacing is also useful for treating facial dyschromias. Dyschromias appear as a result of pigment that is unevenly distributed along the basement membrane. As with other resurfacing techniques, laser resurfacing improves this condition by reducing this clumping of pigment and distributing it more evenly.

Evaluation

When evaluating a patient who is considering laser skin resurfacing, several factors need to be evaluated regardless of the type of laser being used. The patient's skin type, skin thickness, degree of oil content, and the area to be resurfaced are among the most important variables to be considered. Thinner, drier skin in the lower eyelid region of an elderly patient will generally require fewer passes as compared with the thicker, oily skin in the forehead region of a younger patient. Laser treatment should therefore be individualized and the pulse energy selected appropriately. A higher pulse energy will produce more complete ablation and vaporization of the tissue, whereas a lower pulse energy will result in less tissue vaporization. However, lower energies also elicit increased dermal damage secondary to increased conductive thermal injury. For this reason, higher pulse energies are preferred, as greater precision is obtained with fewer passes.

Pretreatment Care

As with other types of skin resurfacing procedures, we prefer to pretreat our patients with a combination of 8% hydroquinone, 1% hydrocortisone, and 0.05% retinoic acid. This regimen offers several advantages, including a shorter healing period and a lower risk of postoperative pigmentary disturbances. In addition, we use an antiviral agent and antibiotic prophylaxis in all our patients. This consists of oral acyclovir 400 mg three times per day, and Keflex 250 mg four times per day, starting 2 days before laser resurfacing and continuing for 5 days postoperatively. We have found that this significantly reduces the risk of developing herpes infections, which may occur in 10% of the population despite a negative herpes simplex history. Prophylactic antibiotics reduce the risk of problems related to bacterial infections. Although rare, we have had instances in which a partial-thickness wound was converted into a full-thickness injury attributable to a bacterial infection that led to scar formation. Meticulous postoperative wound care has helped minimize these potentially devastating complications.

Patient Preparation

In the operating suite, the patient is placed in an upright sitting position and the regions to be resurfaced are marked. Special attention is paid to the natural shadow beneath the mandibular border, where the line of demarcation can be camouflaged. We do not advocate laser resurfacing of the cervical region, as the cervical skin heals more slowly and may display scarring secondary to its reduced number of adnexal structures.

Many types of anesthesia may be used for patients undergoing laser skin resurfacing. When resurfacing the entire face, we prefer IV sedation along with nerve blocks and infiltration of 1% lidocaine as needed. When individual facial subunits or other small regions are resurfaced, local infiltration of 1% lidocaine is preferred. We have not been especially satisfied with the use of EMLA cream, although other physicians advocate its use. Instead, we prefer to use sodium bicarbonate 8.4% mixed with lidocaine, to reduce the pain associated with injection. After local infiltration is completed, tetracaine eyedrops are instilled into the patient's eyes, before protective corneal shields are inserted. Protection of the eye is extremely important when using the laser and should not be disregarded. Other safety precautions must also be employed to avoid intraoperative complications. The patient's hair and surrounding inflammable drapes must be protected with wet towels; the flow of supplemental oxygen must be stopped, as these represent potential fire hazards. To avoid injury to the dental enamel, a moist gauze sponge should be placed over the patient's teeth when resurfacing the perioral region. In addition, all operating room personnel must wear protective eye gear, and a smoke evacuator should be activated to remove laser plume, which may harbor infective agents. Finally, after all necessary precautions have been taken, the laser is tested by firing it at a moistened wooden tongue blade. This ensures that the appropriate settings have been selected and that the laser is functioning properly before laser delivery to the facial skin.

USING THE LASER

As with other skin resurfacing techniques, laser resurfacing of the face is done in a regional fashion. The deepest individual rhytids are generally treated first, using a single pass of the laser. After this localized resurfacing, the remainder of the subunit is treated. When resurfacing the periorbital region, we avoid treating the pretarsal orbicularis region of the upper eyelid. Although it does little for the overall result, it increases postlaser edema and the risk of scarring and webbing significantly, particularly in the medial aspect of the eyelid. The remaining portions of the periorbital region, including the skin of the preseptal area and lateral crow's feet, are then resurfaced with two or three passes as required. The glabella, forehead, nasal, and cheek regions are then treated in a systematic fashion. The skin in these regions is thicker and may therefore be treated with multiple passes with a reduced risk of scarring. The perioral region is treated last. In older patients, this area may exibit significant deep rhytids requiring multiple passes to eradicate. It is not unusual for these patients to require three passes for effective treatment of this area.

Understanding Laser Injury

Understanding the endpoint of laser resurfacing is critical to achieving a safe and effective result. Judging the depth of penetration is a visual art that cannot be determined solely on the basis of the number of passes made with the laser. Treatment must be individualized and should not be performed using a "cookbook" approach. When laser resurfacing, several key visual clues can be observed as the treatment proceeds. The first pass of the CO_2 laser removes the epidermis and penetrates the papillary dermis. The skin color will appear pink, corresponding to the level of the dermal–epidermal blood vessels. The next pass of the laser will generally penetrate the upper reticular dermis, as the skin appears whitish brown. As additional passes are performed, the skin will turn a chamois color. When this color appears, the midreticular dermis has been reached, and resurfacing should not be carried further. Even if residual rhytids remain, resurfacing beyond this point should not be performed, as this will lead to scarring.

Laser Safety and Predictability

The predictability of laser skin resurfacing may be improved by following several guidelines. When laser resurfacing, a certain degree of spot overlap is required to ensure that the result will be satisfactory. However, if the overlap is too great, char builds up and begins to act as a heat sink. When this occurs, increased conductive thermal injury causes additional unpredictable tissue injury, which can lead to postoperative scarring. For this reason, char should always be removed after every pass of the laser. We use a saline-soaked 4 x 4-in. gauze sponge to remove the char before proceeding to the next pass. This allows the necrotic tissue to be removed in a simple manner. After removing the tissue, the skin should be dried before additional resurfacing. If the tissue is wet, the laser will not penetrate the skin in a predictable manner.

Postoperative Wound Care

Although some physicians prefer to use closed-wound dressings after laser skin resurfacing, we currently prefer open-wound dressings. We have used Flexan for regional and full-face laser skin resurfacing in the past but have had some difficulty keeping the dressing in place. Although easier for the patient, closed dressings limit postoperative wound inspection and may increase the incidence of postoperative infections. More recently, we have preferred to use open-wound care consisting of Elta or Eucerin cream for the first 5 to 7 days. This requires more patient compliance as the dressing is reapplied 4 to 5 times per day, but we find that reepithelialization occurs rapidly, with a lower risk of developing postoperative infections. At 7 to 10 days, once reepithelialization has occurred, the Eucerin cream is replaced with Eucerin lotion, which is continued for up to 6 weeks until the sebaceous glands begin to resume their normal functioning. After reepithelialization has occurred, pa-tients may begin using camouflage makeup. Patients are instructed to avoid direct exposure to sun for 6 weeks and are instructed to use a SPF 25 sunscreen during this period.

Complications

Hyperpigmentation Although postinflammatory hyperpigmentation may occur in any patient undergoing skin resurfacing procedures, the risk may be lessened by pretreating the skin with a bleaching agent. We pretreat our patients, especially those with type III skin or greater, with a combination of 8% hydroquinone, 1% hydrocortisone, and 0.05% retinoic acid for up to 4 weeks before they undergo laser resurfacing. By following this preoperative protocol, patients with Fitzpatrick type III or IV skin can undergo laser resurfacing with a reduced risk of postoperative hyperpigmentation. We have also treated patients with type V and VI skin with some success. These patients, however, usually develop transient hyperpigmentation and require prolonged skin care with bleaching agents. Rarely, hyperpigmentation may persist for longer than 6 months. Superficial TCA peels will correct this condition.

Herpes Simplex Infection The most common infection resulting after laser resurfacing is herpes simplex. Similar to other forms of skin resurfacing, herpes simplex infection poses a risk for all patients. We prefer to pretreat all our patients with acyclovir or valacyclovir 400 mg 3 times per day. Despite prophylaxis, some patients will still develop herpes infections during the postoperative period. When this occurs, valacyclovir 500 mg 4 times per day is recommended. These patients need to be followed very closely, as they are at increased risk of postoperative scarring. When treatment is instituted early and aggressively, herpes infection generally will respond well without subsequent complications.

Scarring Hypertrophic scarring after laser resurfacing is most likely to be the result of improper laser techniques, postoperative infections, or poor wound care. Although most experienced surgeons rarely experience this complication, its occurrence is very disconcerting. By following the proper techniques and understanding how to read the laser, postoperative scarring will infrequently occur. If scarring begins to develop, it should be treated aggressively with low-dose intralesional Kenalog injections, starting approximately 4 weeks postoperatively. Patients should be followed up every 2 weeks and additional injections given as needed. Most scars can be treated effectively with this approach. Rarely, a formal scar revision is necessary.

Prolonged Erythema Prolonged erythema is an expected outcome after laser resurfacing. It is related to new collagen formation and angiogenesis and usually lasts several months. In general, the deeper the laser treatment, the greater the degree and duration of erythema. When erythema lasts more than 3 months, we prefer to use 1 to 2.5% hydrocortisone lotion. We have not experienced erythema lasting longer than 6 months.

Hypopigmentation Hypopigmentation after laser resurfacing occurs more often in patients with Fitzpatrick type I or II skin. It becomes more apparent in these patients because they have less pigment in their skin to camouflage the dermal changes that occur after laser therapy. Hypopigmentation may also be noted more readily by the patient who undergoes regional resurfacing because of the contrast in the untreated areas. In general, the deeper the laser penetrates the dermis, the greater the chance of developing hypopigmentation. Unlike hyperpigmentation that can be successfully treated with bleaching agents, this problem is generally more problematic because the only treatment for the patient is camouflage makeup.

Other Potential Laser Complications Lasers are powerful instruments that can potentially be hazardous if proper precautions are not followed. Because the CO_2 laser absorbs water, proper ocular protection must be worn by all personnel and patients in the operating room to avoid serious ocular damage. Reflection hazards, electrical hazards, pollution hazards, and fire hazards also need to be prevented. Only experienced personnel should be allowed to use this equipment.

SUMMARY

Laser resurfacing has already proved a good alternative to other skin resurfacing methods. However, the benefits of laser resurfacing will not be known until long-term results are obtained. Unfortunately, because of the public's high demand and the media's ever-increasing intrigue for laser resurfacing, many physicians now routinely use laser techniques. As a result, patients are victimized by overzealous operators who do not have the proper training with this technology. In well-trained hands, laser skin resurfacing has been an extremely successful tool used to treat photoaged skin.

Conclusion

Facial skin rejuvenation continues to be one of the most popular procedures performed by facial plastic surgeons. Many options are available for the treatment of photoaged skin. As newer technologies continue to develop, the best modality for a given problem may not be obvious. Although it is important that facial plastic surgeons have an understanding of all skin resurfacing procedures, it is even more imperative that they gain experience in the techniques they most commonly use. As no single skin resurfacing procedure can be used for all patients, the most successful outcome will be achieved when the treatment is individualized for each patient. Overall, skin resurfacing procedures remain one of the most rewarding procedures for both the patient and the surgeon.

SUGGESTED READINGS

Mangat and Mendelsohn—CHAPTER 30

Baker TJ, Gordon HL. The ablation of rhytids by chemical means. A preliminary report. *J Florida Med Assoc* 1961;48:451

Baker TJ, Stuzin JM, Baker TM. *Facial skin resurfacing.* St. Louis: Quality Medical Publishing; 1998

Baker TJ, Gordon HL, Seckinger DL. A second look at chemical face peeling. *Plast Reconstr Surg* 1966;37:487

Mangat DM. Chemical peels and dermabrasion. *Facial Plast Surg Clin North Am* 1994;2:1–4, 69–76

Cortez EA. Chemical face peeling. *Otolaryngol Clin North Am* 1990;23:947

Rubin MG. *Manual of Chemical Peels: Superficial and Medium Depth.* Philadelphia: Lippincott-Raven; 1995

Mendelsohn JE, Mangat DS. Deep chemical peeling. In: *Facial Rejuvenation.* (in press)

11

Alloplastic or Homograft Implantation for Nasal Reconstruction

"Although alloplastic implants are plentiful and easy to shape and provide a natural contour under the skin, these materials have the heightened potential for complications and are therefore the least desirable materials to be used as a nasal graft."

Dean M. Toriumi

"Autogenous cartilage is most commonly employed for structural and augmentation grafting in the nasal tip, as well as for dorsal deformities. However, the limited availability and unpredictable resorption of both autologous and homologous implants have made newer alloplastic implants important considerations for dorsal augmentation."

William H. Beeson

"My current thesis is that we should scrupulously avoid placing implants in the nose."

Douglas G. Mann

Alloplastic or Homograft Implantation for Nasal Reconstruction

CHAPTER 31

Matthew D. Mingrone, David B. Lovice, and Dean M. Toriumi

Functional and cosmetic rhinoplasty often mandates the need for implantable materials to change nasal contour or provide improved support for the nasal framework and overlying soft tissues. There are many implant materials, which can be divided into three main categories: autografts, homografts, and alloplasts. Autografts are those harvested from the patient and include, among others, cartilage, bone, dermis, fat, and fascia. Homografts, such as cartilage, bone, and dermis, are materials procured from donors of the same species. Alloplasts encompass a large group of synthetic and semisynthetic materials used as implants. A fourth group of materials, xenografts, are those implant materials harvested from other species, such as bovine collagen. The latter group is relatively small and therefore is not discussed further. Each category of graft maintains notable advantages and disadvantages, as outlined in Table 31–1. The controversy as to which material is superior is not a new one, and will continue to be debated until a group of alloplastic materials are developed that satisfy the basic needs of the ideal implant. A suitable implant must be biocompatible, strong, and elastic. The material should be completely inert, incapable of inducing inflammation or allergy, noncarcinogenic, resistant to mechanical strain, easily modified for shaping, and sterilizable.

Surgical needs, patient selection, and the surgeon's preference and experience are all factors that influence the choice of material for a given circumstance. Most would agree that autografts should remain the primary choice for nasal reconstruction and rejuvenation. Situations do arise, however, in which harvesting a graft is impractical or increases the morbidity of a procedure in a patient with borderline medical status. Additionally, sufficient autogenous material may not exist to satisfy the surgical needs of the patient. For these situations, homograft materials are an adequate substitute to autografts. Graft

TABLE 31–1
Implants in Rhinoplasty: Advantages and Disadvantages

	Autografts	Alloplasts	Homografts
Advantages	1. Biocompatibility 2. Strength (bone) 3. Ability to contour (cartilage) 4. Ability to camouflage (fascia)	1. Strength 2. Elasticity 3. Durability 4. No donor site morbidity 5. Unlimited supply 6. Decreased surgical time	1. Biocompatibility 2. Strength (bone) 3. Ability to contour (cartilage) 4. Ability to camouflage (fascia, AlloDerm) 5. No donor site morbidity 6. Unlimited supply 7. Decreased surgical time
Disadvantages	1. Donor site morbidity 2. Memory (cartilage) 3. Rare resorption 4. Limited material 5. Increased surgical time	1. Higher extrusion rate than autografts 2. Higher infection rate 3. Higher cost	1. Resorption 2. Warping (cartilage) 3. Extrusion 4. Higher infection rate 5. Higher cost 6. Patient confidence with implant safety

SOURCE: Lovice DB, Mingrone MD, Toriumi DM. Grafts and implants in rhinoplasty and nasal reconstruction. *Otolaryngol Clin North Am* 1999; 32:113–41

TABLE 31–2
Implant Materials

Alloplastic Materials	Autologous Materials	Homologous Materials
Metals Titanium Vitalium Stainless steel	Septal cartilage grafts Rib grafts Auricular cartilage grafts	Irradiated and nonirradiated costal cartilage Acellular dermis (AlloDerm)
Ceramics	Calvarial bone grafts	
Polymers Silicone Polyethylene Polytetrafluoroethylene (PTFE) Polyesters Polyamides	Other bone grafts Tissue flaps Cutaneous flaps Mucosal flaps	
Resorbable materials Suture		

location must also be considered when choosing an implant. Grafts for the relatively immobile dorsum may undergo less resorption than those placed in the nasal tip (Table 31–2).

Autografts

Autologous tissue is the most favorable implant material. Biocompatibility is unsurpassed, and the risk of infection and extrusion is far lower with autologous materials as compared with alloplasts.[1] Cartilage to reconstruct the nose can be harvested from the septum, concha, or rib. Bone can also be taken from the septum, calvarium, or rib. Soft tissue can be brought into the area using various pedicle or free flaps as well as dermis and dermal-fat grafts. Autologous materials offer the obvious advantage of unsurpassed biocompatibility, but they do cause donor site morbidity and can resorb over time. Cartilage has the additional disadvantage of potential warping or deformity. The limited supply of cartilage from the septum and ear can also be problematic.

Septal cartilage is the graft of choice for nasal tip grafting.[2-4] Septal cartilage is usually straighter and more rigid than conchal cartilage. It is easier to carve and shape because it is less fragile. Tardy et al.[5] documented a multitude of successful septal cartilage grafts placed during rhinoplasty, with nearly two decades of follow-up. Septal cartilage is commonly used for struts, batten grafts, lateral crural grafts, lateral crural strut grafts, and spreader grafts. This cartilage is also an excellent material for shield tip grafts and buttress grafts adding projection or length and definition to the nasal tip. Dorsal augmentation can be performed using septal cartilage. Single or multiple layered grafts fixed with resorbable suture can be used for differing degrees of augmentation. A radix graft can be fashioned with bruised septal cartilage to improve the deep nasofrontal angle and to increase the acute nasolabial angle in the form of a plumping graft. Crushing cartilage may hasten the onset and severity of cartilage resorption.[6] Septal cartilage is also our choice for strut grafting for tip support and for caudal septal grafting to increase the length and support of the nose.

Septal cartilage can be harvested through a variety of approaches. Regardless of the approach, the amount of cartilage to be removed should be dictated by the amount of cartilage required for grafting. In addition, at least 1.5 cm of dorsal and caudal septal cartilage should be preserved to achieve adequate support of the nose. The degree of cartilaginous hump removal should be contemplated before septum is harvested; if excess cartilage is removed, support may be compromised. The cartilage can then be carved and chamfered for precise contouring to match the surrounding tissue. The graft should be affixed in place with suture material.

Conchal cartilage is an alternative site to harvest an autograft and yields approximately 4 cm^2 of cartilage, as well as perichondrium. Composite grafts including, skin, cartilage, and perichondrium can be used for nasal tip reconstruction, repair of alar retraction, and septal perforation repair (perichondrocutaneous grafts).[7,8] Free perichondrium can be used to camouflage a graft over the nasal tip in thin-skinned patients. Conchal cartilage is an adequate substitute for septal cartilage, grafts when the septum has been harvested previously. Owing to its more brittle nature, conchal cartilage can be more difficult to carve than septal cartilage. In addition, conchal cartilage is curved and less rigid than quadrangular cartilage. Like septal cartilage, conchal grafts can be used as a single-layered implant or sutured together to increase bulk. Conchal cartilage is appropriate for contour improvement of the nasal tip or as an onlay graft. However, septum or rib cartilage is stronger, and provides more support. Previous extensive auricular cartilage harvesting may preclude harvesting of further conchal cartilage. Other contraindications include systemic diseases, such as collagen vascular disease, rheumatic disease, or immunologic disorders involving the auricle, such as lupus, polychondritis, sarcoidosis, and Wegener's granulomatosis. Careful preoperative analysis and questioning will guide the surgeon as to which ear should be used to harvest cartilage. Complete conchal cartilage removal may result in slight medialization of the pinna. Therefore, if asymmetric, the more prominent ear should be harvested. Furthermore, for the patient who has a history of sleeping on only one side of the head, the contralateral conchal cartilage should be harvested.

Several techniques for harvesting conchal cartilage have been described.[9,10] We prefer the posterior approach. The posterior approach avoids an incision on the anterior surface of the auricle and should be used when the postauricular region is to be exposed for other reasons (e.g., during otoplasty or rhytidectomy) or if the patient has a predilection for keloid formation. Conchal cartilage is considered the graft of choice for most nonstructural grafting needs when septal cartilage is unavailable.

Saddle-nose deformities or severe structural deficiencies often require larger grafts, such as rib cartilage. Costal cartilage supplies sufficient amounts of cartilage for almost any structural defect of the nose. Confluent ribs five and six or seven and eight are the preferred ribs to harvest for nasal implantation. The disadvantages of using this graft include the potential for warping and resorption,[11] potential pneumothorax, and postoperative pain.[12] In older patients, cartilage calcification can make carving and shaping nearly impossible. Harvesting rib cartilage in the elderly should therefore be avoided. Carving techniques that attempt to remove equal proportions of cartilage from all surfaces of the rib have been associated with less warping.[12] Despite careful technique unpredictable warping continues to be the primary problem associated with costal cartilage implantation. Costal cartilage should be used primarily as a strut graft for the nose lacking tip support or for dorsal augmentation in patients with saddle-nose deformity. Graft fixation may reduce the risk of malposition and warping.[13] A boat-like configuration is the desired design for carving the graft to re-create the anatomy of the dorsum and allow for camouflage with adjacent nasal anatomy.[14]

Bone is a viable alternative to cartilage for dorsal nasal augmentation.[15,16] Split calvarium (membranous) is less likely to resorb than is iliac crest (endochondral).[17,18] In addition, calvarium can be harvested via the same operative field. The osteotomy required to harvest iliac crest is also associated with significant postoperative pain. For the above reasons, split calvarium is the graft of choice when bone is used for dorsal augmentation. The risks associated with harvesting calvarium include penetration of the cranial cavity, laceration of a major venous sinus, brain injury, and a postoperative depression of the skull.[19,20] Bone used in the nose can create a rigid-appearing structure. Although the graft is usually well tolerated and resorbs minimally, the unnatural nasal appearance and difficulty in shaping the graft make calvarial bone a less desirable implant. Fixation is necessary to maintain graft position and reduce the risk for resorption.[21]

Autologous materials are the implant of choice for many reconstructive surgeons. Situations do arise, however, when harvesting such tissue may be deleterious to the patient, or the tissue is not in a sufficient quantity to correct the given defect. Homografts are a viable alternative. Alloplastic materials have also been used with varying success to augment the nose and serve as an additional, less acceptable, alternative to autografts.

Homologous Grafts

Homologous bone, cartilage, and dermal grafts alleviate donor site morbidity, but significant resorption has been reported. Toriumi et al.[22] studied long-term resorption rates of demineralized bone split rib implants. The average rate of resorption after only 2 years was greater than 80%. The results obtained with homologous tissue can also be unpredictable. The surface structure of the implant material can change with time, leading to distortion of the overlying soft tissue. Despite these potential inadequacies, irradiated cadaveric costal cartilage serves as an adequate substitute for autologous rib cartilage. A number of things can be done to attempt to decrease the risk of warping and distortion. Gunter et al.[13] describe the use of K-wire insertion into grafted cartilage to prevent such changes with time. Shaving equal amounts of cartilage from all surfaces of the graft may reduce the risk of graft distortion and warping. All perichondrium should be removed to further reduce the potential for cartilage distortion. Irradiated costal cartilage grafts have been used by several surgeons for dorsal nasal augmentation with success.[23-25] Use of this material should be limited to the dorsum. Implantation into the mobile nasal tip has been associated with significant resorption.[26]

Cadaveric rib cartilage is obtained from donors who must meet the same criteria required for organ donation, such as screening for VDRL, hepatitis B, human immunodeficiency virus (HIV), tuberculosis, and slow virus testing. The selected donor rib is then exposed to $\leq$ 60,000 Gy γ-waves to destroy cellular and viral pathogens. These grafts are well tolerated because their relative acellular makeup illicits minimal immune response by the host.[1] Cadaveric rib grafts are best reserved for elderly patients who require minimized operative time and donor site morbidity. Moreover, the rib of an older patient may be calcified, making it difficult to shape. Success of implantation and maintenance of graft volume seems to be related to site of implantation. The nasal dorsum appears to tolerate implantation well, most likely because of its relative immobility.[23,25] Rib cartilage, either autologous or homologous, should therefore be reserved for dorsal nasal augmentation where it has the best chance to preserve its volume with time. Longer-term studies are needed for a more accurate determination of the resorption rates of these grafts.

Acellular dermis (AlloDerm) is an excellent camouflage material that has been used as a substitute for skin grafting in burn patients.[27] For rhinoplasty, the material is especially useful for covering dorsal nasal irregularities in the thin-skinned rhinoplasty patient. It has the distinct advantage of being readily available and well tolerated. There are no long-term data on the degree of implant resorption. However, if partially resorbed it may be replaced with a thin layer of scar tissue to maintain a smooth nasal dorsum.[1] AlloDerm can be used as an alternative to fascia or perichondrium for soft tissue camouflage and may serve as an adjuvant in mucosal flap advancement procedures for closing septal perforations. AlloDerm may also be combined with cartilage or bone grafts to facilitate a smooth dorsal nasal contour in patients with thin skin.

Alloplastic Implants

Implantation of synthetic material into the nose must be done with considerable trepidation. Early postoperative or long-term failure is a risk of any implant placed into the nose. In general, synthetic material, if used in the nose, should be reserved for the relatively immobile dorsum and should be considered the last resort after autologous and homologous implants have been considered. Costantino[28] described four concepts to be cognizant of when planning alloplastic implantation: porosity, particle formation, elemental makeup, and location.

Implant materials have pores of varying sizes and can range from less than 20 μm to several hundred μm. Pores permit tissue ingrowth; the larger the pore, the more aggressive the ingrowth. Pores also permit influx of bacteria, which is not necessarily problematic if the pores are sufficiently large enough to allow ingress of macrophages (50 μm) as well.[29] Sufficiently large pores, > 100 μm, will theoretically allow for bony and fibrous ingrowth, which would further stabilize the grafted implant.[28] Solid silicone rubber implants, for example, lack pores and are therefore impenetrable to bacterial invasion and tissue growth. Stabilization is therefore dependent on capsule formation, and infection can occur at any time. Deformation of overlying tissue can be an unfortunate sequelae of silicone rubber implants as a consequence of thick capsule formation.

Particle formation is primarily a concern for implants placed in areas of mobility. Relatively inert particulate materials of 20 to 60 μm can be phagocytized, but ingestion leads to macrophage demise and subsequent release of several inflammatory factors responsible for chronic inflammation. Particles > 60 μm in diameter cannot be phagocytized. Immune complex formation may also be a factor contributing to significant immune reaction in the area.[28]

The ideal implant does not exist. New biomaterials continue to be developed and investigated to meet the rigid criteria necessary to satisfy the needs of a surgeon using implants. An implant should be completely inert, incapable of inducing inflammation or allergy, noncarcinogenic, resistant to mechanical strain, easily modified for shaping, and sterilizable. The most favorable materials are those that most closely resemble the human tissue adjacent to the proposed implant site.[28] Silicone, for example, is close to carbon, one of the main constituents in the body, on the periodic table. Consequently, silicone has been used extensively as an implant because of its relative nonreactivity.

Location of implant placement is critical to success. Regardless of biocompatibility, those areas of the body that are susceptible to movement are at higher risk of implant failure. In the nose, the tip should be considered a mobile unit, and therefore should not undergo alloplastic implantation. The dorsum of the nose and premaxilla are fairly stable areas and are sites that are more appropriate for augmentation with an alloplast. Success even on the dorsum, however, can be difficult to achieve if an adequate amount of skin and soft tissue is not covering the implant, offering sufficient blood supply to the area.

Alloplastic implants for the nose fall into several groups: polymers, metallics, ceramics, and injectables. Polymers comprise the largest group. All these materials discussed have been used with varying success in the nose. We believe, however, that alloplastic implants should be considered the third choice behind autologous or homologous grafts.

Materials

A polymer consists of long chains of repeating subunits. Carbon, hydrogen, and oxygen are the typical constituents, but exceptions are noted in the following discussion. Stability of the material is related to the length of the chains and to the number of cross-bridges between chains. The more stable the material, the less likely it is that the body will break it down.[30] The most common polymers used for nasal implantation include silicone, polytetrafluoroethylene (PTFE), and polyethylenes.

SILICONE

Silicone refers to a group of polymers. Silicon is the fundamental element of this group. Silica, SiO_2, is polymerized with methyl groups to form silicone. Extending the length and cross-linking of the polymer affects the form the material takes. Progressive formation of silicone gel and silicone rubber is the result. The material's form has a significant influence on acceptance by host tissue. Silicone rubber is nonporous and does not form particles. Silicone gel has been used primarily for breast augmentation, but it has also been used in a cured form to improve nasal contour.[31] The risk of migration and significant inflammatory reaction has been documented in the literature and should therefore preclude its use in this form. Because it lacks pores and is relatively stable, silicone rubber or Silastic is less likely to initiate an inflammatory response by the recipient. This material has been used extensively for dorsal, tip, and premaxillary augmentation.[21,32-35] The nonporous nature of silicone reduces the probability for bacterial colonization, but it also impedes tissue ingrowth. Lack of ingrowth may lead to movement of the implant and will induce capsule formation around the implant. The capsule can be a site of bacterial infiltration, acts as a barrier against penetration of antibiotics, and can lead to implant distortion. The risk of extrusion remains for the life of the patient and has been reported as long as 20 years after implantation.[36-38]

The most common use for silicone is for combined dorsum and tip augmentation, and it has been used extensively for Asian nose rhinoplasty.[35] Silicone rubber possesses the advantage of being easily carvable and autoclavable. The method of placement depends on its use. Patients must be informed of the inherent risks of the use of these implants. However, solid silicone should not be lumped into the same category as the breast implant gel and is an excellent material for chin augmentation. Silicone has been used successfully in Asian patients undergoing augmentation rhinoplasty. These patients have thicker skin and are better able to support an alloplastic implant than are thin-skinned patients. However, we prefer to use autologous or homologous materials whenever possible.

POLYTETRAFLUORETHYLENE

Several implant materials fall into the category of PTFE. The most notable are Teflon, Proplast, and Gore-Tex, all of which consist of fluorine–carbon polymers. The bond between these two elements is very strong and therefore stable, despite the lack of fluorine or fluorinelike substances in the body. Gore-Tex is the most widely used PTFE implant material for the nose and, as such, is discussed in detail.

Proplast is a black-colored implant material, which is fairly rigid and easily visible through thin skin, making its use impractical in dorsal nasal augmentation.[39,40] Proplast II was developed 10 years after Proplast. It is composed of PTFE linked to aluminum oxide fibers and hydroxyapatite, to give it a white color and to allow for bone compatibility, respectively.[41] Proplast II is more rigid than Proplast and is more porous, allowing for increased tissue ingrowth. The increased porosity may also be the reason for its propensity for fragmentation and severe inflammatory reactions when subjected to shearing-type forces as demonstrated with replacement of the temporomandibular joint (TMJ).[42-51] Because of the significant problems associated with TMJ reconstruction, Proplast is no longer available as an implant.

Gore-Tex has been the most promising implant in the PTFE group. It has been used extensively as a vascular graft since the early 1970s, and more recently as a facial implant. Subcutaneous augmentation material (SAM) was approved in 1993 for use in facial augmentation, including nasal augmentation.[52] Gore-Tex is a derivative of Teflon, made up of repeating units of carbon bound to fluorine. The material's interweaving fibrillar makeup along with relatively small pores (22 μm) allows for stabilizing tissue ingrowth without significantly inhibiting removal if necessary.[53] Gore-Tex is also hydrophobic, which inhibits bacterial adherence and reduces the severity of tissue ingrowth, again, facilitating its removal. In the rabbit model, Gore-Tex has been shown to elicit minimal inflammation when evaluated grossly and histologically.[54,55] The stability of Gore-Tex is a result of polymerization of repeating units of carbon bound to fluorine. Although fluorine is not found normally within human tissue, the material remains relatively inert as a result of its extremely strong carbon–fluorine bonding.

Indications for the use of Gore-Tex have expanded. The evolution from abdominal wall patch to use in facial augmentation and reconstruction blossomed during the early to mid-1980s. SAM is identical to the soft tissue patch and is used specifically for facial plastic and reconstructive surgery. Gore-Tex implants have been used for a myriad of applications in facial plastic surgery but have found significant success when used to augment the nasal dorsum.[14,56-61] Because of its natural appearance and ease of use as compared with rib cartilage or other autologous implants, Gore-Tex has become popular as a nasal implant.

SAM can be easily carved and shaped to camouflage defects in the nasal dorsum. The material is manufactured in 1-, 2-, and 4-mm thickness, which can be beveled at its periphery to blend with surrounding tissue.[55] Because of its ease of use and natural appearance, it has quickly become the alloplastic implant of choice for many facial plastic and reconstructive surgeons. However, we prefer to use autologous materials whenever possible.

POLYETHYLENES

Polyethylene implants are composed of a group of polymers with different characteristics based on their length, density, and cross-linkages. Three different densities have been described: low-, medium-, and high-density polymers.[62] The high-density polymers are the most often used for reconstructive craniofacial surgery. Medpor (Porex, Fairburn, GA) and Plastipore (Richards Manufacturing Company, Memphis, TN) are examples of high-density polyethylene implant materials. Medpor and Plastipore are flexible but maintain their shape when manipulated.[63] They have pores ranging in size from 100 to 250 μm, which allows for significant soft tissue and bone ingrowth.[64-67] Because of its stiffness, the implant appears unnatural over the nasal dorsum.[21]

POLYESTERS AND POLYAMIDES

Polyethylene terephthalate can be woven into a nonresorbable mesh referred to as Mersilene (Ethicon, Somerville, NJ) for dorsal nasal and subnasal region implantation.[68,69] The implant material allows for significant tissue ingrowth, maintaining implant position, but also making its removal difficult when necessary.[70] The mesh permits bacteria to grow within its network of fibers, leading to significant problems with bacterial colonization, infection, and graft failure.[71] Because of these factors, placement over the nasal dorsum is not recommended. Polyamides include a similar substance to Mersilene mesh with the trade name Supramid (Ethicon) mesh. Both have similar qualities and appearance. Supramid, however will resorb leaving behind a fibrous shell to maintain some of the implant's original volume.[21]

The Future

Autologous, homologous, and alloplastic implants all possess inherent strengths and weaknesses. Tissue-engineered autografts could potentially overcome the biocompatibility issues of alloplasts and the donor site morbidity and limited supply issues associated with autografts. Vacanti et al.[72,73] pioneered the development of xenograft tissue-engineered bovine cartilage grafts placed in immune-depleted mice. More recently, work has been done using autologous bioengineered cartilage grafts in rabbits.[74] Rabbit chondrocytes were harvested and grown in vitro for 5 days, followed by placement on polyglycolic acid nonwoven felt combined with poly-L-lactic acid. This porous, pre-shaped scaffold allowed for directed chondrocyte development into cartilage. Britt and Park demonstrated impressive short-term (4 to 8 weeks) and long-term (6 to 12 months) results using these tissue engineered implants placed into the flank of the donor rabbits. Relatively large amounts of host specific cartilage could be produced in this manner, which would have a significant impact on implantation protocols in the future. Cartilage harvested in this manner would most certainly be more expensive than other alternatives, but the future may also supply more efficient and cost effective methods for producing bioengineered implant materials.

Conclusion

Loss of nasal structure and support often mandates the need for implant materials to improve both form and function of the nose. Autologous implants, most notably septal cartilage, are the nasal grafts to which all others should be compared. Other autologous materials, such as auricular cartilage, costal cartilage, calverial bone, fascia, perichondrium, and dermis, are excellent materials for implantation in the nose. Irradiated rib and acellular dermis are homologous alternatives and should be considered in patients who cannot tolerate the additional morbidity associated with graft harvesting or who do not possess enough autologous material. Although alloplastic implants are plentiful and easy to shape and provide a natural contour under the skin, these materials have the heightened potential for complications and are therefore the least desirable materials to be used as a nasal graft. Their placement should be limited to the relatively immobile nasal dorsum or premaxilla, and the patient should be thoroughly counseled as to the risk of infection or extrusion with these materials. In the not too distant future, bioengineered cartilage may become another option for nasal procedures requiring graft material.

REFERENCES

Mingrone et al.—CHAPTER 31

1. Maas CS, Monhian N, Shah SB. Implants in rhinoplasty. *Facial Plast Surg* 1998;13:279–290
2. Brent B, Ott R. Perichondrocutaneous graft. *Plast Reconstr Surg* 1978;62:1–14
3. Kridel RH, Kraus WM. Grafts and implants in revision rhinoplasty. *Facial Plast Surg Clin North Am* 1995;3:473–486
4. Silver WE, Goldberg J. Nasal grafts and implants. *Facial Plast Surg Clin North Am* 1994;2:477–499
5. Tardy ME, Denneny J, Fritsch MH. The cartilage autograft in reconstruction of the nose and face. *Laryngoscope* 1985;95: 523–533
6. Bujia J. Determination of the viability of crushed cartilage grafts: clinical implications for wound healing in nasal surgery. *Ann Plast Surg* 1994;32:261–265
7. Brent B. The versatile cartilage autograft: current trends in clinical transplantation. *Clin Plast Surg* 1979;6:163–180
8. Johnson CM, Toriumi DM. *Open Structure Rhinoplasty.* Philadelphia: WB Saunders; 1990
9. Baylis HI, Rosen N, Neuhaus R. Obtaining auricular cartilage for reconstructive surgery. *Am J Ophthalmol* 1982;93: 709–712
10. Lusk RP, Kang DR, Muntz HR. Auricular cartilage grafts in laryngotracheal reconstruction. *Ann Otol Rhinol Laryngol* 1993;102:247–254
11. Davis WB, Gibson T. Absorption of autogenous cartilage grafts in man. *Br J Plast Surg* 1957;9:177–185
12. Gibson T, Davis WB. The distortion of autogenous cartilage grafts: its causes and prevention. *Br J Plast Surg* 1958;10:257–273
13. Gunter JP, Clark CP, Friedman RM. Internal stabilization of autogenous rib cartilage grafts in rhinoplasty: a barrier to cartilage warping. *Plast Reconstr Surg* 1997;100:161–169
14. Godin MS, Waldman SR, Johnson CM Jr. The use of expanded polytetrafluoroethylene (Gore-Tex) in rhinoplasty: a six-year experience. *Arch Otolaryngol Head Neck Surg* 1995; 121:1131–1136
15. Powell NB, Riley RW. Facial contouring with outer-table calvarial bone. *Arch Otolaryngol Head Neck Surg* 1980;115: 1454–1458
16. Romo T, Jablonsky RD. Nasal reconstruction using split calvarial grafts. *Otolaryngol Head Neck Surg* 1992;107:622–629
17. Hardesty RA, Marsh JL. Craniofacial onlay bone grafting. *Plast Reconstr Surg* 1990;85:5–12

18. Smith JD, Abramson M. Membranous vs endochondral bone autografts. *Arch Otolaryngol Head Neck Surg* 1974;99: 203–205
19. Cheney ML. Reconstructive grafting by the open nasal approach. *Facial Plast Surg Clin North Am* 1993;1:99–109
20. Kellman RM, Huckins MS, King J, et al. Bioresorbable screws for facial bone reconstruction: a pilot study in rabbits. *Laryngoscope* 1994;104:556–561
21. Staffel G, Shockley W. Nasal implants. *Otolaryngol Clin North Am* 1995;28:295–308
22. Toriumi DM, Larrabee WF, Walike JW, et al. Demineralized bone. *Arch Oto Head and Neck Surg* 1990;116:676–680
23. Kridel RW, Konior RJ. Irradiated cartilage grafts in the nose: a preliminary report. *Arch Otolaryngol Head Neck Surg* 1993;119:24–31
24. Maas CS, Merwin GE, Wilson J, et al. Comparison of biomaterials for facial bone augmentation. *Arch Otolaryngol Head Neck Surg* 1990;116:551–556
25. Schuller DE, Bardach J. Irradiated homologous costal cartilage for facial contour restoration. *Arch Otolarygol Head Neck Surg* 1977;103:12–15
26. Welling DB, Maves MD. Irradiated homologous cartilage grafts: long term results. *Arch Otolaryngol Head Neck Surg* 1988;114:291–295
27. Wainwright DJ. Use of an acellular allograft dermal matrix (AlloDerm) in the management of full-thickness burns. *Burns* 1995;21:243–248
28. Costantino PD. Synthetic biomaterials for soft-tissue augmentation and replacement in the head and neck. *Otolaryngol Clin North Am* 1994;27:223–262
29. Holmes RE, Hagler HK. Porous hydroxyapatite as a bone graft substitute in cranial reconstruction: a histometric study. *Plast Reconstr Surg* 1988;81:662–671
30. Hollinger JO. *Biomedical Application of Synthetic Biodegradable Polymers.* Boca Raton, FL: CRC Press; 1995
31. Han K, Kang J. A custom made nasal implant: prefabrication from curing of silicone adhesive. *Plast Reconstr Surg* 1996;97: 436–444
32. Beekhuis GJ. Use of silicone-rubber in nasal reconstructive surgery. *Arch Otolaryngol* 1967;86:114–117
33. Braley S. The silicones in maxillofacial surgery. *Laryngoscope* 1968;78:549–557
34. Braley S. Use of silicones in plastic surgery. *Arch Otolaryngol* 1963;78:669–675
35. Shirakabe Y, Shirakabe T, Kishimoto T. The classification of complications after augmentation rhinoplasty. *Aesthetic Plast Surg* 1985;9:185–192
36. Fisher AA. Reactions at silicone-injected sites on the face associated with silicone breast implant "inflammation" or "rejection." *Cutis* 1990;45:393–395
37. Peled IJ, Wexler MR, Ticher S, Lax EE. Mandibular resorption from silicone chin implants in children. *J Oral Maxillofac Surg* 1986;44:346–348
38. Shirakabe Y, Shirakabe T, Takayanagi S. A new type prosthesis for augmentation rhinoplasty: our experience in 1600 cases. *Br J Plast Surg* 1981;34:353–357
39. Brown BL, Neel HB, Kern EB. Implants of Supramid, Proplast, Plasti-pore, and Silastic. *Arch Otolaryngol* 1979;105:605–609
40. Kent JN, Homsy CA, Hinds EC. Proplast in dental facial reconstruction. *Oral Surg Oral Med Oral Pathol* 1975;39: 347–355
41. Westfall RL, Homsy CA, Kent JN. A comparison of porous composite PTFE/graphite and PTFE/aluminum oxide facial implants in primates. *J Oral Maxillofac Surg* 1982;40:771–775
42. Berarducci JP, Thompson DA, Scheffer RB. Perforation into middle cranial fossa as a sequel to use of a Proplast-Teflon implant for temporomandibular joint reconstruction. *J Oral Maxillofac Surg* 1990;48:496–498
43. Chuong R, Piper MA. Cerebrospinal fluid leak associated with Proplast implant removal from the temporomandibular joint. *Oral Surg Oral Med Oral Path* 1992;74:422–425
44. Fontenot MG, Kent JN. In vitro wear performance of Proplast TMJ disc implants. *J Oral Maxillofacial Surg* 1992;50: 133–139
45. Gallagher DM, Wolford LM. Comparison of Silastic and Proplast implants in the temporomandibular joint after condylectomy for osteoarthritis. *J Oral Maxillofacial Surg* 1982;40: 627–630
46. Kaplan PA, Ruskin JD, Tu HK, Knibbe MA. Erosive arthritis of the temporomandibular joint caused by Teflon-Proplast implants: plain film features. *AJR* 1988;151:337–339
47. Lagrotteria L, Scapino R, Granston AS, Felgenhauer D. Patient with lymphadenopathy following temporomandibular joint arthroplasty with Proplast. *Cranio* 1986;4:172–178
48. Moriconi ES, Popowich LD, Guernsey LH. Alloplastic reconstruction of the temporomandibular joint. *Dental Clin North Am* 1986;30:307–325
49. Schellhas KP, Wilkes CH, el Deeb M, et al. Permanent proplast temporomandibular joint implants: MR imaging of destructive complications. *AJR* 1988;151:731–735
50. Spagnoli D, Kent JN. Multicenter evaluation of temporomandibular joint Proplast–Teflon disk implant. *Oral Surg Oral Med Oral Pathol* 1992;74:411–421
51. Yih WY, Zysset M, Merrill RG. Histologic study of the fate of autogenous auricular cartilage grafts in the human temporomandibular joint. *J Oral Maxillofac Surg* 1992;50:964–967, discussion 968
52. Gore-Tex, SAM Facial Implant information pamphlet: technical considerations in plastic and reconstructive surgery. Package Insert. Flagstaff, AZ: WL Gore and Associates
53. Schoenrock LD, Chernoff G. Subcutaneous implantation of Gore-Tex for facial reconstruction. *Otolaryngol Clin North Am* 1995;28:325–340
54. Maas CS, Gnepp DR, Bumpous J. Expanded polytetrafluoroethylene (Gore-Tex Soft Tissue Patch) in facial augmentation. *Arch Otolaryngol Head Neck Surg* 1993;119:1008–1014

55. Neel HB. Implants by Gore-Tex. *Arch Otolarynol* 1983;109: 427–433
56. Berman M, Pearce WJ, Tinnin M. The use of Gore-Tex e-PTFE bonded to silicone rubber as an alloplastic implant material. *Laryngoscope* 1986;96:480–483
57. Conrad K, Gillman G. A six-year experience with the use of expanded polytetrafluoroethylene in rhinoplasty. *Plast Reconstr Surg* 1998;101:1675–1683
58. Mole B. The use of Gore-Tex implants in aesthetic surgery of the face. *Plast Reconstr Surg* 1992;90:200–206
59. Owsley TG, Taylor CO. The use of Gore-Tex for nasal augmentation: a retrospective analysis of 106 patients. *Plast Reconstr Surg* 1994;94:241–248
60. Rothstein SG, Jacobs JB. The use of Gore-Tex implants in nasal augmentation operations. *ENTechnology* 1989; Sep: 40–45
61. Waldman SR. Gore-Tex for augmentation of the nasal dorsum: a preliminary report. *Ann Plast Surg* 1991;26: 520–525
62. Lykins CL, Friedman CD, Ousterhout DK. Polymeric implants in craniomaxillofacial reconstruction. *Otolaryngol Clin North Am* 1994;27:1015–1035
63. Wellisz T. Clinical experience with the Medpor porous polyethylene implant. *Aesthetic Plast Surg* 1993;17:339–344
64. Jazayeri MA, Nichter LS, Zhou ZY, et al. Comparison of various delivery systems for demineralized bone matrix in a rat cranial defect model. *J Craniofac Surg* 1994;5:172–178; discussion 179
65. Romano JJ, Iliff NT, Manson PN. Use of Medpor porous polyethylene implants in 140 patients with facial fractures. *J Craniofac Surg* 1993;4:142–147
66. Shaber EP. Vertical interpositional augmentation genioplasty with porous polyethylene. *Int J Oral Maxillofac Surg* 1987; 16:678–681
67. Wellisz T, Dougherty W, Gross J. Craniofacial applications for the Medpor porous polyethylene flexblock implant. *J Craniofac Surg* 1992;3:101–107
68. Ersek RA. Bioplastique: specific technical advice on its use and possible complications. *Aesthetic Plast Surg* 1992;16:67–68
69. McCollough EG, Hom DB, Weigel MT, Anderson JR. Augmentation mentoplasty using Mersilene mesh. *Arch Otolaryngol Head Neck Surg* 1990;116:1154–1158
70. Colton JJ, Beekhuis GJ. Use of mersilene mesh in nasal augmentation. *Facial Plast Surg* 1992;8:149–156
71. Costantino PD, Friedman CD, Jones K, et al. Evaluation of a new hydroxyapatite cement: basic chemistry and biology. *Arch Otolaryngol Head Neck Surg* 1991;117:379–384
72. Vacanti CA, Langer R, Schloo B, Vacanti JP. Synthetic polymers seeded with chondrocytes provide a template for new cartilage formation. *Plast Reconstr Surg* 1991;88:753–759
73. Vacanti CA, Vacanti JP. Bone and cartilage reconstruction with tissue engineering approaches. *Otolaryngol Clin North Am* 1994;27:263–276
74. Britt JC, Park SS. Autogenous tissue-engineered cartilage. *Arch Otolaryngol Head Neck Surg* 1998;124:671–677

CHAPTER 32

Alloplastic or Homograft Implantation for Nasal Reconstruction

William H. Beeson

The use of implants in rhinoplasty is controversial. A variety of materials are commonly employed in nasal surgery for augmentation and for reconstruction. Autogenous tissue has long been advocated as the mainstay for nasal implants. Autogenous cartilage is most commonly employed for structural and augmentation grafting in the nasal tip, as well as for dorsal deformities. However, the limited availability and unpredictable resorption of both autologous and homologous implants have made newer alloplastic implants important considerations for dorsal augmentation.

Selecting the most suitable graft or implant material for soft tissue augmentation is difficult. A wide variety of materials and techniques are employed by outstanding surgeons who have equally compelling arguments for the materials they use. No single material is suitable for all augmentation and nasal reconstruction situations. Each has its advantages and disadvantages (Table 32–1). The surgeon's own experience and personal preference play a large role in the success of the material used.

The indications for soft tissue augmentation in the nose are most commonly associated with depression over the cartilaginous or bony dorsum pyramid—the so-called saddle-nose deformity. This can occur to a variety of degrees and as the result of a variety of causes. This deformity can result from congenital abnormalities such as aplasia of the nasal bones. It can be secondary to trauma, which can produce septal hematoma and cartilaginous necrosis or disarticulation of the upper lateral cartilages and resulting in dorsal depression. It can also be the result of atrogenic causes, such as overresection of the quadrangular cartilage in septoplasty surgery. Studies have shown that 39% of patients undergoing extensive septal reconstructive surgery independent of rhinoplasty surgery exhibited some degree of external deformity with time. Cartilaginous saddle-nose deformity in the middle one-third of the nose is frequently the consequence of radical septal surgery.

In a review of 153 revision rhinoplasties, Stucker[1] noted that 58 patients presented with defects in the bony dorsum and

TABLE 32–1
Summary of Augmentation Materials and Uses

Material	Advantages	Disadvantages	Nose
Bone	Becomes living part Does not warp	Requires precise placement Second surgical site	+
Cartilage	Minimal resorption Minimal displacement Minimal extrusion	Limited quantity available Auricular cartilage may be difficult to contour Rib cartilage warps	++++
Dermis and fat	Minimal extrusion	Significant resorption	0
Zyderm	Injectable	Significant resorption	+
Purified acellular human dermal graft	Readily available Easily sculpted	Possible resorption Long-term effects unknown	++
Silastic	Easily sculpted Low tissue reactivity	Extrusion with superficial placement	+
Mersilene	Facilitates tissue ingrowth Well tolerated by tissues	Soft, potential tissue reactivity	+++
e-PTFE	Readily available Easily contoured Provides for some tissue ingrowth for stabilization	Potential extrusion	++++

91 presented with defects of the cartilaginous vault. Approximately 20% of the defects would be classified as saddle-nose deformities requiring some degree of augmentation. Thus, augmentation of the bony or cartilaginous dorsum is not an infrequent consequence of rhinoplasty surgery.

Types of Grafts

The ideal graft to correct dorsal depressions would exhibit the following qualities: (1) host tolerance, (2) remain unaltered over time, (3) easily carved or molded, (4) no transillumination or discoloration of supervening tissues, (5) pliable, and (6) easily obtainable.

Grafts can be classified as autologous grafts (derived from the host's own tissues), homologous grafts (derived from another individual of the same species), heterologous or xenografts (derived from a different species), and alloplastic or synthetic implants.

Biological materials are called grafts. These living or nonliving tissues are incorporated into the host tissues or are completely replaced by the host tissues. Synthetic or alloplastic materials are synthetic organopolymers that are generally well tolerated by the host's tissues. Synthetic materials are called implants. They retain their characteristic composition within the tissues. Although their structure may be invaded by host tissues, the implant structures are neither altered nor removed by the host.[2]

Autologous Grafts

Autologous grafts have been the preferred choice for implants for nasal augmentation and reconstruction for more than a century.[3] Many surgeons prefer to use the patient's own septal cartilage as the implant of choice for nasal reconstruction.[4,5] This cartilage is particularly useful for tip support and tip augmentation. However, there is often a problem with availability. Alternative sources of autologous cartilage are the auricle and the rib.

There are essentially two types of cartilage for grafting: morphologic and hyaline. Septal cartilage is an example of morphologic cartilage. It has the advantage of maintaining its shape when transplanted. Rib, or costal, cartilage is an example of hyaline cartilage. Hyaline cartilage has a system of interlocking stresses inherent in its molecular structure. There is a balance of internal elastic forces that resist deforming. The protein core and the glycosamine side chain are responsible for this property. Parallel lines of force run through the periphery of the cartilage and counteract the effects of the internal forces. Once the cartilage block is cut, the stress forces on that side of the cartilage are relieved, but they no longer counteract on the opposite side of the graft. This can result in warping of the implant and can be a disadvantage of its use. A technique can be used to minimize warping by shaving only scant amounts from the periphery of the graft, such that the outer restraining forces are not unfettered.

Unlike bone, little remodeling of cartilage takes place in a normal state. Chondrocytes are not replaced during adult life. The ability of cartilage to regenerate remains questionable.

Cartilage does enjoy some immunologic privilege. Cartilage cells possess antigens of the major H-antigen system. Cartilage grafts are antigenic and feebly immunologic because of the matrix proteoglycan that protects the chondrocyte from the afferent arm of the immune response, thereby preventing attack by immunoglobulins. Thus, there is no immune response or biocompatibility problem. Cartilage grafts, as compared with bone grafts, have been reported to have lower absorption rate and lower metabolic requirements for survival.[6] Resorption rates of septal cartilage grafts have been estimated as ranging from 12% to 50%.[7] However, resorbed cartilage is often replaced by host fibrous tissue, making resorption clinically undetectable.

AUTOLOGOUS SEPTAL CARTILAGE GRAFTS

Septal cartilage onlay grafts can be used to correct moderate saddle depressions. Sessions and Stallings[8] reported only 15% resorption after 1 year's experience with this technique. Gunter and Rohrich[9] described an excellent technique of using septal cartilage as a frame graft and inserting autologous cartilage remnants underneath the frame to provide increased dorsal augmentation.

AUTOLOGOUS AURICULAR CARTILAGE GRAFTS

Autologous auricular cartilage grafts can be used when autologous septal cartilage is not available. Auricular cartilage has the disadvantage of requiring the use of a second surgical site. However, incisions can be made in the conchal cavum area with harvesting of the conchal cartilage bowl, which facilitates surgical access and is virtually undetectable when healed. Auricular cartilage can be contoured for use as onlay grafts; its curvature makes it extremely useful for reconstruction of the nasal valve.

In contrast to alloplastic implants, auricular cartilage does not have to be buried deeply in soft tissue. Unlike bone, it does not have to be positioned in direct contact with bone or nasal cartilage. Whether it is advantageous to maintain perichondrium on the surface of the autologous auricular cartilage is debatable. However, it does add a degree of stiffness to the cartilage. As a cautionary note, beyond the age of 45 to 50 years, auricular cartilage becomes more brittle and is easily fractured.

AUTOLOGOUS COSTAL CARTILAGE GRAFTS

Autologous costal cartilage is often used for augmentation of large dorsal nasal defects and for columellar struts. A disadvantage is that it requires a second surgical site and is accompanied by a significant degree of morbidity. Gunter et al.[10] pointed out that the value of the rib as a donor site has been limited by difficulties with postoperative cartilage warping. Stabilizing the graft with longitudinal K-wire appears to eliminate warping and provides internal stabilization of the graft.

Excellent results can be obtained with the use of autogenous costal cartilage to reconstruct the nasal dorsum. Partial resorption is thought to be related to trauma. Smaller implants appear to be more vulnerable to absorption than larger implants. Pressure on the cartilage implant due to tight nasal skin or contracting scar did not seem to alter the behavior or increase the graft absorption rate.

AUTOLOGOUS BONE GRAFTS

The use of septal bone grafts has been reported (H. Smith, personal communication, New Haven, CT; 1993). Multiple small pieces of vomer and perpendicular plate were harvested and placed over the dorsum. Segments were 0.75 to 1.0 cm in length and approximately 2 mm in width. Smith reported on 25 cases with excellent results at 4 years follow-up, with no complications noted and no resorption detected.

Iliac crest grafts had frequently been used for nasal reconstruction when osseous material was required. However, this required a second surgical site that was often painful to patients. In addition, iliac bone grafts diminished in size over time and became more susceptible to fracture as the cancellous portion resorbed, leaving a partially collapsed cortex.

In recent years, split calvarium bone grafts have become popular. These grafts are a large source of material for grafting and have the further advantage of providing excellent structural support and a high level of tolerance.[11] Although it does require a second surgical site, in contrast to iliac bone grafts, the calvarium bone graft is harvested from the same operative field as the rhinoplasty. Hardesty and Marsh[11] demonstrated a difference in resorption between membranous bone such as frontoparietal calvarium and endochondral bone such as iliac crest. Powell and Riley[12] reported resorption rates for calvarium bone within a range of 20 to 30%.

Calvarium bone appears to be an excellent choice for subtotal and total nasal defects and a reasonable alternative when sufficient cartilage is not available. However, it is not without drawbacks. These include increased surgical time and complexity, donor site morbidity, difficulty in shaping the graft, graft warpage, and resorption.[13]

Homologous Cartilage Grafts

The human immunodeficiency virus (HIV) crisis has all but eliminated the use of cartilage banks, where a surgeon would chemically sterilize with methiolate, alcohol, or other chemicals resected septal cartilage for use in subsequent patients. Today, most homograft cartilage is irradiated costal cartilage. Cartilage is obtained from donors who meet the criteria required for organ donation. The specimens are tested for VDRL, hepatitis B, HIV, tuberculosis, and slow viruses. The cartilage is then placed in sterile saline and exposed to 30,000-60,000 Gy γ-waves to destroy cellular elements and pathogens, including viruses.[14] This approach has the advantage of ready availability and does not require an additional surgical harvesting site.

Resorption of homograft cartilage has long been cited as a major drawback to its use. Resorption often depends on the means of preservation of the cartilage. Studies have reported a 42% resorption of methiolate preserved cartilage, whereas irradiated cartilage has provided much greater survival rates.[15]

Schuller et al.[15] reported experience with irradiated homograft costal cartilage implants, 22 of which were nasal; 1.4% had partial resorption, and 0% showed warping. These findings were consistent with those reported by Lefkovits,[16] in which irradiated homograph costal cartilage was used in 27 patients; 83% had good to excellent results, 14% showed warping, and 0% demonstrated resorption.[17]

Resorption is related to granulation tissue surrounding the implant, which undergoes transformation into a fibrous capsule that halts further resorption. For this reason, it may be advantageous to avoid the use of systemic steroids in nasal surgery when homograft cartilage grafts are contemplated.

Advantages to the use of homograft cartilage are that no surgical site is required to harvest the grafts, and it does not preclude the use of autogenous cartilage grafts at a later date. The disadvantages of homograft cartilage are a potential immunologic response (i.e., it is not tolerated as well as host tissue), it must be contoured and shaped, and it is susceptible to warping and resorption.

Heterologous Cartilage Grafts (Xenographs)

Zyplast (Collagen Corporation, Palo Alto, CA) has been used as a temporary implant to camouflage contour abnormalities of the nasal dorsum during the convalescent period of rhinoplasty and to temporize before revision surgery. It also may be helpful to act as a spacer to prevent scar contracture of the nasal tissues before augmenting with a more permanent implant. The expense and transient longevity are negative points for its use. In addition, a skin test is necessary before injection to identify patients who might be sensitive to bovine collagen. Some surgeons recommend two skin tests separated by 30 days to identify additional patients who might demonstrate sensitivity.

Purified acellular human dermal graft (AlloDerm, Life Cell Corporation, Woodlands, TX) is an acellular graft produced from fresh human cadavers by a process that removes the epidermis and the cells from the dermis without altering the extracellular architectures. Although originally used as a dermal scaffolding for skin grafts in burn patients, it has been advocated as a dorsal onlay graft and for use as a draping graft in conjunction with other dorsal implants. The long-term resorption rate is unknown.[17,18]

Alloplastic Implants

Maas et al.[17] pointed out that the clinical efficacy of implant material over the long term is dependent on the stability of the material to chemical degradation such as by hydrolysis and other oxidation–reduction reactions, as well as physiologic cellular activity directed against the material. The porosity of the implant materials plays an important role in host tissue ingrowth and subsequent stability. In addition, such factors as thin skin overlying the implant, scarring of the tissue bed, and the architecture facilitating stabilization of the implant play crucial roles in determining the longevity of the clinical result.[17]

Porous implants have a greater risk of immediate infection, as there is increased surface area for adherence of bacteria. However, porous implants have fewer late-stage infections, as the incorporation of host tissue into the implant pores allows access to the site for immune response mediators.[19]

The great majority of alloplastic implants commonly used in nasal reconstruction are polymeric materials.

SILICONE IMPLANTS

Silicone implants have long been used to correct significant dorsal deformities. Tissue reaction to solid silicone implants is characterized by a moderate fibrous tissue capsule without tissue ingrowth.[20] When a silicone implant is placed in the nasal dorsum, it is subject to trauma and mobilization. Although these implants have been used in large numbers with excellent results, they are subject to moderate to intense ongoing inflammation, seroma formation, and extrusion. Extrusion rates for silicone implants have been reported as high as 10% for dorsal implants and 50% for columellar implants.[21,22]

MERSILENE IMPLANTS

Mersilene (Ethicon, Somerville, NJ) is a polyethyleneterethalate, which is a meshed polymer. It facilitates fibrous tissue ingrowth, making it more difficult to remove. This material can be used as a draping graft over the dorsum or the nasal tip area, or it can be rolled for utilization for dorsal augmentation. The following technical aspects should be considered when using rolled mesh. First, it has tapered ends. Second, the implanted alloplast must be placed away from the incision, to minimize exposure. Third, medial osteotomies can increase fibrosis and help position the rolled mesh. Finally, caution must be exercised in employing this technique in revision rhinoplasties, where there is less vascularity over the nasal dorsum, to prevent difficulties in wound healing and implant extrusion.

Gilmore[23] has recommended using alloplastic mesh as a "draping graft" to cover dorsal implant irregularities and for more uniform contouring.

E-PTFE

Expanded porous polyterrafluoroethylene (e-PTFE) is commonly used for nasal augmentation.[24,25] The 30-μm pore size allows for limited tissue ingrowth. Although the implant is soft, resulting in a natural feel, it provides excellent support over the dorsum and can be used for tip grafts and even in the columellar area. The implant is easily contoured and comes in a variety of thicknesses, making it very applicable to a variety of contouring problems.

I consider e-PTFE the implant of choice for reconstructing moderate to large dorsal defects. This implant has the advantage of being readily available. It also reduces operative time, as no second surgical site is needed to harvest a graft. The implant is easily contoured and very well tolerated by patients. When stacked autologous cartilage implants are used over the nasal dorsum, grafts can become dislodged, and irregularities result when sunglasses or reading glasses are worn. This problem is less likely with the solid alloplastic implant.

I have found that the implant can be easily placed through an internasal incision with the aid of chromic guide sutures affixed to a Keith needle to assist in properly positioning the implants. The implant is first soaked in antibiotic solution before being placed; prophylactic antibiotics are recommended. When such implants are used, it may be appropriate to consider prescribing prophylactic antibiotics for patients who undergo dental work, in order to minimize the possibility of bacteria seeding the implant.

Conclusion

The use of autogenous cartilage material, preferably from the nasal septum, continues to be the graft of choice for nasal reconstruction. However, technical advances in the development of alloplastic implants such as e-PTFE provide an enticing alternative when autogenous cartilage is limited.

Graft and implant materials are very controversial. Their discussion always engenders strong opinions from those who favor one material over another. Figure 32–1 summarizes the author's preferences for selection of implant material. A wide variety of materials can be used successfully in nasal reconstruction when sound surgical principles are employed in conjunction with good surgical technique.

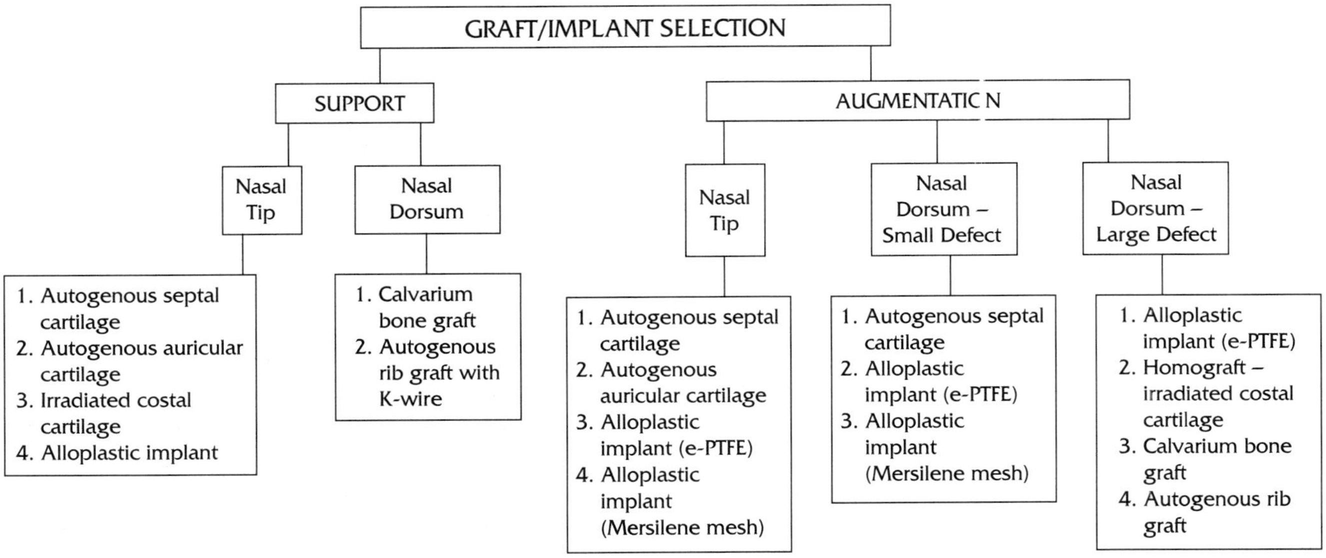

Figure 32–1 Algorithm for selection of implant material representing author's personal preference.

REFERENCES

Beeson—CHAPTER 32

1. Stucker FJ. Use of implantation in facial deformities. *Laryngoscope* 1977;87:1523–1527
2. Adams JS. Grafts and implants in nasal and chin augmentation. *Otolaryngol Clin North Am* 1987;20:913–930
3. Silver WE, Goldberg J. Nasal grafts and implants. *Facial Plast Surg Clin North Am* 1994;2:477–499
4. Tardy ME, Denneny J, Fritsch MH. The cartilage autograft in reconstruction of the nose and face. *Laryngoscope* 1985;95: 523–533
5. Brent B. The versatile cartilage autograft; current trends in clinical transplantation. *Clin Plast Surg* 1979;6:163–180
6. Gibson T, Davis WB. The distortion of autogenous cartilage grafts: its causes and prevention. *Br J Plast Surg* 1958; 10:257
7. Donald PJ. Cartilage grafting in facial reconstruction with special consideration of irradiated grafts. *Laryngoscope* 1986;96: 786–807
8. Sessions DG, Stallings JO. Correction of saddle nose deformity. *Laryngoscope* 1972;82:2000–2007
9. Gunter JP, Rohrich RJ. Augmentation rhinoplasty: dorsal onlay grafting using shaped autogenous septal cartilage. *Plast Reconstr Surg* 1990;86:39–45
10. Gunter JP, Clark CP, Friedman RM. Internal stabilization of autogenous rib cartilage grafts in rhinoplasty: a barrier to cartilage warping. *Plast Reconstr Surg* 1997;100;161–169
11. Hardesty RA, Marsh JL. Cranial facial on-lay bone grafting. *Plast Reconstr Surg* 1990;83:3
12. Powell NB, Riley RW. Facial contouring with outer table calvarium bone. *Arch Otolaryngol Head Neck Surg* 1980;115: 1454–1456
13. Peer LA. The fate of autogenous human bone grafts. *Br J Plast Surg* 1950;3:233–243
14. Brandon GE, Kern EB, Neel BN. Autografts of uncrushed and crushed bone and cartilage. *Arch Otolaryngol Head Neck Surg* 1979;105:75–80
15. Schuller DE, Bardach J, Krause CJ. Irradiated homologous costal cartilage for facial contour restoration. *Arch Otolaryngol Head Neck Surg* 1977;103:12–15
16. Lefkovits G. Irradiated homologous costal cartilage for augmentation rhinoplasty. *Ann Plast Surg* 1990;25:317–327
17. Maas CS, Monhian N, Shah SB. Implants in rhinoplasty. *Facial Plast Surg* 1997;13:279–290
18. Wainwright D, Madden M, Luterman A, et al. Clinical evaluation of an acellular allograft dermal matrix in full-thickness burns. *J Burn Care Rehabil* 1996;17:124–136
19. Maas CS, Monhian N, Shah SB. Implants in rhinoplasty. *Facial Plast Surg* 1998;13:279–290
20. Sclafani AP, Thomas JR, Cox AJ, et al. Clinical and histologic response of subcutaneous expanded polytetrafluoroethylene (Gore-Tex) in porous high-density polyethylene (Medpor) implants to acute and early infection. *Arch Otolaryngol Head Neck Surg* 1997;123:238–336
21. Silver FH, Maas CS. Biology of synthetic facial implant materials. *Facial Plast Surg Clin North Am* 1994;2:241–255
22. Davis PK, Jones SM. The complications of silicone implants. *Br J Plast Surg* 1971;24:405–411
23. Gilmore J. Use of Vicryl mesh in prevention of postrhinoplasty dorsal irregularities. *Ann Plast Surg* 1989;22:105–107.
24. Maas CS, Gnapp DR, Bumpous J. Expanded polytetrafluoroethylene [Gore-Tex] soft tissue patch (in facial augmentation). *Arch Otolaryngol Head Neck Surg* 1993;119:1006–1014
25. Godin MS, Waldman SR, Johnson CM. The use of expanded polytetrafluoroethylene [Gore-Tex] in rhinoplasty. *Arch Otolaryngol Head Neck Surg* 1993;121:1131–1136

Alloplastic or Homograft Implantation for Nasal Reconstruction

CHAPTER 33

Douglas G. Mann

As a conservative surgeon, I believe in creating natural-appearing, well-supported, well-balanced noses. As a result, I not infrequently find the need to add something to create projection, balance, or support. Like everyone else, I try to use autologous septal cartilage wherever possible. There have been times, however, when there just wasn't enough septum to do the job. So I have turned, on occasion, to the use of implants. When academics present at meetings, or write about the successful experience they've had with a new implant material, I am likely to give it a try if it seems to be safe, and sensible, and if their numbers are good. Upon reviewing my own experience, I am glad I took their advice less than half the time, so for me this is a time to reassess this question, and I invite the reader to do the same.

My current thesis is that we should scrupulously avoid placing implants in the nose. My rationale follows.

Definitions

Grafts are biologic materials, either living or nonliving. They may be derived from the host's own tissues (*autologous*), derived from another individual of the same species (*homologous*), or derived from a different species (*heterologous*).

Implants are synthetic materials that have been approved for implantation into the nose, and which maintain their characteristic composition within the tissues.

Notwithstanding the fact that every article ever written about nasal reconstruction indicates that autologous grafts are superior, all the available alternatives, as well as those used not so long ago, which are no longer available, are outlined in Table 33–1.

Literature Experience

GRAFTS

In the most recent comprehensive treatment of the subject of grafts and implants in rhinoplasty, Maas et al.[1] state that "autograft cartilage is the most commonly used material in rhinoplasty and remains the standard against which all others are compared." There is no disagreement with this statement among experts. When used to augment or support the nose, autogenous cartilage has proved to provide long-lasting clinical correction and to be very resistant to infection or extrusion.[2] Tardy[3] reports more than 6000 cartilage autografts implanted over 25 years, with no incidence of rejection or infection: "infrequent complications ... have stemmed from technical errors that diminish with experience .... No significant complications have occurred from the inherent unique properties of the cartilage autograft itself." The issue of the technical errors is

TABLE 33–1
Materials for Nasal Reconstruction

Grafts (autologous unless specified otherwise)
Cartilage
Septal
Other nasal
Ear
Rib
Autologous
Homologous
Heterologous
Bone
Calvarium
Rib
Iliac crest
Dermis
Autologous
Homologous, acellular
Fat
Fascia periosteum
Collagen
Implants
Silastic
Silicone
Mersilene
Supramid
Gore-Tex
Proplast

an important one. Sheen and Tardy spend considerable space discussing technical considerations to ensure adequate blood supply, and avoidance of malposition and visibility, the two most common problems with autografts. I shall return to this issue later.

IMPLANTS

The medical literature is replete with articles advancing the use of one or another kind of new implant material. As time goes on, new implants continue to be advanced, which would suggest that no one has been entirely happy with the materials that were previously advanced. Unfortunately, the failures are not published with the same timeliness as are the initial successes.

Typically, articles that tout the use of one or another implant report complication rates of less than 5%.[4-6] Reports of complications often come from other investigators, citing their own experience with implants inserted by other surgeons. I especially like the wording of a Chinese article that analyzes 349 complications (how much is enough?) of dorsal augmentation using ersatz materials.[7] Tardy says it very well: "The continuing opportunity to care for referred patients suffering from the unpleasant results of nasal implant rejection influences significantly a philosophy of conservatism and patient safety above all else."

Things change pretty quickly on the nasal implant scene. A comparison of two excellent review articles published only 10 years apart points this up very well. A well researched review article in 1987 by Adams[8] can be compared with similarly scholarly reviews by Kridel and Kraus[9] and Maas et al.[1] in 1995 and 1997, respectively. Table 33–2 divides the critiques of these materials into two categories: Then and Now.

Although little, if any, harm has been done by properly performed liquid silicone injections, much legal hay has been made of this substance. Is there an alloplast that is immune from suddenly being declared illegal at some point in time, putting both the manufacturer and the practitioner at great risk?

What about the fact that we continue to use Silastic implants in the nose, even though it is well documented that "in nasal augmentation its use is limited. Thin soft tissue coverage, constant movement of the nose, and frequent midface trauma lead to an unacceptably large incidence of dislodgment and extrusion."[8]

My Personal Experience

I do not perform vast numbers of rhinoplasties. It is for this reason that I believe my experience is potentially most valuable to the majority of practitioners who have similar caseloads.

MERSILENE MESH

I have used Mersilene mesh three times in my career:

Patient 1: Placed through a transfixion incision to augment the premaxillary area, the implant became infected within 1 month of surgery and drained whenever the patient was not on antibiotics. The implant was ultimately removed without difficulty.

Patient 2: Rolled to quickly augment a dorsum that I accidentally overreduced using an osteotome, this implant remained in place but eventually swelled a little, giving the patient the notion that she had wasted her money on a rhinoplasty. The implant was removed with minimal difficulty, and the nose reshaped with satisfactory outcome.

TABLE 33–2
Nasal Implants: Then and Now

Implant Material	Then[a]	Now[b,c]
Supramid	"For more than 35 years ... proved ... to be a stable, reliable, implant material."	"Clinical trials have shown resorption and loss of material substance ... [and] have made this mostly of historical interest with respect to rhinoplasty."
Mersilene	Was not yet on the radar screen	"Removal of infected implants very difficult ... nearly impossible ... and reported infection rates between 4 and 9%."
Proplast	"Has found it very useful for augmentation of the nasal dorsum and nasal tip support."	"Because of this disastrous outcome (in the jaw) ... Proplast is no longer approved by the FDA for any implantation uses."
Silicone fluid	"A very safe product that gives excellent results.... Highly versatile."	Not even mentioned by either author (probably on advice of their attorneys).

[a] Adams JS. Grafts and implants in nasal and chin augmentation—a rational approach to material selection. *Otol Clin North Am* 1987;20:913–930.
[b] Maas CS, Monhian N, Shah SB. Implants in rhinoplasty. *Facial Plast Surg* 1997;13:279–290.
[c] Kridel RWH, Kraus WM. Grafts and implants in revision rhinoplasty. *Facial Plast Surg Clin North Am* 1995;3:473–486.

Patient 3: Placed to correct a slight mid–third unilateral depression, this implant began to exude a foul odor noticed by the patient. Athough clinically there was no infection, one could see the graft fibers protruding through the intercartilaginous incision site. At the first revision, I reopened the incision and removed any graft within 3 mm of the incision. The problem recurred after many months, and I had to return to remove the remainder. The excisions were technically difficult in both instances. The final result was acceptable.

SILASTIC

I knew that Silastic could be problematic in the tip and the dorsum, but I allowed myself to be convinced that it might be acceptable in the premaxilla. Two such implants were placed. Both lasted about 5 years:

Patient 1: Placed in a secondary rhinoplasty to project a nasal tip complex, the implant accomplished this task beautifully. Over the course of years, however, beginning months after insertion, foul drainage would occur from a small portion of the incision. Antibiotics worked for a time, but infection would always recur. Because the patient loved the appearance, the implant was removed long after I would have wanted to remove it otherwise. The tip remained in good position, and no further surgery was needed.

Patient 2: This patient had not undergone surgery but did have a drug-induced septal perforation, and resultant loss of premaxillary support. Placement was similar to that used in patient 1. This patient did well until 5 years later, when she presented with asymptomatic exposure from the region of the hemitransfixion incision. The implant was removed; no further surgery was needed.

GORE-TEX

Gore-Tex is currently in fashion in our literature. Eight implants have been placed. Three have required removal, with the following results:

Patient 1: A 2-mm piece of reinforced Gore-Tex was placed into the nose of a man who had injured his nose in Vietnam. He had undergone a rhinoplasty for an acute condition, leaving him with an overreduced dorsum and valve collapse. The implant was placed through endonasal incisions. He did well, with his airway as well as his appearance improved for 1 year. At that time he began to experience episodes of nasal swelling. The implant could be seen protruding from the intercartilaginous region on the left side. The area was explored and the graft was shortened. He was placed on oral, intravenous antibiotics consistent with cultures obtained at the time. After several months without symptoms, the nasal swelling and erythema recurred. The implant was removed. So far, he has not needed any further surgery.

Patient 2: Rolled Gore-Tex was used to augment the premaxilla in a primary rhinoplasty. After an initial good result, the material spontaneously became infected, resulting in foul drainage from the transfixion incision. The implant was removed after two temporarily successful courses of antibiotics. The nose has maintained its position.

Patient 3: Reinforced Gore-Tex was used as a spreader in a 55-year-old man who had had previous septoplasty, who had internal valve collapse and needed support in conjunction with his cosmetic/functional rhinoplasty. The grafts functioned nicely for about 12 months, after which a foul odor alerted us to the extrusion of one of the grafts through the septal mucosa. He had a great deal of nasal dorsal and columellar swelling with these infections, and this was his greatest concern. Ultimately, despite antibiotics and graft trimming, the implants required removal. The swelling has resolved, and he has been satisfied with the result.

Although no serious sequelae have resulted from my implant experiences, the trouble resulting does not seem to be worth the time saved or donor site morbidity saved. What about recipient site morbidity?

Why We Want to Use Implants—Even Though They Aren't Good for Us

There are times when, after getting all one can get out of the septum, one just doesn't have enough material to build the nose one is looking for. One may not want to open the ear and try to fuss with crooked cartilage. One wants to be able to open a box and pull something out that one can easily shape into what one needs, that won't take a lot of additional time, that will give the nose the volume or the support needed, and that will complete the procedure before the vasoconstrictor wears off, and the bleeding starts.

There is nothing wrong with that logic, as it stands, but it is short sighted. It will get you out of the operating room with a happy patient, but you could very well return some day with one who is not as happy. What we need, I believe, is an alternative set of possibilities, things that we can turn to when we might otherwise be opening a box of something.

Clinical Situations Calling for Implants

The following five cases present specific situations in which grafts may be needed.

Case 1: A revision rhinoplasty has been performed in a patient who has had a dorsal overreduction, but nothing is left in the septum.

Case 2: A primary rhinoplasty does not have enough good pieces of septum to make the big dorsal graft you wanted or to make the tip grafts.

Case 3: You'd like to augment the premaxilla.
Case 4: You need structure and lengthening, but there is not enough septum.
Case 5: You need to make a slight contour correction after a rhinoplasty has been performed.

Graft Alternative Strategies

Several alternative strategies for the use of graft material can be considered. The following suggestions are recommended for specific cases, such as the five described above.

1. *Plan to take some other tissue:* Let the patient know that you will need an alternative and plan to take what you think you will need.
   Applies in cases 1, 3, and 4.
2. *Stretch two pieces of septum into one:* Godfrey[10] presents a technique for splicing two lengths of septal cartilage together.
   Could work for cases 2 or 4.
3. *Try a pericranial graft:* Ioannides and Fossion[11] report this technique in which a hidden incision can provide large quantities of easily stackable firm tissue.
   For all cases in which mesh would have worked, such as 1, 2, and 3.
4. *Use an autogenous rib:* An excellent report by Sherris and Kern[12] details the harvesting techniques as well as some of the uses for rib for dorsal grafts, columellar struts, and tip grafts. The extra incision should be no problem if your patient is prepared for it.
   Excellent choice for cases 1, 3, and 4. Overkill, perhaps, for cases 2 and 5.
5. *Try alloderm:* Is it a graft or an implant? Yes, it comes in a box, but it *is* a biologic material and is incorporated into the host tissue. Although "the jury is still out" on this, I believe it could be useful for premaxillary augmentation, dorsal augmentation, lateral wall fill, and possibly tip grafting as well. It is not a structural graft.
   Applies to cases 1, 2, 3, and 5.
6. *Use autologous fat:* Coleman[13] and others have refined the techniques of autologous fat transplantation to the point where long-term corrections of volume deficiency can be reliably corrected. Fat is harvested by syringe and small cannulae, handled minimally, and injected through small needles or cannulae.
   A wonderful technique for case 5, possibly an alternative to revision rhinoplasty in case 1.
7. *Possibly try auricular cartilage:* This material has not been mentioned until now. Because you have already thought of it, I include it for the sake of completeness and because we should be reconsidering it. Endo et al.[14] report 1200 cases of augmentation rhinoplasty in Japanese and detail their methods for getting rid of that troublesome cartilage spring. Tardy[3] and Sheen[2] go into great detail on their handling of auricular cartilage so that it can provide either structure or contour replacement.
   Very useful for cases 1, 2, and 5. May work to provide length (case 4) for Sheen, but this is perhaps a stretch for the ordinary surgeon.

Conclusion

We have tried to make the case that grafts are highly superior to implants in the nose, and that the use of implants should be assiduously avoided. We have tried to understand the thinking that goes into selection of an implant and interrupt that thought process with some alternative grafting suggestions.

REFERENCES

Mann—CHAPTER 33

1. Maas CS, Monhian N, Shah SB. Implants in rhinoplasty. *Facial Plast Surg* 1997;13:279–290
2. Sheen JH, Sheen AP. *Aesthetic Rhinoplasty.* 2nd Ed. St. Loius, MO: CV Mosby; 1987
3. Tardy ME Jr. *Rhinoplasty—The Art and the Science.* Philadelphia: WB Saunders; 1997
4. Conrad K, Gillman G. A 6 year experience with the use of expanded polytetrafluoroethylene in rhinoplasty. *Plast Reconstr Surg* 1998;101:1675–1683
5. Romo T III, Sclafani AP, Sabini P. Use of porous high density polyethylene in revision rhinoplasty and in the platyrrhine nose. *Aesthetic Plast Surg* 1998;22:211–221
6. Juraha LZ. Experience with alternative material for nasal augmentation. *Aesthetic Plast Surg* 1992:16:133–140
7. Wu ZQ. Complications of hump nose after transplantation of tissue ersatz materials. *Chin J Surg* 1992;30:50–64
8. Adams JS. Grafts and implants in nasal and chin augmentation—a rational approach to material selection. *Otol Clin North Am* 1987;20:913–930
9. Kridel RWH, Kraus WM. Grafts and implants in revision rhinoplasty. *Facial Plast Surg Clin North Am* 1995;3:473–486
10. Godfrey NV. Augmentation rhinoplasty with mortised septal cartilage. *Aesthetic Plast Surg* 1993;17:31–35
11. Ioannides C, Fossion E. The role of free pericranium grafts in augmentation rhinoplasty. *J Craniomaxillofac Surg* 1995;23: 105–108
12. Sherris DA, Kern EB. The versatile autogenous rib graft in septorhinoplasty. *Am J Rhinol* 1998;12:221–227
13. Coleman S. Facial recontouring with lipostructure. *Clin Plast Surg* 1997;24:347–367
14. Endo T, Nakamaya Y, Yuukuo I. Augmentation rhinoplasty: observations in 1200 cases. *Plast Reconstr Surg* 1991;87:54–59

12

Management of the Draining Pressure Equalization Tube

"Probably less than 5% of all patients with chronic draining PE tubes, have underlying localized mucosal or temporal bone disease, or upper respiratory immunologic, allergic, or bacterial disease that perpetuates tube drainage."

Gordon B. Hughes

"Dry or serous effusions are rarely associated with PTOs, whereas mucoid or mucopurulent effusions and/or middle ear mucosal disease is statistically correlated with PTO. An enormous literature has been dedicated to surgical PTO prophylaxis. Although contradictory, consensus appears to refute the efficacy of drop therapy or canal preparation."

C. Gary Jackson

"At tympanostomy tube placement, we like to obtain mesotympanic fluid for bacteriologic assessment (Gram stain, and culture and sensitivity). Not only are the data a preemptive guide to the antimicrobial treatment of postoperative otorrhea, but also a measure of clinically significant respiratory bacteria in the community."

N. Wendell Todd

Management of the Draining Pressure Equalization Tube

CHAPTER 34

Gordon B. Hughes

Pressure equalization (PE) tube placement is one of the most commonly performed surgical procedures, and purulent drainage through the tube is the most common complication of tube insertion. Fortunately, drainage usually quickly resolves with initial treatment. Occasionally, drainage persists and requires more aggressive therapy, including tube removal or chronic ear surgery (tympanomastoidectomy). Because management of acute and chronic drainage is distinctly different, discussion is divided into these two categories. In this chapter, acute drainage refers to new drainage, rather than a specific duration. Chronic drainage refers to persistent drainage after initial treatment has failed.

Acute Drainage

Frequently, the cause of acute drainage is either a recent viral upper respiratory infection (URI) or water contamination into the ear canal. Of these two, viral URI is far more common because a small amount of water in the canal is rarely harmful. Note that most URIs are viral whereas most middle ear drainage is bacterial. It is well known that acute bacterial otitis media most often results from a viral URI, usually within 2 weeks of onset. Inflammation and swelling of the eustachian tube and middle ear mucosa impair the protective mucociliary clearance and aeration of the middle ear, encouraging bacterial infection. In the same way, viral URI can initiate bacterial purulent discharge through a PE tube. The point is that drainage through a PE tube is presumed bacterial, even though it often results from a viral URI. The bacteria are similar to those of acute otitis media: *Streptococcus pneumoniae*, *Hemophilus influenzae*, and *Moraxella catarrhalis*. Treatment consists of broad-spectrum oral antibiotics such as amoxicillin (Amoxil) 40 mg/kg/day, amoxicillin-clavulanate (Augmentin) 40 mg/kg/day, cefpodoxime (Vantin) 10 mg/kg/day, or clarithromycin (Biaxin) 15 mg/kg/day for 10 days. The patient is instructed to keep water out of the ear (dry ear precautions).

Although water contamination of the middle ear through the canal and tube is usually harmless, it occasionally causes inflammation and bacterial discharge. If the history suggests water contamination, topical antibiotics alone often are sufficient to treat infection. Polymyxin–neomycin–hydrocortisone (Cortisporin, Colymycin) or a similar suspension is given in 3 drops tid, left in the ear each time for 5 min. A 5-day course of treatment is usually sufficient.

When the history suggests neither water contamination nor viral URI, often both a topical and an oral antibiotic are given for 10 days. A routine culture of the drainage at this point is not needed because infection usually clears quickly with this simple combined treatment.

Chronic Drainage

After topical or oral antibiotics, or both, have been given for initial treatment, the patient is reexamined at 10 days. If drainage is greatly improved but not yet resolved, the same antibiotics can be continued for another 10 days. However, if drainage is no better, several causative factors must be considered.

First, chronic drainage can persist because the bacteria are resistant to the antibiotic. Frequently this implies that the infection is caused by *Pseudomonas aeruginosa*, which is resistant to all oral antibiotics except ciprofloxacin. Moreover, even though most topical antibiotics will cover *Pseudomonas*, sometimes drainage is so profuse that the drop cannot penetrate the tube to the middle ear. If the ear is still draining without improvement after initial antibiotic treatment, the drainage should be cultured to determine whether *Pseudomonas* infection is present. Preliminary results often are known in 36 h.

After the culture is obtained, the ear canal is cleaned and the tube suctioned. Often pulsating pus quickly exudes again through the tube to fill the ear canal. One helpful additional treatment is to irrigate the canal with 2% acetic acid before instilling the drops. The mechanical flush of the canal gets rid of most of the drainage and debris long enough for the antibiotic drop to reach the tube and middle ear. A simple inexpensive wash can be prepared by mixing equal parts of white vinegar and tap water, boiling the solution for 5 min for sterilization, and preserving it at room temperature. A small bulb syringe is used to flush the solution into the canal with the ear turned downward. The ear is then dried off and turned upward, and the drops are instilled for 5 min. These steps are repeated three times daily. The patient is reminded about dry ear precautions.

Another change of treatment for *Pseudomonas* is oral ciprofloxacin hydrochloride (Cipro). Ciprofloxacin is routinely used in adults, but its use is more controversial in children. Initial publications suggested that bone growth in children might be impaired by ciprofloxacin. However, these data were based largely on animal research, and many clinicians now believe that ciprofloxacin can be given safely to children without impairing bone growth.[1] The dose of ciprofloxacin is 250 to 500 mg bid, depending on body weight.

After the canal is carefully cleaned down to the tube, the relationship among the tube, eardrum, and middle ear mucosa is determined. An operating microscope is very helpful for this, and the child should be restrained as needed to get a clear view of the tube. If granulation tissue surrounds the tube, if myringitis is present, or if the tube lumen is completely obstructed with mucosal disease, removing the tube right away is the most helpful step. Any foreign-body irritation is removed, and topical drops then penetrate better into the middle ear through the residual myringotomy/perforation. The very same topical and oral antibiotics that failed to help in the initial treatment with the tube in place, often quickly clear the infection now with the tube out. Thus, ciprofloxacin can be avoided in children. Removing the tube requires no anesthesia in the youngest children, general anesthesia in older children, and local anesthesia in adults.

Sometimes the tube appears in good position, no granulation surrounds the flange, and no mucosal disease obstructs the lumen. In this case the culture report determines the treatment. If the causative organism is *Pseudomonas* and the patient is an adult, oral ciprofloxacin 500 mg bid is added to topical drops. If the organism is *Pseudomonas* and the patient is a child, the fastest, safest treatment still is tube removal, even though the tube appears normal. The patient then is scheduled to return for follow-up examination in another 10 days. If the tube has been removed, the eardrum usually is healed and the active infection is resolved. Residual effusion may be present in the middle ear. The patient is seen again in several weeks depending on hearing in the opposite ear. If middle ear effusion becomes chronic, a new tube is reinserted.

Probably 80% of acutely draining PE tubes clear with initial treatment, and another 80% of chronically draining tubes clear with anti-*Pseudomonas* treatment with or without tube removal. The remaining few patients, probably less than 5% of all patients with chronic draining PE tubes, have underlying localized mucosal or temporal bone disease, or upper respiratory immunologic, allergic, or bacterial disease that perpetuates tube drainage. A careful history and examination at the first office visit usually identifies these patients. Does the patient have "allergy" or "sinus" disease, especially inhalant allergy with rhinitis and sinusitis? Does the patient have frequent bronchitis or pneumonia, perhaps associated with sinusitis and recurrent otitis? Consider immunoglobulin G (IgG) subclass deficiency, immotile cilia syndrome, iatrogenic immunosuppression, human immunodeficiency virus (HIV) infection, tuberculosis, and Wegener's granulomatosis. Does chronic ear pain suggest neoplasm, particularly squamous cell carcinoma? Has the patient received radiation therapy within recent months? Is there evidence of osteoradionecrosis? If any of these underlying disorders is suspected, appropriate consultation and studies are indicated, including consultation for allergy, immunodeficiency, and recurrent respiratory disease; computed tomography (CT) for sinusitis, neoplasm, or osteoradionecrosis; magnetic resonance imaging (MRI) as indicated clinically; and tissue culture for tuberculosis and histology for malignancy and Wegener's granulomatosis.

If the initial history and examination do not suggest any of these problems, and appropriate antibiotics have been given based on the culture and sensitivity report, yet drainage persists despite removal of the PE tube, the middle ear mucosa is assumed to be irreversibly diseased. Treatment consists of intravenous antibiotics or chronic ear surgery, or both. Hospitalization and intravenous antibiotics are appropriate for patients, particularly children, who have chronic middle ear mucosal disease, and who have persistent fever, pain, or other symptoms suggesting possible complication of infection. The child is admitted for several days of intravenous antibiotic(s) based on culture, with consultation with a pediatric infectious disease specialist. If there is prompt clinical improvement within several days, surgery is postponed indefinitely and home intravenous antibiotic therapy (HIVAT) is continued as an outpatient. If there is no clinical improvement, tympanomastoidectomy is performed, middle ear tissue is sent for histology and culture, and antibiotics are continued as an outpatient after recovery from surgery.

Management of the draining PE tube is usually straightforward; antibiotics, dry ear precautions, and occasional tube removal will cure almost all patients. Persistent chronic drainage, however, requires evaluation for underlying disease, intravenous antibiotics, and/or surgery. Table 34–1 provides a summary of management.

TABLE 34–1
Management of Acute and Chronic Draining PE Tubes

- Acute drainage
  - Etiology
    - Upper respiratory infection/inflammation
    - Water/other contamination of ear canal
  - Treatment
    - Canal cleaning and examination of PE tube
    - Topical/oral antibiotics
    - Dry ear precautions
- Chronic drainage (persists after initial treatment)
  - Etiology
    - Resistant bacterial infection
    - Different causative organism (fungus, tuberculosis)
    - PE tube foreign body reaction/myringitis
    - Underlying upper respiratory/temporal bone disease
      - Sinusitis
      - Osteoradionecrosis
      - Neoplasm
    - Underlying systemic disease
      - IgG subclass deficiency/immunosuppression
      - Inhalant allergy
    - Irreversibly diseased mucosa (serous mastoiditis)
  - Treatment
    - Dry ear precautions
    - Different antibiotic based on culture and sensitivity
    - Different antimicrobial therapy to cover fungus, tuberculosis
    - Sinus/temporal bone CT
    - Allergy/immunology workup as indicated clinically
    - Tube removal and topical/oral antibiotics
    - Intravenous antibiotics
    - Chronic ear surgery

REFERENCES

1. Sabella C, Goldfarb J. Editorial. Fluoroquinolone therapy in pediatrics: where we stand. *Clin Pediatr* 1997;36(8):445–448

Management of the Draining Pressure Equalization Tube

CHAPTER 35

C. Gary Jackson

First conceived by Politzer and Cassells[1] in 1868, ventilating tubes were not popular until the 1950s, when Armstrong[2] introduced them in 1954. The tympanostomy tube has since become one of the most commonly employed yet contentious devices in modern medicine. In children, otitis media is the most frequent reason for nonwell visits to a physician. Often it is recurrent and medically refractory. Vent tube placement has become an important weapon in the otolaryngologist's war on this problem. In fact, myringotomy with vent tube placement has become the most common operation in children requiring general anesthesia in the United States. Enthusiasm for the procedure has been moderated, however, in both otolaryngologists and pediatricians by complications, the most common of which is post-tympanostomy otorrhea (PTO).

Although vent tube placement is a safe and effective treatment strategy that has significantly reduced the incidence of chronic mastoiditis and acquired cholesteatoma, PTO occurs within a range of 3.1 to 37.9%. Luxford and Sheehy's[3] reported incidence of 21% is typical. This literature is well summarized by Goldstein et al.[4] Higher rates of PTO have been associated with large-bore vent tubes (41% and 69% in two studies[5,6]). PTO is not thought to be more common in patients who have undergone prior myringotomy with intubation.[7] In children with cleft palates, reflux of nasopharyngeal secretions into the middle ear has been associated with higher rates of PTO (67%).[8,9] Patients undergoing concomitant adenoidectomy do not represent higher PTO risks.[10]

PTO can occur early, at 2 weeks after surgery, or at some time later. The etiology of both scenarios is different.[11] Early PTO is thought to be a function of the underlying disease or to represent surgical contamination. Early PTO is clearly related to the conditions in the middle ear cleft at surgery.[12] Dry or serous effusions are rarely associated with PTOs, whereas mucoid or mucopurulent effusions and/or middle ear mucosal disease is statistically correlated with PTO. An enormous literature has been dedicated to surgical PTO prophylaxis. Although contradictory, consensus appears to refute the efficacy of drop therapy or canal preparation. Younger children appear to be more susceptible than older children.[7,10] Late PTO is more frequently associated with extrinsic contamination of the middle ear and otitis media associated with upper respiratory infection or allergic disorders.[11] Late PTO occurs more commonly during the summer months with water contamination.[13] Intubation abolishes the air cushion of the middle ear. In young children, this may make bacterial reflux from the nasopharynx and eustachian tube more problematic.[14] Adenoidectomy does not appear to influence late PTO.

PTO bacteriology has been reviewed by Schneider.[15] In young children under age 3 years, isolates were similar to those found in acute otitis media, except that *Hemophilus influenzae* is more common than *D. pneumoniae.* The presence or absence of concurrent upper respiratory infection is significant in choosing a treatment strategy. In children older than age 3 years and in whom infectious causes are more common, *Pseudomonas* sp. is a common isolate (in 25%). Gram-positive species (*Staphylococcus*) are even more common (in 45%), many of which are penicillin resistant, even in nonhospital communities (80%). PTO management in this population is somewhat more problematic.

Most cases of PTO arise from extensive contamination of the middle ear through the open tube. The risk of otorrhea after tympanostomy tube placement is three times higher than after myringotomy alone.

Treatment Strategies

My strategy for managing PTO is based on a condition driven escalation of therapeutic invasion. I try to reserve complicated solutions for complicated problems. In most cases, PTO can be successfully managed by topical or systemic antibiotics, or both. In children younger than age 3 years, bacteriology is similar to that of acute otitis media (AOM). For minor cases, the application of steroid-containing antibiotic drops (SCAD), 3 drops in the affected ear on a t.i.d. schedule is effective. As a general rule, my endpoint is 7 days or at any time the child reacts to drop application as if it were painful. Even with the milder ophthalmic preparations, the pH can elicit pain when it comes in contact with normal mucosa. Meyerhoff's 1983 study[16] in chinchillas clearly demonstrated drop ototoxicity when applied through tubes in ears with normal eustachian tubal function and middle ear mucosa. Infected mucosa offers a barrier to this ototoxicity, the absence of which is heralded by the pain elicited in ears with "healed" mucosa. If the PTO is the only site of infection, drop therapy should suffice. However, in this toddler population, upper respiratory infection is often concomitant. In such cases I add an appropriate oral antibiotic or enlist the help of the child's pediatrician to do so.

For the older child, extensive sources of contamination are more common and the bacteriology more complicated. *Pseudomonas* species are more common. In such cases, oral preparations are not realistic, except for ciprofloxacin, which is contraindicated in this population. For these cases, I rely on SCAD therapy.

This protocol is effective in most cases. When PTO is persistent, antennae should go up and treatment be advanced. First, what is "persistent"? If PTO continues beyond 2 to 3 weeks or recurs within a week or so after cessation of treatment, rarer disorders or immunologic compromise should be considered. This is one of the few times I will culture a draining ear and consider the results in specific therapy. Rare disorders, such as diabetes, cystic fibrosis, tuberculosis, the histiocytoses, or immunodeficiency syndromes, should be addressed. I do so by means of pediatric consultation.

Based on the cultures and the pediatric evaluation, I then begin to treat these children with intravenous antibiotics supervised by a pediatric infectious disease colleague. Hospital admission for at least 24 h to 72 h for culture specific intravenous therapy is usually necessary, the course completed by administration of home health care. The PTO usually resolves promptly within 5 days. The duration of treatment is generally 10 days to 2 weeks. If the PTO is not clinically under control in 5 days or so, I consider the tube a foreign body corrupting control of infection and remove it. Replacement is determined by the subsequent clinical course.

Failing this strategy or, again, if PTO recurs in the absence of external contamination after seemingly successful conservative therapy, the situation is adjudicated to be medically refractory. The implication is that infected tissue is retained, mastoiditis has been established, or purulent material has been sequestered, not eliminated; that is, a surgical disease exists. A tympanoplasty with mastoidectomy is executed. Granulation tissue is extensively derided, diseased mucosa evacuated, and a very complete mastoidectomy performed, employing a canal wall-up strategy.

I generally do not drain the mastoid bowl postoperatively unless acute mastoiditis is the problem. This is rare. Because of the infrequency with which this protocol is prescribed and the condition encountered, a final search for the unexpected should prompt preoperative imaging. High-resolution temporal bone computed tomography (CT) both with and without contrast is warranted. The chaos of the prolonged infection precludes even competent otomicroscopic assessment of ears in customers small enough to defy compliance. Even examinations under anesthesia are confounded by the overwhelming picture of infection. Congenital cholesteatoma, masked intratemporal or intracramal complication, temporal bone abnormality, aberrant carotid artery, or even infratemporal fossa disease affecting eustachian tube should declare themselves on imaging. Don't forget the nasopharynx!

With this strategy of treatment outlined, perhaps a word on prevention as a management structure is in order. What instructions do I give my patients with tubes, as well as their parents, to prevent post-tympanostomy complications? I am convinced that medicine has created a society of cripples by restriction. I practice a medicine of involvement, with only notable cautions:

- Office visits every 6 months while tubes are in place
- Swimming and bathing with water exclusion
  - For bathing, Vaseline and cotton or custom plugs/molds
  - For swimming, custom molds, again Vaseline under a snug-fitting swim cap or other commercial device
  - Taking care with soapy water and, in my region, lakes, rivers, creeks, or ponds.
  - Swimming in moderation
- Aggressive treatment of allergy and upper respiratory episodes

Conclusion

PTO is a common complication of the most common operation performed in the United States today. Treatment strategy should be prophylactic but, once PTO occurs, aggressive protocols only proceed once conservative efforts fail. Etiology and bacteriology of patients younger than 3 years of age are different than patients older than age 3. These features should be recognized in therapy for PTO in these groups.

REFERENCES

Jackson—CHAPTER 35

1. Politzer A, Cassells JP. *Diseases of the Ear*. Philadelphia: Henry C. Lea's Son; 1883:375–377
2. Armstrong BW. A new treatment for chronic secretory otitis media. *Arch Otolaryngol* 1954;69:653
3. Luxford WM, Sheehy JL. Myringotomy and ventilation tubes: a report of 1568 ears. *Laryngoscope* 1982;92: 1293–1297
4. Goldstein NA, Roland JT Jr, Sculerati N. Complications of tympanostomy tubes in an inner city population. *Int J Pediatr Otolaryngol* 1996;34:87–89
5. Holt JJ, Harner SG. Effects of large bore middle ear ventilation tubes. *Otolaryngol Head Neck Surg* 1980;88:581–585
6. Per-Lee JH. Long-term middle ear ventilation. *Laryngoscope* 1981;91:1063–1072
7. Balkany TJ, Barkin RM, Suzuki BH, Watson WJ. A prospective study of infection following tympanostomy and tube insertion. *Am J Otol* 1983;4:288–291
8. Bluestone CD, Klein JO. Otitis media with effusion, atelectasis, and eustachian tube dysfunction. In: Bluestone CD, Stool SE, Arjona SK, eds. *Pediatric Otolaryngology*. Vol. I. Philadelphia: WB Saunders; 1983:399–400
9. Paradise J, Bluestone CD. Early treatment of the universal otitis media of infants with cleft palate. *Pediatrics* 1974;53:48–54
10. Gates GA, Avery C, Holt GR, Prihoda TJ. Post tympanostomy otorrhea. *Laryngoscope* 1986;96:630–634
11. Baldwin RL, Aland JL. The effects of povidone-iodine preparation on the incidence of post tympanostomy otorrhea. *Otolaryngol Head Neck Surg* 1990;102:631–634
12. Scott BA, Strunk CL. Post tympanostomy otorrhea: a randomized clinical trial of topical prophylaxis. *Otolaryngol Head Neck Surg* 1992;106:34–41
13. Bluestone CD. Status of the tympanostomy tube. In: Shambaugh GE Jr, Shea JJ, eds. *Proceedings of the Sixth Shambaugh–Shea International Workshop in Otomicrosurgery and the Third Shea Fluctuant Hearing Loss Symposium*. Huntsville, AL: Strode; 1981:85–95
14. Gates GA, Avery C, Prihoda TJ, Holt RG. Delayed onset post-tympanostomy otorrhea. *Otolaryngol Head Neck Surg* 1988; 98:111–115
15. Schneider ML. Bacteriology of otorrhea from tympanoplasty tubes. *Arch Otolaryngol Head Neck Surg* 1989;115:1225–1226
16. Meyerhoff WL, Morizono T, Shaddock LC, et al. Tympanostomy tubes and otic drops. *Laryngoscope* 1983;93:1022–1026

Management of the Draining Pressure Equalization Tube

CHAPTER 36

Philomena Mufalli Behar and N. Wendell Todd

Tympanostomy tube insertion is one of the most commonly performed surgical procedures in children. Otorrhea is a frequent complication of tympanostomy tubes, occurring in 6 to 68% some time after tube insertion.[1-5] Persistent or recurrent otorrhea is reported in approximately 3 to 38% of patients.[5,6] Otorrhea may occur during the immediate postoperative period, or later, and persist for weeks or months.

Measures useful in diminishing tympanostomy tube otorrhea are widely discussed and debated among otolaryngologists. The safety and effectiveness of these measures are controversial. Factors considered, at least by some physicians, to decrease the incidence of postoperative tympanostomy tube otorrhea include control of environmental and behavioral risk factors for otitis media, antiseptic preparation of the ear during tympanostomy tube insertion, tube material, topical antibiotics at tube insertion, and perhaps for a few days later, and "water precautions" (i.e., keeping water out of the ear).

Background

Astley Cooper, an Englishman born in 1768, promoted myringotomy for indications that would be acceptable today. However, the challenge was maintaining the patency of the myringotomy. Before the 1860s, when Politzer introduced a hard rubber eyelet to keep a myringotomy open, catgut string, fishbone plugs, and lead wires had been tried. These techniques were abandoned because of "the high failure rate coupled with a high infection rate."[7] Thus, postoperative otorrhea was a problem long before Armstrong reintroduced tympanostomy tubes in 1954.

Factors Related to Tympanostomy Tube Otorrhea

The development of otorrhea after tympanostomy tube insertion is probably of multifactorial etiology. These factors can be considered to overlap those for otorrhea in chronic otitis media patients. Preoperatively recognizable patient characteristics and comorbidities, the surgeon's operative findings, the surgeon's operative choices, and the postoperative management may all influence the development of drainage through the tube.

PATIENT CHARACTERISTICS, COMORBIDITIES, AND BEHAVIORS

There is little doubt that some patients with tympanostomy tubes are susceptible to otorrhea. But why do some patients, operated and managed in each practitioner's routine, have bothersome ear drainage, whereas other seemingly similar patients do remarkably well with their tympanostomy tubes?

Age of Patient

Infants have a greater propensity to develop post-tympanostomy otorrhea than do older children and adults. In addition, there may be a difference in the bacteriology of the otorrhea when comparing younger with older patients. Pathogens of acute otitis media seem to be more common in patients less than 3 years of age compared with those older than 3 years, where *Pseudomonas aeruginosa* and *Staphylococcus aureus* are more common.[2]

Cleft Palate

Tympanostomy tube otorrhea in cleft palate children is such a problem (68% of patients with open clefts; otorrhea of at least 1 month's duration in 38% of patients[5]) that some authorities prefer to ignore the otitis and delay tympanostomy tube placement until the cleft has been repaired.[8] Even after palate repair, in comparison with noncleft "normal" children, these patients have an increased rate and severity of tympanostomy tube otorrhea.

Tympanostomy tube placement is often done at age 2 or 3 months, with the intention of improved hearing and better speech and language development.[9] Conversely, some advocate delaying the insertion of tympanostomy tubes until a few months after palate closure, arguing that (1) after cleft palate closure, the otitis may resolve so that tympanostomy tubes are not needed; and (2) those who receive tympanostomy tubes have less otorrhea.[8]

Immune Deficiency

Immune problems, both congenital and acquired, humoral and T-cell mediated, are associated with an increased occurrence of tympanostomy tube otorrhea. Masin et al.[10] report that in children who received tympanostomy tube placement because of recurrent otitis media, those with isolated IgG2 deficiency have a threefold increase in occurrences of otorrhea, in contrast to IgG2-competent controls. Anecdotal information supports the idea that patients with immotile cilia syndrome (e.g., Kartagener syndrome), or acquired immunodeficiency syndrome (AIDS), or who have had radiation to the ear, have a worse problem with tympanostomy tube otorrhea than do immune-competent patients.

Dermatitis of External Ear Canal

Eczematoid dermatitis involving the external ear canal is associated with such problematic tympanostomy tube otorrhea that many otolaryngologists prefer to manage the effusion with the combination of observation and amplification not requiring an ear mold (e.g., auditory trainer assistive listening device, or bone oscillator hearing aid).

Bottle Feeding, Especially in the Supine Position

The observation of middle ear fluid that resembles carbonated strawberry soda pop is convincing evidence of reflux from pharynx through the eustachian tube into the middle ear when the patient's mother proceeds to exhibit a baby bottle containing such soda pop. Presumably the eustachian tube architecture that allows such reflux in noncleft palate patients is the same architecture that permits reflux in cleft patients.

Day Care

Children in day care are at increased risk of needing tympanostomy tube insertion (and reinsertion).[11] This may be related to increased exposure to viral and bacterial pathogens. That children in day care have an increased occurrence of tympanostomy tube otorrhea is anecdotal.

Mastoid Opacification

Valtonen et al.[12] report that in children aged 5 to 16 months, early postoperative otorrhea correlates more ($P < 0.001$) with radiographically determined opacification of the mastoid air cell system than with finding a pathogenic bacteria ($P < 0.01$). As the mesotympanum connects via the epitympanum to the mastoid air cell system, radiographically normal mastoids are to be expected in patients with rather minimal otitis media.

OPERATIVE FINDINGS

Middle Ear Fluid

The presence of middle ear fluid and the type of effusion at tympanostomy may be indicative of whether postoperative otorrhea will develop.[3,12] Patients with effusions of any type seem to have a higher rate of postoperative otorrhea than do those with dry middle ears, 21.1% vs 6%.[12] Patients with mucoid and purulent effusions at surgery seem to have an even higher rate of otorrhea during the early postoperative period than that of patients with serous fluid.[13-15]

Middle Ear Mucosa

The intraoperative findings of edematous or granular middle ear mucosa are probably important in predicting postoperative otorrhea.[3,15] Although an increased proportion of patients with inflamed middle ear mucosa have bacterial pathogens in the middle ear fluid, Giebink[3] found inflamed mucosa and mesotympanic pathogens independently to increase the risk of postoperative otorrhea approximately twofold.

Eustachian Tube Caliber

The caliber (internal diameter) of the eustachian tube can be measured intraoperatively by sounding with increasingly larger bougies through the myringotomy into the eustachian tube. Ears with bougie-determined large caliber eustachian tube lumens (i.e., ≥4 Fr) are more likely to have persistent otitis. The bougie-determined caliber of a normal eustachian tube is 2 Fr (0.67 mm). Otitis patients have calibers as large as 6 Fr (2.0 mm). Eustachian calibers are bilaterally symmetric and apparently do not change with patient age or growth. Intraoperative bouginage of the eustachian tube may provide useful information.[16]

OPERATIVE CHOICES OF THE SURGEON

Antiseptic Preparation of the Ear Canal

It has been suggested that bacteria within the ear canal may contribute to postoperative otorrhea. Antiseptic preparation of the external ear canal has been advocated to decrease postoperative otorrhea. Baldwin and Aland[15] reviewed 111 children who underwent canal preparation of one ear, with the contralateral ear acting as a control. Postoperative otorrhea (by report on postoperative days 3 through 6 and by otolaryngologist's observation on day 7) developed in 6.3% of the treated ears and in 10% of the control ears—not a statistically significant difference. These investigators concluded that preparing the ear canal with povidone-iodine had no demonstrable effect on early postoperative otorrhea.[15] Interestingly, all patients with otorrhea had had either mucoid or purulent fluid in the middle ear: 19% who had mucoid fluid, 29% who had pus. None of the patients who had dry middle ears or serous fluid had otorrhea. Giebink et al.[3] performed a prospective study preparing the ear canal with 70% alcohol or povidone-iodine and found again that there was no difference in early postoperative otorrhea. Scott and Strunk[17] similarly reported no difference in early postoperative otorrhea in children with and without canal preparation with povidine-iodine and alcohol.

Benefits other than perhaps reducing early postoperative tympanostomy tube otorrhea may prompt antiseptic preparation of the ear canal. These benefits may include (1) a better view of the tympanum to identify vexations (e.g., cholesteatoma, retraction pocket, dehiscent jugular bulb); (2) minimizing the dilemma of deciding whether a microorganism identified at culture was of external ear canal origin; and (3) minimizing the question of iatrogenic infection.

Middle Ear Irrigation

Middle ear irrigation with saline at tympanostomy tube insertion reduces postintubation otorrhea by one-half.[18] The irrigation presumably decreases the microbial burden in the mesotympanum.

Intraoperative Cultures

There are conflicting data in the literature regarding the usefulness of intraoperative culture results and postoperative otorrhea.

The overall incidence of positive cultures at surgery is probably 20%[13] to 35%.[3] Reports are contradictory as to whether patients with positive middle ear cultures at tube insertion do not[13] or do[3,12,19] have a higher rate of immediate postoperative otorrhea. These reports are not comparable due to differing durations of otitis, ages of patients, external ear canal preparations, and topical antimicrobial prophylaxis. The early postoperative otorrhea rates, for patients with middle ear pathogens versus sterile ear cultures, ranged from 5.4% versus 2.9%[19] to 37 versus 17%.[12]

Choice of Tube Material

A wide variety of tympanostomy tubes are available for insertion. Tubes for short-term and long-term use are manufactured from various biocompatible materials, including stainless steel, titanium, plastics such as silicon elastomer (Silastic), polytetrafluoroethylene (Teflon), and hydroxyapatite.

The type of tympanostomy tube chosen may influence postoperative otorrhea. A study of the scanning electron microscopic characteristics of fluorocarbon versus silicon tubes showed that fluorocarbon tubes had a smoother surface and a lower rate of early postoperative otorrhea.[20] Hester et al.[14] report that of five tympanostomy tubes (Reuter Bobbin, Paparella, Armstrong, T, and Shepard), the incidence of postoperative otorrhea was highest with the Shepard and lowest with the Reuter Bobbin tubes, but the difference was not statistically significant. Recently, silver oxide-coated tubes have been developed with the premise of lowering postoperative otorrhea. Analysis of 125 patients by Chole and Hubbell[21] demonstrated a significant decrease in otorrhea, between 1 week and 1 year postoperatively, in ears with silver oxide-impregnated tubes compared with plain Silastic tubes.

Large-bore tympanostomy tubes and long-term tubes tend to have a higher rate of otorrhea. Rates as high as 40 to 70% are reported.[1] However, this high rate of otorrhea may be a function of the disease process, rather than of the tube itself (patients with more severe and/or recalcitrant disease generally get the larger tubes, that reside longer) or of the larger surface area of the larger tubes.

Nontouch Technique

That this intuitively appealing technique makes no difference in the occurrence of postintubation otorrhea is intriguing. The premise of this technique is to avoid contacting the tympanostomy tube with the gloved hand. The rationale is that, "unless the operative field is sterilized and the patient, surgeon and microscope are fully draped," the glove itself may contaminate the tube.[22]

Contrast the nontouch technique with a maneuver sometimes used to clear the debris-filled tympanostomy tube: push the plug of debris into the mesotympanum. Interestingly, acute otitis is an uncommon aftermath. These reports lend further support to the idea that early postoperative otorrhea is most related to the patient's middle ear status.

Prophylactic Topical Antibiotics

The use of prophylactic antibiotic drops at the time of tympanostomy tube insertion is widely debated. The possible benefit of topically applied antibiotic drops must be weighed against the practical risks of ototoxicity (cochlea and vestibular, i.e., hearing and balance), allergic reaction, and direct monetary costs. It seems inherently counterintuitive to administer ototoxic drugs topically in the vicinity of the oval and round window membranes. The type of ototopical preparation, the duration of therapy, and the effectiveness of the therapy are debated.

Some studies support intraoperative and/or postoperative use of topical antibiotic therapy. Hester et al.[14] performed a prospective study of 587 tubes, 10.2% had postoperative otorrhea. Ears with mucoid or purulent effusions had the highest rate of postoperative otorrhea. All ears that received a prophylactic single intraoperative dose of Cortisporin drops (polymyxin B, neomycin, hydrocortisone) had a decreased rate of postoperative otorrhea compared with controls. If the topical antibiotic was continued for 5 days, ears with mucoid or purulent effusion had a further decrease in postoperative otorrhea. However, Giebink et al.[3] report that prophylactic topical cortisporin drops applied intraoperatively and postoperatively did not significantly alter otorrhea rates.

A study of topical gentamicin prophylaxis showed no statistically significant difference in early postoperative otorrhea.[13] As others have found, patients with mucoid effusion had a higher rate of otorrhea. However, Salam and Cable[23] report early postoperative otorrhea rate of 8.6% when no antibiotic drops were given, significantly more ($P < 0.01$) than 1.85% when Betnesol-N (betamethasone and neomycin) was given for 3 days postoperatively.

Prophylactic Systemic Antimicrobial Agents

Although systemic antimicrobial agents in children with inflamed middle ear mucosa or middle ear effusion containing bacterial pathogens had been suggested to decrease the incidence of postoperative otorrhea,[3] this was not substantiated.[24]

POSTOPERATIVE MANAGEMENT

Early (within 2 Weeks) Postoperative Otorrhea

Early postoperative otorrhea may be the result of the middle ear disease itself or of contamination through the external ear canal occurring at the time of tube insertion.[24] The data usually reveal pathogens of acute otitis media (*Streptococcus pneumoniae*, *Hemophilus influenzae*, *Moraxella catarrhalis*, and *Streptococcus pyogenes*), suggesting that the microorganisms were not introduced with the operative procedure.

If mesotympanic fluid was found at the operative procedure, and Gram stain and culture and sensitivity data are available, the patient-specific evidence-based systemic management is antimicrobial therapy, usually per os. Lacking such bacteriologic information, if the patient does not have systemic symptoms or signs of toxicity, or both (i.e., if the patient is not "sick"), some physicians only prescribe topical antimicrobial(s), and some treat both topically and systemically.

Late (More Than 2 Weeks) Postoperative Otorrhea

Delayed-onset otorrhea, defined by some[25] as more than 7 weeks postoperative, is reported to occur in 26.4%[25] to 68%[5] of cases. In general, children younger than 6 years of age have organisms typical of acute otitis media, whereas older patients have organisms typical of chronic otitis media. Late-onset post-tympanostomy otorrhea is increased during the summer months.[19] Mandel et al.,[2] who acquired specimens by swabbing the external ear canal, found pathogens of acute suppurative otitis to predominate, but *Pseudomonas aeruginosa* and *Staphylococcus aureus* were found more than in early-onset otorrhea. However, Brook et al.,[26] who demonstrate that specimens collected from the external auditory canal can be misleading, found 50% of ears to have only aerobes (mostly *Pseudomonas aeruginosa* or *Staphylococcus aureus*), 13% to have only anaerobes (mostly *Peptostreptococcus* sp.), and 36% to have both both aerobes and anaerobes. Only 26% of their patients had early-onset otorrhea. Thus, delayed-onset otorrhea is often related to microorganisms that enter from the external ear canal.

The spectrum of managements, often without benefit of patient-specific laboratory data, ranges from observation alone to systemic antimicrobial agents. Systemic antimicrobial agents are more often prescribed for younger children and for those with symptoms and signs of systemic toxicity.

Topical Therapy

The use of topical antibiotic therapy for chronic otorrhea is the cause of much rumination among otolaryngologists. The ruminations relate to efficacy and to untoward effects (ototoxicity, allergic reactions, and costs).

The ototoxicity of topically applied drops containing aminoglycosides has been studied in various animal models, and in humans. In cats, cochlear damage was demonstrated by Smith and Myers,[27] in which penetration of perilymph with gentamicin and neomycin occurred across the round window membrane. Wright and Meyerhoff[28] reported hair cell and stria vascularis damage in chinchillas after application of cortisporin.

Whereas intratympanic and intravenous administration of aminoglycosides has been associated with ototoxicity in humans, there is little information documenting hearing loss from topical application of drops onto an open tympanostomy tube.[29] One would expect high-frequency hearing loss more commonly, as a result of round window penetration of an ototoxic drug and its effects on the basal turn of the cochlea (high-frequency hearing region). Insufficient evidence for ototoxicity may be the result of poor penetration of the drug through the tympanostomy tube into the middle ear, minimal drug getting into the cochlea because inflammation (e.g., edema of the middle ear mucosa and of the round window membrane) limits drug access, or inadequate audiometric testing to document the temporal relationship of dosing and hearing loss, or simply failure to report an untoward consequence of therapy. In a 1992 survey (response rate 30%) of 7463 otolaryngologists in the United States, 3.4% reported presumed inner ear damage from ototopical medications.[30] Merifield et al.[29] recorded pre- and post-treatment bone conduction thresholds at 3000, 4000, and 6000 Hz in 70 ears and found no difference in sensorineural hearing in any ear. Welling et al.[31] similarly recorded pre- and postoperative air and bone conduction and speech reception thresholds for patients who received one dose of topical cortisporin injected into the middle ear at tube insertion. Again, there was no statistically significant difference in any patient, regardless of the middle ear findings (dry vs effusion).[31]

In patients with chronic suppurative otitis media (open tympanic membrane, with otorrhea for at least 1 month), aminoglycosides (e.g., gentamicin, neomycin, and tobramycin) have been popular choices for topical therapy. These drugs are chosen to treat infection presumed to involve *Pseudomonas aeruginosa*. However, other topical preparations such as boric or acetic acid, as well as topical quinolones (ciprofloxacin and ofloxacin), are useful in treating such otorrhea. These preparations have no known ototoxic effects. Indeed, ofloxacin is the only antimicrobial-containing topical ear preparation that has package insert endorsement for use in the patient with an opening in the tympanic membrane. Nevertheless, the American Academy of Otolaryngology—Head and Neck Surgery in 1998 "recognizes the appropriateness of using currently available topical preparations, including those containing aminoglycosides, in the treatment of external and middle ear disorders."[32]

Allergic reactions to ototopicals are common, especially after chronic usage. More than one-half of chronic otorrhea patients may have allergy to topical medications.[33] The most common offending agent is neomycin, with polymyxin B and gentamicin less common offenders. Allergic reactions occur even to topical corticosteroids.[34]

Swimming and Water Getting into the Ears

Recommendations for water precautions after tympanostomy tube insertion are variable among otolaryngologists. Many advise avoidance of swimming and water exposure to the ears presumably to prevent middle ear contamination. The manufacturers' package insert with tympanostomy tubes used in the United States recommend avoidance of water exposure. If water exposure is anticipated at an intubated ear, many physicians recommend ear plugs. Some report that there is no difference in the rate of otorrhea despite swimming.[35] In another in vitro study, Hebert et al.[36] concluded that water precautions are not necessary for surface (depth <60 cm) swimming. However, because soapy water has a surface tension lower than that of pool water, bath water may enter a tympanostomy tube more readily. An important limitation of the hydraulic study of Hebert et al.[36] is the assumption that all tympanostomy tube patients have eustachian tube lumens similar to that of an 18-gauge needle (i.e., about 0.7 mm), which is much more flow resistant than the 1- or 2-mm diameter lumens of otitis patients. As patients with more impressive otitis media often have functionally patulous (at least intermittently) eustachian tubes, they may be at greater risk of water entering through a tympanostomy tube than the patient with lesser disease that manifests just as recurring otitis media during infancy.

Granulation Tissue

This pink-red vascularized connective tissue that forms granular projections on the surface of a wound, is especially common at a foreign body. When exuberant, it is often termed "proud flesh." (Confusingly, the term "granuloma" is sometimes used, provoking thoughts of "granulomatous" diseases, e.g., tuberculosis). Although anecdotally small granulations may be eradicated by topical antimicrobials or anti-inflammatory corticosteroids, in practice the control of granulation tissue necessitates the removal of the foreign body tympanostomy tube. The draining ear is often found to have granulation tissue in the mesotympanum.

Tube Removal

Removing the offending tympanostomy tube may be necessary to control otorrhea. Offenses occur in two ways that sometimes interrelate. One offense is to have microbes persisting on the surface, this is especially a problem, at least theoretically, with rough surfaces that involve pits and crevices. The other offense is for the tympanostomy tube to be a nidus for granulation tissue. In a report about operative removal of tympanostomy tubes, Cunningham et al.[37] removed 22% because of otorrhea, and 20% because of granulation tissue; one-third of these ears had both otorrhea and granulation tissue.

Recidivistic Otorrhea

Despite all the precautions and managements mentioned, some patients continue to have purulent otorrhea—even after the presumably offending tympanostomy tube has been removed. These perplexing problems are analogous to persistently active chronic suppurative otitis media. Some practitioners have advocated weeks of intravenous antimicrobial therapy based on laboratory bacteriologic data obtained from the purulent specimen that is presumably representative of the deeper infectious process. Others, mentioning the menagerie of problems including foreign body lost somewhere in the middle ear, tumor (rhabdomyosarcoma, granulocytic sarcoma, histocytosis X), osteomyelitis sequestered in the mastoid, unrecognized cholesteatoma, and mycobacterial or fungal infections, advocate mastoid and middle ear surgical exploration. Lastly, consider Munchausen's syndrome, including by proxy.

Authors' Perspective

We minimize the risks of tympanostomy tube otorrhea by (1) addressing patient characteristics, comorbidities, and behaviors; (2) considering practical ear characteristics (mesotympanic fluid and mucosa, and eustachian caliber); and (3) antiseptic ear cleansing, and irrigating until accessible mesotympanic fluid is cleared. In infants with cleft palate, assuming that behavioral audiometry has not revealed worse than a mild loss (in the better-hearing ear), we like to defer tympanostomy tube placement until the anesthetic at which the cleft is repaired, typically at 9 to 12 months of age. In acquired immunodeficiency syndrome (AIDS) patients, and in patients with immotile cilia syndrome, we try to avoid placing tympanostomy tubes; for persistent nonsuppurative fluid with clinically significant bilateral hearing loss, amplification seems appropriate. Bottle feeding in the supine position is discontinued before tympanostomy tube insertion. Graduation from the bottle by the first birthday is encouraged. The otitis-exaggerating effects of day care and smoke exposure are discussed with the family.

At tympanostomy tube placement, we like to obtain mesotympanic fluid for bacteriologic assessment (Gram stain, and culture and sensitivity). The data are not only a preemptive guide to the antimicrobial treatment of postoperative otorrhea, but also a measure of clinically significant respiratory bacteria in the community. For example, the finding of highly resistant *Streptococcus pneumoniae* in the mesotympanum in a generally healthy 18-month-old day care attendee may prompt a discussion of the risks versus benefits of the child being in that particular day care scenario. If the microbe burden in the mesotympanic fluid is low, as evidenced by absence of organisms on Gram stain, and the culture reveals *Hemophilis influenzae* or *Moraxella catarrhalis*, otorrhea usually does not manifest. By contrast, if Gram-positive diplococci are found in the smear, purulent otorrhea is likely, and antimicrobial treatment is advised.

We like to prepare the ear with povidone-iodine and rinse with sterile saline. We like to irrigate the mesotympanum with saline, until all available mucoid or purulent fluid is removed. Information on eustachian caliber is helpful in deciding which patients should avoid water into the ears, as well as prognostically.

If otorrhea occurs, we prefer to examine the patient, perform aural suctioning while viewing with a microscope, and obtain a specimen (through the tympanostomy tube[26]) for Gram stain, culture, and sensitivity. The ear is examined for a malpositioned tube, granulation tissue, cholesteatoma, and smoldering mastoiditis. A hydrocellulose wick is placed and expanded with nonototoxic nonallergenic Domeboro otic drops. Domeboro otic solution is well tolerated onto a wick. We advise 4 gtts q.i.d. for 4 days. By day 4, bacteriologic data are available: if *Streptococcus pneumoniae* are found, an appropriate antimicrobial is prescribed by mouth, and Domeboro gtts continued an additional 4 days. If the bacteriologic data are negative, or show other microorganisms, the parent removes the wick on day 4, stops the Domeboro gtts, and keeps water and Q-tips out of the ear. The wick serves three purposes: (1) assists in delivery of the pH-normalizing medication into the ear; (2) helps calm the often-concomitant inflammation of the external ear canal; and (3) prevents the patient from placing fingers or other objects into the ear.

A practical alternative to seeing the patient is to prescribe ofloxacin drops; we typically do this for the otherwise healthy patient. We avoid topical aminoglycosides, unless the case is recalcitrant and bacteriologic data endorse their use.

Conclusion

A stepwise approach, graded or balanced in reference to the severity, risks, and costs of the otorrhea problem, is advised. Typically, the initial management includes topical and/or oral medications directed at likely pathogens. In recalcitrant cases, antimicrobial therapy guided by Gram stain, culture, and sensitivity data acquired from a representative specimen obtained through the lumen of the tympanostomy tube is helpful. If otorrhea persists for several weeks despite these usual treatment measures, additional causative factors should be considered. Such additional factors include resistant or unusual microorganisms, susceptible microorganisms sequestered in a reservoir (e.g., smoldering mastoiditis, or a previously placed unwittingly retained tympanostomy tube) not accessible to topical or systematically administered drugs, granulation tissue, eustachian tube reflux, immunodeficiency, cholesteatoma, and systemic or neoplastic disorders.

REFERENCES

Behar and Todd—CHAPTER 36

1. Per-Lee JH. Long-term middle ear ventilation. *Laryngoscope* 1981;91:1063–1072
2. Mandel EM, Casselbrant ML, Kurs-Lasky M. Acute otorrhea: bacteriology of a common complication of tympanostomy tubes. *Ann Otol Rhinol Laryngol* 1994;103:713–718
3. Giebink GS, Daly K, Buran DJ, et al. Predictors for postoperative otorrhea following tympanostomy tube insertion. *Arch Otolaryngol Head Neck Surg* 1992;118:491–494
4. Luxford WM, Sheehy JL. Myringotomy and ventilation tubes: a report of 1,568 ears. *Laryngoscope* 1982;92:1293–1297
5. Paradise JL, Bluestone CD. Early treatment of the universal otitis media of infants with cleft palate. *Pediatrics* 1974;53: 48–54
6. Debruyne F, Jorissen M, Peolmans J. Otorrhea during transtympanic ventilation. *Am J Otol* 1988;9:316–317
7. Alberti PW. Myringotomy and ventilating tubes in the 19th century. *Laryngoscope* 1994;84:805–815
8. Crysdale WS. Closure of the soft palate for persistent otorrhea after placement of pressure equalization tubes in cleft palate infants (Braganza et al., 1991) (letter). *Cleft Palate Craniofacial J* 1992;29:97
9. Braganza RA, Kearns DB, Burton DM, et al. Closure of the soft palate for persistent otorrhea after placement of pressure equalization tubes in cleft palate infants. *Cleft Palate Craniofacial J* 1991;28:305–307
10. Masin JS, Hostoffer RW, Arnold JE. Otitis media following tympanostomy tube placement in children with IgG_2 deficiency. *Laryngoscope* 1995;105:1188–1190
11. Postma DS, Poole MD, Wu SM, Tober R. The impact of day care on ventilation tube insertion. *Int J Pediatr Otorhinolaryngol* 1997;41:253–262
12. Valtonen H, Qvarnberg Y, Puhakka H, Nuutinen J. Early post-tympanostomy otorrhea in children under 17 months of age. *Acta Otolaryngol (Stockh)* 1997;117:569–573
13. Scott BA, Strunk CL. Post-tympanostomy otorrhea: a randomized clinical trial of topical prophylaxis. *Otolaryngol Head Neck Surg* 1992;106:34–41
14. Hester TO, Jones RO, Archer SM, Haydon RC. Prophylactic antibiotic drops after tympanostomy tube placement. *Arch Otolaryngol Head Neck Surg* 1995;121:445–448
15. Baldwin RL, Aland J. The effects of povidone-iodine preparation on the incidence of post-tympanostomy tube otorrhea. *Otolaryngol Head Neck Surg* 1990;102:631–634
16. Todd NW. Otitis media and eustachian tube caliber. *Acta Otolaryngol (Stockh)* 1983;404:1–17
17. Scott BA, Strunk CL Jr. Posttympanostomy otorrhea: the efficacy of canal preparation. *Laryngoscope* 1992;102:1103–1107
18. Gross RD, Burgess LP, Hall DJ, et al. Middle ear irrigation in the prevention of otorrhea after tympanostomy tube placement. *Laryngoscope* 1999;110:246–249
19. Gates GA, Avery C, Prihoda TJ, Holt GR. Post-tympanostomy otorrhea. *Laryngoscope* 1986;96:630–634
20. Karlan MS, Skobel B, Grizzard M, et al. Myringotomy tube materials: bacterial adhesion and infection. *Otolaryngol Head Neck Surg* 1980;88:783–795
21. Chole RA, Hubbell RN. Antimicrobial activity of silastic tympanostomy tubes impregnated with silver oxide: a double-blind randomized multicenter trial. *Arch Otolaryngol Head Neck Surg* 1995;121:562–565
22. Kinsella JB, Fenton J, Donnelly MJ, McShane DP. Tympanostomy tubes and early post-operative otorrhea. *Int J Pediatr Otorhinolaryngol* 1994;30:111–114

23. Salam MA, Cable HR. The use of antibiotic/steroid ear drops to reduce post-operative otorrhoea and blockage of ventilation tubes. A prospective study. *J Laryngol Otol* 1993;107:188–189
24. Daly KA, Giebink GS, Lindgren B, et al. Randomized trial of the efficacy of trimethoprim-sulfamethoxazole and prednisone in preventing post-tympanostomy tube morbidity. *Pediatr Infect Dis J* 1995;14:1068–1074
25. Gates GA, Avery C, Prihoda TJ, Holt GR. Delayed onset post-tympanostomy otorrhea. *Otolaryngol Head Neck Surg* 1988; 98:111–115
26. Brook I, Yocum P, Shah K. Aerobic and anaerobic bacteriology of otorrhea associated with tympanostomy tubes in children. *Acta Otolaryngol (Stockh)* 1998;118:206–210
27. Smith BM, Myers MG. The penetration of gentamycin and neomycin into perilymph across the round window membrane. *Otolaryngol Head Neck Surg* 1978;87:888–891
28. Wright CG, Meyerhoff WL. Ototoxicity of otic drops applied to the middle ear in the chinchilla. *Am J Otolaryngol* 1984;5: 166–176
29. Merifield DO, Parker NJ, Nicholson NC. Therapeutic management of chronic suppurative otitis media with otic drops. *Otolaryngol Head Neck Surg* 1993;109:77–82
30. Lundy LB, Graham MD. Ototoxicity and ototopical medications: a survey of otolaryngologists. *Am J Otol* 1993;14:141–146
31. Welling DB, Forrest LA, Goll F 3rd. Safety of ototopical antibiotics. *Laryngoscope* 1995;105:472–474
32. American Academy of Otolaryngology—Head and Neck Surgery. Policy statement 1420 Topical Antibiotic Drops, adopted 7/9/94, reaffirmed 3/1/98, Alexandria, Virginia, AAO-HNS Bulletin, October 1998.
33. Van Gickel CJW, Bruintjes TD, Huizing EH. Allergy due to topical medications in chronic otitis externa and chronic otitis media. *Clin Otolaryngol* 1995;20:326–328
34. Lauerma AI, Reitamo S. Contact allergy to corticosteroids. *J Am Acad Dermatol* 1993;28:618–622
35. Parker GS, Tami TA, Maddox MR, et al. The effect of water exposure after tympanostomy tube insertion. *Am J Otolaryngol* 1994;15:193–196
36. Hebert RL II, King GE, Bent JP III. Tympanostomy tubes and water exposure: a practical model. *Arch Otolaryngol Head Neck Surg* 1998;124:1118–1121
37. Cunningham MJ, Eavey RD, Krouse JH, Kiskaddon RM. Tympanostomy tubes: experience with removal. *Laryngoscope* 1993;103:659–662

13

Management of Cholesteatoma

"Most otologic surgeons prefer to avoid operating on an only hearing ear. Preoperative scanning can not only help determine the risk of observation, but if no evidence of disease is seen in the middle ear space, a modified radical mastoidectomy (without tympanoplasty) can be justified. Some surgeons believe that avoiding surgery in the middle ear space reduces the risk of postoperative hearing loss."

Peter S. Roland

"The added safety of a second look procedure, however, does not preclude primary reconstruction of the ossicular chain in most cases. Thus it is not necessary to commit the patient to months of a large or maximal conductive loss just because a second look procedure may be indicated at a later time. It is the author's practice to delay ossicular reconstruction in only certain circumstances such as cases in which the middle ear mucosa has been replaced by granulomatous disease in which time is necessary to achieve a mucosalized and aerated middle ear compartment, or in such cases in which the footplate is fixed and stapedectomy will be necessary for hearing reconstruction."

Joseph B. Nadol, Jr.

"Residual cholesteatoma is not related to recurrent cholesteatoma. Recurrent cholesteatoma rarely develops in canal wall down procedures. Recurrent cholesteatoma is preventable: residual cholesteatoma is not. The incidence of residual cholesteatoma in the middle ear is the same (in our hands), CWU or CWD."

James L. Sheehy

Management of Cholesteatoma

Peter S. Roland

CHAPTER 37

Several areas of controversy persist in the management of cholesteatoma. All these controversies must be evaluated in the light of clearly established treatment goals. The goals for the removal of cholesteatoma are listed succinctly in Table 37–1.

TABLE 37–1
Goals of Surgery for Cholesteatoma

1. To remove all potentially erosive or invasive disease
2. To create a smooth, exteriorized cavity that can be completely cleaned in the office
3. To create a cavity lined with normal skin that tolerates the usual activities of daily living, including swimming
4. To conserve residual hearing
5. To improve hearing, if possible
6. To provide acceptable cosmetics

Preoperative Imaging

There is little question about which imaging techniques should be used for the preoperative evaluations of individuals known or suspected to have cholesteatoma. Computed tomography (CT) scanning is the modality of choice.[1] Contrast is rarely necessary. While plain film radiographs can provide a limited amount of useful information, they have generally been abandoned for use with cholesteatoma. Magnetic resonance imaging (MRI) scanning should be used only when very specific problems involving surrounding soft tissues are expected, including dural involvement or invasion, sub- or epidural abscess, the presence of herniated brain into the mastoid cavity, inflammation of the membranous labyrinth or facial nerve, or sigmoid sinus thrombosis.[1]

Because CT scanning provides excellent bony resolution, it can detect subtle defects such as: scutal erosion, labyrinthine fistula, defects in the tegmen, details of ossicular involvement, erosion or discontinuity, and anomalies or invasion of the fallopian canal.

However, CT scanning cannot always distinguish between granulation tissue and cholesteatoma and/or effusion. Therefore, CT scans cannot reliably determine the full extent of disease and, consequently, the surgeon cannot predict precisely what will need to be done in the operating room. Both the operating surgeon and the patient or parent must understand the limitations of this imaging technique and be prepared for intraoperative surprises.

Although there is wide agreement among physicians about the use of CT scanning as the technique of choice, there is little agreement as to which patients should receive preoperative imaging. Some surgeons believe that all individuals scheduled for tympanomastoid surgery should have CT imaging preoperatively. These physicians believe that useful information is obtained in every circumstance; consequently, the expense and radiation exposure are always justified. Other surgeons reserve preoperative imaging for special cases and are quite comfortable performing surgery without preoperative imaging in most patients with cholesteatoma. The following special cases would qualify for CT scans:

1. *When the diagnosis is in doubt:* The diagnosis may be in doubt in individuals with small attic retractions. CT scanning may show only a retraction without soft tissue extension into the epitympanic space and without bony erosion. In some of these circumstances, it may be permissible simply to observe the patient carefully. If bony erosion or an extensive soft mass is seen, operation is probably advisable. The diagnosis is frequently in doubt in individuals who have already had tympanomastoid surgery. In this group of patients, a white mass behind the tympanic membrane could represent tympanosclerosis, cartilage, or recurrent cholesteatoma, and CT scanning can frequently resolve such questions.
2. *When a patient wishes to avoid operation:* If an individual is a poor surgical candidate or for other reasons wishes to avoid operation, CT scanning can help assess the risk of conservative management. The presence of extensive disease, labyrinthine fistula, encroachment around the fallopian canal, and involvement of the oval window niche, increase the risk of expectant management, and the patient should be so advised. Most otologic surgeons prefer to avoid operating on an only hearing ear. Preoperative scanning can not only help determine the risk of observation, but if no evidence of disease is seen in the middle ear space, a modified radical mastoidectomy (without tympanoplasty) can be justified. Some surgeons believe that avoiding surgery in the middle ear space reduces the risk of postoperative hearing loss.[2]

3. *For preoperative risk assessment:* In some circumstances, it may be especially important to patients or parents to have some assessment of the risk of ossicular involvement and postoperative conductive hearing loss. This is especially true in children with cholesteatoma who have normal hearing. Preoperative scanning can often help determine the likelihood of ossicular involvement. If ossicular involvement is apparent on preoperative CT scans, parents can be counseled that ossicular removal may be necessary and that significant postoperative conductive hearing loss should be expected.
4. *In revision cases:* When the underlying anatomy is indeterminate and the extent of the disease is unclear.
5. *In cases in which congenital anomalies might be reasonably expected:* These include cases of atresia or individuals with craniofacial anomalies.
6. *When there is concern about the presence of complicating factors:* If labyrinthine fistula or erosion of the fallopian canal is suspected, CT scanning remains the procedure of choice. If intracranial invasion, dural inflammation, meningitis, abscess, or sigmoid sinus thrombosis is suspected, MRI should be used.
7. *To help identify associated conditions:* These conditions include nasal septal deviation and chronic sinusitis.

Open versus Closed Cavity Techniques

Although controversy over "open" versus "closed" cavity techniques has cooled down considerably during the last decade or two, and despite the fact that most surgeons are now willing to use either technique depending on circumstance, there are still some surgeons who favor closed techniques and others who favor open ones.[3-5]

The characteristics of the two techniques are illustrated in Table 37–2. It is now generally recognized and is widely accepted that there is no significant difference in the hearing results between the two techniques.[5-8]

Sometimes the decision whether to use a canal wall-up or canal wall-down technique can be made preoperatively. If there have been several episodes of recurrence and the patient wishes to avoid a future operation, the canal wall-down technique is chosen. For individuals unwilling or unable to be followed-up regularly and be available for a second "stage" procedure, canal wall-down is preferable. Some patients may refuse to accept a meatoplasty under any circumstances, and such individuals should be treated with closed (canal wall-up) techniques. These patients must understand that the disease can recur, and they may require multiple serial procedures.

In individuals who have known irremediable auditory tube dysfunction (on the basis of congenital anomalies or previous surgical procedures which have destroyed the eustachian tube), a canal wall-down procedure is best.[3,5,9]

It is generally best to reserve the decision as to how to manage the canal wall until the time of operation because intraoperative findings are frequently important in making that decision. Findings that favor a canal wall-down or an open technique include the following:

1. Involvement of the sinus tympani
2. Involvement of the medial end of the canal wall with cholesteatoma wedged laterally between the heads of the ossicles and the medial canal wall
3. Osteitis or irremovable cholesteatoma in the pro-tubal area or hypotympanum, which generally calls for a true radical mastoidectomy
4. Substantial destruction of the canal wall, with small defects in the canal wall readily repaired (however, if the defect is large, the better part of valor may be to remove it completely[3])
5. The presence of labyrinthine fistula,[5,10] especially if the labyrinthine fistula is large and one wishes to leave the matrix down (it is not possible to leave the cholesteatoma matrix down and perform a closed or canal wall up technique[5]).

More important than the technique actually chosen is how well the operation is performed. The requirements for a

TABLE 37–2
"Open" versus "Closed" Cavity Techniques

Closed Cavity	Open Cavity
1. Normal appearance	1. Enlarged meatus
2. Easy-to-fit hearing aid	2. Difficulty to fit hearing aid
3. No routine cleaning required	3. Annual or semiannual canal cleaning needed
4. Relatively high rate of recurrent or persistent cholesteatoma	4. Low rate of persistent or recurrent cholesteatoma
5. High tolerance for water exposure	5. Occasional problem with water exposure
6. Usually staged	6. Usually single procedure

TABLE 37–3
Creation of a Well-Functioning Open Cavity

1. Remove all air cells, including those within the retrofacial, retrolabyrinthine, and subarcuate air cell tracts.
2. Remove the lateral and the posterior walls of the epitympanum so that the tegmen mastoid and tegmen tympani are a smooth, featureless plane.
3. Amputate the mastoid tip.
4. Saucerize the lateral margins of the cavity.
5. Lower the posterior bony external auditory wall to the level of the facial nerve.
6. Exteriorize the anterior epitympanic recess by removing the "cog."
7. Enlarge the meatus (at least twice as large) by removing conchal cartilage.
8. Lower the medial end of the EAC toward the floor of the hypotympanum.

good open or closed cavity are listed in Table 37–3. Closed cavities must be followed regularly to detect recurrences. Open cavities must be followed regularly for annual or semi-annual "cleaning."

Primary Versus Secondary Ossicular Reconstruction

Whether to repair the ossicular chain at the time of primary cholesteatoma removal or to delay that reconstruction for some months is frequently debated. In reality, most practicing otologists use both strategies depending on circumstances.[3,11] If a second exploration is planned, delaying the ossicular reconstruction is more appealing. A second procedure does permit the middle ear space and tympanic membrane to heal up well in advance of reconstruction and provides additional motivation for the patient to return for the second stage of his or her procedure.

If there is concern about postoperative aeration because of suspected eustachian tube dysfunction, it is often better to wait and make sure an appropriate middle ear space has developed and that the tympanic membrane has healed before attempting to reconstruct the ossicular chain. If there have been failed ossicular reconstructions in the past, or previous operations have been followed with severe postoperative retraction, staging a reconstruction is prudent. Often, the decision to delay ossicular reconstruction is made on the basis of the severity of the disease encountered at the time of primary cholesteatoma removal. If the mucosa has been seriously damaged, is thick, edematous, and large amounts of middle ear mucosa need to be removed, postoperative scarring, fibrosis, and retraction are more likely. The timing of ossicular chain reconstruction is a judgment call that requires significant amounts of experience.

Intraoperative Monitoring

Facial nerve injuries are the most feared untoward consequence of cholesteatoma surgery. The necessity of intraoperative facial nerve monitoring when performing cholesteatoma surgery remains controversial. A survey of practicing otologists performed in 1990 showed that most experienced otologists do not believe that facial nerve monitoring is obligatory, and many experienced otologists use it only occasionally.[12] They do not believe the extra expense and time required to use the technique is justified and expressed concern that the device can be misleading. "Silent" transections do occur, and the use of a facial nerve monitor does not ensure against facial nerve injury. They recognize that intraoperative monitoring can be begun in the middle of a case when difficult circumstances that justify its use are encountered.

Other surgeons argue that one can never predict the cases in which facial nerve monitoring may be useful and that the expense and time required to set it up is justified in every case. They see it as a "safety net," much like electrocardiographic (ECG) monitoring, that is always potentially useful.[13] Most surgeons who use facial nerve monitoring do not feel compelled to do so by medical/legal considerations. However, they would feel uncomfortable about a case in which the facial nerve was injured and monitoring was omitted.[13] An effective use of facial nerve monitoring techniques requires experience. Some surgeons justify routine use of the facial nerve monitor as a method of developing and retaining experience in its use.[14]

Some surgeons pursue an intermediate course and do not use facial nerve monitoring on a regular basis, but only for selected cases. These cases may include revision operations, circumstances in which the patient had previous postoperative facial nerve paralysis, or, for patients who have preoperative facial nerve involvement, either paresis or hyperirritability, or cases in which preoperative scanning shows anomalies or dehiscence of the fallopian canal.[14]

REFERENCES

Roland—CHAPTER 37

1. Mancuso A, Harnsberger H, Dillon W. MRI and CT of the head and neck. 2nd Ed. Baltimore: Williams & Wilkins; 1989
2. Sheehy J, Brackmann D, Graham M. Complications of cholesteatoma: a report of 1024 cases. In: McCabe B SJ, Abramson M, eds. *Cholesteatoma, First International Conference*. Birmingham, AL: Aesclapius, 1977:420
3. Sheely J. Mastoidectomy: the intact canal wall procedure. In: Brackmann D, Shelton C, Arriaga M, eds. *Otologic Surgery*. Philadelphia: WB Saunders; 1997
4. Paparella M, Meyerhoff W, Morris M, DaCosta S. Mastoidectomy and tympanoplasty. In: Parparella MM, Shumrick DA, Gluckman JL, Meyerhoff WL, eds. *Otolaryngology*. Vol 2. Philadelphia: WB Saunders, 1991:1405–1439
5. Smyth G, Tower J. Mastoidectomy: canal wall down techniques. In: Brackmann D, Shelton C, Arriago M, eds. *Otologic surgery*. Philadelphia: WB Saunders, 1997
6. Cook J, Krishnan S, Fagan P. Hearing results following modified radical versus canal-up mastoidectomy. *Ann Otol Rhinol Laryngol* 1996;105:379–383
7. Whittemore K Jr, Merchant S, Rosowski J. Acoustic mechanisms: canal wall-up versus canal wall-down mastoidectomy. *Otolaryngol-Head Neck Surg* 1998;118:751–761
8. Dodson E, Hashisaki G, Hobgood T, Lambert P. Intact canal wall mastoidectomy with tympanoplasty for cholesteatoma in children. *Laryngoscope* 1998;108:977–983
9. Bhatia S, Karmarkar S, DeDonato G, et al. Canal wall down mastoidectomy: causes of failure, pitfalls, and their management. *J Laryngol Otol* 1995;109:583–589
10. Law K, Smyth G, Kerr A. Fistula of the labyrinth treated by staged combined approach tympanoplasty. *J Laryngol Otol* 1975;89:471–478
11. Sheehy J, Shelton C. Tympanoplasty: to stage or not to stage. *Otolaryngol Head Neck Surg* 1991;104:399–407
12. Roland PS, Meyerhoff WL. Intraoperative facial nerve monitoring: what is its appropriate role? (Editorial.) *Am J Otol* 1993;14:I
13. Pensak M, Willging J, Keith R. Intraoperative facial nerve monitoring in chronic ear surgery: a resident training experience. *Am J Otol* 1994;15:108–110
14. Silverstein H, Rosenberg S. Intraoperative facial nerve monitoring. *Otolaryngol Clin North Am* 1991;24:709–725

Management of Cholesteatoma

CHAPTER 38

Joseph B. Nadol, Jr.

The primary objectives of management of chronic otitis media with and without cholesteatoma include (1) elimination of infection or cholesteatoma; (2) prevention of recurrent disease; and (3) reconstruction of the tympanic membrane and ossicular chain to minimize the postoperative air bone gap. As judged by published success rates in achieving a dry, safe ear over time and in reconstruction of the middle ear, surgical management of the chronic ear remains one of the more challenging disease processes in otology. In chronic otitis media with cholesteatoma, combined rates of either residual or recurrent cholesteatoma occur in up to 50% of patients.[1-3] In general, most series suggest a lower recidivism rate for cholesteatoma in cases managed by canal wall-down technique as compared with canal wall-up.[3-6] However, even without recurrent cholesteatoma, the canal wall-down technique appears to predispose the patient to persistent or recurrent intermittent drainage requiring revision surgery[7-9] in up to 60% of cases.

Hearing results have been likewise disappointing in chronic otitis media as compared with other middle ear reconstructive problems. Thus, postoperative air bone gaps ≥20 dB were reported in 38%,[10] and ≥30 dB in 30%.[11] In 400 second-stage procedures of chronic otitis media, closure of the air bone gap to ≤20 dB occurred in 68% of patients with intact stapes. In general, postoperative air bone gaps are even larger when the stapes superstructure is not intact.[5,12-14]

Although some authors a priori prefer either the canal wall-up technique[2,15] or canal wall-down technique,[16] it is this author's opinion that each case should be individualized to minimize recurrence of disease.

Factors Involved in Treatment Algorithm for Chronic Otitis Media

INITIAL EVALUATION

The initial evaluation of patients with chronic otitis media should include a thorough otologic and general medical history. The otologic history must include careful documentation of symptoms and previous treatment, both medical and surgical. The general medical history should include documentation of potential predisposing factors including upper respiratory allergy, smoking, diabetes mellitus, and possible immunologic compromise.

Examination should include a thorough otologic and complete head and neck examination. Audiometry is essential. Bacteriologic cultures, including anaerobes in cases of chronic otitis media with otorrhea may be helpful. Computed tomography (CT) of the temporal bones, in both the axial and coronal planes, will provide valuable information concerning pneumatization of the mastoid, extent of cholesteatoma and granulation tissue, potential complications such as dehiscence of a semicircular canal or the facial nerve, or unexpected findings such as extension of disease to the petrous apex. In chronic otitis media with impending complications, CT is particularly useful.

CATEGORIZATION OF CHRONIC OTITIS MEDIA

As part of the initial evaluation of the patient with chronic otitis media, an attempt should be made to assign the disease process to one of the categories shown in Table 38–1. In the author's hands, such subcategorization of disease will suggest a management strategy selected from a medical and/or surgical algorithm. Failure to control chronic otitis media can be attributed to the improper selection of a medical or surgical strategy at least as often as inadequate execution of that procedure.

REVIEW OF ALGORITHM FOR MANAGEMENT OF PRIMARY CHRONIC OTITIS MEDIA

After initial evaluation, including ancillary studies and assignment to a subcategory of disease (Table 38–1), possible contributory disease processes such as allergic rhinosinusitis, smoking, obesity and/or diabetes mellitus, immunocompromise, should be assessed and controlled if possible (Fig. 38–1).

Chronic otitis media with cholesteatoma almost always requires surgical intervention. In those cases without otorrhea,

TABLE 38–1
Categories of Chronic Otitis Media

Chronic active otitis media
With cholesteatoma
With otorrhea
Without otorrhea
Without cholesteatoma
With otorrhea
Chronic inactive otitis media
With frequent reactivation
Without frequent reactivation

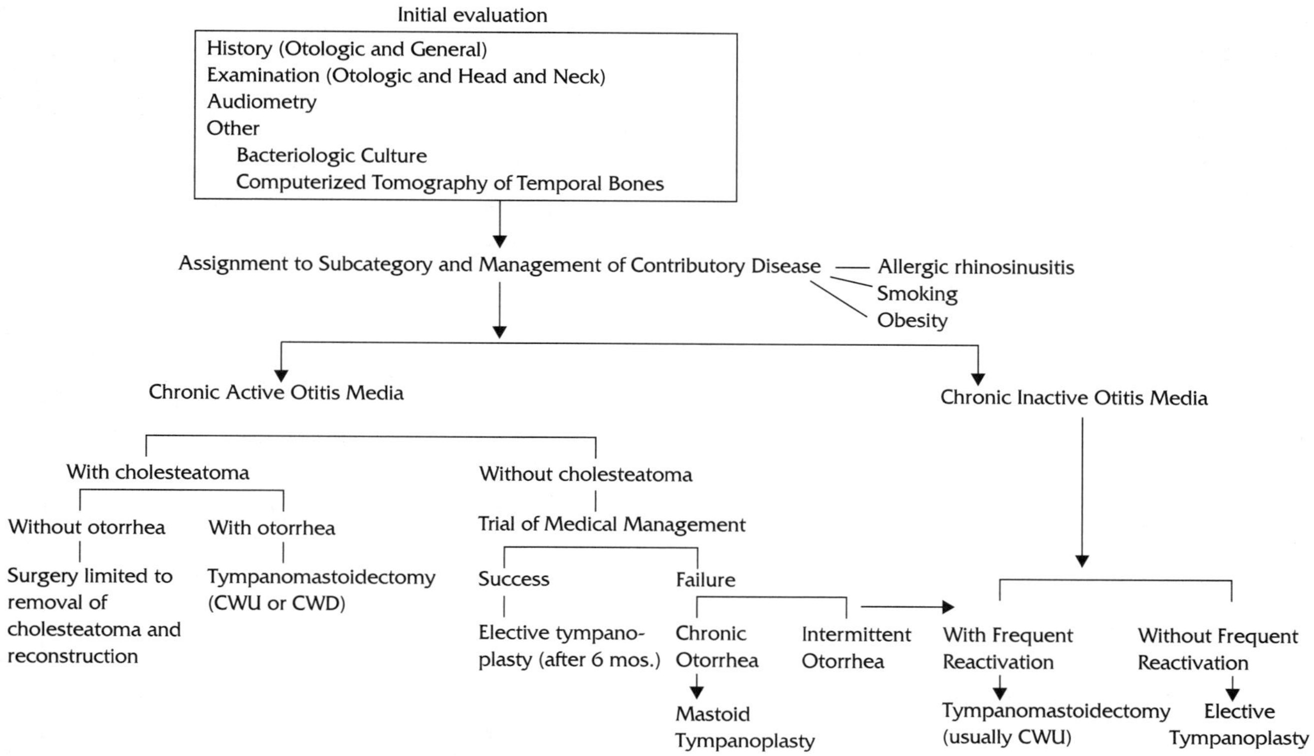

Figure 38–1 Algorithm for management of primary chronic otitis media. CWU, canal wall-up; CWD, canal wall-down.

surgery may be limited to the removal of cholesteatoma and reconstruction of the ossicular chain and tympanic membrane. However, in those with otorrhea, even with limited cholesteatoma, a complete tympanomastoidectomy, either canal wall-up or canal wall-down, should be performed. For example, chronic active otitis media with cholesteatoma limited to the attic with no history of otorrhea may be managed successfully with atticotomy and reconstruction without mastoidectomy, whereas chronic active otitis media with cholesteatoma, limited to the attic, but with a history of recurrent or chronic infection, mandates mastoidectomy as well as atticotomy. Similarly, chronic inactive otitis media without frequent reactivation represents an elective surgical candidacy for reconstruction of the tympanic membrane and ossicles and does not require mastoidectomy. By contrast, chronic inactive otitis media with frequent reactivation, that is spontaneous recurrent otorrhea after adequate medical management, generally requires rnastoidectomy. In many of these cases, the recurrent otorrhea may be explained by obstruction of the aditus ad antrum and sequestration of the mastoid air space by "aditus block."[17]

In those cases with chronic active otitis media without cholesteatoma, a trial of medical management should be undertaken. This includes management of potential contributing diseases, and knowledge of the bacteriology of the suppuration. In most patients in whom otorrhea has stopped for at least 6 months, elective tympanoplasty and ossiculoplasty may be considered. For those who fail medical management, those with persistent chronic suppuration should undergo tympanomastoidectomy. Cases in which the suppuration temporarily clears only to recur promptly after cessation of medical management should be reassigned to the category "chronic inactive otitis media with frequent reactivation."

FACTORS AFFECTING CHOICE OF CANAL WALL-UP OR CANAL WALL-DOWN APPROACH

The selection of the canal wall-up versus the canal wall-down approach should be individualized based on the experience of the surgeon and details of the clinical variables of the case in question. Examples of preoperative clinical variables that frequently have an influence on this decision are shown in Table 38–2. For example, a very poorly pneumatized mastoid as determined by preoperative physical examination and imaging is a relatively negative indicator for the canal wall-up approach. Similarly, a unilateral nonhearing ear (dead ear) with chronic otitis media, is a good candidate for canal wall-down surgery and tympanomastoid obliteration. In patients who have had multiple previous procedures, particularly those in whom the canal has been partially or totally removed, I prefer the canal wall-down technique with mastoid obliteration. Individuals with bilateral longstanding chronic otitis media are generally managed by canal wall-down technique.

Intraoperative findings that will suggest selection of the canal wall-down technique include inadequate surgical access with preservation of the canal wall, extensive cholesteatoma, and the presence of complications such as facial paresis or labyrinthine fistula.

TABLE 38–2
Factors Affecting Choice of CWU or CWD Approach

Preoperative	
	Bilateral disease
	Multiple previous procedures
	Only hearing ear
	Pneumatization of mastoid and temporal bone
	Nonhearing ear ("dead ear")
Intraoperative	
	Inadequate surgical access
	Extensive cholesteatoma
	Presence of complication
	Facial paresis
	Labyrinthine fistula

CWU, canal wall-up; CWD, canal wall-down.

TREATMENT ALGORITHM FOR MANAGEMENT OF RECURRENT CHRONIC OTITIS MEDIA (SURGICAL FAILURE)

Although there is obvious similarity in the management of recurrent chronic otitis media with that of primary chronic otitis media, nevertheless there are some differences (Fig. 38–2). I find it useful to categorize these patients into those who have had previous canal wall-up versus those who have had previous canal wall-down surgery. In general, in previous surgical failures, CT imaging in axial and coronal planes is a valuable tool. Recurrent cholesteatoma with or without otorrhea almost always requires revision surgery. However, management of chronic or recurrent otorrhea without cholesteatoma differs significantly between canal wall-up and canal wall-down groups. Thus, those who have had previous canal wall-up surgery are treated in a similar manner as those with primary chronic otitis media without cholesteatoma, but with otorrhea. Depending on the bacteriology of the otorrhea, medical management with topical and oral antibiotics may prove successful. Those with continued or recurrent drainage undergo CT scanning and a revision tympanomastoidectomy, either canal wall-up or canal wall-down. In patients who have undergone previous canal wall-down technique, but who have persistent or recurrent otorrhea (the problematic mastoid bowl), bacteriology is essential. The prevalence of anerobes as pathogens in persistent chronic otitis media after canal wall-down surgery has been estimated to be in the range of 50%.[18-21] The use of antibiotics with good anerobic coverage may result in a dry ear. Mastoid bowls with persistent or recurrent otorrhea, despite otic drops, may become candidates for a diagnostic/therapeutic trial of split-thickness skin grafting, which can be done in the office with minimal morbidity, and may well result in a dry ear. Those with persistent or recurrent otorrhea should undergo CT imaging and revision canal wall-down tympanomastoidectomy with thorough exenteration of residual contaminated air cells, both in the mastoid and in the hypotympanum, with a mastoid obliteration to facilitate postoperative long-term management of the mastoid bowl.

Clinical and Surgical Pitfalls and Tips for Canal Wall-Up and Canal Wall-Down Approaches

It is not the purpose of this essay to go through a step-by-step detailing of the technique of canal wall-up and canal wall-down mastoid surgery. However, based on the author's experience, some very commonly encountered pitfalls are worth considering in both the planning and execution of these techniques.

1. *Inadequate surgical objectives:* Despite total elimination of cholesteatoma, persistent or recurrent otorrhea may ensue. In cases of chronic active otitis media with cholesteatoma, the principal focus of the operating surgeon may be the cholesteatoma itself. However, it should be recognized that the surrounding reaction, including granulation, suppuration, or sequestration of air cells, in both the mastoid and the middle ear, may result in persistent or recurrent drainage.[22] Analysis of failed mastoid tympanoplasty, particularly those without cholesteatoma, provide insight to common locations for residual disease.[11,23-25] In my experience, residual suppurative disease occurs commonly in sequestrated tegmental and sinodural cells, mastoid tip, facial recess, and the hypotympanum.[23,24]
2. *Remember the hypotympanum:* A common cause for failure of tympanomastoidectomy may be residual disease in the hypotympanum. Despite the name chronic "otitis media," it is commonly assumed that the principal site of persistent otorrhea is infection in the mastoid compartment. Although classic training would suggest that edematous mucosa in the middle ear should be preserved in mastoid surgery and that inflammatory changes will subside during the postoperative period, nevertheless, suppuration in hypotympanic and infralabyrinthine cells may be contributory or, in some cases, is the sole cause of persistent otorrhea, particularly in revision cases.[24,26,27]
3. *Adequate intraoperative exposure is not sufficient, particularly in the canal wall-down technique:* Overlooking important ancillary procedures designed primarily for postoperative rather than intraoperative exposure can result in failure. Thus, Sade et al.[28] found a direct correlation between persistent postoperative otorrhea and the size of the mastoid cavity, height of the facial ridge, and adequacy of meatoplasty. A high facial ridge may make it impossible to clean the mastoid cavity thoroughly during the postopera-

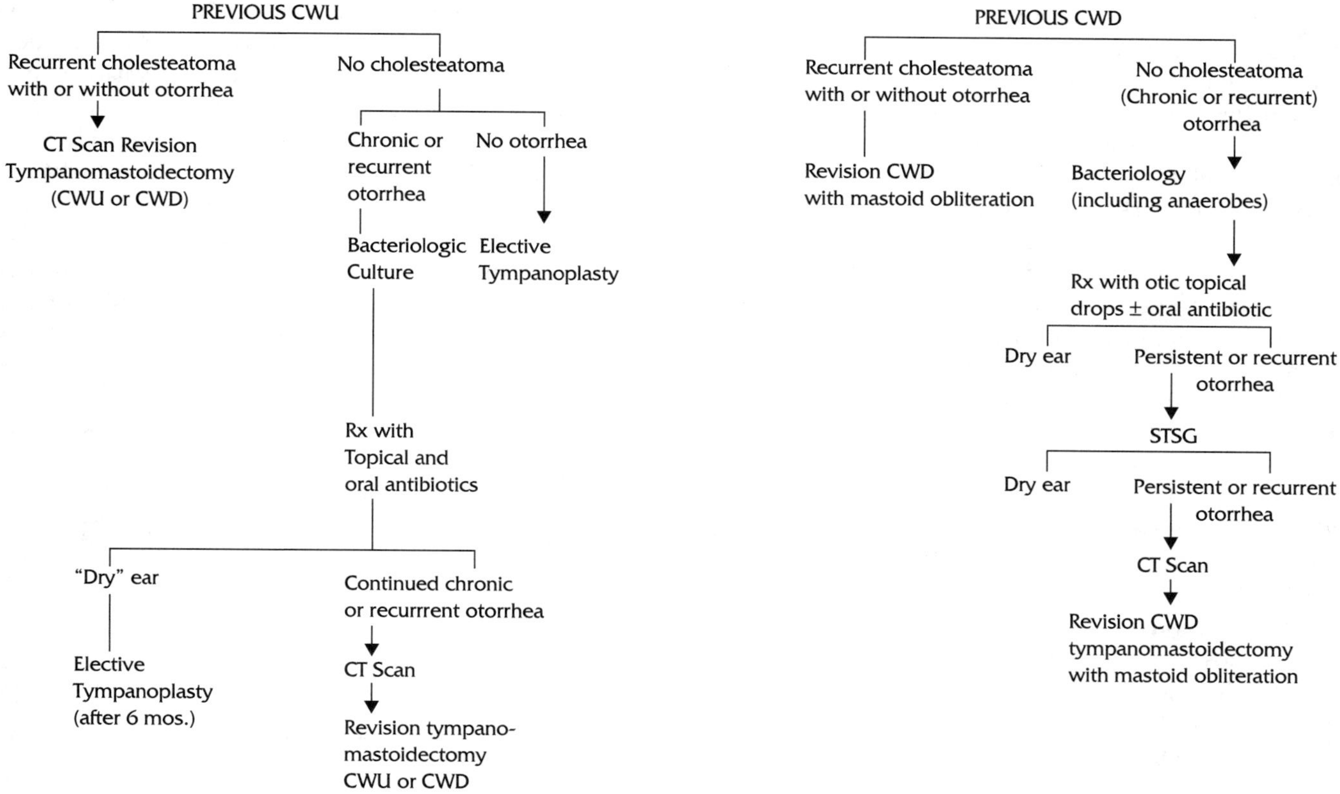

Figure 38–2 Algorithm for management of recurrent chronic otitis media (surgical failure). CWU, canal wall-up; CWD, canal wall-down.

tive period. In chronic otitis media with suppuration, it is probably more important to do a thorough exenteration of residual air cells in the canal wall-down technique than in the canal wall-up approach because the healing phase in the two approaches is fundamentally different. In the canal wall-up technique after complete exenteration of disease, a mucosalized and aerated mastoid air space is the objective. However, in the canal wall-down technique, residual air cells, even if not previously infected, may become subject to suppuration because of surgical sequestration. This is clearly demonstrated in fenestration surgery. In these cases, despite the fact that none had preoperative infection, postoperative residual air cells may become chronically infected due to surgical sequestration of air cells and inability to clean the mastoid cavity because of a high facial ridge or stenotic meatus.

4. *Utility of mastoid obliteration:* In the canal wall-down technique, obliteration of the mastoid cavity serves several important functions with the objective of achieving a dry ear. Even in the most extensive exenteration, residual air cells that are mucosalized still persist. Although this may not be a problem in the canal wall-up technique, it certainly may become a problem in the canal wall-down technique if these residual air cells become sequestrated and infected. Thus, obliteration prevents surface contamination. Second, a healthy soft tissue layer between bone in the outside world results in a more suitable and stable substrate for skin grafts and healthy skin. Third, hygiene of the mastoid bowl is markedly improved by reducing volume and hidden and troublesome crannies.
5. *Remember the limitations imposed by the dysfunctional auditory tube:* Most cases with chronic otitis media have abnormal eustachian tube function that will persist after active suppuration has been controlled. As previously stated, an important objective of mastoid surgery is the prevention of recurrent disease, which is best accomplished by altering the anatomy to avoid recurrence of retraction, cholesteatoma, and suppuration. The restoration of normal-appearing anatomy may fall short of achieving this goal. Thus, in limited attic cholesteatoma, in which an anterior atticotomy is all that is necessary to remove the disease, an attempt should be made to prevent re-retraction of the tympanic graft into the attic and aditus, for example, by the use of cartilage grafts.
6. *Remember the utility of skin grafting:* A mastoid procedure is not fully healed until the canal, tympanic membrane, and bowl, if any, are fully epithelialized with squamous epithelium. It is my practice to use split-thickness skin grafts intraoperatively in almost all cases, in an effort to speed this epithelialization and to lessen the chance of postoperative stenosis and blunting of the anterior angle between the tympanic membrane and the anterior canal wall. In addition,

split-thickness skin grafting may be helpful during the postoperative period and, in some cases, may control chronic suppuration in the problematic mastoid bowl. Thus, despite skin grafting used during the course of mastoid surgery, the recipient bed, including exposed bone and an avascular tympanic graft, may not be suitable recipients for a split-thickness skin grafting until a number of weeks postoperatively. In the problematic mastoid bowl, removal of the pyogenic granulation tissue and the application of split-thickness skin grafts, which can easily be done in the office under local anesthesia, may be curative. At the very least, this approach serves to separate those cases in which the infection is superficial from those with sequestrated disease in residual mastoid cells for which revision surgery is indicated.

7. *Remember the limitations placed by the histologic changes that occur in the tympanomastoid compartment after long-standing suppuration:* Fibrous tissue deposited in the submucosal plane, or "fibrocystic sclerosis," is a consequence of chronic suppuration, and may produce loculation of pneumatized spaces, in both the middle ear and mastoid and limit the reconstructive potential for hearing improvement, especially when this disease occurs in the round window niche.[29] Similarly, tympanosclerosis is common in chronic active otitis media. Not only can it produce changes in the tympanic membrane, it may fix one or more of the ossicles.
8. *Hearing reconstruction: staged versus unstaged:* When the canal wall-up approach is used for chronic otitis media with cholesteatoma, it is the author's practice to perform a second-look procedure approximately 8 to 12 months after the first procedure, as has been advocated by others[15,30-32] with the exception of limited middle ear or attic cholesteatoma.[33] The added safety of a second-look procedure, however, does not preclude primary reconstruction of the ossicular chain in most cases. Thus, it is unnecessary to commit the patient to months of a large or maximal conductive loss just because a second-look procedure may be indicated at a later time. It is my practice to delay ossicular reconstruction only in certain circumstances, such as cases in which the middle ear mucosa has been replaced by granulomatous disease, in which time is necessary to achieve a mucosalized and aerated middle ear compartment, or in such cases in which the footplate is fixed and stapedectomy will be necessary for hearing reconstruction. When the ossicular chain is incomplete, necessitating an interposition, the author prefers autologous bone grafts, except when the superstructure of the stapes is missing. In such cases, a hydroxyapatite TORP is generally used.

Future Research

The entire landscape of surgery for chronic otitis media will change significantly with new insights in restoration of normal eustachian tube function. In addition, most reconstructive procedures that are done in the middle ear are based more on intuition than scientific proof. Research in the area of middle ear mechanics and reconstruction[34,35] is most welcome and will undoubtedly provide better methods of reconstruction in the future.

REFERENCES

Nadol—CHAPTER 38

1. Smyth GDL. Postoperative cholesteatoma in combined approach tympanoplasty. *J Laryngol Otol* 1976;90:591–621
2. Sheehy JL, Brackmann DE, Graham MD. Cholesteatoma surgery: residual and recurrent disease: a review of 1,024 cases. *Ann Otol* 1977;86:451–462
3. Edelstein DR, Parisier SC. Surgical techniques and recidivism in cholesteatoma. *Otolaryngol Clin North Am* 1989;22:1029–1039
4. Abramson M, Lachenbruch PA, Press BH, McCabe BF. Results of conservative surgery for middle ear cholesteatoma. *Laryngoscope* 1977;87:1281–1287
5. Schmid H, Dort JC, Fisch U. Long-term results of treatment for children's cholesteatoma. *Am J Otol* 1991;12:83–92
6. Hirsch BE, Kamerer DB, Doshi S. Single-stage management of colesteatoma. *Otolaryngol Head Neck Surg* 1992;106: 351–354
7. Beales PH. The problem of the mastoid segment after tympanoplasty. *J Laryngol Otol* 1959;73:527–531
8. Palva T. Operative technique in mastoid obliteration. *Acta Otolaryngol (Stockh)* 1973;75:289–290
9. Saunders JE, Shoemaker DL, McElveen JT Jr. Reconstruction of the radial mastoid. *Am J Otol* 1992;13:465–469
10. Vartiainen E, Kansanen M. Tympanomastoidectomy for chronic otitis media without cholesteatoma. *Otolaryngol Head Neck Surg* 1992;106:230–234
11. Veldman JE, Braunius WW. Revision surgery for chronic otitis media: a learning experience. Report on 389 cases with long-term follow-up. *Ann Otol Rhinol Laryngol* 1998;107:486–491
12. Shelton C, Sheehy JL. Tympanoplasty: review of 400 staged cases. *Laryngoscope* 1990;100:679–681
13. Brackmann DE. Tympanoplasty with mastoidectomy: canal wall up procedures. *Am J Otol* 1993;14:380–382
14. Vartiainen E, Vartiainen J. Hearing results of surgery for chronic otitis media without cholesteatoma. *Ear Nose Throat J* 1995;74:165–166, 169

15. Glassock ME III, Miller GW. Intact canal wall tympanoplasty in the management of cholesteatoma. *Laryngoscope* 1976;86:1639–1657
16. Smyth GDL. Cholesteatoma surgery: the influence of the canal wall. *Laryngoscope* 1985;95:92–96
17. Proctor B. Attic-aditus block and the tympanic diaphragm. *Ann Otol Rhinol Laryngol* 1971;80:371–375
18. Jokipii AMM, Karma P, Ojala, K, et al. Anaerobic bacteria in chronic otitis media. *Arch Otolaryngol* 1977;103:278–280
19. Harker LA, Koontz FP. Bacteriology of cholesteatoma: clinical significance. *Trans Am Acad Ophthalmol Otolaryngol* 1977;84:683–686
20. Brook I. Aerobic and anaerobic bacteriology of cholesteatoma. *Laryngoscope* 1981;91:250–253
21. Erkan M, Aslan T, Sevuk E, et al. Bacteriology of chronic suppurative otitis media. *Ann Otol Rhinol Laryngol* 1994;103:771–774
22. Merchant SN, Wang P, Jang CH, et al. Efficacy of tympanomastoid surgery for control of infection in active chronic otitis media. *Laryngoscope* 1997;107:872–877
23. Nadol JB Jr. Causes of failure of mastoidectomy for chronic otitis media. *Laryngoscope* 1985;95:410–413
24. Nadol JB Jr, Krouse JH. The hypotympanum and infralabyrinthine cells in chronic otitis media. *Laryngoscope* 1991;101:137–141
25. Vartiainen E, Virtaniemi J. Findings in revision operations for failures after cholesteatoma surgery. *Am J Otol* 1994;15:229–232
26. Proctor B. Chronic middle ear disease. *Arch Otolaryngol* 1963;78:276–283
27. Savic D, Djeric D. Surgical anatomy of the hypotympanum. *J Laryngol Otol* 1987;101:419–425
28. Sade J, Weinberg E, Berco M, et al. The marsupialized (radical) mastoid. *J Laryngol Otol* 1982;96:869–875
29. Nadol JB Jr. Chronic otitis media. In: Nadol JB Jr, Schuknecht HF, eds. *Surgery of the Ear and Temporal Bone.* New York: Raven Press; 1993:155–170
30. Sheehy JL, Crabtree JA. Tympanoplasty: staging the operation. *Laryngoscope* 1973;83:1594–1621
31. Smyth GDL. Surgical treatment of cholesteatoma: the role of staging in closed operations. *Ann Otol Rhinol Laryngol* 1988;97:667–669
32 Tos M, Lau T. Attic cholesteatoma: recurrence rate related to observation time. *Am J Otol* 1988;9:456–464
33. Austin DF. Single-stage surgery for cholesteatoma: an actuarial analysis. *Am J Otol* 1989;10:419–425
34. Rosowski JJ, Davis PJ, Merchant SN, et al. Cadaver middle ears as models for living ears: comparisons of middle ear input immittance. *Ann Otol Rhinol Laryngol* 1990;99:403–412
35. Merchant NS, Rosowski JJ, Ravicz ME. Middle ear mechanics of type IV and type V tympanoplasty II. Clinical analysis and surgical implications. *Am J Otol* 1995;16:565–575

Management of Cholesteatoma*

CHAPTER 39

James L. Sheehy

There have been very few changes in the techniques of management of cholesteatoma since the mid-1970s, but controversies remain. It is not uncommon to attend a scientific meeting, listen to three presentations on a subject, and hear that each (different) technique or prosthesis is "the only way to do it." "It gives perfect results." "If you do it my way you will get results just like mine."

Of course, none of these statements is true. There are many ways to accomplish a desired result, but nothing works perfectly. The results you obtain will depend on your personal ability to use your hands and instruments and on your judgment. There's an old saying that judgment comes from experience, and experience comes from bad judgment! So what any of us do, or teach, is based on having had problems and learning how to avoid them: *what* to do, *how* to do it, and *what not* to do: judgment!

This chapter summarizes the many factors involved in making a decision on management of cholesteatoma, particularly the management of the mastoid. I leave it up to the reader to review articles mentioned in the Suggested Readings for in-depth discussion on various aspects of management.

Aims and Objectives

There were two aims or objectives in the management of cholesteatoma long before the introduction of tympanoplasty: to obtain a safe ear and, one hoped, a dry ear. These were accomplished by a radical or modified radical mastoidectomy. With the introduction of tympanoplasty during the mid-1950s, a third objective was added: a hearing ear. This also introduced a controversy: how hard do you try to improve the hearing? This led to much controversy unrelated to the manner of management of the mastoid. How hard should you try to improve the hearing? To stage or not to stage?

The aims and objectives of surgery on the ear with cholesteatoma, then, are (1) eliminate the disease: obtain a safe, dry, ear; and (2) restore the function: obtain a good hearing ear.

Type of Operation

The number one aim of cholesteatoma surgery is to obtain a safe, dry ear. The classic radical mastoidectomy accomplished the safety factor. When preservation of hearing was deemed feasible, the operation used was a modified radical mastoidectomy, a procedure that involved preservation of the tympanic membrane and ossicles while exteriorizing the epitympanum and mastoid to the ear canal. (The modified radical mastoidectomy is not a tympanoplasty, contrary to the way the term is often used today by some people.)

With the advent of tympanoplasty during the mid-1950s, it became possible, in many cases, to restore function rather than to just preserve whatever function remained. The mastoidectomy was canal wall-down (CWD), as it had been with a modified radical or radical. But a problem developed: a narrow middle ear space. And the space often collapsed, of course, blamed on the eustachian tube. There was no help for the hearing.

To avoid this narrowing of the middle ear space the canal wall-up (CWU) procedure was developed, also called the intact canal wall tympanoplasty with mastoidectomy, combined approach tympanoplasty, and posterior tympanotomy approach. This was similar to a simple (or cortical) mastoidectomy, as had been done for more than 50 years for the treatment of acute mastoiditis.

The middle ear space was much wider, so prostheses were needed to transfer the sound vibrations from the tympanic membrane to the inner ear. This worked fine in some cases: a dry ear, no mastoid cavity, and improved hearing. But problems developed early on, leading many otologists to decide that the CWU procedure was not wise. If the middle ear was not mucosal lined, and air containing, the tympanic membrane retracted. Any ossicular prosthesis might well extrude. More important, a postero-superior retraction pocket might develop leading to *recurrence* of cholesteatoma, requiring a second operation, usually a CWD procedure.

Add to this the fact that bits of cholesteatoma matrix may have been left behind gave trouble, requiring further surgery to remove this *residual disease* in the mastoid, epitympanum, and middle ear. Was there any good reason to use the CWU rather than the CWD procedure?

Many otologists felt there was not a good reason to use the CWU rather than the CWD procedure. A major reason was the need to perform the operation in two stages, at times, to avoid the problem of *residual* and *recurrent* cholesteatoma.

Counseling the Patient

Counseling the patient is an individual matter. It relates to the surgeon's personal experience, the status of the ear and the patient's ability to understand what you are saying. Let us assume this is a patient with a draining ear and cholesteatoma with a 30-dB conductive deficit. Using our chronic ear patient discussion booklet, we explain how a normal ear functions and then show a

* This work was supported by funds from the House Ear Institute, affiliated with the University of Southern California.

second drawing of the ear with skin growing into the ear and forming a cholesteatoma. The explanation usually proceeds in the following way, and is the same for CWU and CWD:

> Cholesteatoma is an in-growth of skin into the mastoid. This forms a skin lined cyst called a cholesteatoma. It is not a tumor, but does tend to get larger as time goes on if the ear continues to drain.
>
> There are three reasons why your ear should have surgery. In the first place, the cholesteatoma is potentially dangerous. If the drainage continues over a long period of time about 10 to 20% of individuals may eventually develop severe dizziness because of the cholesteatoma breaking into a balance canal. This could also result in a total loss of hearing. There's also the possibility the cholesteatoma could break into the nerve to the face or break into the covering of the brain. The likelihood of these certainly is less than 1%.
>
> Secondly, the longer the problem goes on, the more damage there may be to the hearing. Finally, there is a matter of the drainage.
>
> So the objectives of the surgery are to obtain a safe ear, a dry ear, and a hearing ear. Getting a safe, dry ear is almost certain. Unfortunately, to obtain a good hearing result it may be necessary to do the operation in two steps. The hearing is often worse following the first operation. There is a 60 to 70% chance you will end up with good hearing following the second operation.
>
> I have made some notations of all this in the booklet. In the back of the booklet there is an area called Risks and Complications of Surgery. The only complication that happens with any degree of regularity, and is serious, is a total, 100%, loss of hearing in the operated ear. The likelihood of this is no more than 1 to a 2% chance; all of the other things listed here are either very remote or are temporary.

The Risks and Complications sheet appears as an appendix to this chapter. If the patient has a labyrinthine fistula, the patient should be told that there is a 10% chance of a total loss of hearing as a result of the surgery. Prolonged dizziness that would eventually subside may also occur.

Making Decisions

IS SURGERY NECESSARY?

If surgery is necessary, how soon should it be performed? Unless there is some clear-cut indication of an impending complication there is usually no reason to treat the active cholesteatoma as urgent. The exception is when the discharge is through a small attic perforation, and/or there is night pain, or a positive fistula test or facial weakness.

When the cholesteatoma has developed from a posterior superior retraction pocket (has a "large" opening) and there are no symptoms other than discharge (and hearing loss), then it may be treated electively. Explain that it is best to operate sometime to avoid any complications or further loss of hearing, and let the patient decide. In such cases, frequent follow-up is indicated.

The exception to the above comments is when dealing with an only hearing ear: the indication for surgery (modified radical mastoidectomy—not a tympanoplasty) is to prevent further loss of hearing.

TYPE OF SURGERY?

Canal wall-up or canal wall-down? If CWD, a tympanoplasty or a modified radical mastoidectomy? For those who prefer the CWU procedure (as we do at House Ear Clinic), there are some clear-cut indications to use the CWD technique, decisions made preoperatively. Most of these would be a modified radical mastoidectomy: only hearing ear (or by far the better hearing ear), labyrinthine fistula in a sclerotic mastoid, or elderly patient.

Why CWD in the above situations? Is it a safer procedure? The reason for a classic modified radical mastoidectomy is to avoid "disturbing" the hearing and to avoid the need for a second-stage procedure. Leave it as it is.

TO STAGE OR NOT TO STAGE?

Staging the operation is a controversial subject, even in the hands of some of those who use a CWU procedure. The absence of mucosa is a major factor, but I shall limit discussion to the extent of cholesteatoma and the certainty of its removal.

In noncholesteatoma cases staging is not usually needed. In cholesteatoma cases we stage 70% or more of the tympanoplasties because of both mucosal disease problems and the certainty (or uncertainty) of removal of cholesteatoma—the possibility of residual cholesteatoma.

Residual cholesteatoma is not related to recurrent cholesteatoma. Recurrent cholesteatoma rarely develops in CWD procedures. Recurrent cholesteatoma is preventable: residual cholesteatoma is not. The incidence of residual cholesteatoma in the middle ear is the same (in our hands) for CWU and CWD.

PREOPERATIVE TESTING

What tests one does preoperatively is an individual matter. At House Ear Clinic, we do not routinely take radiographs (CT scans) nor do we test eustachian tube function or culture the draining ear. Hearing tests (air, bone, and speech), are done immediately before surgery.

AGE OF THE PATIENT

We are more likely to encourage early surgery in children with active cholesteatoma. Often their mastoids are well developed, and they have extensive cholesteatosis; in these cases, we are more likely to use the CWU. We are more likely to use a CWU in children because this avoids the problem that could come about with getting water in the ear.

In elderly patients, particularly if there is a major health problem, a CWD procedure, usually a modified radical mastoidectomy, is the best choice. "Simple and safe," and no need for staging.

FACIAL NERVE MONITORING

In most cases, we do not monitor the facial nerve unless there is an impending complication or this is revision of an operation performed elsewhere.

Conclusion

The management of cholesteatoma remains controversial. The major issues are whether to leave the CWU and whether to stage the procedure. At the House Ear Clinic, we prefer the CWU technique in most cases. This often requires a staged procedure in extensive cholesteatoma and badly diseased ears. We do not hesitate to do a CWD procedure when indicated.

In either case, a safe and dry ear is achieved in more than 90% of patients. Hearing improvement can be achieved in most, regardless of the severity of the disease, but this will often require a second-stage procedure.

Appendix: Risks and Complications of Tympanoplasty

EAR INFECTION

Ear infection, with drainage, swelling, and pain, may persist after surgery or, on rare occasions, may develop after surgery due to poor healing of the ear tissue. Were this to be the case, additional surgery might be necessary to control the infection.

LOSS OF HEARING

Further permanent impairment of hearing develops in 3% of patients due to problems in the healing process. In 2% of cases, this loss of hearing may be severe or total in the operated ear. Nothing further can be done in these instances. When a two-stage operation is necessary, hearing is usually worse after the first operation.

TINNITUS

If the hearing is worse after surgery, tinnitus (head noise) may be more pronounced as well.

DIZZINESS

Dizziness can occur immediately after surgery due to irritation of the inner ear structures. Some unsteadiness may persist for 1 week postoperatively. Prolonged dizziness is rare unless there was a problem with dizziness before surgery.

TASTE DISTURBANCE AND MOUTH DRYNESS

Taste disturbance and mouth dryness are not uncommon for a few weeks after surgery. In some patients, this disturbance is prolonged.

FACIAL PARALYSIS

A rare postoperative complication of ear surgery is temporary paralysis of one side of the face. This can occur as the result of an abnormality or can be caused by swelling of the nerve. It usually subsides spontaneously. On very rare occasions, the nerve may be injured during surgery, or it may be necessary to excise it in order to eradicate infection. When this happens, a skin sensation nerve is removed from the upper part of the neck to replace the facial nerve. Under these circumstances, paralysis of the face lasts 6 months to 1 year and there would be a permanent residual weakness. Eye complications, requiring treatment by a specialist, could develop.

SUGGESTED READINGS

Committee on Conservation of Hearing of the American Academy of Ophthalmology and Otolaryngology: Standard Classification for Surgery of Chronic Ear Infection: I. Of the Technical Procedures in Surgery for Chronic Ear Infection: II. Of the Gross Pathology Found at Such Operations: III. For the reporting of Postoperative Results of the Surgical Procedures Mentioned. *Arch Otolaryngol* 1965;81:204–210

House JW, Sheehy JL. Cholesteatoma with intact tympanic membrane: a report of 41 cases. *Laryngoscope* 1980;90: 70–76

Kohut RI. Cholesteatoma: the advantages of modified radical and radical mastoidectomy. In: Snow JB Jr, ed. *Controversy in Otolaryngology.* Philadelphia: WB Saunders; 1980: 223–227

Litton WB, Krause CJ, Anson BA, et al. The relationship of the facial canal to the annular sulcus. *Laryngoscope* 1969;79: 1584–1604

Sheehy JL. Intact canal wall tympanoplasty with mastoidectomy. In: Snow JB Jr, ed. *Controversy in Otolaryngology.* Philadelphia: WB Saunders; 1980:213–222

Sheehy JL. Testing eustachian tube function. *Ann Otol Rhinol Laryngol* 1981;90:562–565

Sheehy JL. Cholesteatoma surgery in children. *Am J Otol* 1985; 6:170–172

Sheehy JL. Cholesteatoma surgery: canal wall down procedures. *Ann Otol Rhinol Laryngol* 1988;97:30–35

Sheehy JL. Mastoidectomy: the intact canal wall procedure. In: Brackmann DE, Shelton C, Arriaga MA, eds. *Otologic Surgery.* Philadelphia: WB Saunders; 1994:211–224

Sheehy JL, Brackmann DE. Cholesteatoma surgery: management of the labyrinthine fistula—a report of 97 cases. *Laryngoscope* 1979;89:78–87

Sheehy JL, Brackmann DE. Surgery of chronic ear disease: what we do and why we do it. *Instructional Courses* C.V. Mosby; 1993; 6:349–353

Sheehy JL, Brackmann DE. Surgery of chronic otitis media. In: English GM, ed. *Otolaryngology.* Philadelphia:1994

Sheehy JL, Robinson JV. Cholesteatoma surgery at the Otologic Medical Group: residual and recurrent disease: a report on 307 revision operations. *Am J Otol* 1982;3:209–215

Sheehy JL, Shelton C. Tympanoplasty: to stage or not to stage. *Otolaryngol Head Neck Surg* 1991;104:399–407

Sheehy JL, Brackmann DE, Graham MD. Complications of cholesteatoma: a report on 1,024 cases. In: McCabe BF, Sade J, Abramson M, eds. *Cholesteatoma: First International Conference.* Birmingham, AL: Aesculapius; 1977:420–429

14

Acute Facial Paralysis

"Surgical treatment of Bell's palsy is controversial. A clear efficacy of this surgery must be achieved because the complications of subtemporal middle fossa surgery, although infrequent, include epidural hematoma, seizure, cerebrospinal fluid leakage, meningitis, facial nerve injury, deafness, and vertigo."

Samuel H. Selesnick

"Surgical decompression of the facial nerve has been shown to be highly effective in restoration of normal facial function."

Jack L. Pulec

"Anatomic disruption of the facial nerve is an absolute indication for exploration and possible grafting. Determining the extent of injury preoperatively with CT scans and electrical testing can be difficult. Even with direct inspection during surgery, an accurate determination can be difficult because of disease, traumatic anatomic distortion, and surgeon bias."

Douglas A. Chen

Acute Facial Paralysis

Samuel H. Selesnick

CHAPTER 40

Like many topics in otology, the diagnosis and management of acute facial paralysis generate controversy. Acute facial paralysis can be idiopathic, traumatic, iatrogenic, infectious, or inflammatory, whereas facial paralysis of gradual onset is most often attributed to a neoplastic or chronic inflammatory process and should therefore be considered separately. Facial paralysis can be complete or partial; it may be global, involving all branches, or segmental, involving fewer than all branches. Generally, segmental facial paralysis occurs as a result of a peripheral, nonotologic pathology, distal to the stylomastoid foramen.

This chapter addresses issues in the diagnosis and management of complete, global, and acute-onset paralysis, by far the most common type. The most common type of complete, global, and acute-onset facial paralysis is Bell's palsy, the primary focus of this chapter which acounts for 75% of all facial palsies.[1] However, the management of other etiologies of acute facial paralysis is controversial as well. For example, blunt temporal bone trauma may result in temporal bone fracture and facial paralysis. Immediate and complete facial paralysis in this setting should be surgically explored, whereas partial delayed facial paralysis should be observed. There are patients, however, who sustain a temporal bone fracture and then go on to develop a complete but delayed facial paralysis. In the care of these patients, some investigators suggest that surgical decompression of the facial nerve after electroneuronography (ENOG) falls below 90% degeneration improves outcome, whereas others suggest that intervention does not improve ultimate facial function in this group. A large recent study addressing temporal bone fracture conducted by Brodie and Thompson[2] in 1997 followed 820 patients with temporal bone fractures, 58 of whom had facial nerve injuries. All patients with partial facial paralysis recovered completely. Of the 58 patients with facial nerve injuries, 9 had a delayed complete facial paralysis. Six of the 9 patients were observed, and all fully recovered. Three of the 9 patients underwent surgical decompression. Two of these patients recovered, and one remained paralyzed. McKennan and Chole[3] reported in 1992 reported on the outcome of 19 patients who developed delayed complete facial paralysis. In this series, 94% returned to normal without intervention. Our institution also follows a conservative course for this controversial group of patients with posttraumatic delayed facial paralysis.

Acute facial paralysis may also result from acute infectious ear disease such as otitis media. In these cases, urgent myringotomy and pressure-equalizing tube placement in conjuction with intravenous antibiotics is indicated. In some cases, however, the facial paralysis does not resolve; it remains controversial whether and when a mastoidectomy should be performed. Some investigators recommend mastoidectomy as early as 2 days after myringotomy, and some as late as 10 days.[4,5] Because aggressive drainage has been accomplished by myringotomy, cultures have been acquired, and intravenous antibiotics instituted, our institution adopts a less aggressive posture toward early mastoidectomy, waiting at least a full week. At the time of mastoidectomy in these patients, the epineurium should be left intact over the facial nerve because it acts as a protective barrier against further spread of infection, and the risk to facial nerve injury is high, as it is edematous, erythematous, friable, and polypoid in the face of acute infection.

Whereas acute iatrogenic postoperative facial nerve paralysis is most common after cerebellopontine angle surgery for acoustic neuroma, no immediate surgical intervention is indicated, as the facial nerve is already decompressed. However, in otologic surgery, unanticipated acute postoperative facial paralysis may occur, requiring removal of ear canal packing and dressings. If no return of facial function occurs, it is often wise to seek a consultation with another otologic surgeon, to gain additional insight in both operative and nonoperative management. The adage "the sun should never set on an acute postoperative facial paralysis after otologic surgery," although not entirely true, does impart the urgency of this problem, and the need for intervention as soon as possible, once more innocuous etiologies of facial paralysis have been excluded, such as facial paralysis due to effects of local anesthesia. A wide decompression of the facial nerve should be performed at reexploration. Splitting the epineural sheath can further decompress an edematous and traumatized nerve.

As noted earlier, Bell's palsy is the most common cause of acute-onset complete, global facial paralysis, and typically presents as an abrupt onset facial paralysis that may be accompanied by otalgia, hyperacusis, or in some cases, other cranial neuropathies.

Although the etiology of Bell's palsy has been attributed to vascular, autoimmune, and inflammatory causes, evidence for a herpes simplex virus (HSV) infection is most compelling. In the past, only indirect evidence for HSV-1 infection was available, but in 1996 Murakami et al.[6] clarified the role of this virus in Bell's palsy. These investigators pro-spectively assessed endoneurial fluid from 14 patients with Bell's palsy, 9 with herpes zoster oticus, and 12 with normal controls. These investigators then went on to use the polymerase chain reaction (PCR) and Southern blot analysis in an attempt to identify the viral genomes of the HSV-1, herpes zoster virus (HZV), and Epstein-Barr virus (EBV). Although 79% of patients with Bell's palsy were found to have HSV-1 DNA in their endoneurial fluid, none of the patients with herpes zoster oticus or normal controls were found to have HSV-1 DNA in their fluid samples. The presence of HSV-1 infection of the facial nerve is thought to lead to inflammation and edema. In 1983, Fisch and Felix[7] proposed the entrapment theory, which states that the narrowest portion of the bony fallopian canal of the facial nerve is the meatal foramen where the facial nerve leaves the internal auditory canal and enters the labyrinthine segment and, that at this segment, edema leads to compression of the nerve itself and of its local blood supply, resulting in clinical facial nerve dysfunction. Electrophysiologic conduction studies have confirmed the meatal foramen as the site of conduction block, thus supporting the entrapment theory.[8,9]

Bell's palsy has a favorable prognosis, as demonstrated in the often cited study by Pietersen from 1982. This study followed 1011 patients with complete or partial Bell's palsy and found that 85% recovered to normal within 1 year without treatment.[10] Patients who recovered fully began their recovery within the 3 weeks after onset of facial nerve dysfunction. Good prognostic indicators were early onset of recovery, young age, and incomplete paralysis.

Formulation of a treatment plan is dependent on identification of the 15% of patients with Bell's palsy who do not fully recover. Both imaging studies and electophysiologic studies of the facial nerve have been used in this aim. Computed tomography (CT) scan of the temporal bone cannot demonstrate subtle facial nerve inflammation; MRI assessment of the facial nerve has been disappointing as well. Although magnetic resonance imaging (MRI) often shows enhancement of the facial nerve in Bell's palsy, no correlation with site of enhancement or degree of enhancement and ultimate facial nerve outcome has been made.[11,12] The primary role for MRI in Bell's palsy is to exclude the possibility of other mass lesions that can lead to facial nerve paralysis. Topognostic testing has no role in the assessment of facial paralysis due to its inadequate ability to predict clinical outcome.

ENOG does have predictive power. Nerve excitability testing and maximal stimulation testing are electrophysiologic tests that are subjectively interpreted by the examiner and that have, by definition, poor objectivity. Electromyography (EMG) becomes most useful after 3 weeks, at a point when the opportunity for effective aggressive intervention has passed. Also known as evoked EMG in the neurology literature, ENOG is performed by applying suprathreshold electrical excitation of the facial nerve transcutaneously at the stylomastoid foramen, and recording the electrical waveforms generated by muscles innervated by the facial nerve, at the nasolabial groove. Comparison is made between the affected side and the contralateral, and presumably normal, side. If there is greater than 90% degeneration of the amplitude of the ENOG waveform on the affected side, the prognosis worsens. The study that established ENOG as a reliable prognostic tool was published in 1977 by Esslen.[13] He found that of those patients with 90 to 97% degeneration, 30% recovered fully; of those patients with 98 to 99% degeneration, 14% recovered fully; and of those with 100% degeneration, none recovered fully. In comparison, all patients with <90% degeneration recovered fully. A larger and more recent study conducted by Tojima et al.[14] in 1994 found that 80% or less degeneration was the criterion for complete recovery. In their study of 551 patients, Tojima and colleagues found that of patients with 80 to 89% degeneration, 85% recovered fully; of patients with 90 to 99% degeneration, 50% recovered fully; and of patients with 100% degeneration, none recovered fully. Tojima et al. found the ENOG nadir to occur on day 8 of paralysis, whereas Esslen found the ENOG nadir to occur on day 10.[13,14] Disadvantages of ENOG include cost, discomfort, and test–retest variability of up to 11.2% of cases.[15-17]

Treatment of Bell's palsy should be instituted early. In 1990, a retrospective study of 1235 patients found that the administration of oral steroids, traditionally used to treat Bell's palsy, had no siginificant effect on ultimate clinical facial nerve outcome.[18] It was not until 1993 that a well-constructed double-blind placebo-controlled but unmatched study of 76 patients found that oral steroids did improve outcome after Bell's palsy.[19] This study by Austin and coworkers, used the House–Brackmann grading scale of I–VI. All patients treated with steroids were in the good outcome group of grades I and II, whereas 17% of patients not treated with steroids fell into grade III. None of the patients in the study had poor outcomes of grades IV, V, or VI. These results were statistically significant. A double-blind randomized controlled study in 1996 found that the addition of acyclovir to a steroid regimen led to no improvement in patients whose condition deteriorated to complete facial paralysis; however, it led to significant improvement in patients with milder forms of paresis, a group that already has a good prognosis.[20]

It is imperative that any patient with facial weakness, and who lacks the inability to blink effectively, be treated with hourly saline eye drops in the affected eye, and that nightly ophthalmic ointment be placed on the eye as well. The use of an eye patch at night carries the risk that the upper lid will open slightly beneath the patch, exposing the cornea to direct contact with the patch itself, leading to a conjunctivitis or corneal abrasion. Hermetically sealed eye bubbles circumvent the problem of direct contact with a foreign object during sleep, but bubbles are effective only if they are hermetically sealed around the eye with an adhesive. Natural skin oils can keep the adhesive from maintaining a hermetically sealed chamber, thereby negating any benefit of this device.

Surgical treatment of Bell's palsy is controversial. The rationale of surgical therapy goes back to the entrapment theory proposed by Fisch,[21] in which edema of the nerve leads to direct nerve compression and to ischemia of the local vasculature at the site of greatest narrowing of the bony fallopian canal, the meatal foramen, and the labyrinthine segment. A clear efficacy of this surgery must be achieved because the complications of subtemporal middle fossa surgery, although infrequent, include epidural hematoma, seizure, cerebrospinal fluid (CSF) leakage, meningitis, facial nerve injury, deafness, and vertigo. The original work supporting middle fossa facial nerve decompression in Bell's palsy was put forth by Fisch in 1981.[21] In an earlier small study, Fisch[22] found that when ENOG deteriorated to 90% degeneration, it had a very good chance of deteriorating further; if this occurred, one-half of patients would have unsatisfactory outcomes based on a facial nerve grading system that he used at that time. Fisch found that maximal degeneration occurred by day 14 after paralysis: thus, his criteria for surgical intervention were complete facial paralysis and ENOG degeneration of 90% within 14 days of paralysis. Only 6% of patients with Bell's palsy followed by Fisch met these criteria. Fisch used a 0 to 100% facial nerve function scale at that time. Of the 14 patients offered surgery, 7 accepted and had a facial nerve score of 79%, whereas the 7 patients who met criteria but refused surgery had a score of 64%. The improvement with surgery was statistically significant but, as shown by the data, the numbers in this study are small.

Several other investigators have tried to corroborate these findings using the same criteria for surgical intervention. Rubinstein and Gantz,[23] reported on the combined data from three centers: the University of Iowa,[23] the University of Michigan,[24] and Baylor University.[25] The pooling of data was necessary to accrue adequate numbers to gain statistical power. In this collation, Rubinstein and Gantz found that 92% of patients who underwent surgical decompression of the facial nerve by a middle fossa route had grade I or II function, whereas a second group of pooled patients meeting criteria for surgical intervention who were instead treated with steroids had a grade I or II outcome in 45%. These new data underscore an important point: the number of patients presenting to an otolaryngologist during the first 2 weeks after facial paralysis who are willing to undergo ENOG testing and ultimately elective craniotomy surgery for a disease entity with an overall good prognosis, are few in number, as the cumulative institutional experiences at three centers were necessary to make an important statement about the efficacy of surgical intervention.

Herpes zoster oticus, also know as Ramsey–Hunt syndrome, is similar in pathophysiology to Bell's palsy, but is caused by HZV. This has been demonstrated in specimens from patients with herpes zoster octicus by identifying herpes zoster DNA from archival temporal bone DNA using PCR and cloning.[26] The classic presentation of this entity includes a vesicular eruption of the concha bowl, as well as facial paralysis and sensorineural hearing loss. The principles of treatment are similar to those of Bell's palsy, but the prognosis for return of normal facial function is far more grave. In a study by Devriese and Moesker,[27] only 10% of patients with complete facial paralysis went on to recover fully. As in the case of Bell's palsy, MRI is unable to predict outcome. Steroids are used in treatment but, when an antiviral agent is employed, valcyclovir is used instead of acyclovir, due to its greater action on HZV. The arguments for surgical decompression are much the same as those in Bell's palsy.

It is clear that the management of acute facial paralysis is still evolving, with many unresolved issues being investigated. Scientific inquiry may lead to healthy controversy until superior diagnostic or treatment methods have been established.

REFERENCES

Selesnick—CHAPTER 40

1. Adour KK. Current concepts in neurology: diagnosis and management of facial paralysis. *N Engl J Med* 1982;307: 348–351
2. Brodie HA, Thompson TC. Management of complications from 820 temporal bone fractures. *Am J Otol* 1997;18: 188–197
3. McKennan KX, Chole RA. Facial paralysis in temporal bone trauma. *Am J Otol* 1992;13:167–172
4. Pollock RA, Brown LA. Facial paralysis in otitis media. In: Graham MD, House WF, eds. *Disorders of the Facial Nerve.* New York: Raven, 1982:175–205
5. Goldstein NA, Casselbrant ML, Bluestone CD, et al. Intratemporal complications of acute otitis media in infants and children. *Otolaryngol-Head Neck Surg* 1998;119:444–454
6. Murakami S, Mizobuchi M, Nakashiro Y, et al. Bell palsy and herpes simplex virus: identification of viral DNA in endoneurial fluid and muscle. *Ann Intern Med* 1996;124:27–30
7. Fisch U, Felix H. On the pathogenesis of Bell's palsy. *Acta Otolaryngol (Stockh)* 1983;95:532–538
8. Fisch U, Esslen E. Total intratemporal exposure of the facial nerve. Pathologic findings in Bell's palsy. *Arch Otolaryngol* 1972;95:335–341
9. Gantz BJ, Gmur A, Fisch U. Intraoperative evoked electromyography in Bell's palsy. *Am J Otolaryngol* 1982;3: 273–278
10. Peitersen E. The natural history of Bell's palsy. *Am J Otol* 1982;4:107–111
11. Murphy TP, Teller DC. Magnetic resonance imaging of the facial nerve during Bell's palsy. *Otolaryngol Head Neck Surg* 1991;105:667–674
12. Korzec K, Sobol SM, Kubal W, et al. Gadolinium-enhanced magnetic resonance imaging of the facial nerve in herpes zoster oticus and Bell's palsy: clinical implications. *Am J Otol* 1991;12:163–168

13. Esslen E. Investigation on the localization and pathogenesis of meato-labyrinthine facial palsies. In: Esslen E, ed. *The Acute Facial Palsies*. Berlin: Springer-Verlag; 1977:41–91
14. Tojima H, Aoyagi M, Inamura H, Koike Y. Clinical advantages of electroneurography in patients with Bell's palsy within two weeks after onset. *Acta Otolaryngol* 1994;511(suppl):147–149
15. Hughes GB, Josey AF, Glasscock ME, et al. Clinical electroneurography: statistical analysis of controlled measures in twenty-two normal subjects. *Laryngoscope* 1981;91: 1834–1846
16. Hughes GB, Nodar RH, Williams GW. Analysis of test-retest variability in facial electroneurography. *Otolaryngol Head Neck Surg* 1983;91:290–293
17. Fisch U. Maximal nerve excitability testing vs electroneuronography. *Arch Otolaryngol* 1980;106:352–357
18. Devriese PP, Schumacher T, Scheide A, at al. Incidence, prognosis and recovery of Bell's palsy. A survey of about 1000 patients (1974–1983). *Clin Otolaryngol* 1990;15:15–27
19. Austin JR, Peskind SP, Austin SG, Rice DH. Idiopathic facial nerve paralysis: a randomized double blind controlled study of placebo versus prednisone. *Laryngoscope* 1993;103: 1326–1333
20. Adour KK, Ruboyianes JM, Von Doersten PG, et al. Bell's palsy treatment with acyclovir and prednisone compared with prednisone alone: a double-blind, randomized, controlled trial. *Ann Otol Rhinol Laryngol* 1996;105:371–378
21. Fisch U. Surgery for Bell's palsy. *Arch Otolaryngol* 1981;107: 1–11
22. Fisch U. Diagnostic studies on idiopathic facial palsy. In: *Shambaugh Fifth International Workshop on Middle Ear Microsurgery and Fluctuant Hearing Loss.* Chicago: Strode; 1997, 1977
23. Rubinstein JT, Gantz BJ. Facial nerve disorders. In: Hughes GB, Pensak ML, eds. *Clinical Otology*. New York: Thieme Medical; 1997:367–380
24. Sillman JS, Niparko JK, Lee SS, Kileny PR. Prognostic value of evoked and standard electromyography in acute facial paralysis. *Otolaryngol Head Neck Surg* 1992;107:377–381
25. Marsh MA, Coker NJ. Surgical decompression of idiopathic facial palsy. *Otolaryngol Clin North Am* 1991;24:675–689
26. Wackym PA. Molecular temporal bone pathology. II. Ramsay Hunt syndrome (herpes zoster oticus). *Laryngoscope* 1997; 107:1165–1175
27. Devriese PP, Moesker WH. The natural history of facial paralysis in herpes zoster. *Clin Otolaryngol* 1988;13:289–298

Acute Facial Paralysis*

CHAPTER 41

Jack L. Pulec

There is probably no benign ailment that causes patients more physical and emotional suffering than facial palsy.[1-4] The curse of permanent facial disfigurement is a burden to patients who sustain it and, for most, it is difficult to accept. Bell's palsy can result in a lifetime of facial disfigurement if not treated promptly and properly. The sudden development of facial paralysis constitutes a medical and surgical emergency. The patient must consult an otologist immediately so that medical treatment is initiated within the first few hours after the onset of palsy. Thorough diagnostic evaluation must be completed within a few days and surgical decompression of the nerve accomplished before the 6th day of complete paralysis. In the year 2000, management in this manner of acute facial palsy, one type of which is Bell's palsy, is the only way that normal facial function can be routinely restored in almost every patient.[3] Once irreparable damage to the facial nerve has occurred because of delayed or inadequate treatment, normal facial expression is seldom attained. Unfortunately, few physicians are knowledgeable about Bell's palsy, and fewer still are trained to perform surgery of the nerve. In addition, most physicians minimize the significance of facial disfigurement to the patient. Although the facts regarding Bell's palsy have been known and published for several decades, they have been ignored and obscured by unsubstantiated, unscientific misleading opinions. This chapter reviews the known facts, the author's analysis of the implications of these facts, and the best treatment of acute facial palsy.

Established Facts about Acute Facial (Bell's) Palsy

1. *No* test is available to determine prognosis before it is too late to avoid risk of a poor result.[5]
2. Without treatment, 29% of patients with acute facial palsy have permanent disfigurement.[1]
3. The cause of acute facial palsy is edema of the facial nerve in the fallopian canal.[3,5]
4. Recovery beginning within 5 days of the onset results in 100% recovery.[1]
5. Surgery performed while nerve excitability tests are normal results in 100% recovery.[5]
6. In Bell's palsy, edema involves only the mastoid and tympanic portions of the nerve in 85%; the labyrinthine portion is also involved in 15%. Herpes zoster oticus involves the labyrinthine segment in 66% of cases.
7. Facial nerve decompression surgery can be performed:[3,5-8]
    a. To reach the entire facial nerve
    b. With no injury to the facial nerve
    c. Without making a mastoid cavity
    d. Without causing hearing loss nor vestibular loss
8. In 15% of patients with acute facial palsy, the cause is a neoplasm, and not Bell's palsy.[9-11]

Real Examples of Results

RESULTS WITH ADEQUATE TREATMENT

A 24-year-old woman awoke one morning with a complete right facial palsy and right ear pressure. She had had a cold 1 week before for which she was taking tetracycline, 250 mg qid. She immediately consulted an otologist, who treated her with prednisone, 20 mg tid, and told her that recovery would be good. On the 9th day of palsy, another physician obtained an electromyelogram (EMG), which demonstrated facial nerve degeneration. At the direction of her uncle, a neurosurgeon, she was referred to the author. She was found to have a complete right facial palsy. Hilger nerve excitability test showed no activity on the right. The Schirmer tear test had 1.5-cm saturation of paper on the right. The electric taste test showed no reaction on the right. Audiogram for pure tones and speech discrimination was normal bilaterally.

Electronystagmography (ENG) showed a second-degree left-beating spontaneous nystagmus with normal caloric reactions. Impedance audiometry demonstrated absent stapedius reflexes on her right. Petrous pyramid imaging was within normal limits. The diagnosis of right Bell's palsy was made. On the 13th day postpalsy, a right facial nerve decompression from the stylomastoid foramen to the cochleariform process was performed. Edema 3+++ of the facial nerve was found extending from the tympanic segment near the midpoint of the footplate to the stylomastoid foramen. Facial motion began to return 7 weeks later. The face moved normally with no evidence of synkinesis when she was examined 14 weeks after surgery. Follow-up examination 9 months later indicated a perfect result, and she was very happy. This patient was very fortunate to have a good result despite delaying surgical decompression until nerve excitability had been lost.

* This investigation was supported in part by Ear International, Los Angeles, California

The window of opportunity between the stage of neuropraxia and the development of degeneration and scarring is fleeting and of uncertain length. The availability of a prognostic test to determine which patient will develop axon degeneration before it occurs would be ideal. As much as everyone would like to have such a test, unfortunately none exists. Surgical decompression performed when nerve excitability is normal will eliminate the risk of residual facial deformity. Decompression performed after loss of nerve excitability has occurred will minimize, but not always avoid, permanent poor results. The earlier surgery is done, the better the result, even in cases where the delay is months or years from the onset of complete palsy.

RESULTS WITHOUT EFFECTIVE TREATMENT

A significant number of patients (29% of Bell's palsy patients who develop complete palsy) who do not obtain surgical decompression of the nerve within 5 days of onset will have permanent disfigurement. The author has examined hundreds of patients with complaints of residual facial deformity years after their acute facial palsy. No surgery had been performed. For example, in one case, excessive closure of the eye was noted when she pursed her lips. When she attempted to close her eyes, the left side of her face simultaneously pulled strongly into an involuntary smile. Other patients have recovered good strength of all muscles but have significant synkinesis with excessive closure of the involved eye and distortion of the lower facial muscles. In some patients the eye fails to close.

Treatment for patients with these deformities involves the use of special training and facial exercises, as well as the judicial use of repeated Botox injections to paralyze unwanted facial muscle function. Most of these patients are unhappy with results of this type, but many physicians dismiss the problem as inconsequential and recommend neither thorough examination nor prompt surgical treatment at a time when surgery could prevent a bad result. It is human nature that patients wish to avoid or delay surgery until they are convinced that it is necessary. They are commonly advised to wait several weeks by a well-meaning relative, friend, or neighbor who made a good spontaneous recovery without treatment; 71% will. The problem is that 29% of all patients with untreated acute facial palsy will have not be so fortunate.[1] Table 41–1 presents an algorithm for evaluating such cases of acute facial palsy.

TABLE 41–1
Algorithm for the Evaluation and Management of All Patients with Acute Facial Palsy

First 3 h of palsy
- History
  - Neuro-otologic examination
  - Topognostic testing
  - Photographic or video documentation
- Medical treatment to be started immediately
  - Vasodilator
    - Histamine IV (2.75 mg in 250 ml saline) daily
    - Nicotinic acid 100 mg every hour when awake
  - Antiviral agents
    - Famvir (famiciclovir) 500 mg qid
  - Steroids (prednisone 20 mg qid)
  - Eye care

First 4 days
- Audiometry: air conduction, bone conduction, stapedius reflex and auditory evoked potentials (AEP)
- Vestibulography: ENG
- Imaging
  - Magnetic resonance imaging (MRI) with gadolinium infusion of brain and facial nerve
  - Thin-section computed tomography (CT) of the temporal bone
- Electrical tests (nerve excitability)

Fifth day of facial palsy
- Incomplete palsy
  - Continue medical therapy and observation
- Complete palsy with good tearing
  - Surgical facial nerve decompression of the mastoid and tympanic portions
- Complete palsy with a dry eye, no tearing
  - Total surgical decompression of the entire intratemporal portions of the facial nerve

After the fifth day of complete facial palsy
- Thorough examination and surgical decompression as soon as possible

Discussion

Acute facial palsy is a true medical emergency. Failure to identify the nature of the problem and to offer prompt and timely treatment can lead to permanent facial disfigurement. Accurate diagnosis and effective medical and surgical treatment of acute facial palsy can almost always prevent permanent facial deformity. Incomplete facial paralysis rarely results in permanent disfigurement but requires a thorough examination, including audiometric, vestibular, and imaging studies using CT and MRI with gadolinium enhancement. The MRI should include the entire brain, cerebellopontine angle, temporal bone portion of the facial nerve, and parotid gland. Imaging can detect lesions such as multiple sclerosis, strokes, brain tumors, and primary facial nerve tumors such as facial nerve neuroma, facial nerve angioma, and facial nerve sarcoma. Chloroma, cholesteatoma, infectious disease, bone diseases, congenital anomalies, metastatic tumors, and a variety of other conditions can be detected. Enhancement of the nerve gives some indication of the area of edema. A determination of facial function in all branches for both function and synkinesis is best accomplished by recording in percentage (where 100% is normal facial function, and 0% is no motion, and where 100% involves all branches of the facial nerve, and 0% is no synkinesis), cine, or video.[11-13]

Attention to the eye to protect the cornea from damage is of paramount importance. Most commonly, lubricating eyedrops and simple taping together of the eyelids at night affords satisfactory protection. Should there be any redness or obvious irritation, immediate ophthalmologic consultation should be obtained. An eye patch is never to be used.

Medical treatment, unless contraindicated for other medical reasons, includes prednisone, at least 20 mg qid;[14] Famvir, 500 mg qid; daily administration of intravenous histamine; 2.75 mg of histamine phosphate in normal saline given over 30 to 40 minutes in the office; as well as oral administration of 100 mg niacin every hour while the patient is awake. The patient experiences red hot tingly skin all day long. The author has found this innocuous treatment to be helpful.

A Schirmer tear test is performed initially and again before surgery is to be considered. The presence of dry eye indicates that a total facial nerve decompression through the mastoid and middle cranial fossa approaches is required. As a total decompression is a significantly more extensive procedure than decompression of the mastoid tympanic portion, patients who require it may prefer to take the greater risk of reduced recovery by waiting until there is deterioration of electroneuronography (EnoG) or nerve excitability. Either of these tests is equally effective and useful.

If this intensive therapy fails to achieve noticeable facial motion, facial nerve decompression is indicated on the 5th day after onset of complete palsy. All patients who have undergone surgical decompression by the author when the nerve excitability test is normal have experienced complete recovery.[3-5] Patients whose decompression is performed after loss of nerve excitability will have a delayed recovery and run a much greater risk of permanent deformity.

The early stages of herpes zoster oticus may be indistinguishable from Bell's palsy, generally thought to be caused by herpes simplex virus. Herpes zoster oticus is treated in the same manner as Bell's palsy. The difference between these two conditions is the involvement of the nerve. In Bell's palsy, 15% required total decompression. Herpes zoster oticus indicates involvement of the labyrinthine and internal auditory canal portions in 66% of cases; these patients require total decompression much more frequently.

It is interesting to reflect on the recommendations of Jonkees, who performed decompression only of the mastoid segment. Jonkees found that performing that type of surgery for herpes zoster oticus patients was associated with a high failure rate—certainly expected—now that we know that two-thirds of those cases require total facial nerve decompression and would not be significantly helped by decompression of the mastoid segment alone. Nevertheless, the extent of surgery required is determined by topognostic testing in these two diseases. It is primarily the Schirmer tear test for crying that makes this determination. In the case of tumors and fractures, topognostic tests are much less reliable.

Surgical decompression of the facial nerve has proved highly effective in restoring normal facial function.[2-6, 15] When accurately performed, the procedure carries low morbidity and, in most patients, requires an operation of 1-h duration, performed as outpatient surgery. A local anesthetic may be used if desired. The combined mastoid and middle cranial fossa approach needed to accomplish total decompression of the nerve in cases with no tearing requires 2 h to perform and a general anesthetic. Hospitalization is generally for 3 days.

Most patients have great concern about their facial expression and appearance. Prompt diagnosis, intensive medical therapy, and surgical decompression of the facial nerve within 5 days will provide the best opportunity to restore normal facial motion.

Exceptions and Special Situations

There are exceptions to the comments of the preceding discussion. In a small number of patients with acute facial palsy (less than 5%), it is known that the cause is a demyelinating disease similar to Guillain-Barré syndrome. Patients with palsy of this type will have complete loss of nerve excitability, suggesting an unsatisfactory result. Complete recovery without treatment within 1 month indicates the true nature of the problem. In addition, surgery performed on patients with this problem reveals no edema and has no effect on the outcome, one way or the other.

Most patients will sustain progressive deterioration of the nerve over a period during which no recovery occurs. However, a small number of patients will maintain normal nerve excitability for months or even years after the onset of palsy. Surgical decompression in such cases usually results in prompt, complete recovery within 3 or 4 weeks. Surgical decompression of the facial nerve for long-term idiopathic hemifacial spasm with facial nerve edema and partial weakness can also provide complete recovery after the myelin sheath of the nerve regrows.

Conclusion

Permanent facial disfigurement is often the source of great misery and suffering to the patient. Most physicians treat patients with facial palsy in a cavalier manner, not appreciating the seriousness of the problem from the patient's point of view. Unfortunately for most patients, thorough examination is not performed and adequate treatment is delayed or not provided at all. Prompt medical and surgical treatment as well as thorough evaluation including audiometric, vestibular, topognostic tests and imaging by MRI with gadolinium and CT scan of the temporal bone needs to be done. Neoplasms and tumors are the cause of paralysis in 15%. To avoid the risk of lasting facial deformity, surgical decompression of the entrapped edematous portion of the facial nerve must be performed before loss of nerve excitability occurs. This means that, for the best results, surgical facial nerve decompression must be performed within the first 5 days of onset of facial palsy.

REFERENCES

1. Peitersen E. The natural history of Bell's palsy. *Am J Otol* 1982;4:107–111
2. Yanagihara N, Mehle B. *New Horizons in Facial Nerve Research and Facial Expression.* Krueger.
3. Pulec J. Early decompression of the facial nerve in Bell's palsy. *Ann Otol Rinol Laryngol* 1981;90:570–577
4. Kettle K. *Peripheral Facial Palsy: Pathology and Surgery.* Copenhagen: Munksgaard; 1959
5. Pulec JL. Bell's palsy: diagnosis, management and results of treatment. *Laryngoscope* 1975;84:483–492
6. Pulec JL. Total decomprsesion of the facial nerve. *Laryngoscope* 1966;76:1015–1028
7. Pulec JL. Total facial nerve decompression: technique to avoid complications. *ENT J* 1996;7:410–415
8. Pulec JL. Facial nerve: how to find it. *ENT J* 1993;10:677–682
9. Pulec JL. Facial nerve neuroma. *ENT J* 1994;10:1–20
10. Pulec JL. Facial nerve angioma. *ENT J* 1996;75:225–238
11. Pulec JL. Aggressive fibromatosis (fibrosarcoma) of the facial nerve. *ENT J* 1993;72:460–467, 470–472
12. Neely JG, Jekel JF, Chueng JY. Variations in maximum amplitude of facial expressions between and within normal subjects. *Otolaryngol Head Neck Surg* 1994;110:60–63
13. Helling TD, Neely JG. Validation of objective measures for facial paralysis. *Laryngoscope* 1997;107:1345–1349
14. Adour KK. Combination treatment with Acyclovir and prednisone for Bell palsy. *Arch Otolaryngol Head Neck Surg* 1988;124:824
15. Gantz BJ, Rubinstein JT, Gidley P, Woodworth GG. Surgical management of Bell's palsy. *Laryngoscope* 1999;109: 1177–1188

Acute Facial Paralysis

CHAPTER 42

Douglas A. Chen and Moisés A. Arriaga

The most common causes of acute unilateral facial paralysis include Bell's palsy and trauma to the temporal bone. The physical as well as emotional liability it produces can be devastating. Accurate evaluation and proper management can reduce the sequelae the patient may sustain. Because most facial palsies are associated with some spontaneous resolution, the evaluation of various treatment modalities has been problematic.

Important prognostic and management implications can be determined by means of accurate observation at the time of initial physical examination, with documentation of any degree of facial function that subsequently deteriorates. The House–Brackmann classification grading facial paralysis has been widely accepted and is recommended by the American Academy of Otolaryngology—Head and Neck Surgery (AAO-HNS).[1]

By definition, patients with Bell's palsy have idiopathic facial paralysis with no other identifiable cause. Fortunately, most patients with Bell's palsy have a satisfactory recovery, but 15 to 20% will have significant sequelae. Facial paralysis associated with the unilateral auditory or vestibular symptoms should be evaluated to rule out retrocochlear pathology. In addition, recurrent ipsilateral Bell's palsy, or one that has a poor outcome after 6 months, should be imaged. Whether all patients with Bell's palsy require an imaging procedure is debatable.

Patients with facial paralysis secondary to temporal bone trauma frequently have other life-threatening injuries, making facial nerve evaluation a low priority, and simply not possible in other cases. Frequently, the otolaryngologist is consulted several days after the initial trauma, confounding the important assessment of whether the facial paralysis was complete, of immediate onset, or a partial delayed progressive paralysis. The timing of this assessment is critical, especially in extratemporal facial nerve injuries, because surgical exploration is facilitated substantially by intraoperative electrical stimulation, which can only be done up to approximately 3 days after injury.

Temporal bone imaging after traumatic facial paralysis, especially for intratemporal injuries, provides important information required for subsequent decision making. Although axial computed tomography (CT) scan of the head has usually already been performed, it is usually inadequate for evaluation of the temporal bone. CT scan of the temporal bone should be done in 1-mm-thin cuts in axial and coronal planes. The full course of the nerve should be evaluated. Cervical spine injury may prevent coronal CT scanning of the temporal bone. Magnetic resonance imaging (MRI) for evaluation of facial nerve trauma has not been helpful in our experience.

Electrodiagnostic Testing

Electrodiagnostic testing has been advocated as an important element in diagnostic evaluation of facial paralysis. It is used to determine the extent of facial nerve injury and to provide prognostic information for the use of treatment planning. The electrical tests that we have found the most helpful include electroneuronography (ENOG), volitional motor unit potentials on electromyelogram (EMG), spontaneous EMG responses, and Hilger nerve stimulation minimum nerve excitability test (NET). ENOG is used to document the extent of facial nerve degeneration in comparison with the contralateral side. It should not be performed until approximately 3 to 4 days after the development of a complete unilateral paralysis. ENOG provides valuable information up to 21 days after injury. Degeneration to less than 10% function compared with the contralateral side is considered significant and is considered to be the threshold for possible surgical exploration.[2] Sources of error do occur in ENOG, including electrode placement, skin impedance, masseter muscle artifact, equipment variability, and lack of standardization. Consequently, ENOG results alone should not be considered sufficient in selecting patients for surgery.

In NET, a 2–3$\frac{1}{2}$ mA difference between sides of stimulation threshold is considered significant. Hilger NET testing is used to collaborate findings on ENOG as well as a possible substitute for ENOG in good prognostic situations. Hilger stimulation is usually quicker, easier to perform, and more economical to the patient than is ENOG testing. The test, however, introduces subjectivity in that it relies on visual detection of response.

EMG responses reflect postsynaptic membrane potentials that may be either initiated at the neuromuscular junction voluntarily or spontaneously across the membrane potential. The presence of voluntary EMG facial motoring unit potentials early on after an acute facial paralysis was noted by Granger[3] to be associated with ultimate recovery from a facial paralysis. Motor unit potentials in four or five muscle groups during the first 3 days after onset of an acute facial paralysis was associated with satisfactory outcome in more than 90% of the patients. Thus, the presence of EMG voluntary facial motor unit potentials despite clinically absent motion has important prognostic implications. Spontaneous EMG activity has prognostic implications at 6 months after a major intratemporal facial nerve injury. Fibrillation potentials in the muscle are considered evidence of continuing complete denervation. Polyphasic potentials are considered evidence of regeneration, as well as a good prognostic finding. Reevaluation with EMG at the 6-month point has been selected because this provides adequate time for an intratemporal facial nerve injury to regenerate at the expected 1-mm/day growth rate to the facial periphery.

Bell's Palsy

The clinical course of patients with Bell's palsy varies from rapid early complete recovery to a more debilitating course of permanent disfiguring facial nerve dysfunction. Fortunately, most Bell's palsies recover completely and spontaneously, with 85% of patients with Bell's palsies having a full or near full recovery. Those patients who have a complete paralysis persisting for 8 weeks are likely to develop sequelae. All patients, however, regain some function within 6 months and, if no motion returns, a vigorous search for another origin should begin.

The pathogenesis of Bell's palsy is obscure. Histologic and clinical data exist to establish that injury to the nerve and loss of impulse conduction result from edema and constriction in an unexpandable bony canal. Prolonged or increased constriction leads to Wallerian degeneration. Viral etiology has been proposed as a cause for Bell's palsy. In 1975, Adour et al.[4] found elevated viral antibody titers in 40 patients with Bell's palsy and deduced that reactivated herpes simplex virus (HSV) was the probable cause of Bell's palsy. Subsequent information has also added to the validity that viral etiology is a cause of Bell's palsy. Animal studies have shown that herpes virus inoculation can produce facial paralysis in animals.[5] Other studies have shown viral DNA in endoneural fluid and muscle in patients with Bell's palsy and HSV.

The use of corticosteroids to treat the patients with Bell's palsy has been widely accepted.[6] Several studies show more favorable outcome with steroid therapy. It may reduce the risk of denervation if initiated early on. It may prevent synkinesis and progression of incomplete to complete paralysis; it may also hasten recovery. Patients presenting within the first week of facial paralysis are administered corticosteroid therapy consisting of prednisone, 1 mg/kg over three equal divided doses for the first week. Patients are then reevaluated during the second week after onset of facial paralysis. If their symptoms are resolving, the prednisone is tapered over the following week. The side effects of steroids are well documented, including hyperglycemia, emotional changes, fluid and electrolyte disturbances, gastrointestinal tract hemorrhage, and aseptic necrosis of the hip.

Adour et al.[7] examined the empirical use of acyclovir and steroids for patients with Bell's palsy. This double-blind study compared 99 patients with Bell's palsy who were treated with either acyclovir–prednisone or placebo–prednisone. The outcome in the acyclovir–prednisone-treated patients was superior to that of patients who received placebo–prednisone. Dosages of acyclovir were administered at 400 mg 5 times daily.

Surgical decompression of the facial nerve remains a controversial and emotional subject. Historically, the vertical and horizontal segments of the facial nerve in the mastoid were recommended for decompression. The preferred route was a transmastoid approach. Little if any therapeutic effect was observed in the ultimate outcome of patients with acute facial paralysis after decompression.

Anatomic and electrophysiologic evidence of a specific anatomic site of lesion in Bell's palsy emerged focusing on the meatal segment of the facial nerve. Both transmastoid and middle fossa approaches have been advocated to gain access to this region. The transmastoid approach to the geniculate ganglion and labyrinthine segment avoids a craniotomy. It does require the removal of the incus in poorly pneumatized mastoids. In our opinion, it is impossible to achieve adequate exposure of the labyrinthine segment consistently because the ampulated end of the superior canal prevents complete exposure of the proximal labyrinthine segment. May[8] used the transmastoid approach for facial nerve decompression and found decompression to improve recovery in patients whose maximal nerve stimulation responses were reduced by 75% or more. However, long-term follow-up evaluation of these patients failed to show any significant benefit as compared with patients who didn't have surgery, and was ultimately abandoned.

The meatal foramen is most adequately approached by the middle cranial fossa.[9] Fisch[9] performed decompression of the facial nerve in Bell's palsy via the middle fossa approach when ENOG was less than 10% of the normal side. All patients who underwent decompression demonstrated satisfactory return of facial function. The 90% of satisfactory outcome with surgery compared favorably with a 50% chance of satisfactory turn noted in unoperated patients matched by EMG profile.

Surgery performed on eight patients during the third week after the onset of palsy, when degeneration exceeded 90%, did not significantly improve the return of facial function. However, two patients in this group demonstrated exceptional return of facial motion after decompression. Although this experience suggests that middle fossa craniotomy for decompression of the meatal portion of the facial nerve may have some beneficial affects in reducing the sequelae of Bell's palsy, it is only suggestive. Further studies are needed and are being performed. Because these studies are not completed, we have used medical therapy consisting of, prednisone–acyclovir as our mainstay of treatment of Bell's palsy. We have reserved middle fossa craniotomy decompression of the facial nerve for the patient at high risk of sequelae, and only after the patient has been informed of possible risks and complications of the procedure.

Traumatic Facial Paralysis—Intratemporal Injury Closed-Head Trauma

Closed-head trauma is a very common etiology of traumatic facial paralysis. These patients can have numerous life-threatening injuries with other systemic problems. Often the management of these patients is shifted to rehabilitation facilities, so that otolaryngologists must coordinate serial evaluation of these patients with such facilities. In general, a patient who has a partial paralysis, House–Brackmann, grade II–V, is managed with observation. The only medical intervention available for post-traumatic facial paralysis is steroid therapy. Prednisone 1 mg/kg/day, equally divided doses over 10 days, is recommended in the absence of medical contraindications. The patient with the minimal grade function, House grade V, must be viewed with circumspection. This is a setting in which contralateral function or nearby muscle groups such as masseter motion may mislead the clinician. Accordingly, EMG is helpful for confirming voluntary motor action potentials if there is any doubt of residual function.

For the patient with complete facial paralysis, grade VI, medical therapy with steroids can be combined with surgical treatment as an option for either facial nerve decompression or grafting. Table 42–1 shows an algorithm for managing complete facial paralysis in the patient who has closed head trauma. Although it is generally assumed that delayed paralysis has a better prognosis than immediate paralysis, reliable information concerning the timing of facial paralysis is often difficult to obtain.[10] The typical scenario is generally one in which the timing of the development of facial paralysis is unknown. Both CT imaging and electrical facial nerve testing are used to guide the management of these patients. Significant CT findings include a temporal bone fracture through the course of the facial nerve with diastasis of >1 mm or an apparent bone spicule along the course of the facial nerve. Electrical testing includes volitional EMG beginning after the first 3 days of injury if there is any question of retained motion. Hilger nerve excitability testing is also helpful if there was a suggestion that the paralysis was delayed in onset or if there is no evidence of fracture or bone spicule on CT scan. ENOG testing is also helpful in the face of a significant fracture on CT and loss of Hilger excitability. Surgical exploration of the course of the facial nerve is advocated in patients who have a complete facial paralysis with evidence of significant diastasis along the course of the facial nerve or bone spicule along the course of the facial nerve on CT scan, and electrical degeneration within 3 weeks of their injury to less than 10% of the normal side. In contrast, patients who have temporal bone fractures on CT, but without significant findings along the facial nerve, or with electrical degeneration within the 3-week period, are encouraged to await spontaneous recovery for 6 months. In addition, steroid therapy is implemented. The possible value of a facial nerve exploration and decompression is mentioned because there is some evidence to support decompression and exploration in this setting.[11]

Patients who develop any motion during this time are observed and are not candidates for temporal bone facial nerve surgery. Patients in whom spontaneous activity does not develop during this time are restudied with EMG for spontaneous muscle fibrillation or polyphasic potentials. Patients who demonstrate fibrillation potentials have not experienced reinnervation of their facial muscle so surgical exploration of the temporal course of the nerve should be considered. Patients who develop polyphasic potentials are undergoing reinnervation of their facial muscule and should be managed with additional observation[12] (Table 42–2).

TABLE 42–1

Closed-Head Trauma Paralysis: 3-Week Decision Algorithm

CT[a]	Electrical Testing[b]		Therapy
+	—	→	Observe
+	+	→	Surgery
—	—	→	Observe
—	+	→	Observe[c]

[a] CT +, 1-mm diastasis along course of facial nerve, or spicule in nerve.

[b] Electrical testing +, <10% residual function on electroneuronography.

[c] Patients are informed that some anecdotal evidence supports facial nerve exploration and decompression. However, I encourage these patients to await the 6-month point.

TABLE 42–2

Closed Head Trauma—Complete Paralysis: 6-Month Decisions

Motion	→	Observe		
No motion	→	EMG		
		Fibrillations	→	Surgery
		Polyphasic	→	Observe

EMG, electromyography.

Penetrating Temporal Bone Trauma

The management of patients who have facial paralysis after penetrating trauma to the temporal bone is more straightforward than in closed-head trauma. The timing of the paralysis is usually immediate onset, and the location of the injury can be evaluated with CT scan. Surgery is recommended to patients who have CT evidence of penetrating trauma on their temporal bone through the facial nerve and electrical evidence of degeneration. If the CT scan does not indicate a direct penetrating injury to the facial nerve, but electrical degeneration reaches less than 10% function, these patients are also offered surgery, unlike the closed-head trauma patients, because heat or associated trauma from a missile injury may be responsible for delayed paralysis.[13] (Table 42–3).

TABLE 42–3

Management of Patients Who Have Facial Paralysis from Penetrating Trauma

CT[a]	Electrical Testing[b]		Therapy
+	—	→	Observe
+	+	→	Surgery
—	—	→	Observe
—	+	→	Surgery

[a] CT +, 1-mm diastasis along course of facial nerve, or spicule in nerve.

[b] Electrical testing +, <10% residual function on electroneuronography.

Iatrogenic Trauma

The patient who has iatrogenic facial paralysis is usually noted to have facial paralysis in the recovery room immediately after surgery. The temporal relationship between the surgery and the onset of paralysis obviously suggests that the surgical procedure is the cause of paralysis.

The first step in the management of these patients is to consider each step of the procedure and the possible involvement of the facial nerve. Reasonable time should be given for the effects of local anesthesia to dissipate. In addition, if the ear or mastoid cavity was packed with firm material, this should be loosened to provide an opportunity for any direct pressure on the nerve to dissipate as well. After a few hours to allow these maneuvers to take effect, if the paralysis persists, consideration should be given to exploration of the facial nerve. Volitional EMG potentials may be helpful at this time. Evidence of volitional motor action potential corroborates an intact nerve that will recover with time.

Immediate postoperative facial paralysis is an emotionally charged situation for the patient as well as the surgeon. The surgeon should readily seek consultation in this situation and should preferably perform the facial nerve exploration in conjunction with another surgeon who has particular expertise in the facial nerve surgery. This provides the additional objectivity of another observer, as well as a surgeon who is less emotionally involved in the decision-making process. The presence of another surgeon acting as a co-observer to record findings and decision making in a more objective fashion also has potential medicolegal ramifications. In addition, although prompt exploration is indicated, waiting until the next morning for a complete fresh surgical team is preferable to subjecting the patient to a same-day operation with a team that is either tired or incomplete.

Surgical Repair of the Traumatized Facial Nerve

Radiographic findings are extremely important in the guidance of the surgical exploration in repair of a traumatized facial nerve. Most injuries are in the vicinity of the geniculate ganglion, specifically, the proximal tympanic segment, the geniculate ganglion, or the labyrinthine segment.[14] Surgical exploration of the facial nerve after temporal bone trauma is initially performed as a transmastoid approach. Canal wall-up mastoidectomy with facial recess is often adequate for surgical exploration and decompression of the facial nerve from the proximal tympanic segment through the distal vertical segment. Exploration of the geniculate ganglion or labyrinthine internal auditory canal segment can be performed via a middle fossa craniotomy. If the patient has suffered total sensorineural hearing loss from trauma, a translabyrinthine approach is preferable to the middle fossa approach to obtain total facial nerve exposure without temporal lobe retraction in the acute head injury scenario.

If the nerve is anatomically intact, it is widely decompressed around the fracture site, and the sheath is opened. Only spicules are removed from the facial nerve if present. A large diastasis in the course of the facial nerve usually requires facial nerve interposition graft. The greater auricular nerve is an excellent source for a grafting material. If this is unavailable, the sural nerve is another option. Interposition grafts can be placed in the trough of the fallopian canal that are held in place with absorbable hemostatic material. Sutures are required such as in the labyrinthine or proximal tympanic segments, two or three 10-0 monofilament sutures are then used. Damage in the perigeniculate region of the nerve can require middle fossa exposure for complete visualization if hearing is intact. In cases in which hearing is not intact, the tympanic segment may be rerouted directly to the labyrinthine or internal auditory canal (IAC) portion. Suture repair or grafting of the IAC facial nerve can be technically difficult. Usually only one suture can be placed to approximate the ends of the nerves and the anastomosis is reinforced with absorbable hemostatic material.

Partial transections of the facial nerve require a difficult decision as to whether facial nerve grafting is indicated. Most surgeons would agree that if 50% or more of the facial nerve is transected, the nerve should be grafted.[15] Obtaining an accurate estimation can be difficult in the face of anatomic constraints or granulation tissue. Especially in the presence of an iatrogenic injury, and because of the inability to determine the extent of injury adequately, some investigators have suggested that if the facial nerve appears to be transected greater than one-third of its diameter, it should be grafted.

If an injury to the sheath is identified with herniation of nerve fibers through the damaged sheath, a segment of the nerve on either side of the injury is decompressed, and the sheath is opened to prevent strangulation of the nerve.

Conclusion

The case of an anatomically intact facial nerve, but with evidence of electrical degeneration, presents a therapeutic dilemma, regardless of whether trauma or Bell's palsy is the cause. Some degree of spontaneous recovery without any therapy would be expected in this setting, and so arises the controversy in treatment. Although treatment with steroids or antiviral agents, or both, depending on etiology, may improve outcomes in high-risk patients, the literature is still incomplete. In our opinion, the possible benefits of treatment despite potential side effects are worth the risk. Until further research is completed, however, we remain cautious in our recommendations of the possible benefits of facial nerve decompression.

Anatomic disruption of the facial nerve is an absolute indication for exploration and possible grafting. Determining the extent of injury preoperatively with CT scans and electrical testing can be difficult. Even with direct inspection during surgery, an accurate determination can be difficult because of disease, traumatic anatomic distortion, and surgeon bias.

REFERENCES

Chen and Arriaga—CHAPTER 42

1. House JW, Brackmann DE. Facial nerve grading systems. *Otolaryngol Head Neck Surg* 1985;93:146–147
2. Fisch U. Prognostic value of electrical tests in acute facial paralysis. *Am J Otol* 1984;5:494–498
3. Granger C. Prognosis in Bell's palsy. *Arch Phys Med Rehabil* 1976;57:33–35
4. Adour KK, Bell DN, Hilsinger RL. Herpes simplex virus on idiopathic facial paralysis (Bell palsy). *JAMA* 1975;233:527–530
5. Kumagani H. Experimental facial nerve paralysis. *Arch Otolaryngol* 1972;95:305–312
6. Stankiewicz JA. A review of published data on steroids and idiopathic facial paralysis. *Otolaryngol Head Neck Surg* 1987;97:481
7. Adour KK, Ruboyianes JM, Von Doersten PG, et al. Bell's palsy treatment with acyclovir and prednisone compared with prednisone alone: a double-blind, randomized controlled trial. *Ann Otol Rhinol Laryngol* 1996;105:371–378
8. May M. Total facial nerve exploration: transmastoid, extralabyrinthine and subtemporal. *Laryngoscope* 1979;89:906–917
9. Fisch U. Surgery for Bell's palsy. *Arch Otolaryngol* 1981; 107:1–11
10. Brodie HA, Thompson TC. Management of complications from 820 temporal bone fractures. *Am J Otol* 1997;18: 188–197
11. Fisch U. Facial paralysis in fractures of the petrous bone. *Laryngoscope* 1974;82:2141–2154
12. Arriaga MA. Traumatic facial paralysis. *Curr Ther Otolaryngol Head Neck Surg* 1998;121–125
13. Duncan NO, Coker NJ, Jenkins HA, Canalis RF. Gunshot injuries of the temporal bone. *Otolaryngol Head Neck Surg* 1986;94:47–55
14. Green DJ, Shelton C, Brackmann DE. Iatrogenic facial nerve injury during otologic surgery. *Laryngoscope* 1994;104: 922–926
15. Green DJ, Shelton C, Brackmann DE. Surgical management of intragenic facial nerve injuries. *Otolaryngol Head Neck Surg* 1994;606–610

15

Otosclerosis Management

"The size of the footplate fenestra or amount of footplate removed during stapedectomy for optimal performance and minimal complication has been evaluated by several studies. The general consensus is that there are probably no significant differences for overall performance in speech frequencies between stapedectomy and stapedotomy (fenestra size), but there may be a lower incidence of SNHL with stapedotomy."

William H. Lippy

"In a revision operation, it is important to avoid (1) penetrating the lining membrane of the vestibule to open the oval window, (2) removing a wire from beneath the lining membrane of the vestibule, or (3) reopening the oval window if closed by regrowth of otosclerotic bone."

John J. Shea, Jr.

"Use of a laser for refenestration of the oval window permits precise, controlled, atraumatic removal of connective tissue without mechanical forces being exerted into the inner ear. We feel strongly that the benefit of modern otologic lasers to revision stapes surgery is so great that we would not begin a revision procedure without the availability of a laser."

Karl L. Horn

Otosclerosis Management

CHAPTER 43

William H. Lippy and Robert L. Daniels

Otosclerosis is a disease that has seen its share of controversy over the past 40 years. It now represents a readily diagnosable and treatable process in which the surgical techniques for correction with some variability have been nearly perfected. Even now, however, some areas of controversy remain in the management of otosclerosis, specifically in patient selection for therapy, in treatment options, and in surgical techniques. Controversies in patient selection include determining the candidacy of groups that have unique issues that define the limits of intervention, such as children, the elderly, aviators and pilots, patients with small air–bone gaps, and patients with coexisting endolymphatic hydrops. Other issues include selecting patients for revision stapedectomy and anticipating problems that can be encountered in these cases. Differing opinions exist with regard to prosthesis choice, use or nonuse of tissue grafts, laser instrumentation, management of a mobile footplate, type of anesthesia, and amount of footplate removed. Finally, for some the medical management of otosclerosis and the use of fluoride or biphosphonates remains controversial. We present a discussion of these topics and our management of otosclerosis.

Background

Controversy in the management of otosclerosis began in 1876 with the first attempt at surgery for otosclerosis with total stapedectomy by Kessel. Unsuccessful largely due to a lack of sterile technique and antibiotics, otosclerosis surgery was abandoned until 1923, when Holmgren performed a three-stage lateral semicircular canal fenestration, a technique later improved by Lempert. The next era of controversy paralleled advances in surgical technique. Very controversial at the time, the first modern successful stapedectomy technique was performed and described by Shea in 1956.[1,2]

Several modifications of the technique and prostheses have since evolved, with the overall success rates (four frequency average of conductive gap closure within 10 dB) in experienced hands climbing to more than 90%. Laser applications have added the ability to achieve hemostatic and atraumatic access to the footplate/oval window interface. This has become most useful during revision procedures when working with unknown footplate status, mucosal scarring at the oval window (OW) and the potential of intralabyrinthine adhesions. In recent series, laser revision techniques have demonstrated improved results, due to this ability to open the OW seal atraumatically and allow the surgeon to reestablish ossicular chain continuity.[3-6] Before laser revision techniques, reopening of the OW was associated with a high rate of sensorineural hearing loss (SNHL) and was avoided. Lasers, of both visible and nonvisible wavelengths, have been shown to be safe and effective in primary and revision stapes surgery. With all laser types performing equally well, choice is determined by cost, availability, and delivery system preference.[3-10]

Discussion

INDICATIONS FOR PATIENT SELECTION

Bone conduction greater than air (negative Rinne), using a 512-Hz tuning fork with appropriate masking, should be reproducible on at least two separate occasions. Audiometric data should demonstrate a predominant low-frequency conductive gap that averages ≥ 10 dB in the speech frequencies, which may narrow with a mild sensorineural notch at 2000 Hz (Carhart notch). Acoustic reflexes must be absent with normal compliance tympanometry. Ideally, speech discrimination scores (SDS) should be greater than 80%, unless the loss is severe. Patients with poor SDS may have other neural disease, including cochlear otosclerosis, portending a suboptimal surgical result.

INDICATIONS BY AGE

Age is not a contraindication to surgery. If the individual is in reasonable health, both the elderly and children can be appropriate candidates for surgery. The elderly can tolerate local anesthesia without difficulty when counseled appropriately. In our experience with 154 patients ranging in age from 70 to 92 years, these patients were as likely to obtain a successful hearing result (93%) with improvement in SDS and to avoid vestibular symptoms as were patients under age 70.[11] Studies have documented the safety of stapedectomy in children with appropriate evaluation.[12,13] Children older than 5 years of age who are not susceptible to otitis media do well with a general anesthetic. Surgery can be delayed in this group if otitis confuses the clinical picture or delayed until the child is older and mature enough to cooperate with local anesthesia. We are much more likely to delay surgery in unilateral losses. In our experience with 47 ears of children aged 17 or younger, successful results were obtained in 92%. These children were less likely to obtain overclosure and were three times more likely to require a drillout. Long-term results were stable with minimal decay.[12]

MENIERE'S DISEASE AND OTOSCLEROSIS

Patients with concomitant otosclerosis and Meniere's disease can be difficult to manage. In patients with active Meniere's disease, stapedectomy has a high rate of severe or total sensorineural hearing loss (SNHL). Some have attributed this to an enlarged saccular or Reissner's membrane abutting the under surface of the footplate, which is traumatized at footplate fenestration. Although some otosclerotic patients have transient dysequilibrium made worse by sudden movements, few rarely describe rotatory vertigo. The patients who have episodic vertigo or other symptoms suggestive of Meniere's disease should undergo a formal vestibular work-up and treatment as necessary prior to stapes surgery. Only patients who have had symptoms of Meniere's disease inactive for several years, and with bone conduction levels of ≥ 35 dB at 500 Hz and no high-frequency loss, as well as good discrimination, should be considered for stapedectomy.[14]

AIRCREW AND COMBAT PILOTS

Aircrew and pilots with otosclerosis also pose an interesting dilemma. As it progresses, hearing loss is burdensome. However, performing a procedure that opens the OW may put them at risk of fistula and untimely vestibular symptoms, which would disqualify them from flight status. The Federal Aviation Administration (FAA) policy is to grant waivers from disqualification due to stapedectomy on an individual basis, pending clearance from the surgeon. Up to 1994, no waived commercial pilot has had any mishaps or complications from a stapedectomy; recent studies have also shown that stapedectomy in military flight team members can be safe and successful.[15,16] Data compiled from combat pilots in the Israeli Air Force have demonstrated that pilots undergoing stapedectomy with a large vein graft and Robinson prosthesis can safely return to combat-intensity flying without concern for malfunction of the stapedectomy. Nine pilots operated on by the senior author obtained successful hearing results and have safely logged more than 4160 hours of high-performance flying without vestibular symptoms. The senior author recommends only procedures using a vein or tissue graft and comprehensive postoperative vestibular and altitude chamber testing at 3 months, before approval for return to flight status.[16]

SMALL AIR–BONE GAPS

Because some otosclerotic patients retain a small conductive hearing loss for years, whereas others progress rapidly, many surgeons prefer to wait for a larger conductive loss to improve the risk/benefit ratio for stapedectomy. Current guidelines have been reported that advocate a 20-dB pure-tone average air–bone gap.[17] However, for experienced stapedectomy surgeons with high rates of success and low rates of complication, a high rate of overclosure in recovering cochlear reserve has occasionally allowed surgery to correct air–bone gaps as small as 10 dB.[18] In our experience with 136 patients, almost all had a family history or previous diagnosis of otosclerosis in the opposite ear. All had appropriate tuning fork tests and absent acoustic reflexes. Only if otosclerosis was surgically confirmed did the surgeon proceed with a stapedectomy. These patients had rejected hearing aids but desired improved hearing. Mean hearing improvement was 16.7 dB with mean overclosure of 8.1 dB. More than 89% of patients in that study overclosed their air–bone gap.[18]

INDICATIONS FOR REVISION STAPEDECTOMY

The decision to revise a stapedectomy is made on the basis of information from the patient, the operative report if available, and pre- and postoperative audiograms. The operative note may be unreliable, but it may contain information that, with corresponding audiograms, could be used to predict chances of success and anticipate problems. The length of the surgical procedure may indicate increased difficulty or an inexperienced surgeon. Prosthesis type should be noted and problems anticipated for that particular prosthesis. Anatomic abnormalities that could potentially impact successful stapedectomy in the first ear may have a significant chance of occurring in the second ear. These include obliterative otosclerosis requiring an OW drillout and dehiscent and overhanging facial nerves.[19] Those patients whose hearing initially improved (air–bone gap closure) and then deteriorated over time (gap reappearing) are the best candidates for revision. Early failure may be more common among less experienced surgeons, whereas late failures are more likely due to ossicular erosion.[6] Also, patients who have a fluctuating, progressive SNHL, or who remain dizzy after the first surgery, are candidates for revision in hope of repairing an OW fistula or finding a long prosthesis.[20-22]

Surgical Algorithms

The surgical algorithm for primary stapedectomy in either routine or problem cases is essentially the same. Our technique has been described elsewhere as have techniques for specific problems encountered at both primary and revision stapedectomy.[20-29] Six general principles in our partial stapedectomy technique have served the senior author successfully for more than 38 years in more than 15,000 stapedectomies: the use of local anesthesia, vein graft for OW coverage, partial stapedectomy technique, Robinson prosthesis, intraoperative audiometry, and laser assistance when necessary.

Stapedectomy under local anesthesia has been widely acknowledged as having the added safety and benefit of active feedback from the patient. This is most important during manipulation of the OW–footplate interface and in positioning the prosthesis to monitor for any vestibular symptoms and to allow audiologic testing at the end of the procedure.

A tissue graft is a key element to the success of the technique for protection of the vestibule and prevention of fistulae and also for the mechanical advantage of this self-centering and self-height-adjusting Robinson prosthesis. Causse et al.[10] have argued in favor of "reconstructing the acoustic impedance of the annular ligament" with a vein graft, a tissue of similar thickness, resistance, and elasticity. Causse and colleagues eloquently explain biophysically what many have noted clinically. A tissue graft can and should be used with any technique or prosthesis and is easily accessible above the wrist. We prefer the vein for its texture, thickness, translucency, elasticity, and lack of memory.

The size of the footplate fenestra or amount of footplate removed during stapedectomy for optimal performance and minimal complication has been evaluated by several studies.[29-33] The general consensus is that there are probably no significant differences for overall performance in speech frequencies between stapedectomy and stapedotomy (fenestra size), but there may be a lower incidence of SNHL with stapedotomy.[30] Review of our own cases varying only fenestra size demonstrated no significant differences for hearing (including 4 kHz). However there was a significant difference for overclosure with a medium to large vs. small fenestra (80% vs 64%; $P = 0.0018$).[29] Causse et al.[10] reason in favor of a medium sized fenestra, suggesting that a fenestra of medium size, located posteriorly with a vein graft gives a "more balanced response from low to high frequencies," simulating best the natural acoustic impedance transfer of the ossicular chain. We recommend removing the portion of the footplate that comes most easily, usually the posterior third to half. A stout, short, footplate hook (Lippy) is useful for this maneuver.

Prosthesis choices are numerous, each having individual nuances, technical benefits, and difficulties. Our selection of the Robinson prosthesis for use in stapedectomy for the past 38 years is based on a combination of sensible mechanics, ease of use, and reproducibility of results. The mechanical advantages are that the prosthesis is self-centering in the fenestra and self-adjusting for height. A large-well, 0.4-diameter shaft, 4-mm-length prosthesis is used in more than 98% of cases. The distance from the incus to the OW is not measured. The position of the prosthesis is determined by an equalization of forces from the natural tension of the incudal ligaments levering the incus long process down on the prosthesis and the elastic resistance of the vein graft covering the OW. The piston end of the prosthesis naturally migrates to the center of the fenestra, whereas the cup end is held in place by the lenticular process. The Robinson prosthesis has several advantages in dealing with special problems encountered during stapedectomy and revisions.[20-29]

The use of intraoperative audiometry (IOA) in the operating room offers several advantages: (1) it can provide instant, quantifiable, objective feedback to the surgeon; (2) improvement in hearing defines the endpoint of surgery; (3) it dictates attempts in repositioning the prosthesis to maximize hearing gains; and (4) in difficult revision cases, it permits testing with different reconstructive solutions to determine the best option for optimal hearing results. Preoperative air level is tested at either 500 or 1000 Hz, wherever the gap is wider. Improvement of the same test frequency to within 10 to 15 dB of the preoperative bone threshold is considered a satisfactory end result. Further improvement is seen postoperatively. If test performance does not fall within the expected range, the prosthesis is reexamined, and adjustments are made until retesting determines that the best possible result has been obtained. If a satisfactory result is not achieved in the primary procedure, a revision procedure is not indicated. In revision cases, IOA has become especially invaluable.[34]

The final principle is the use of laser assistance, when necessary. For example, in primary cases in which a "blue" footplate is mobilized, the laser is used to safely fenestrate or incise the footplate and allow completion of the procedure. If a laser is unavailable, successful results in 94% of cases can be achieved by placing a Robinson vein graft over the mobile footplate.[28] In revision cases, a laser allows us to atraumatically ablate soft tissue at the OW membrane–prosthesis interface to verify or re-create patency of the fenestra and also facilitate removal of the failed prosthesis. We prefer the argon laser for its hemostatic qualities and method of delivery, a hand-held "otoprobe" that gives the surgeon control to manipulate and defocus the beam easily as needed.[10]

Revision Stapedectomy Algorithm

The overriding principles for revision stapedectomy include the following: (1) perform the surgery in a properly selected patient under local anesthesia, (2) monitor for dizziness, (3) use the vein graft and Robinson prosthesis technique, (4) use a laser to open the OW seal (only when absolutely necessary), and (5) perform IOA. The surgical algorithm is as follows. First, previous curetting is assessed and improved if needed. Next, the middle ear is explored for more obvious etiologies of failure (i.e., incus necrosis, displaced prosthesis). The ossicular chain is then carefully palpated to determine the mobility and position of the prosthesis and rule out undiagnosed malleus (incus) fixation. Abnormal movements, such as side-to-side motion or rotation of the prosthesis, should be noted and may be indicative of the prosthesis impinging on adjacent bone in the OW or on intact footplate. Next, the prosthesis is removed or pushed aside if the patient becomes dizzy, and a vein graft and Robinson prosthesis are placed. The IOA algorithm is then followed.

If the hearing remains unimproved despite repositioning of the prosthesis and the footplate area seems firm to palpation, the laser is used to expose the footplate area by gently vaporizing tissue overlying the fenestra. The argon laser power is set at 1 W and pulse duration at 0.1 s. A 26-gauge suction evacuates smoke, and a cooling interval of at least 2 s is used after each pulse to avoid caloric stimulation from the heated tissue. Vestibular symptoms that occur during OW exploration are monitored to eliminate any potential for inner ear trauma. The laser is used to create a fenestra away from the original fenestra if possible, so that ideally the posterior portion of the footplate can be removed. A vein graft and Robinson prosthesis are placed and the IOA algorithm followed. Using the laser in this fashion for revision stapedectomy, we have achieved success (10-dB closure) in 80% of cases, with overclosure in 36%. In cases of otosclerosis regrowth with an obliterated footplate, if the regrowth is not too severe, the laser can be used similarly to vaporize regrowth and open the OW. A slightly longer prosthesis (4.5 mm) may be used to retard reclosure of the OW.

Medical Treatment Algorithm

Medical treatment of otosclerosis using fluoride has historically been used to treat patients thought to have cochlear involvement manifested by progressive audiologic and vestibular symptoms. The scientific basis for using fluoride is thought to be in its ability to inhibit osteoclasts and promote bone maturization. This deactivates the lesions and removes the toxic effect of the biochemical products produced during bone turnover on the hair cells.[35] Several studies have suggested some benefit in stabilizing SNHL by using fluorides in these patients.[36-39] We have used a fluoride/calcium mixture (Fluorical) in almost all of our postoperative stapedectomy patients since the early 1970s, as well as any nonsurgical patient in whom the diagnosis of cochlear otosclerosis has been made. We generally maintain these patients on Fluorical for at least 2 years. If, after years of stability, the sensorineural function begins to deteriorate they can be restarted. In some cases, with an only hearing ear, medical treatment with Fluorical has been used for many years in lieu of surgery.

Recently another drug has shown some promise for use in treating neurologic symptoms in otosclerotic patients. Etidronate (Didronel) a bisphosphonate, mimics the function of pyrophosphate, having similar if not more profound effects than fluoride by inhibiting osteoclasts, osteoblasts, and their enzymes and by promoting bone stabilization.[40,41] In our limited 2-year experience using etidronate, we have seen in many patients a remarkable decrease of tinnitus and a definite decrease in vestibular symptoms. We are in favor of further studies to document its role in treating otosclerosis.

Conclusion

Management of otosclerosis remains challenging even in an era with more than 90% success rates and advancing technology and research. The controversial issues will always be defined by how different management and treatment improve our results and change our indications for therapy. Our management of these issues may not yet be through its final modifications but it currently provides a high degree of success and satisfaction for both patients and surgeons.

REFERENCES

Lippy and Daniels—CHAPTER 43

1. House HP. The evolution of otosclerosis surgery. *Otolaryngol Clin North Am* 1993;26:323–333
2. Shea J Jr. Fenestration of the oval window. *Ann Otol Rhinol Laryngol* 1958;67:932–951
3. McGee TM, Diaz-Ordaz E, Kartush J. The role of KTP laser in revision stapedectomy. *Otolaryngol Head Neck Surg* 1993;109:839–843
4. Haberkamp TJ, Harvey SA, Khafagy Y. Revision stapedectomy with and without the CO_2 laser: an analysis of results. *Am J Otol* 1996;17:225–229
5. Lundy LB. Otosclerosis update. *Otolaryngol Clin North Am* 1996;29:257–263
6. Langman AW, Lindeman RC. Revision stapedectomy. *Laryngoscope* 1993;103:954–958
7. Perkins R. Laser stapedotomy. In: Brackmann DE, ed. *Otologic Surgery.* Philadelphia: WB Saunders; 1994:314–329
8. Kodali S, Harvey SA, Prieto TE. Thermal effects of laser stapedectomy in an animal model: CO_2 vs KTP. *Laryngoscope* 1997;107:1445–1450
9. Wong BJ, Neev J, van Gemert MJ. Surface temperature distributions in carbon dioxide, argon, and KTP (Nd:Yag) laser ablated otic capsule and calvarial bone. *Am J Otol* 1997; 18:766–772
10. Causse JB, Gherini S, Horn KL. Surgical treatment of stapes fixation by fiberoptic argon laser stapedotomy with reconstruction of the annular ligament. *Otolaryngol Clin North Am* 1993;26:395–415
11. Lippy WH, Burkey JM, Fucci MJ, et al. Stapedectomy in the elderly. *Am J Otol* 1996;17:831–834
12. Lippy WH, Burkey JM, Schuring AG, Rizer FM. Stapedectomy in children: short- and long-term results. *Laryngoscope.* 1998;108:569–572
13. Millman B, Giddings NA, Cole JM. Long-term follow-up of stapedectomy in children and adolescents. *Otolaryngol Head Neck Surg* 1996;115:78–81
14. Issa TK, Bahgat MA, Linthicum FH Jr, House HP. The effect of stapedectomy on hearing of patients with otosclerosis and Meniere's disease. *Am J Otol* 1983;4:323–326
15. Thringer JK, Arriaga MA. Stapedectomy in military aircrew. *Otolaryngol Head Neck Surg* 1998;118:9–14
16. Katzav J, Lippy WH, Shamiss A, Davidson BZ. Stapedectomy in combat pilots. *Am J Otol* 1996;17:847–849
17. Clinical Indicators Compendium. Annual Meeting of the American Academy of Otolaryngology–Head and Neck Surgery Foundation, Inc., Washington, D.C. *Otolaryngol Head Neck Surg* 1992;107:141–145

18. Lippy WH, Burkey JM, Schuring AG, Rizer FM. Stapedectomy in patients with small air–bone gaps. *Laryngoscope* 1997;107:919–922
19. Daniels RL, Lippy WH. The other ear—findings and results in 3600 bilateral stapedectomies. COSM 1999
20. Lippy WH, Schuring AG. Stapedectomy revision of the wire-Gelfoam prosthesis. *Otolaryngol Head Neck Surg* 1983;91: 9–13
21. Lippy WH, Schuring AG. Stapedectomy revision following sensorineural hearing loss. *Otolaryngol Head Neck Surg* 1984;92:580–582
22. Lippy WH. Schuring AG, Ziv M. Stapedectomy revision. *Am J Otol* 1980;2:15–21
23. Rizer FM, Lippy WH, Schuring AG. Partial footplate removal in stapedectomy. *Operative Techniques Otolaryngol Head Neck Surg* 1998;9:13–19
24. Lippy WH. Special problems in otosclerosis surgery. In: Brackmann DE, ed. *Otologic Surgery.* Philadelphia: WB Saunders; 1994:347–355
25. Lippy WH, Schuring AG. Solving ossicular problems in stapedectomy. *Laryngoscope* 1983;93:214–216
26. Lippy WH, Schuring AG. Prosthesis for the problem incus in stapedectomy. *Arch Otolaryngol* 1974;100:237–239
27. Lippy WH, Schuring AG, Ziv M. Stapedectomy for otosclerosis with malleus fixation. *Arch Otolaryngol* 1978;104: 388–389
28. Lippy WH, Fucci MJ, Schuring AG, Rizer FM. Prosthesis on a mobilized stapes footplate. *Am J Otol* 1996;17:713–716
29. Rizer FM, Lippy WH. Evolution of techniques of stapedectomy from the total stapedectomy to the small fenestra stapedectomy. *Otolaryngol Clin North Am* 1993;26: 443–451
30. Sedwick JD, Louden CL, Shelton C. Stapedectomy vs stapedotomy: do you really need a laser? *Arch Otolaryngol* 1997; 123:177–180
31. McGee TM. Comparison of small fenestra and total stapedectomy. *Ann Otol Rhinol Laryngol* 1981;90:633–636
32. Fisch U. Stapedotomy vs stapedectomy. *Am J Otol* 1982;4: 112–117
33. Cremers W, Beusen J, Huygen P. Hearing gain after stapedotomy, partial stapedectomy, or total stapedectomy for otosclerosis. *Ann Otol Rhinol Laryngol* 1991;100:959–961
34. Lippy WH, Schuring AG, Rizer FM. Intraoperative audiometry. *Laryngoscope* 1995;105:214–216
35. Causse JR, Causse JB, Uriel J, et al. Sodium fluoride therapy. *Am J Otol* 1993;14:482–490
36. House HP, Linthicum FH Jr. Sodium fluoride and the otosclerotic lesion. *Arch Otolaryngol* 1974;100:427–430
37. Shambaugh GE Jr, Causse J. Ten years experience with fluoride in otosclerotic (otospongiotic) patients. *Ann Otol Rhinol Laryngol* 1974;83:635–642
38. Forquer BD, Linthicum FH Jr, Bennett C. Sodium fluoride: effectiveness of treatment for cochlear otosclerosis. *Am J Otol* 1986;7:121–125
39. Bretlau P, Salomon G, Johnsen NJ. Otospongiosis and sodium fluoride: a clinical double-blind, placebo-controlled study on sodium fluoride treatment in otospongiosis. *Am J Otol* 1989;10:20–22
40. Kennedy DW, Hoffer ME, Holliday M. The effects of etidronate disodium on progressive hearing loss from otosclerosis. *Otolaryngol Head Neck Surg* 1993;109:461–467
41. Brookler KH, Tanyeri H. Etidronate for the neurologic symptoms of otosclerosis: preliminary study. *Ear Nose Throat J* 1997;76:371–381

Otosclerosis Management

CHAPTER 44

John J. Shea, Jr.

Controversies about the management of otosclerosis, which began with the first report by Johannes Kessel in Jena in 1876[1] on stapedectomy, through the fenestration era, beginning in 1910,[2] did not end with the resurrection of the stapedectomy operation by John Shea, Jr., in 1956.[3] Once stapedectomy and reconstruction of the sound-conducting mechanism of the middle ear were demonstrated by surgeons all over the world to restore hearing in most patients (with only a small number made worse), the question of what operation to do was settled. Mobilization of the stapes and fenestration of the lateral semicircular canal were no longer performed, and everyone began to perform the stapedectomy operation. Now the controversies concern on whom to perform stapedectomy, at what age, what degree of hearing loss, whether to perform the procedure on the only hearing ear, how much of the footplate of the stapes to remove, how to seal the oval window, and how to reconstruct the sound-conducting mechanism of the middle ear. What to do after a good hearing improvement, whether or not to give sodium fluoride, when and if to operate on the other ear, when to recommend a hearing aid rather than stapedectomy, and other questions continue to be debated.

Background

Controversies about the management of otosclerosis are now influenced by a dramatic change in the patient population coming for operation. When stapedectomy was resurrected in 1956, there were many patients with all degrees of hearing loss that previously had not been operated on, but that were suitable for stapedectomy. As the number of stapedectomies performed increased each year, the number performed peaked in 1962; it has since undergone a gradual decline but has not yet reached a plateau. As a result, the number of patients coming for stapedectomy is now so small that many residents do not perform even one stapedectomy during their residency, and the teachers of these residents have done so few stapedectomies as to lack sufficient experience to teach them properly. Many of the patients coming for operation now have localized anterior otosclerosis with slight or moderate hearing loss or have had one or more prior unsuccessful stapedectomy operations. There is less likelihood of achieving a good result in these previously operated ears and, more important, the chance of further hearing loss is much greater. Accordingly, the likelihood of a good result after revision operation is less, which must be explained to the patient in great detail, with a witness present, and documented in writing given to the patient.

Most importantly, failed stapedectomy, especially a bad result from revision stapedectomy, is one of the most important causes of malpractice lawsuits against otolaryngologists. Therefore, the risk of having a worse outcome must be explained to the patient in great detail, and the protocol to conduct the operation must be followed very carefully to avoid litigation. Several inflexible rules must be followed. Do not remove a wire loop from the vestibule. Do not reopen bony closure of the oval window. If a perilymph fistula is present, do not enlarge the fistula, but seal it with a living oval window seal, such as vein or fascia, and insert a prosthesis.

More than 43 years after the resurrection of the stapes operation, the sad fact is that about one-third of those who attain a good initial hearing gain, with closure or overclosure of the air–bone gap, will develop sensorineural hearing loss in excess of what would be expected from presbyacusis and therefore must return to the use of a hearing aid. This further hearing loss is due to the invasion of the margins of the cochlea by the otosclerotic focus, as in cochlear otosclerosis. To prevent this problem, we give 7.6 mg of sodium fluoride (Florical; Mericon Industries, Peoria, IL) with 200 mg of calcium carbonate with the two largest meals to all patients with extensive otosclerosis or severe sensorineural hearing loss. This is administered especially in the young or female patient to prevent invasion of the margins of the cochlea by otosclerosis.

Diagnosis

To make the diagnosis of otosclerosis suitable for operation, the following conditions must be present: (1) a history of progressive hearing loss; (2) a normal ear canal, drum, and middle ear; (3) conductive hearing loss with air–bone gap of $\geq$ 20 dB and an air conduction level of $\geq$ 30 dB for the three speech frequencies with good speech discrimination; and (4) a type A (stiff) impedance audiogram with absent stapedial reflexes.

Discussion

Stapedectomy constitutes the only proper management of the hearing loss of otosclerosis, except in that very small group (about 1%) who have a fibrous, but not bony, fixation of the stapes. In such an ear, gentle mobilization of the stapes, by pushing down on the margins of the footplate in the areas of the fibrous fixation, to loosen the stapes footplate and preserve the annular ligament of the stapedial oval window joint so no perilymph is lost should be done. These ears almost always achieve a good permanent hearing gain.

In those ears with localized anterior otosclerosis, the crura of the stapes are cut across with a hand-held probe delivering low-power argon laser bursts, and the arch of the stapes is removed. The lining membrane of the middle ear is removed for about 2 mm around the oval window and bleeding controlled. The footplate is cut across the middle with the argon laser from top to bottom by connecting a series of openings, and the posterior half of the footplate is removed. A 2 × 2-mm piece of compressed vein from the back of the hand is then put in place over the oval window opening, adventitia down, intima up, to make a living oval window seal. Fascia, perichondrium, and compressed earlobe fat can be used, but they are not as effective as compressed vein. A living oval window seal must be used to prevent perilymph fistula, which does occur in a small number of ears in which Gelfoam (Upjohn, Kalamazoo, MI), blood clot, or other material is packed around the shaft of the prosthesis, to seal the oval window opening. With all the reports in the literature of perilymph fistula when a living oval window seal is not used, and all the complications that can occur when this happens, I believe it to be a "departure from the standard of care expected of the surgeon to prevent such a leak" if a living oval window seal is not used to cover the oval window opening after all or part of the stapes is removed. For this reason, I strongly recommend the use of a living oval window seal, such as vein, fascia, perichondrium, and even compressed earlobe fat.

The tip of a platinum Teflon cup piston prosthesis, or other such prosthesis, with a 0.6-mm diameter shaft and 4 mm long (Smith & Nephew ENT, Memphis, TN) is then placed on the invaginated oval window vein graft, and the shaft is depressed about 0.5 mm into the oval window, while the incus is lifted up 0.5 mm with a delicate right-angle hook, and the lenticular process of the incus inserted into the cup in the head of the prosthesis. The platinum loops on the prosthesis are then closed around the end of the incus to hold it into the cup of the prosthesis. Gelfoam pieces moistened in blood are then positioned around the shaft of the piston prosthesis on the vein to hold it in place in the center of the oval window opening until it heals.

If the lenticular process of the incus is past the center of the oval window opening, so the platinum Teflon cup piston will not come down into the center of the oval window opening, an original Teflon piston is used rather than the platinum Teflon cup piston, 0.6 mm in diameter and 4 mm long, which fits onto the shaft of the incus above the lenticular process.

The patient is advised to remain quiet, but not necessarily in bed, for 2 or 3 days after operation with the operated ear up. There is usually no pain, dizziness, nausea, vomiting, or loss of balance. Most hearing returns during the first 30 days after operation, but complete recovery of hearing continues for 1 year.

When the otosclerosis is more widespread, obliterating the margins of the oval window, a 1-mm-diameter opening is made in the thin center of the footplate, which is usually not invaded by otosclerosis, with the hand-held argon laser. The opening is then covered with a compressed vein graft, and the platinum Teflon cup piston prosthesis is inserted. If the lenticular process of the incus is past the center of the oval window opening, a 0.6-mm-diameter Teflon piston can be used. The loop in the head fits around the shaft long process of the incus.

Results with these two variations in primary stapedectomy have been good, with 90% closure of the air–bone gap; in only 1% of cases is the patient's hearing made worse.[4] In about 10% of cases, the initial hearing gain is lost, usually due to incus necrosis and/or dislocation of the prosthesis out of the oval window or off the incus, most often due to eversion of the lining membrane of the vestibule. These ears are usually suitable for revision stapedectomy.

Revision of these failures after your own (or after others') operations is difficult. First, one must warn the patient, both by word and in writing, that the chance of a good hearing gain is less, not 90% but 50%, and the chance of a further sensorineural hearing loss is greater, not 1% but 10% or more. When properly informed, many patients, will not choose a revision operation.

The most common cause of failure to obtain a good hearing gain is incorrect diagnosis; that is, the patient does not have otosclerosis. Commonly made mistaken diagnoses are epitympanic fixation of the incus and/or malleus, indistinguishable preoperatively from otosclerosis, inner ear conductive hearing loss of unknown cause in which the stapedial reflex is not absent and the round window reflex is not present, and congenital abnormalities of the middle ear and ossicles. One must be careful to test the mobility of the incus and malleus and to verify the presence of a round window reflex and the continuity of the ossicular chain. It is also important to identify the extent of the otosclerotic focus, to verify the diagnosis of otosclerosis, before beginning the operation.

The next most common cause of failure to get a good hearing gain, or loss of a hearing gain, when achieved, is failure to reconstruct the sound-conducting mechanism of the middle ear properly and failure of that reconstruction, when achieved, by bony closure of the oval window, dislocation of the prosthesis and/or eversion of the lining membrane of the vestibule with necrosis of the tip of the incus.[5] The loop at the lower end of a wire prosthesis has a tendency to migrate after being put into place and to become bound to the margins of the oval window. When Gelfoam or clotted blood is used to seal the oval window, the membrane may form lateral to the loop at the lower end of the wire prosthesis; this tends to prevent a good (or any) hearing gain. The loop at the upper end of the wire prosthesis may cause necrosis of the incus tip and become loose.

In a revision operation, it is important to avoid (1) penetrating the lining membrane of the vestibule to open the oval window, (2) removing a wire from beneath the lining membrane of the vestibule, or (3) reopening the oval window if closed by regrowth of otosclerotic bone.

I have found the best way to reconstruct the sound-conducting mechanism of the middle ear after eversion of the lining membrane of the vestibule with dislocation of the prosthesis and necrosis of the incus tip is with a total ossicular replacement prosthesis (TORP) with a porous hydroxyapatite head and Teflon shaft with a wire. This will hold it under the drum in contact with the malleus handle and tip of the incus.

Over time, about one-third of these good results are lost due to the inevitable hearing loss of advancing age, as well as additional sensorineural hearing loss as a result of otosclerotic invasion of the margins of the cochlea. Most of these patients can return to the use of one or two of the new digital programmable hearing aids very successfully.

Conclusion

Stapedectomy, with reconstruction of the sound-conducting mechanism of the middle ear, is one of the most successful operations ever devised. It has stood the test of time, almost unchanged since it was first described in 1956.

Recently, measles virus invasion of the otic capsula has been implicated in the etiology of otosclerosis, in addition to the genetic tendency for this otosclerotic focus to occur in the fissula ante fenestrium region of the otic capsula. With measles vaccine inoculation almost universal in developed countries, we are likely to see much less otosclerosis in the future. Although the role of measles virus in the etiology of otosclerosis has not yet been fully explained, preliminary evidence is very convincing and, after all the facts are known, it should soon be accepted by everyone.

Now at the beginning of the twenty-first century, this most common and devastating cause of conductive hearing loss has been virtually eliminated by modern medical and surgical advances, measles vaccination, and stapedectomy with reconstruction of the sound-conducting mechanism of the middle ear. The profound hearing loss that afflicted Beethoven, Edison, and numerous less well-known people has been all but completely eliminated.

REFERENCES

1. Kessel J. Über das Mobilisieren des Steigbügels durch Ausschneiden des Trommelfells, Hammers und Ambosses bei Undurchgängigkeit der Tube. *Arch Ohrenh*, 1878;13:69–88
2. Shea JJ, Jr. A personal history of stapedectomy. *Am J Otol* 1998; 19(suppl):S1–S12
3. Meltzer PE, Lindsay JR, Goodhill V, et al. Symposium. The operation for the mobilization of the stapes in otosclerotic deafness. *Laryngoscope* 1956;66:729–784
4. Shea JJ, Jr. Stapedectomy—a long-term report. *Ann Otol Rhinol Laryngol* 1982;91:516–520
5. Shea JJ, Jr. Eversion of the lining membrane of the vestibule. *Laryngoscope* 1974;84:1122–1134

SUGGESTED READINGS

Shea—CHAPTER 44

Rosen S. Palpation of stapes for fixation: preliminary procedure to determine fenestration suitability in otosclerosis. *AMA Arch Otolaryngol* 1952;56:610–615

Schuknecht HF. *Stapedectomy*. Boston: Little, Brown, and Co.; 1971

Otosclerosis Management

CHAPTER 45

Karl L. Horn and Stuart G. Gherini

In 1958, John J. Shea, Jr., revived the long abandoned concept of stapedectomy for the surgical treatment of otosclerosis.[1] Unlike Blake and Jack earlier in this century, Shea covered the opened oval window with connective tissue and reconstructed the impedance transfer of the ossicular chain with a polyethylene prosthesis from the incus to the oval window. Like the pioneering work of Lempert and Rosen, Shea's original surgical procedure was soon followed by many modifications of his technique. The common goal of all these subsequent stapes procedures is to restore the impedance transfer of the ossicular chain. Controversy for contemporary otosclerosis surgery is concerned primarily with the choice of surgical technique for bypassing the otosclerotic focus. It is our belief that there is no one correct way to perform stapes surgery for the treatment of otosclerotic stapes fixation. However, advances in instrumentation, particularly the introduction of microdrills and fiberoptic visible light laser hand pieces, have enabled surgeons to accomplish this goal in a more precise and delicate fashion.

Lasers in Otology

Stahle and Hogberg first proposed the use of surgical lasers for otologic surgery in 1965.[2] Unfortunately, this study and others using powerful pulsed lasers had distinctly chilling effects on early enthusiasm for otologic and neurologic laser surgery.[3-5] These studies demonstrated the devastating damage of pulsed lasers on the ear and brain. Unlike the "studies in biologic overkill" using pulsed lasers, an early study by Sataloff[6] demonstrated the clinical potential of lasers in otosclerosis surgery. In 1967, using a neodymium-glass laser, Sataloff[6] discretely fenestrated a cadaver stapes footplate. In 1979, Escudero et al.[7] excited the otologic world by reporting the use of an argon laser in seven patients undergoing tympanoplasty. Perkins[8] and DiBartolomeo and Ellis[9] first reported the application of a surgical laser to clinical stapes surgery in 1980. Both DiBartolomeo and Perkins used the argon laser to create a small fenestra in the stapes footplate. Numerous reports have since outlined the use of argon, KTP-532, and CO_2 lasers for otosclerosis and other middle ear disorders.[10-31]

While discussing the use of an argon laser in acoustic tumor surgery, Glasscock et al.,[32] in 1981, pointed out the practical problems associated with microscope-mounted micromanipulator delivery systems, including increased working distance, decreased available light, the need to "bounce the laser off of small mirrors to reach inaccessible areas," and the necessity of keeping one hand out of the operative field on the joystick of the micromanipulator. In 1986, we began to experiment with hand-held fiberoptic systems for the argon laser. The initial system consisted of a 200-μm fiber taped to a Rosen needle. In 1987, we developed several fiberoptic hand pieces for the argon laser. The hand pieces consist of a 200-μm fiber housed in a 24-gauge graduated needle hand piece designed to be held and used in a manner similar to a traditional otologic instrument. Fiberoptic hand pieces have eliminated the practical problems described by Glasscock. Fiberoptic hand pieces for both argon and KTP-532 lasers have since been used in otosclerosis, middle ear, and acoustic tumor surgery.

Laser Safety

Laser damage to the inner ear structures or the facial nerve has been a concern since both before and after lasers proved clinically effective in otologic surgery. Silverstein et al.[33] reported adverse results in their first two cases using an argon laser fiberoptic hand piece. In a revision stapes procedure, their first patient developed a discrimination loss of 40%. In a second case, a total hearing loss resulted when a large granuloma of the tympanomeatal flap filled the middle ear and grew into the oval window.

In a study using model vestibules and thermocouples to monitor temperature changes, Lesinski and Palmer,[13] questioned the safety of both argon and KTP-532 lasers in primary and revision stapes surgery. Lesinski and Palmer's experimental model showed minimal (0.4°C) temperature elevations recorded by a large (0.5-mm) black thermocouple within a model vestibule with careful argon and KTP-532 laser stapedotomies but marked temperature elevations with direct laser irradiation of the thermocouple.

In 1992, we repeated the experiments of Lesinski and Palmer, using a model vestibule with a small (0.025-mm) silver thermocouple and a 200-μm optical fiber delivery system for an argon laser.[34] No significant changes in temperature within the vestibule were noted with vaporization of the stapes crura, footplate, or open vestibule. A temperature elevation was only obtained in an open vestibule when using a large thermocouple (0.5-mm) painted black and after saline was aspirated from the model vestibule. An interesting observation in our study was an 80°C temperature elevation in a second thermocouple placed at the level of the facial nerve. Kodali et al.[35] recently performed a similar thermocouple study in the chinchilla and found no significant difference between fiberoptic KTP-532 and CO_2 lasers. These investigators concluded that there was no contraindication, in terms of thermal injury to the inner ear, for the use of a visible light laser with a hand-held probe delivery system as compared to the CO_2 laser for stapedotomy.

There is a theoretical advantage to an optical fiber visible light laser system for stapes surgery. A micromanipulator system produces a highly focused beam. When using a 250-mm lens, the laser beam in a micromanipulator system has an angle of convergence of approximately 3 degrees; beyond the focal point, the beam has an angle of divergence of approximately 3 degrees. The rate of power density fall-off on either side of the focal point is small, and structures both proximal and distal to the target tissue are at potential risk to laser damage. This also means that a micromanipulator system must be checked before each use to ensure that the laser beam is focused properly on the target tissue. By contrast, with a fiberoptic hand piece, the angle of divergence of energy at the tip of the optical fiber is approximately 14 degrees. Because of the larger angle of divergence and subsequent rapid power density fall-off inherent with a optical fiber, the risk of damage to a distal structure, such as the saccule in stapedotomy, is less likely to occur.

The safety of fiberoptic visible light laser use in an open vestibule is further implied by a recent series of publications on inner ear laser surgery. In 1990, Okuna et al.[36] reported using the argon laser through the oval window after stapedectomy in guinea pigs and monkeys. These workers noted acute elevation of the supporting and sensory epithelium from the basement membrane in the irradiated area of the utricular macula. Two weeks after irradiation, the otoliths of the macula had disappeared; by 10 weeks, the entire macula had disappeared. In these experimental animals, there was no change in the structure of the membranous labyrinth, sensory epithelium of the cochlea or nonirradiated vestibular organs. Both Nomura et al.[37] and Anthony[38] have reported safe use of the fiberoptic argon laser for utricular macula ablation.

In the series of Anthony, 13 of 14 patients were treated without loss of auditory function with a power setting of 3.5 W for 0.5 s. In this procedure, the laser is directed at the utricule through a fiberoptic probe placed through the oval window. Anthony attributed the loss of auditory function in his one patient to opening the footplate in an ear with endolymphatic hydrops.

In summary, experimental data presented during the past decade do not support the concept of thermal damage to the inner ear using either argon, KTP-532, or CO_2 lasers. Clinically, the use of otologic lasers over the past two decades has proved safe and effective for the surgical treatment of otosclerosis as well as other otologic disorders.

Advantages of Lasers for Stapes Surgery

Early enthusiasm for lasers in stapes surgery was far from unanimous. In the discussion of Perkin's first presentation, Frances Sooy cited Kaplan's law, "When you give a kid a hammer, everything he sees needs pounding."[39] Similarly, the fiberoptic argon laser hand pieces have been described as a gimmick and fad by more than one nationally recognized otologist. One may question whether surgical lasers are little more than technological bravado for an operation considered by many the quintessence of otologic surgery. We believe that surgical lasers offer several worthwhile advantages to the stapes surgeon. The most significant benefit is elimination of mechanical trauma. In our experience, the high-frequency notch occasionally seen after mechanical stapedectomy is avoided with use of the argon laser. The absence of mechanical trauma is particularly important during revision stapes. The small spot size of the CO_2, KTP-532, and argon lasers allows precise and controlled removal of both bone and soft tissue in the oval window. Finally, the CO_2, KTP-532, and argon lasers all have hemostatic qualities that virtually eliminate bleeding during fenestration of the stapes footplate. In our hands, we believe that these advantages have increased the speed, efficiency, and safety of the small fenestra stapes procedure.

From a practical point of view, the use of a fiberoptic hand piece avoids a cumbersome micromanipulator that must be attached to the microscope and increases the working distance from the surgeon to the operative field. The fiberoptic hand piece may be held similar to a traditional surgical instrument and avoids removal of the surgeon's dominant hand from the operative field to control the joystick on the micromanipulator. By moving the tip of the optical fiber closer or farther from the target, the power density may be changed instantaneously from a high-power density for cutting or vaporization to a low-power density for coagulation. Fiberoptic hand pieces can be used around corners by simple movement of the instrument in the surgeon's hand rather than moving the entire micromanipulator/microscope system to a different visual axis or using micromirrors. Finally, the protective shutter may be left on the microscope at all times, and laser use is accomplished by turning on the system and attaching the fiberoptic hand piece. This avoids time-consuming micromanipulator calibration and testing.

Patient Selection and Evaluation

Although we believe that surgical lasers offer significant advantages to the surgeon, it is important to remember that a successful stapes operation is predicated on much more than the technique of footplate management. When asked to list the 20 fine points of otosclerosis surgery, J. Bernard Causse[40] related 9 of these 20 fine points to preoperative evaluation and patient selection. We feel that a brief review of preoperative considerations is important.

A family history of otosclerosis is helpful in making the diagnosis of otosclerotic stapes fixation, but it is not present in most patients, and it is not necessary to determine candidacy for surgery. A history of otitis media is important to elicit in order to anticipate lateral ossicular chain pathology. Patients with a history of fluctuating hearing loss, progressive hearing loss after head trauma, or congenital anomalies of the ear and head and neck, particularly in the young, should be considered for an associated inner ear anomaly. High-resolution computed tomography (CT) of the temporal bone is suggested for these patients. Large vestibular aqueduct syndrome frequently presents with a mixed hearing loss and is not improved with surgery. A large cochlear aqueduct or widened internal auditory canal suggests the possibility of a perilymph gusher, and these patients are best treated with hearing amplification.

A history of dizziness should be explored thoroughly, but it is not necessarily a contraindication for surgery. Patients with benign paroxysmal positional vertigo who benefit from vestibular exercises or an otolith repositioning maneuver are not contraindicated for surgery. Patients with active Meniere's disease are not considered appropriate for surgery. Vague or nonspecific dizziness is treated as labyrinthine otosclerosis with fluoride for 12 to 24 months. These patients are considered for surgery if they remain free of dizziness for 6 months.

Preoperative evaluation should include a complete audiologic, otologic, head and neck examination. The ear canal should be free of inflammation or infection. The ear canal should be large enough to allow the use of at least a 4-mm speculum. The tympanic membrane should be intact and the middle ear free of middle ear effusion. A short or misshapen malleus may indicate an inner ear anomaly and is an appropriate indication for a preoperative CT scan of the temporal bone. The nasal vaults and pharynx should be free of any suppuration.

Tuning fork testing, is still an important and inexpensive part of the preoperative evaluation. The Weber test, either audiologic or tuning fork, lateralizing to the poorer hearing ear is a good criterion for patient selection for surgery. A negative Rinne tuning fork test at 256, 512, and 1024 Hz strengthens the diagnosis of conductive hearing loss.

Audiologic evaluation routinely includes pure tone air and bone conduction, speech testing, and impedance testing. A Carhart notch and absence of the stapedius reflex on impedance testing with a negative history of otitis media argues strongly for a diagnosis of otosclerosis. An on–off response on impedance testing implies partial stapes fixation and surgery should be deferred for complete fixation. Surgery need not be limited to patients with a very large conductive hearing loss. However, an average air–bone gap of 10 dB in the speech frequencies (500 to 3000 Hz) is considered a minimum for surgery. Patients with advanced otosclerosis resulting in a severe to profound mixed hearing loss can also benefit from stapedotomy. Closure of the air–bone gap in these patients greatly improves their ability to benefit from hearing amplification.

Surgical Technique

Surgery is performed with the patient in the supine position. The operating table may be manual or electrical, but must rotate from side to side, as well as Trendelenburg. The surgeon sits at the head of the operating table with the operating nurse sitting on the opposite side of the table. An audiologist monitors the facial nerve in patients with known anomalies of the facial nerve and in patients with a congenital hearing loss. The anesthesia equipment and anesthesiologist sit at the foot of the table.

General anesthesia or local anesthesia supplemented with intravenous sedation is employed, depending on the patient preference. The ear is cleaned with povidone-iodine solution and sterile self-adhering drapes are applied. The skin of the external auditory canal is injected with a solution of 1% lidocaine with 1:100,000 epinephrine. The injections are placed in the four quadrants of the external auditory canal at 1 to 2 mm lateral to the bony–cartilaginous junction.

While waiting for the vasoconstriction effect of the epinephrine, a vein graft is harvested. In men, a distal superficial vein from the dorsum of the hand provides a graft of proper thickness. In women, a more proximal vein, such as the cephalic vein or a vein from the volar surface of the wrist proximal to the flexor crease, may be chosen. The incision is closed with an absorbable subcuticular suture. The loose adventitia of the vein is removed by running a wire (or a Barbara needle) through the vein, grasping the adventitia with forceps and running a No. 15 scalpel blade along the sulcus between the vein and the adventitia. The vein is incised lengthwise, trimmed to a 5 × 5-mm square, and set aside in saline. If the vein graft is too thick, it may be placed in a Gelfoam press until used.

Speculums of increasing sizes are used to dilate and compress the skin of the ear canal, thus improving exposure and reducing bleeding at the incision. The speculums used are relatively soft and malleable, made of nickel–silver alloy. Only the posterior half of the tympanic membrane needs to be visualized.

The ear canal incision is made parallel to the annulus at the end of the speculum, not perpendicular or tangential to the annulus. This incision avoids tearing the tympanic membrane and reduces bleeding. The incision must not be made with the laser, which would result in a several millimeter shrinkage of the flap. The flap is elevated with a Merocel microsponge and the middle ear space is entered. The microsponge prevents direct trauma to the flap from the microsurgical instruments, aids in hemostasis, and prevents introduction of loose cotton fibers when cotton pledgets are used.

The bone over the chorda tympani is outfractured using a strong hook or is removed with a stapes curette. Adequate removal of the bony canal for the chorda tympani nerve is important to permit mobilization of this nerve inferior to the oval window The posterior scutum is removed with either a mallet and gouge or a stapes curette. The amount of the scutal bone that is removed is limited, but one needs to visualize the pyramidal eminence and the inferior aspect of the facial nerve clearly. Care is taken to maintain adequate scutal bone over the incus to avoid postoperative retraction of the tympanic membrane onto the incus and the prosthesis. The mobility of the lateral ossicular chain is tested for attic fixation.

Mesenchymal middle ear adhesions are removed with the laser (1.5 W × 0.1 s). The stapedius tendon is vaporized with three to five laser pulses. A No. 3 suction in the surgeon's nondominant hand aspirates the laser plume. Alternately, the stapedius tendon may be preserved and separated with a small hook from the stapes for later attachment to the stapes prosthesis.

With the suction stabilizing the incus, the incudostapedial joint is separated using a small, flat, right-angled hook or incudostapedial joint knife. The mobility of the malleus, incus, and stapes is checked again to rule out attic fixation or a mobile stapes. The posterior crus is vaporized (1.5 W × 0.1 s) as close as possible to its junction with the footplate. Care must be taken to avoid direct laser irradiation of the facial nerve and to aspirate the laser plume. Waiting 10 to 15 s for cooling between laser pulses lessens the risk of thermal injury to the facial nerve. Vaporization of the posterior crus is complete when bone turns to a white or gray char. The anterior crus is then vaporized at its junction to the footplate. In approximately one-fourth of cases, this step may be accomplished under direct vision. In the remaining cases, the junction of the anterior crus and the footplate cannot be seen. The fiberoptic tip is placed by palpation on the junction of the anterior crus and the footplate. Vaporization is complete after three to four pulses. The superstructure remnant is removed. The remnant of the posterior crus is removed to the level of the stapes footplate using a 0.7-mm diamond burr and microdrill.

The distance between the incus and the stapes is determined using a measuring instrument or by the use of "dummy" prostheses trimmed to a known length. A dummy prosthesis is placed on the posterior half of the stapes footplate and against the long process of the incus. With a Causse prosthesis, the proper size to select is one in which the lower portion of the ring sits approximately half above and half below the medial edge of the incus. This additional prosthesis length provides extension of the prosthesis 0.2 to 0.3 mm into the fenestra.

The fenestra is placed in the posterior half of the footplate. The tip of the optical fiber is placed directly on the footplate to create the laser rosette for the stapedotomy. A 0.8-mm rosette is made by connecting 0.2-mm laser spots (1.5 W × 0.1 s). Once again, care is taken to allow 10 to 15 s between pulses for cooling. The laser char of the rosette is gently brushed away with microdrill using a 0.7-mm diamond burr. Alternatively, the char may be removed with an oval window rasp.

The fenestra is placed in the posterior half of the footplate for several reasons. Placing the fenestra posteriorly minimizes the chance of damaging the saccule. Any adhesions between the saccule and footplate will be found at the level of the anterior annular ligament. Avoiding the anterior otosclerotic focus reduces the risk of releasing proteolytic enzymes into the inner ear and reduces the chance of bleeding. Finally, placing the fenestra posteriorly allows reconstruction of the annular ligament with restoration of the proper acoustic impedance.

The prosthesis is trimmed 0.2 to 0.3 mm longer than the distance from the incus to the footplate. The ring of the prosthesis is opened by placing it between the thumb and index finger, placing a Barbara or Rosen needle instrument through the ring, and gently rolling the needle away from the shaft. Alternatively, the ring of the piston may be opened by placing the cup forceps within the ring of the piston and spreading the jaws of the instrument several times. With either method, the ring will remain open for several minutes because of the memory of the Teflon.

Before placing the vein graft in position, the surgeon notes the location of the fenestra relative to nearby landmarks. Alternatively, a single laser spot on the promontory may be used as a point of reference to the fenestra. The vein is placed over the tip of a No. 3 suction with the intimal surface facing the suction tip. With the suction in the surgeon's nondominant hand and a needle in the dominant hand, the vein is placed over the fenestra, and the edges are unfurled with the intimal surface facing the tympanic membrane and adventitial surface facing the vestibule.

Placement of the prosthesis into the vein-covered fenestra and over the incus may be accomplished with cup forceps, but for finer control, a suction to hold the prosthesis and needle to stabilize the incus are used. Alternatively, a Barbara needle is used to impale the prosthesis and a suction to stabilize the incus is used. With the prosthesis is in place, the vein graft puckers around the shaft of the prosthesis. The position of the prosthesis may be adjusted on the long process of the incus so that the shaft is perpendicular to the fenestra. The ring of the prosthesis is gently crimped over the incus with cup forceps. To ensure that the prosthesis is engaged into the fenestra, a small hook is used to apply lateral pressure to the shaft. If the prosthesis is not secure in the fenestra, it will swing out of position. If the prosthesis is properly positioned in the fenestra, the shaft will bend. The tympanomeatal flap is returned to the normal anatomic position and is held in place with a thin layer of Gelfoam that is covered with a Merocel otowick sponge expanded with saline. The expanded otowick applies gentle pressure to the flap and limits bleeding. The otowick also acts as aural protection for the immediate postoperative period.

Postoperative Care

Stapedotomy for otosclerosis is usually performed as an outpatient procedure with patients leaving the hospital several hours after surgery. Using the operative technique that we have outlined, most patients have little postoperative dizziness, and true vertigo is unusual. Vestibular suppressants are not given routinely postoperatively but may be used for several days for patients who have true postoperative vertigo. Although patients are asked to avoid strenuous activity, most routine daily activities may be resumed the day following surgery. Patients may travel by automobile or air the day after surgery.

A broad-spectrum intravenous antibiotic, such as a cephalosporin, is administered intravenously during the perioperative period, and a broad-spectrum oral antibiotic is prescribed for 7 to 10 days postoperatively. The packing is removed 7 to 10 days postoperatively and an audiometric evaluation is performed 6 weeks after surgery. Patients are routinely asked to return for annual follow-up visits.

Results

The argon laser has been used for stapes surgery for two decades, and the fiberoptic argon laser has been used for more than one decade. The question of visible light laser safety has been answered by the paucity of reported clinical complications in the literature. In a review of more than 2200 cases, there were no cases of significant sensorineural hearing loss or facial nerve injury.[34] In the report of our first 43 patients undergoing fiberoptic argon laser stapedotomy, 72% of patients had closure of the air–bone gap to within 5 dB, 19% had closure to within 10 dB, and 9% had closure to within 15 dB.[14] In our review of 300 patients, our results had changed very little. Closure of the air–bone gap to within 5 dB was found in 73%, 20% had closure to within 10 dB, and 7% had closure to within 15 dB.[21] These results are similar to those reported for the CO_2 laser (91% within 10 dB) and the KTP-532 (90% within 10 dB).[27,29]

Revision Stapes Surgery

Otologists have grown accustomed to quoting 90% or more air-bone gap closure and less than 1% sensorineural hearing loss for primary stapes surgery. Unfortunately, revision stapes surgery offers neither the safety nor success generally associated with primary surgery. The explanation for this apparent conundrum lies in the pathologic imparity that exists between otosclerotic stapes fixation and a failed stapes procedure. In primary stapes surgery, stapes fixation is the only abnormality in the ossicular chain that must be corrected by the surgeon. However, with revision stapes surgery, a variety of ossicular abnormalities may cause failure of impedance transfer, and frequently more than one of these abnormalities may be present. In addition, greater risk is associated with mechanical refenestration of oval window connective tissue as compared with primary surgery of the stapes footplate. The combination of more surgical variables and increased difficulty in refenestration of the oval window has resulted in overall decreased air–bone gap closure to approximately 50% and sensorineural hearing loss of greater than 1% in most series using mechanical revision techniques.[41-45]

The most hazardous and difficult step in revision stapes surgery is refenestration of the oval window. This is particularly true when the primary procedure was a total stapedectomy. Histologic studies by Linthicum[46] showed adhesions between the membrane in the oval window and the saccule and utricle. Sheehy et al., recognizing the danger of revision of the oval window, suggested not removing the soft tissue membrane in the oval window.[47] Modern otologic lasers have largely alleviated concern that manipulation of the prosthesis or membrane in the oval window may rupture the endolymphatic space resulting in sensorineural hearing loss and vertigo. Use of a laser for refenestration of the oval window permits precise, controlled, atraumatic removal of connective tissue without mechanical forces being exerted into the inner ear. We feel strongly that the benefit of modern otologic lasers to revision stapes surgery is so great that we would not begin a revision procedure without the availability of a laser.

Patient Selection

Revision stapes surgery is reserved for patients who continue to have conductive hearing loss after primary stapes surgery or who develop recurrent conductive hearing loss after initial improvement in hearing. Nonprogressive sensorineural hearing is not considered an indication for revision surgery. However, progressive or fluctuating sensorineural hearing loss or incapacitating balance disturbance may be an indication for surgical exploration. Surgical exploration is performed in these patients to look for a perilymphatic fistula. In the absence of a visible perilymphatic fistula, the oval window and prosthesis should not be disturbed. Vague or nonspecific dizziness is treated as labyrinthine otosclerosis with fluoride for 12 to 24 months.

Because revision stapes surgery does not yield the same rate of success achieved in primary surgery, a larger preoperative air–bone gap is required. More than 90% of our primary stapedotomy patients have closure of the air–bone gap to ≤ 10 dB. In this group of patients, a 10-dB preoperative air–bone gap in the speech frequencies (500 to 3000 Hz) is considered the minimum indication for surgery. More than 90% of our revision stapes surgeries have closure to ≤ 20 dB.[48] Therefore, we use a 20-dB air–bone gap as a minimum for revision surgery.

Surgical Technique

Patient positioning and operating room setup are the same as described for primary stapes surgery. Early in our experience with revision stapes surgery, all cases were performed under local anesthesia to have constant patient feedback. However, the absence of intraoperative complications have led us to use general anesthesia or local anesthesia supplemented with intravenous sedation, depending on patient preference. The ear is prepared, draped, and injected as noted for primary surgery. Speculums of increasing size are inserted into the external canal to dilate and compress the skin of the ear canal, in order to improve exposure and reduce bleeding from the canal incision.

The ear canal incision is made parallel to the annulus at the end of the speculum. Elevation of the tympanomeatal flap with a Merocel microsponge reduces flap trauma and swelling. The elevated flap is everted into the anterior tympanomeatal sulcus to avoid obscuring the surgical field. If not previously removed, the posterior scutum is curetted to expose the oval window, pyramidal eminence and the inferior aspect of the facial nerve. Special care is taken to avoid removing excess scutal bone over the incus. Adhesions around the chorda tympani are removed and if necessary, the bone over the chorda tympani is outfractured to allow displacement of the nerve inferior to the oval window. Mesenchymal adhesions are vaporized with the laser by holding the tip of the optical fiber directly on the tissue and using one or more pulses with a power setting 1 to 1.5 W and pulse duration of 0.1 s. A No. 3 suction in the nondominant hand is used to aspirate the laser plume. The adhesions are removed until the status of the malleus, incus, prosthesis, and oval window can be established.

In patients who have undergone a small fenestra procedure, the piston is usually displaced from the stapedotomy and bound down to adjacent bone with mesenchymal tissue. Adhesions around the piston may be removed with the laser at the lower power setting. After the connective tissue has been removed from the piston, the prosthesis is removed from the incus. This procedure is performed with a small right angle hook in the dominant hand, while the incus is steadied with the suction in the nondominant hand.

When a platinum ribbon/Teflon piston prosthesis has been used, the displaced prosthesis may also have been displaced from the incus and, not infrequently, may be found free in the mesotympanum. In this situation, it is important to examine the incus for necrosis. Soft tissue may obscure incus necrosis, and a fibrous union of the long process may be overlooked.

After the prosthesis has been removed from the middle ear, the stapes fenestra is inspected. The stapedotomy is usually filled with fibrous connective tissue that obscures the limits of the fenestra. The edges of the stapedotomy are defined with the laser at a power setting of 1 to 1.5 W and pulse duration of 0.1 second. After the circumference of fenestra has been established, the connective tissue filling the stapedotomy is thinned using the laser. Connective tissue is removed until the endosteum is identified. The endostium is loosened from the edges of the stapedotomy with an oval window rasp. The distance from the incus to the fenestra is measured and the new prosthesis is cut approximately 0.3 mm longer. The new prosthesis, a Causse 0.6-mm (K.L.H.) or 0.4-mm (S.G.G.), is either placed through the endosteum and sealed with fibroadipose tissue (KLH) or the prosthesis is placed onto a vein graft used to seal the fenestra (S.G.G.).

In patients who have undergone total stapedectomy, the most common finding is a displaced prosthesis. If a wire/Gelfoam or wire/tissue technique was used, the prosthesis is usually lateralized to the inferior edge of the oval window. Soft tissue in the oval window is removed around the shaft of the prosthesis until the knotted end has been exposed. In cases in which a wire/Gelfoam prosthesis was used, the tissue covering the knot is usually quite thin, and a power setting of 1 W with a pulse duration of 0.1 s is typically used. The cases with wire/tissue frequently have thick tissue surrounding and fixing the shaft and knot of the prosthesis. The power setting is increased to 1.5 W for removal of this thick tissue. The tissue is slowly vaporized around the circumference of the prosthesis until the knot is exposed. It is not uncommon to remove several millimeters of tissue until the knot of the prosthesis is encountered. After the prosthesis has been freed from the connective tissue in the oval window, the prosthesis is removed from the incus as noted previously. The remaining connective tissue in the oval window is inspected. If the patient has undergone a wire/Gelfoam procedure, the oval window membrane is quite thin and the new prosthesis is placed on or through the membrane without further manipulation (K.L.H.). If connective tissue, such as fascia, vein, or fat, has been used to seal the oval window, the connective tissue remaining in the oval window after removal of the prosthesis may be several millimeters thick. This membrane is thinned in the posterior third of the oval window with the laser at a power setting of 1 to 1.5 W and pulse duration of 0.1 s. The membrane is thinned until the endosteum is identified and the fenestra in the connective tissue enlarged to a diameter of 0.6 mm (K.L.H.) or 0.8 mm (S.G.G.). The distance from the outer surface of the incus to the fenestra is measured and the prosthesis is cut 0.3 mm longer. A 0.6-mm Causse stapes prosthesis is placed on or through the endosteum and sealed with fibroadipose tissue (K.L.H.) or a 0.4-mm Causse prosthesis is placed over a vein graft to seal the fenestra (S.G.G.). The tympanomeatal flap is returned to the normal anatomic position and held in place with gelfoam and Merocel otowick expanded with saline solution.

Lateral Ossicular Chain Problems

Although surgical lasers have improved the safety and ease of tissue removal from the oval window, lateral chain problems continue to complicate revision stapes surgery. Abnormalities of the incus and malleus include erosion of the long process of the incus and incus/malleus fixation.

Pathology of the lateral ossicular chain in most cases of revision stapes surgery is due to necrosis of the long process of the incus. In our experience, necrosis of the incus is usually encountered in cases with a lateralized wire prosthesis that becomes firmly adherent to the edge of the oval window or in small fenestra cases with a displaced platinum ribbon/Teflon piston prosthesis. A less frequently encountered, but equally difficult, lateral ossicular chain problem is attic fixation of the incus and/or malleus. This finding requires removal of the incus and, if also fixed, the malleus neck is cut.

In patients with incusor necrosis attic fixation, the prosthesis is removed as discussed previously. The eroded incus is disarticulated from the malleus and removed from the attic with a large right-angle hook. Using the argon laser, the connective tissue in the oval window is removed to the level of the endosteum to create a new fenestra. The fenestra is covered with either a vein or a perichondrial graft. This graft is necessary to prevent migration of the new prosthesis into the vestibule. In cases of previous total stapedectomy, ossicular reconstruction is accomplished using a Brackmann modified total ossicular prosthesis covered with tragal cartilage. The Brackmann prosthesis is trimmed to a total length of the distance from the fenestra to the edge of the scutum. The prosthesis is packed in place to prevent either lateral or medial displacement. The platform of the prosthesis is covered with tragal cartilage to prevent the prosthesis from contacting the tympanic membrane. In cases of small fenestra, ossicular reconstruction is performed with a Causse malleus to footplate prosthesis. This prosthesis has a narrow shaft that is more suited to a small fenestra.[48] The Causse prosthesis is trimmed to a total length of the distance from the long process of the malleus to the fenestra. The Causse prosthesis is placed on a vein graft over the fenestra to prevent medial displacement of the prosthesis.

Results

In 1994, we reported the results of 32 patients who underwent argon laser revision stapectomy.[49] Closure of the air–bone gap to ≥10 dB was noted in 75% of these patients. Closure of the air–bone gap was worse when there was necrosis of the long process of the incus. In these six patients, only three had closure of the air–bone gap to ≥10 dB. There was no sensorineural hearing loss, facial palsy, or permanent complaint of dysequilibrium or vertigo.

REFERENCES

1. Shea JJ. Fenestration of the oval window. *Ann Oto Rhinol Laryngol* 1958;67:932–951
2. Stahle J, Hogberg L. Laser and labyrinth: some preliminary experiments on pigeons. *Acta Otolaryngol (Stockh)* 1965;60: 367–374
3. Kelemen G, Laor Y, Klein E. Laser irradiation and hearing organ. In: *Proceedings of the Pan American Congress on Otolaryngology*, Mexico, 1966
4. Kelemen G, Laor Y, Klein E. Laser-induced ear damage. *Arch Otolaryngol* 1967;85:58–60
5. Sugar J, Stahle J, Hogberg L. Laser irradiation of the stria vascularis. *Arch Otolaryngol* 1974;99:330–336
6. Sataloff J. Experimental use of laser in otosclerotic stapes. *Arch Otolaryngol* 1967;85:614–616
7. Escudero LH, Castro AO, Drummond M, et al. Argon laser in human tympanoplasty. *Arch Otolaryngol* 1979;105(5):252–253
8. Perkins RC. Laser stapedotomy for otosclerosis. *Laryngoscope* 1980;90:228–241
9. DiBartolomeo JR, Ellis M. The argon laser in otology. *Laryngoscope* 1980;90:1786–1796
10. McGee TM. The argon laser in surgery for chronic ear disease and otosclerosis. *Laryngoscope* 1983;93:1177–1183
11. Palva T. Argon laser in otosclerosis surgery. *Acta Otolaryngol (Stockh)* 1987;104:153–157
12. McGee T. Lasers in otology. *Otolaryngol Clin North Am* 1989;22:233–238
13. Lesinski SG, Palmer A. Lasers for otosclerosis. *Laryngoscope* 1989; 99(suppl):46:1–24
14. Horn KL, Gherini SG, Griffin GM. Argon laser stapedectomy using an endo-otoprobe system. *Otolaryngol Head Neck Surg* 1990;102:193–198
15. Gherini S, Causse JB, Griffin G, et al. Sonde de Gherini-Causse et laser argon HGM. Intérêt dans la chirurgie des malformation d'oreilles. *Ann Otolaryngol (Paris)* 1990;107: 418–422
16. Gherini S, Horn KL, Bowman CA, et al. Small fenestra laser stapedectomy utilizing a hand held argon laser in obliterative otosclerosis. *Laryngoscope* 1990;100:1276–1282
17. Bartels L. KTP laser stapedotomy: is it safe? *Otolaryngol Head Neck Surg* 1990;103:685–692
18. Palva T, Ramsay H. Revision surgery for otosclerosis. *Acta Otolaryngol (Stockh)* 1990;110:416–420
19. Thedinger BS. Applications of the KTP laser in chronic ear surgery. *Am J Otol* 1990;11:79–84
20. Hodgson RS, Wilson DF. Argon laser stapedectomy. *Laryngoscope* 1991;101:230–233
21. Horn KL, Gherini SG. Use of the fiberoptic argon laser in middle ear surgery. *Oper Tech Otolaryngol Head Neck Surg* 1992;3:243–245
22. Rauch SD, Bartley ML. Argon laser stapedectomy: comparison to traditional fenestration techniques. *Am J Otol* 1992;13: 556–560
23. Perkins RC, Curto FS. Laser stapedotomy: a comparative study of prosthesis and seals. *Laryngosope* 1992;102:1321–1327
24. Causse JB, Gherini S, Horn KL. Surgical treatment of stapes fixation by fiberoptic argon laser stapedotomy with reconstruction of the annular ligament. *Otolaryngol Clin North Am* 1993;26:395–416
25. McGee TM, Diaz-Ordaz EA, Kartush JM. The role of KTP laser in revision stapedectomy. *Otolaryngol Head Neck Surg* 1993;109:839–843
26. Strunk CL, Quinn FB. Stapedectomy surgery in residency: KTP 532 versus argon laser. *Am J Otol* 1993;14:113–117
27. Lesinski SG, Newrock R. Carbon dioxide lasers for otosclerosis. *Otolaryngol Clin North Am* 1993;26:417–441
28. Silverstein H, Bendet E, Rosenberg S, et al. Revision stapes surgery with and without laser: a comparison. *Laryngoscope* 1994;104:1431–1438
29. Perkins R. Laser stapedotomy. In: Brackmann DE, Shelton C, Arriaga MA, eds. *Otologic Surgery*. Philadelphia: WB Saunders; 1994:313–329
30. Haberkamp TJ, Harvey SA, Khafagy Y. Revision stapedectomy with and without the CO_2 laser: an analysis of results. *Am J Otol* 1996;17:225–229
31. Vernick DM. A comparison of results of KTP and CO_2 laser stapedotomy. *Am J Otol* 1996;17:221–224

32. Glasscock ME, Jackson CG, Whitaker SR. The argon laser in acoustic tumor surgery. *Laryngoscope* 1981;91:1405–1416
33. Silverstein H, Rosenburg S, Jones R. Small fenestra stapedotomies with and without KTP laser: a comparison. *Laryngoscope* 1989;99:485–488
34. Gherini S, Horn KL, Causse JB, et al. Fiberoptic argon laser stapedotomy: is it safe? *Am J Otol* 1993;14:283–289
35. Kodali S, Harvey SA, Prieto TE. Thermal effects of laser stapedectomy in an animal model: CO_2 versus KTP. *Laryngoscope* 1997;107:1445–1450
36. Okuna T, Nomura Y, Hara M. Argon laser irradiation of the otolithic organ. *Otolaryngol Head Neck Surg* 1990;103: 926–930
37. Nomura Y, Okuna T, Mizuno M. Treatment of vertigo using laser labyrinthectomy. *Acta Otolarynogol (Stockh)* 1993;113:261–262
38. Anthony PF. Laser applications in inner ear surgery. *Otolaryngol Clin North Am* 1996;29:1031–1048
39. Sooy FA. In Discussion of Perkins RC: laser stapedotomy for otosclerosis. *Laryngoscope* 1980;90:228–241
40. Causse JB. The twenty fine points of otosclerosis surgery. *Am J Otol* 1989;10:75–76
41. Feldman BA, Schuknecht HF. Experiences with revision stapedectomy procedures. *Laryngoscope* 1972;80:1281–1291
42. Dawes JDK, Curry AR. Types of stapedectomy failure and prognosis of revision operations. *J Laryngol Otol* 1974;88: 213–226
43. Shah N. Revision stapedectomy for late conductive deafness. *J Laryngol Otol* 1974;88:207–212
44. Crabtree JA, Britton BH, Powers WH. An evaluation of revision stapes surgery. *Laryngoscope* 1980;90:224–227
45. Han WW, Incesulu A, McKenna MJ, et al. Revision stapedectomy: intraoperative finding, results, and review of the literature. *Laryngoscope* 1997;107:1185–1192
46. Linthicum F. Histologic evidence of the cause of failure in stapes surgery. *Ann Otol Rhinol Laryngol* 1971;80:67–77
47. Sheehy JL, Nelson RA, House HP. Revision stapedectomy: a review of 258 cases. *Laryngoscope* 1981;91:43–51
48. Horn KL, Gherini SG, Franz DC. Argon laser revision stapedectomy. *Am J Otol* 1994;15:383–388
49. Causse JB, Horn KL. Correction of incus necrosis during revision stapes surgery using the Causse malleus prosthesis. *Oper Tech Otolaryngol Head Neck Surg* 1998;9:98–102

16

Management of the Meniere's Patient

"If medical therapy of diuretics and steroids fails to alleviate symptoms, intratympanic aminoglycoside injection is the treatment of choice. I have not had to operate on a patient for Meniere's disease since using intratympanic aminoglycoside treatment. Less than 5% of patients progress to the stage where destructive treatment is indicated."

Brian W. Blakley

"Remission procedures include steroid perfusion of the round window and endolymphatic sac surgery. The term *remission* is used to indicate that these procedures attempt to restore function to the inner ear rather than destroy or decrease function. Also, this term clearly explains that the remission may be short-lived and that symptoms may then recur."

Mitchell K. Schwaber

"Despite the obvious conflicting beliefs concerning the benefits of endolymphatic sac surgery in Meniere's disease, most otologists routinely perform the procedure. The nondestructive nature of the surgery, low complication rate, minimal morbidity, and ability to perform the procedure as an outpatient are obvious advantages over labyrinthectomy or vestibular nerve section. For these reasons, and with a success rate approaching 80%, endolymphatic sac surgery remains a valuable option for treating the vertigo of Meniere's disease."

William L. Meyerhoff

Management of the Meniere's Patient

CHAPTER 46

Brian W. Blakley

Diagnosis

Diagnosis precedes treatment. It's a simple concept, yet diagnostic uncertainty is a major frustration in treating Meniere's patients. A complete diagnosis includes estimates of the severity of symptoms, medical and nonmedical influences, and assessment of previous therapy. Each of these can affect treatment decisions. The literature about Meniere's disease is not very helpful either. Although Meniere's disease is uncommon—some even say it is rare—there are many single-author reports in the literature with huge numbers of patients. How is this possible? Clearly there is doubt about the diagnosis. Great results occur if the disease is absent.

The diagnosis is made on the basis of the history. The official definition of the American Academy of Otolaryngology–Head and Neck Surgery (AAO–HNS) seems reasonable.[1] A good, classic history with the criteria as outlined is adequate proof of Meniere's disease, even if another disorder is found. The following symptoms must be present for a confident diagnosis of Meniere's disease:

1. The principal symptom must be vertigo at some point in the disease. Vertigo is a spinning sensation. Overdiagnosers include any sensation of movement (swaying, weaving, veering) under the term vertigo, but these symptoms alone do not suggest an otologic cause. Acute vertigo often becomes less severe over time, so that dizziness symptoms like veering and swaying result. This description identifies how "dizziness" and "vertigo" are used in this chapter.
2. Sensorineural hearing, and aural fullness or tinnitus, particularly of a low tone type, must be present. Hearing may fluctuate.
3. Spells must be recurrent. A single spell of vertigo does not constitute Meniere's disease.
4. The spells must last 20 min or more, at least sometime in the disease. Actually it is unlikely that the pathophysiologic events[2,3] that are attributed to Meniere's disease could occur within 20 min. A minimum time of 1 h seems stronger, but the official AAO-HNS definition suggests 20 min.

Some further diagnostic points to consider are that the physical examination is usually normal, and tests are optional. Many tests are interesting for research purposes, but no test proves or disproves the diagnosis of Meniere's disease. Vestibular testing for clinical purposes is poor. An audiogram should be done; an electronystagmogram (ENG) is usually perfomed as well, to confirm the presence of function in the other ear. Destroying the only functioning ear would result in disaster. The summating potentials from electrocochleography and other tests are interesting but should not alter clinical treatment decisions. Figure 46–1 presents a flowchart for a treatment plan for Meniere's disease.

Treatment

Once we have a firm diagnosis, what is the next step? This chapter considers only the treatment of vertigo spells. Meniere's disease patients frequently have varying degrees of imbalance, which is not treated in the same way as vertigo. First we consider the effect on the patient's activities of daily living. Once again, we have to ask the patient: How frequent is the dizziness? How severe? Does it prevent him or her from going out? Driving? Walking? Working? Specific treatment may not be needed.

The first step in treatment is explanation. The patient must understand as much as possible about the unpredictability of the prognosis. Symptoms may resolve. Although effective treatment can usually be found, the fix may not be quick. The risks and alternatives of treatment should be discussed. Even patients with mild disease should be aware of the range of treatment options from the conservative to aggressive surgery.

Nonspecific factors that exacerbate most dizziness should be addressed: (1) avoidance of stress if possible, (2) inadequate sleep (consider getting an hour more sleep per night), (3) inadequate irregular meals, (4) side effects of medications, and (5) high caffeine intake (some dizzy patients drink 20 cups of coffee a day. No wonder they are dizzy!).

Adequate explanation is all some patients need. For others, a temporary sedative will ease their anxiety over the disabling period. In treating this disorder, it is important to remember that people do not die of Meniere's disease. We are treating a symptom. The patient will help decide if and when more aggressive therapy is desired.

If more than a weekly average of an hour of dizziness occurs, most people will want help. This may be either a single spell or multiple spells. Of course, this guideline should be individualized. Many patients will demand treatment for lesser degrees of vertigo and, if the treatment is safe and inexpensive, it may be reasonable. Any treatment should be continued for at least 1 month, if possible.

There are many treatment options. Some are placebos, but we don't know which ones, and patients may love them. Some treatments that I do not use because of lack of evidence and/or poor clinical results include hypnosis, lipoflavinoids,

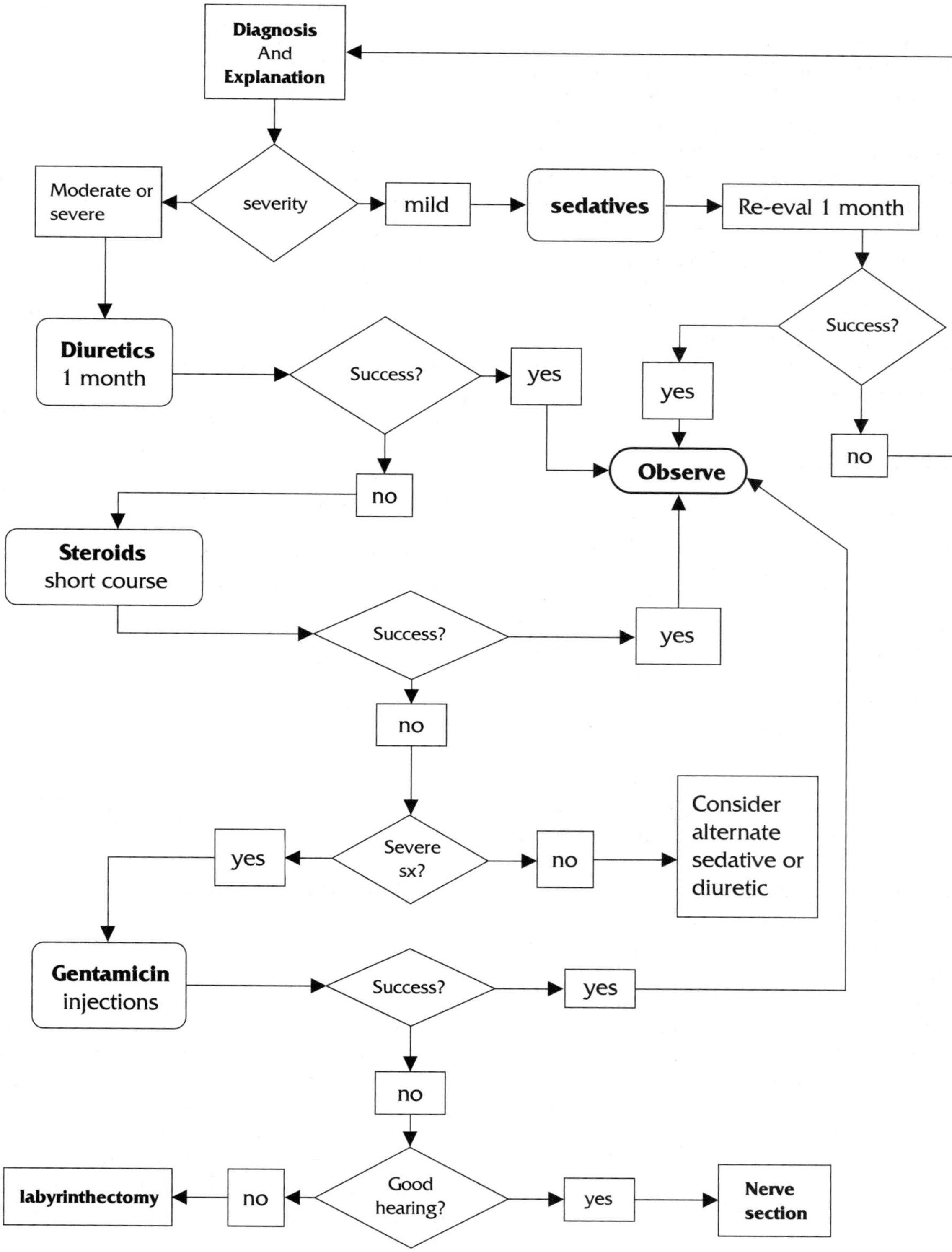

Figure 46–1 Meniere's disease decision flowchart.

megavitamins, nicotinamide, nicain, allergy injections, dietary glucose manipulation for hypoglycemia, and glycopyrrolate. The use of vestibular rehabilitation or habituating exercises to treat intermittent symptoms is illogical. Accepted treatments include sedatives, diuretics, steroids, intratympanic gentamicin, and surgery.

SEDATIVES

Although sedatives are not a good long-term solution, they are frequently adequate to cover brief (up to 2 weeks) periods of difficulty with dizziness. The patient should be told about side effects, such as sleepiness. The list of interactions with other medications is considerable. There are many sedatives on the market. With some general principles in mind, the specific choice is probably not critical. Most patients with mild dizziness achieve adequate relief from meclizine taken up to three times per day. Meclizine is not more effective than many other drugs but because it has fewer side effects, it is popular. For severe vertigo, one of the benzodiazepines such as diazepam is reasonable. Most patients do not need these. It is important to moderate the dose in the elderly or frail. Alprazolam or dimenhydrinate are useful as well.

The key is to use sedatives briefly. Prolonged use of sedatives impairs compensation, prolongs symptoms, and produces a suboptimal result. Also, patients frequently become psychologically or physically dependent on sedatives if they experience initial relief. Persistent use causes reduced efficacy and shorter effect, necessitating increasing amounts.

DIURETICS AND SALT RESTRICTION

I rarely recommend one of these without the other. The salt restriction is not severe. I simply instruct patients not to add salt to their food and to avoid salty foods such as potato chips and salted crackers. Hydrochlorothiazide is the most commonly used diuretic, but differences in efficacy among different diuretics have not been shown. Potent diuretics such as furosemide are not more effective. I usually use a combination of hydrocholorothiazide/triamterene to avoid potassium loss.

That is standard procedure, but I have a new wrinkle. Some research papers[4-6] have reported high numbers of receptors for aldosterone in the inner ear. What are they doing there? We know that aldosterone is involved in renal sodium/potassium metabolism. Perhaps upregulation of aldosterone receptors contributes to the electrolyte imbalances in Meniere's disease. Spironolactone blocks aldosterone receptors and has been available for many years. I have successfully used spironolactone in some Meniere's patients who failed treatment with other diuretics, but more data are needed to be confident of these results. After all, many people's symptoms of Meniere's disease improve spontaneously. It is also possible that we want to enhance, rather than block, the receptor if it is active in Meniere's disease.

Spironolactone can cause hyperkalemia, whereas most diuretics cause hypokalemia; this agent can also cause abdominal cramps and gynecomastia in men and breast tumors in women, although a review article disputed this.

STEROIDS

Some papers in the literature suggest an allergic and/or immune-mediated basis for Meniere's disease in some patients,[7,8] but the relationship is poorly understood. There is no test of blood, or anything else, that proves or disproves autoimmune ear disease, so an empirical short course of steroids is reasonable if diuretics fail. Often a single course provides long-lasting relief of symptoms. Prednisone is the usual steroid of choice. In the literature, the recommended dose of prednisone varies, so how much should one use?

My approach to dosing is to compromise between a large dose that has an effect and a smaller one that is unlikely to result in side effects. Examination of the general medical literature and experience leads to the impression that the incidence of side effects increases when daily doses of prednisone approach 60 mg/day. In my experience, the most common complications of a short dose of prednisone are gastric irritation (so the medication should be taken with food or milk) fluid retention, weight gain, and psychosis. Other reported complications include aseptic necrosis of the hip, gastric bleeding, and diabetic complications. Even unsophisticated patients are aware that the use of steroids may produce complications.

I instruct patients to discontinue the medication if they have gastric irritation, if they feel weird or goofy, or if they have joint pains or severe symptoms. Diabetics should be aware that while they are taking steroids their blood sugar will be higher, but this is transient and frequently does not require changes in insulin. Patients who are aware of the possible side effects are able to recognize them. Stopping the medication early can avoid big problems.

I typically recommend the following 15-day prednisone regimen using 5-mg tablets:

2 tabs qid for 7 days (40 mg/day), then
2 tabs tid day for 2 days (30 mg/day), then
2 tabs bid for 2 days (20 mg/day), then
1 tab bid for 2 days (10 mg/day), then
1 tab daily for 2 days (5 mg/day)

This regimen is modified for elderly or small people or for people in whom the suspicion of immune disorder is weak.

INTRATYMPANIC AMINOGLYCOSIDES

If medical therapy of diuretics and steroids fails to alleviate symptoms, intratympanic aminoglycoside injection is the treatment of choice. I have not had to operate on a patient for Meniere's disease since using intratympanic aminoglycoside treatment. Less than 5% of patients progress to the stage where destructive treatment is indicated. Streptomycin and gentamicin are the two most reasonable agents to inject into the ear. Of these, gentamicin seems to be safest and least uncomfortable.[9] Risks include persistent tympanic membrane scarring or perforation, ossicular trauma, allergic or idiosyncratic reactions to the medication (which I have not seen from gentamicin injection), and possible hearing loss. Ataxia may become a problem.

Advantages and Disadvantages

Intratympanic gentamicin has advantages and disadvantages compared with destructive surgery. Advantages include avoidance of surgery and all its risks, pain, and expense; simplicity; probability of preserving hearing at the pretreatment level; and possibility of fine-tuning treatment so that the vestibular response is reduced, but not destroyed. If doubts arise, treatment can be reinstituted later.

There are several disadvantages to the use of intratympanic gentamicin. The first concern is uncertainty about the dose to be injected—how much medication remains in the middle ear, for how long, and what the desired amount needed to affect the inner ear should be. There is also a known genetic predisposition to aminoglycoside toxicity. The dose uncertainty is addressed by using multiple small doses over several weeks and assessing effect between each. Effects may take many days to become fully expressed. A second disadvantage to the use of intratympanic aminoglycosides is the inconvenience in having to return to the physician's office several times, and have tests and needle pokes. Third, patients must be informed that they will experience imbalance while receiving the injections. However, this imbalance is much less severe than that experienced after a vestibular nerve section because the lesion is created more slowly and permits compensation between injections.

Technique

Buffering the standard 40 mg/ml solution of gentamicin with $NaHCO_3$ results in a final solution of about 30 mg/ml. Most hospitals have a pharmacist who can do this. I inject with a 1-ml tuberculin syringe with a 25-gauge spinal needle, through the tympanic membrane while viewing with a microscope using an otologic speculum. The spinal needle is bent so that the view of the tympanic membrane is unimpeded. The injections are repeated on a weekly basis. Hearing is tested prior to each injection if good hearing is present.

Unless research data are being collected, repeated vestibular testing is not currently essential, but this could change in the future if reliable data are collected. Some investigators have used serial caloric tests to determine a treatment endpoint. This overshoots the amount of aminoglycoside needed for control of symptoms and often causes hearing loss.

So when is the last injection? The endpoint may occur when the patient indicates that the spells are gone and when six injections have been given and some physiologic effect (usually imbalance) has been noted. What if the patient's spells are so infrequent that he/she cannot tell if they are gone? If spells are that infrequent, intratympanic injection may not be justified. Some patients in the literature have required 12 injections, but this is unusual. If 10 or more injections are needed, an obstruction or other factor may be present. Even if such a factor is present, it does not necessarily preclude injection as a rational treatment.

Intratympanic steroids have been advocated by some, although support for this modality is weaker than for aminoglycosides.[9]

Surgery

There can be little doubt that vestibular surgery has been overdone. Nevertheless, surgery has a role in Meniere's disease. There are two main types of operation for Meniere's disease: destructive and nondestructive. The destruction is done to hearing. There are also some procedures that may or may not be destructive.

NONDESTRUCTIVE SURGERY

There are two types of nondestructive surgery for Meniere's disease:

1. *Repair of presumed perilymphatic fistula* (PLF): Some investigators believe that the symptoms of Meniere's disease are similar to those of PLF, so this may be a diagnostic, rather than a treatment, decision. The diagnostic criteria of PLF are uncertain and vary from investigator to another, and from day to day. Although some patients may have fistulae, we don't know who they are. The early overenthusiasm for surgery has caused the reputation of PLF surgery to fall into disrepute. Fortunately, the heyday for PLF surgery is over.
2. *Endolymphatic sac surgery:* Although some investigators report subtle differences between different endolymphatic sac operations and the type of shunt or prosthesis used, there is little reason to believe that these differences are real. The principal involved is the use of a plastic shunt to drain the sac into the mastoid cavity. Although the role of endolymphatic sac surgery for treatment of vertigo remains controversial, the literature indicates no support for improvement of hearing.[10,11] Endolymphatic sac surgery should not be performed to improve hearing. Patients with Meniere's disease have poor and/or fluctuating hearing before surgery, so we should expect that some will experience improvement and some will experience deterioration. Of course we can actually measure hearing, and compensation does not occur as it does for vestibular problems.

Patients should be told about the risks of ear surgery, but risks should be small in this group of patients. In addition, patients should be told that there is considerable doubt as to the efficacy of the procedure. If symptoms are not improved other destructive procedures are still feasible.

DESTRUCTIVE SURGERY

Labyrinthectomy

For many years, labyrinthectomy has been a standard weapon against Meniere's disease. The goal is to destroy the vestibular portions of the inner ear while sacrificing the cochlear portion (hearing). Although this seems odd, the notion of destroying hearing is not foolish in patients for whom the disease has destroyed most auditory function anyway. There are generally two techniques:

1. *Transcanal labyrinthectomy:* The oval and round windows are connected by drilling the bone away between them. Streptomycin or gentamicin is usually placed in the ear as well. The semicircular canals remain intact.
2. *Transmastoid labyrinthectomy:* This approach allows more thorough destruction of the inner ear by drilling the semicircular canals, opening the vestibule, and destroying the saccule and utricle. Many surgeons place streptomycin or gentamicin in the inner ear as well.

Vestibular Nerve Section

Vestibular nerve section is the "gold standard" for control of severe vertigo spells, but not for imbalance. This procedure should be performed infrequently because it is destructive. Most patients experience some imbalance afterward. The goal is to totally abolish vestibular function in one ear. The only reason that we can do this and get away with it relates to the tremendous compensatory power of the vestibular system. Compensation works best when the brain and the other ear are normal. There's the rub! Even perfectly normal patients could develop Meniere's disease in the other ear.

Nerve sections are a bad idea in patients whose contralateral ear is abnormal or who cannot compensate. Poor compensation is hard to predict.[12] The elderly and patients whose main symptom is chronic imbalance rather than episodic spinning vertigo tend to be poor compensators. Uncompensated vestibular neuritis is a central nervous system CNS problem and is a contraindication to vestibular nerve section. (The term *uncompensated vestibular neuritis* means different things to different people. Frequently the term is applied to patients with chronic imbalance in whom an unanticipated caloric loss is found. The diagnosis of vestibular neuritis is highly presumptive. *Idiopathic caloric loss* is a more honest term.) Patients with CNS disease (e.g., multiple sclerosis, strokes, degenerative disease) should generally not undergo vestibular nerve sections.

In this procedure, the vestibular nerve is cut or sectioned proximal to the geniculate ganglion, but it is hoped that the cochlear nerve is not damaged. The operation is appropriate in patients who require a destructive procedure, but who have good hearing. There are two popular approaches: the retrolabyrinthine, which I favor, and the retrosigmoid.

The main risks of vestibular nerve section are loss of hearing, chronic imbalance, and all the other risks of ear and intracranial surgery. Facial weakness is not likely after vestibular nerve section. The facial nerve is a few millimeters away, but this is akin to miles in skull base surgery.

Strange as it may seem, some patients experience return of symptoms and even regain a caloric response a year or so after labyrinthectomy or even after the vestibular nerve has been cut. This may result from hair cell re-growth, nerve or axon sprouting, repair, or incomplete sectioning; so many surgeons remove a segment of nerve rather than just cut the nerve. There is no justice! When we don't want an organ to work, we can't stop it. When we do want it to work right, we can't start it!

Combined Labyrinthectomy and Nerve Section

Do you wear a belt and suspenders? Some do so to be safe. Some otologists extend their transmastoid labyrinthectomy so that the internal auditory canal is explored and the vestibular nerve sectioned. The hope is that by sectioning and destroying the end organ, return of symptoms cannot occur. Maybe.

Other Surgery

Every year another operation or two is advocated for Meniere's disease. Many procedures for Meniere's disease have come and gone. The Cody tack operation, the Fick procedure, cryosurgery, and ultrasound proved less reliable than other methods.

REFERENCES

1. Monsell EM, Balkany TA, Gates GA, et al. Committee on hearing and equilibrium guidelines for the diagnosis and evaluation of therapy in Meniere's disease. Committee on hearing and equilibrium. *Otolaryngol Head Neck Surg* 1995;113:181–185
2. Gibson WP, Arenberg IK. Pathophysiologic theories in the etiology of Meniere's disease. *Otolaryngol Clin North Am* 1997;30:961–967
3. Wackym PA, Sando I. Molecular and cellular pathology of Meniere's disease. *Otolaryngol Clin North Am* 1997;30:947–960
4. Pitovski DZ, Drescher MJ, Kerr TP, Drescher DG. Aldosterone mediates an increase in [^{3}H]ouabain binding Na^+ K^+-ATPase sites in the mammaliam inner ear. *Brain Res* 1993;601:273–278
5. Ferrary E, Bernard C, Teixeira M, et al. Hormonal modulation of inner ear fluids. *Acta Otolaryngol (Stockh)*1996;116:244–247
6. Freeman S, Geal Dor M, Sohmer H. The role of adrenocortical steroid hormones in the development of hearing. *J Basic Clin Physiol Pharmacol* 1996;7:167–177
7. Derebery MJ. Allergic and immunologic aspects of Meniere's disease. *Otolaryngol Head Neck Surg* 1996;114:360–365
8. Soliman AM. A subpopulation of Menière's patients produce antibodies that bind to endolymphatic sac antigens. *Am J Otol* 1996;17:76–80
9. Blakley BW. Clinical forum: a review of intratympanic therapy. *Am J Otol* 1997;18:520–526
10. Grant IL, Welling DB. The treatment of hearing loss in Meniere's disease. *Otolaryngol Clin North Am* 1997;30: 1123–1144
11. Quaranta A, Onofri M, Sallustio V, Iurato S. Comparison of long-term hearing results after vestibular neurectomy, endolymphatic mastoid shunt, and medical therapy. *Am J Otol* 1997;18:444–448
12. Blakley BW, Barber HO, Tomlinson RD, et al. On the search for markers of poor vestibular compensation. *Otolaryngol Head Neck Surg* 1989;101:572–577

Management of the Meniere's Patient

Mitchell K. Schwaber

CHAPTER 47

Perhaps the most controversial subject in neurotology concerns the diagnosis and management of patients with Meniere's disease. There is uncertainty regarding not only the etiology and pathophysiology, but also the role of medical management, particularly because the precise cause is unknown, the illness has frequent periods of remission, and only anecdotal reports of efficacy exist for most treatments. Furthermore, there is a perception that many of the surgical procedures used to control the disorder may merely be inducing a remission phase or may have no effect at all. Much of the conventional wisdom regarding Meniere's disease merely reflects the opinion of experienced clinicians, rather than scientific fact.

With such a controversial subject, it is easy to extrapolate that certain findings, symptoms, or responses to treatment are indicative of the nature of the problem. The reader should be reminded that neither an apparent response to therapy nor postmortem histopathologic findings represent scientific evidence of the exact pathophysiology of a condition. Plainly stated, Meniere's disease is a chronic condition characterized by a progressive dysfunction of the inner ear or the cochleovestibular nerve, or both. Beyond this basic description, the precise etiology of the problem remains to be clearly elucidated.

As a consequence, to manage Meniere's syndrome patients successfully, the physician must assume their care for many years, albeit the need for services may vary considerably. This is particularly true in light of the long periods of remission as well as the cyclic nature of this condition in some patients. Therefore, management of these patients should be done with the mindset of a long-term chronic disorder, much like adult-onset diabetes mellitus, chronic pain, or hypertension. Although treatment may modify the clinical course of Meniere's disease patients somewhat, cures are indeed rare. Patients must be followed and therapy adjusted as clinical circumstances warrant. Also, measuring the effects of therapy can be extremely difficult, and the physician should never assume that the recommended intervention or treatment has actually stopped the progression of this disorder. Rather, the condition may simply have entered a remission phase.

Having stated that the exact etiology is unknown, what do we know of Meniere's disease? Meniere's disease is a clinical disorder associated with the histopathological finding of endolymphatic hydrops. Most of the hydropic distention found in postmortem specimens is seen in the cochlea and the saccule, although occasionally the utricle and the ampullae are involved. Other histopathologic features include ruptures or fistulae, collapse of membranes, and vestibular fibrosis. Minimal histopathologic changes are seen in the sensory epithelia, although the loss of ganglion and neuronal cells, inner and outer hair cells, and strial vascularity has been reported. Recognized causes of Meniere's syndrome include idiopathic, post-traumatic, postinfectious (i.e., delayed onset after a viral illness), late-stage syphilitic, and Cogan's syndrome or one of its variants.

One theory of Meniere's disease is that increased endolymphatic pressure causes the symptoms as well as the histopathologic features. According to this theory, pressure buildup leads to membrane ruptures, so that potassium-rich endolymph gains access to the sensory and neural structures, causing sudden or fluctuant hearing loss and episodic vertigo. This theory also suggests that pressure buildup develops as a result of altered resorption of fluid by the endolymphatic sac. Abnormalities that lead to this altered resorption include perisaccular and vestibular epithelial fibrosis, altered glycoprotein metabolism, viral infection of the inner ear, and autoimmune-mediated dysfunction of the sac. Bony narrowing of the endolymphatic duct might also contribute to the obstruction and dysfunction of the sac.

A number of studies from the Massachusetts Eye and Ear Infirmary refute the pressure theory and suggest that endolymphatic hydrops is an epiphenomenon. These studies propose that Meniere's disease develops as a result of a problem with altered biochemical gradients within the endolymphatic space. Findings in support of this theory include a number of biochemical alterations found in hydropic inner ears. These alterations include a decrease in endocochlear potential, an increase in intracochlear calcium, alterations in potassium permeability, inhibition of electrogenic transport processes, and increased endolymph fluid protein content.

It seems likely that Meniere's disease can be caused by a number of factors, each resulting in an alteration that leads to similar clinical features. It also seems likely that, at some point, idiopathic endolymphatic hydrops will no longer be an appropriate description of this syndrome. Rather, the specific biochemical or cellular abnormality will be identified and treated by the clinician.

In this era of managed care with declining health care revenues, most clinicians are uncertain as to which studies are needed for proper evaluation of patients with suspected Meniere's disease. The history can be helpful, specifically with regard to fluctuating hearing loss, ear pressure, hearing distortion or hypersensitivity, and severe episodic vertigo accompanied by increased tinnitus or hearing loss. Physical findings that should be elicited include spontaneous or gaze-evoked nystagmus (usually away from the affected ear), fistula test, Dix-Hallpike maneuver, and Romberg and gait tests. The otologic examination, although usually unremarkable, occasionally indicates other causes, such as cholesteatoma or middle ear tumor. A comprehensive audiogram is also essential, with particular attention to the presence of a low-frequency sensorineural hearing loss. Unexpectedly low speech discrimination scores or abnormal acoustic reflexes may be helpful in determining the need for additional testing.

Additional audiovestibular testing, including otoacoustic emissions, electrocochleography, and electronystagmography, should be obtained if there is a need for further supporting data for the diagnosis of Meniere's disease. An elevated summating potential may raise the clinician's suspicion of bilateral dysfunction, but medical judgments based on this study should be made conservatively. Auditory brainstem response testing can be used to screen for retrocochlear disorders masking as Meniere's syndrome, although an imaging study such as a magnetic resonance imaging (MRI) scan is much more definitive and should be obtained before any surgical procedure. Other studies indicated in the evaluation of Meniere's syndrome patients include syphilis screening tests, rheumatoid factor, sedimentation rate, antinuclear antibody titers, blood glucose levels, cholesterol, and triglyceride levels. In cases of bilateral Meniere's syndrome, in cases with rapidly progressive hearing loss, or in cases of suspected Cogan's syndrome, specific studies for autoimmune inner ear antibodies (heat shock protein) should be obtained.

The diagnosis of Meniere's disease has been formalized by the American Academy of Otolaryngology—Head and Neck Surgery and is detailed in Table 47–1. A single episode of severe vertigo with hearing loss is classified as probable Meniere's disease, whereas multiple episodes of vertigo associated with hearing loss represent definite Meniere's disease.

Staging the disease currently depends on the severity of the hearing loss, as noted in Table 47–2. This staging system is in contrast to prior staging systems that depended on the frequency of the vertigo episodes. Stages 1 and 2 are considered representative of early, reversible disease (i.e., susceptible to remission). Stage 1 and 2 cases are more likely to be amenable to remission-type therapies, including endolymphatic sac surgery or steroid perfusion. Stage 3 is considered fixed or not reversible; these patients might be considered for deafferentation procedures, including aminoglycoside perfusion of the round window or retrosigmoid vestibular nerve section. Stage 4 cases are usually considered candidates for destructive procedures, such as transmastoid labyrinthectomy or triple canal ablation with laser.

The medical management of Meniere's disease is directed at either decreasing the fluid volume of the endolymph, increasing the circulation of the inner ear, or altering the immune reactivity or blockage of the endolymphatic duct. None of these proposed regimens has ever been shown to be effective in a double-blind controlled study. Despite that fact, most clinicians use one or more of these strategies in an effort to alter the natural history of the disorder. The most common management strategy is the use of a low-sodium diet and diuretic to decrease endolymph volume. It is entirely possible that if this treatment works, it is through an unrecognized indirect mechanism, such as altering the ionic balance in some way. Recent reports indicate that the epithelial cells of the endolymphatic sac have a large number of receptors that specifically bind with antidiuretic hormone (ADH, or vasopressin [AVP]). One can only speculate whether this explains the action of diuretics and low-salt diet on this condition. However, if this is the case, dehydration and hypovolemia should be avoided, as these would tend to

TABLE 47–1
Diagnosis of Meniere's Disease

Certain Meniere's disease
- Definite Meniere's disease, plus histopathologic confirmation

Definite Meniere's disease
- Two or more definitive spontaneous episodes of vertigo ≤ 20 min
- Audiometrically documented hearing loss on at least one occasion
- Tinnitus or aural fullness in the treated ear
- Other causes excluded

Probable Meniere's disease
- One definitive episode of vertigo
- Audiometrically documented hearing loss on at least one occasion
- Tinnitus or aural fullness in the treated ear
- Other causes excluded

Possible Meniere's disease
- Episodic vertigo of the Meniere's type without documented hearing loss, or
- Sensorineural hearing loss, fluctuating or fixed, with disequilibrium but without definitive episodes
- Other causes excluded

TABLE 47–2
Staging of Definite and Certain Meniere's Disease*

Stage	Four-Tone Average (dB)
1	≤25
2	26–40
3	41–70
4	> 70

* Staging is based on the four-tone average (arithmetic mean rounded to the nearest whole number) of the pure-tone thresholds at 0.5, 1, 2, and 3 kHz of the worst audiogram during the interval 6 months before treatment. This is the same audiogram that is used as the baseline evaluation to determine hearing outcome from treatment. Staging should be applied only to cases of definite or certain Meniere's disease.

raise AVP levels. Simply stated, to keep AVP levels low, the most effective route would be a mild diuretic, a modest 2000- to 2500-mg salt diet, and plenty of water.

Vasodilator therapy is based on the belief that Meniere's disease is related to decreased blood flow in the inner ear. In this treatment strategy, the patient is instructed to avoid caffeine and nicotine completely. A vasodilator drug such as niacin, B-histamine, or papaverine is prescribed to improve blood flow. The patient is asked to avoid stress and to begin an exercise program for conditioning and stress reduction. Although the efficacy of this regimen can be questioned, it is extremely beneficial to the patient both physically and psychologically, and it has few side effects.

A third medical regimen is to alter the immune response with either steroids, methotrexate, cytoxan, or allergic desensitization. Steroids are usually recommended first for patients with severe vertigo unresponsive to low salt diet, diuretics, and vestibular suppressants and for patients with a sudden decline in hearing. Patients with bilateral Meniere's disease or with suspected autoimmune inner ear syndrome may also be candidates for steroid therapy. If the patient is initially responsive to steroids, other immunosuppressive therapies can be tried, usually with success. If the symptoms can be stabilized for 1 year, the immunosuppressive drug can be tapered and discontinued.

If a patient continues to have episodic vertigo in spite of an adequate trial of medical therapy, surgical management should be considered. Episodic vertigo occurring once a month or more often is considered life-altering. These patients are usually prepared to have a procedure if the clinician recommends it. The type of procedure recommended depends on the duration and stage of the Meniere's disease and the desires of the patient.

In explaining the available surgical options to the patient, it is helpful to divide the procedures into three types: remission procedures, deafferentation procedures, and destructive procedures.

Remission procedures include steroid perfusion of the round window and endolymphatic sac surgery. The term *remission* is used to indicate that these procedures attempt to restore function to the inner ear rather than destroy or decrease function. Also, this term clearly explains that the remission may be short-lived and that symptoms may then recur. Patients are much more understanding of this concept, rather than predicting the duration of relief. Remission procedures are recommended for stage 1 or 2 disease, particularly with a history of long remissions in the past. These procedures are particularly appropriate in patients with relatively short histories of the illness, that is, less than 2 to 3 years.

Few procedures in otologic surgery have been as controversial as endolymphatic sac surgery. Opinions vary from those who conclude the procedure is effective in more than 80% of cases to those who believe it is nothing more than a placebo procedure. Endolymphatic sac surgery offers the possibility of vertigo control with little risk of morbidity; theoretically, surgery improves the function of the sac or opens a blocked endolymphatic duct. Alternatively, endolymphatic sac surgery might cause a temporary subclinical labyrinthitis that perhaps alters the natural history of the Meniere's disease.

Steroid perfusion, like endolymphatic sac surgery, is a controversial procedure. This procedure can be performed alone in the office or in conjunction with endolymphatic sac surgery. Theoretically, the drug penetrates the round window membrane and then, through an unknown mechanism, leads to improvement in the function of the labyrinth. This improvement is reflected by a period of remission with improved hearing and relief from vertigo, which often lasts for months. Like endolymphatic sac surgery, this transient improvement may be a placebo effect or quite possibly a result of the induction of a mild labyrinthitis.

Deafferentation procedures are those that remove the vestibular nerve function without necessarily destroying the end organ or decreasing the cochlear function. These include retrosigmoid vestibular nerve section and gentamycin perfusion of the round window. Although either procedure might be appropriate for stage 1 or 2 disease with hearing fluctuation, they are more often applied in stage 3 disease. Each has advantages and disadvantages. Gentamicin perfusion can be performed in the office under local anesthesia and it effectively decreases vestibular function in the treated ear in approximately 80 to 85% of patients. In these cases, patients either have no vertigo episodes, or very mild ones. This treatment is associated with hearing loss and persistent unsteadiness in 10 to 15% of patients. Recently, some clinicians have recommended gentamicin perfusion as the surgical treatment of choice in Meniere's disease, using retrosigmoid vestibular nerve section only in cases of gentamicin failure.

Retrosigmoid vestibular nerve section also has a role in the surgical management of Meniere's disease. Its advantages include a more complete deafferentation of the vestibular nerve, leading to much less postoperative unsteadiness and only rare episodic vertigo. Also cochlear function can be more certainly preserved with this approach. The disadvantages of this procedure are its higher cost, the patient's loss of gainful employment during recovery, and, because it is an intracranial procedure, the risk of severe neurologic complication. Even so, retrosigmoid vestibular nerve section is appropriate in gentamicin failures, in patients who want a single definitive surgical procedure for control of the vertigo, and in patients who want to preserve their hearing if at all possible.

Destructive procedures, specifically transmastoid labyrinthectomy, are used to destroy the entire vestibular end-organ to cure the vertigo. This procedure is appropriate in stage 4 disease and in cases for which other surgical treatments have failed. Episodic vertigo can be controlled in more than 90% of patients undergoing this procedure, although this may reflect the careful selection used before this procedure. The major disadvantage of this procedure is total hearing loss, although several clinicians have reported hearing preservation in some cases in which the laser was used to seal the canals prior to the bony exenteration. This has not been sufficiently reproducible to recommend as a treatment alternative.

SUGGESTED READINGS

Schwaber—CHAPTER 47

Arriaga MA, Goldman S. Hearing results of intratympanic steroid treatment of endolymphatic hydrops. *Laryngoscope* 1998;108(11 pt 1):1682–1685

Gibson WP, Arenberg IK. Pathophysiological theories in the etiology of Meniere's disease. *Otolaryngol Clin North Am* 1997;30(6): 961–967

Harner SG, Kasperbauer JL, et al. Transtympanic gentamicin for Meniere's syndrome. *Laryngoscope* 1998;108:1446–1449

Kerr AG, Toner JG. A new approach to surgery for Meniere's disease: talking about surgery. *Clin Otolaryngol* 1998;23:263–264

Kumagami H, Loewenheim H, Beitz E, et al. The effect of anti–diuretic hormone on the endolymphatic sac of the inner ear. *Pflugers Arch* 1998;436:970–975

Pensak ML, Friedman RA. The role of endolymphatic mastoid shunt surgery in the managed care era. *Am J Otol* 1998; 19:337–340

Schwaber MK. Vestibular disorders. In: Hughes GB, Pensak ML, eds. *Clinical Otology*. 2nd Ed. New York: Thieme Medical Books, 1997;345–365

Takeda T. Computed radiographic measurement of the dimensions of the vestibular aqueduct in Meniere's disease. *Acta Otolaryngol (Stockh)* 1997(suppl);528:80–84

Thomsen J, Bonding P, Becker B, et al. The non-specific effect of endolymphatic sac surgery in treatment of Meniere's disease: a prospective, randomized controlled study comparing "classic" endolymphatic sac surgery with the insertion of a ventilating tube in the tympanic membrane. *Acta Otolaryngol (Stockh)* 1998;118: 769–773

Management of the Meniere's Patient

William L. Meyerhoff and Jennifer Jordan

CHAPTER 48

No treatment has proved effective in reversing the pathophysiologic process of Meniere's disease. Further, no known treatment of Meniere's disease will consistently reverse the hearing loss or eliminate the aural fullness and tinnitus that often accompany this disorder. Most treatments are directed toward eliminating the often incapacitating symptom of vertigo with its associated vegetative symptoms (Fig. 48–1). It is axiomatic that before treating the symptoms of Meniere's disease, one must make the diagnosis. Most clinicians recognize the classic quadrad of fluctuating hearing, tinnitus, aural fullness, and incapacitating vertigo. The symptoms of Meniere's disease, however, are frequently evolutionary, and any one of the four symptoms may precede the others by months to years.[1] A high index of suspicion and the judicious use of diagnostic aids such as electrocochleography and, when hearing loss is present, dehydration audiometry can facilitate early diagnosis when doubt exists.[2] Treatment may then be instituted avoiding unnecessary delay and morbidity.

To complicate matters, some patients with the symptoms of Meniere's disease (Meniere's syndrome) will actually have a local, regional, or systemic cause for their symptoms.[3] Failure to identify these causes may lead to inappropriate treatment and additional morbidity. Therefore, patients suffering the symptoms of Meniere's syndrome should be evaluated for inhalant and food allergies, immune disease, syphilis, cerebellopontine angle lesions, and demyelinating disease. If any of these disorders are identified, their treatment takes priority. If no underlying cause can be identified, or if auditory and vestibular symptoms persist despite specific successful treatment of an identified abnormality, the cause of the patient's symptoms is presumed to be idiopathic (Meniere's disease).

Histologic study of ears harvested from patients with Meniere's disease has demonstrated distention of Reissner's membrane into the vestibular scala, suggesting either overproduction of endolymph within the scala media of the cochlea or decreased absorption (endolymphatic hydrops).[4] Most treatments have therefore been directed toward reducing endolymph volume pressure or bypassing the proposed pathophysiology of the disorder and directing treatment toward eliminating the symptoms of vertigo.

Treatment for the vertigo that often accompanies acute spells of Meniere's disease is designed to eliminate, or significantly reduce, this symptom and its associated nausea and vomiting. This objective is best accomplished using intravenous diazepam or droperidol if the patient can be carefully monitored. Promethazine hydrochloride (an antihistamine) in suppository form may be helpful in less controlled situations. Reassurance that the patient is not suffering a cerebrovascular accident or other life-threatening disease is essential if it is the initial attack and fluid repletion may be needed.[5]

Treatments used for the chronic condition of Meniere's disease with recurrent incapacitating vertigo basically fall into the two categories of invasive and noninvasive therapy. Noninvasive treatments directed toward reversing the pathophysiologic process include low-salt diet (<2 g of sodium per day) and diuretics. Sodium causes fluid retention and has been implicated in the exacerbation of symptoms, presumably by increasing endolymphatic hydrops. It is hoped that low-salt diet and diuretics will have the opposite effect.[6] It is proposed that some diuretics have a direct effect on ion transport in the stria vascularis and spiral ligament. Acetazolamide (a carbonic anhydrase inhibitor) and hydrochlorothiazide are commonly used. Acetazolamide appears somewhat more effective but also has a greater rebound effect when discontinued. Furosemide, a loop diuretic, may also be used but is more likely to require potassium supplementation.

Vasoconstriction has never been convincingly shown to contribute to the pathophysiology of Meniere's disease; therefore, vasodilators (e.g., niacin, histamine, papaverine hydrochloride, histamine analogues) probably do not play a role in its treatment. Other noninvasive treatments used theoretically to reverse the pathologic process, such as lipoflavonoid (proposed to improve microvascular integrity of the stria vascularis), also appear to play little role in altering the pathophysiology of this disease.[7,8]

Noninvasive treatments directed toward eliminating vertigo without addressing the inner ear disease process are legion. They include those treatments designed to produce temporary symptomatic relief and those designed to permanently ablate the vestibular neuroepithelium (e.g., streptomycin). Anticholinergic drugs are known to suppress activity within the vestibular system and, on occasion, reduce the vertigo associated with attacks of Meniere's disease. They also reduce peristalsis and gastric secretion, which helps reduce nausea and vomiting, and they inhibit sweat gland activity or diaphoresis. Scopolamine and probanthine are the two most commonly used drugs in this class. Occasionally, however, the side effects of these drugs, especially scopolamine, are worse than the symptoms of Meniere's disease, and the drugs may need to be discontinued.

Antihistamines, especially those with strong anticholinergic effects, also seem to reduce the severity of the vertigo spells by suppressing the activity within the central nervous system. The precise mechanisms, however, are not totally clear. Meclizine, a piperazine derivative, is the most commonly employed antihistamine, and the side effect of drowsiness is

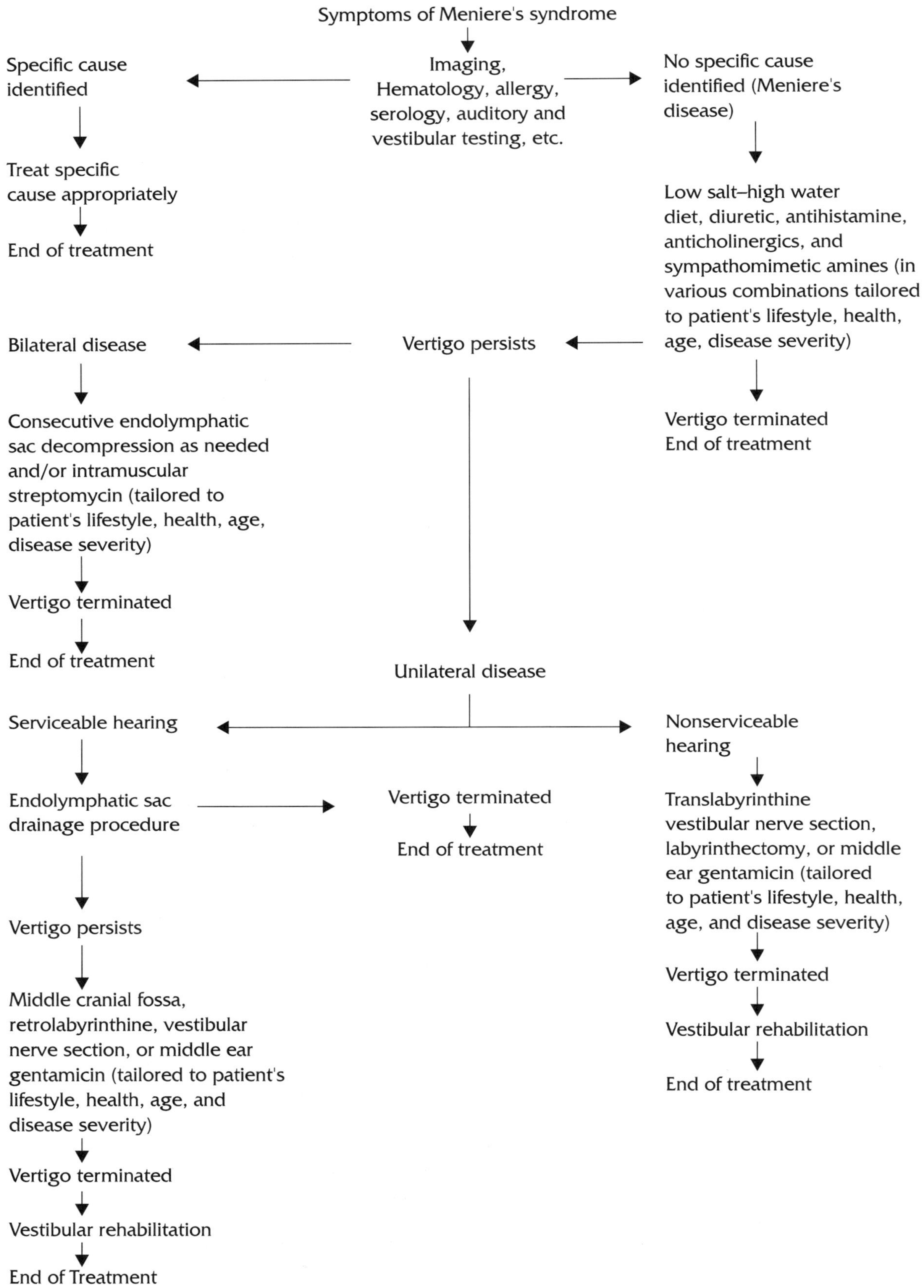

Figure 48–1 Treatment for the vertigo of Meniere's disease.

uncommon. Amitriptyline, a dibenzazepine derivative, has not only been used to treat depression but may also reduce vertigo through its anticholinergic action.

Sympathomimetic amines have long been used for suppression of vestibular symptoms. Amphetamines are notorious for substance abuse and are now under strict control by the Drug Enforcement Agency. The effects of ephedrine are similar to amphetamines but less pronounced. Ephedrine depolarizes and then blocks cells in the autonomic ganglia and appears to have the capacity of suppressing activity within the vestibular nuclei. It should be used judiciously in patients with hypertension.

Psychotropic drugs, such as the benzodiazepines, have been used to treat the vertigo of Meniere's disease. Benzodiazepines (diazepam, lorazepam, and clonazepam) either directly or indirectly enhance hyperpolarization and inhibition of neuronal firing. They are extremely effective in "crisis intervention" but their tendency to cause psychological and physical dependency argues against prolonged use.

Parenteral streptomycin has been used to ablate peripheral vestibular function in patients suffering vertigo secondary to bilateral Meniere's disease since the late 1940s.[9] Streptomycin treatment is particularly useful when the offending ear is unclear and can often be titrated to eliminate vertigo while avoiding oscillopsia and further hearing loss.[10] This treatment modality is an essential component of the therapeutic armamentarium for physicians treating patients with the vertigo of Meniere's disease.

Invasive therapy is reserved for patients who are not good candidates for or who fail noninvasive therapy. Invasive therapy can be chemical or mechanical. The most contemporary treatment is chemical and involves infusion of gentamicin into the inner ear either by intratympanic injection or the use of a microcatheter. Gentamicin is an aminoglycoside antibiotic that appears to be preferentially toxic to the vestibular hair cells; it may also be toxic to the dark cells of the inner ear. Treatment in therapeutic doses presumably ablates the peripheral vestibular end organ and may decrease endolymphatic hydrops by its action on the dark cells. It is primarily used for patients with unilateral Meniere's disease and carries the risk of sensorineural hearing loss. Although most investigators report a 70 to 90% success rate for control of vertigo with a 20 to 40% likelihood of additional hearing loss, the number of doses, concentration of drug, and total dose vary significantly between reports leaving the physician in a bit of a quandary regarding the best methodology.[11] Streptomycin has been used in a similar manner but has fallen out of favor because of a perceived narrower therapeutic window and the difficulty in obtaining it.[12]

Steroids have also been placed in the middle ear of patients suffering Meniere's disease, presumably to reduce immune-mediated inflammation. Although evidence exists to support the association between immune-mediated inflammation and the symptoms of Meniere's disease, inflammation is conspicuously absent in histologic studies of temporal bones harvested from patients suffering from Meniere's disease. Data regarding intratympanic steroids for the treatment of Meniere's disease are inadequate, and personal experience is extremely inconclusive.[13]

Various agents have also been directly perfused through the inner ear by surgically fenestrating the horizontal semicircular canal. The results of this form of treatment have been extremely capricious and it has never gained widespread popularity. Although profusion of the horizontal semicircular canal with streptomycin appears to have some efficacy in ablating the peripheral vestibular end organ in treating the vertigo of Meniere's disease, the high incidence of associated hearing loss is unacceptable.

Of the invasive procedures used to eliminate the vertigo of Meniere's disease that are purely mechanical, there are those designed to ablate the end organ response and those designed to decompress the endolymphatic system. The ablative procedures are usually limited to patients with unilateral disease because of the risk of postoperative hearing loss and oscillopsia, and they include vestibular nerve section through either the middle cranial fossa, posterior cranial fossa, or retrolabyrinthine approach. These procedures eliminate vertigo in 85 to 90% of patients and complications such as sensorineural hearing loss, cerebrospinal fluid leak, facial nerve injury, and meningitis are uncommon, although sensorineural hearing loss can approach 15%. Translabyrinthine vestibular nerve section is extremely successful in ablating the peripheral vestibular response in the treatment of vertigo secondary to Meniere's disease when there is no useful hearing in the involved ear. Labyrinthectomy is similarly useful in elderly patients, as long-term ataxia seems less problematic than with translabyrinthine vestibular nerve section.[14] All ablative therapy, whether invasive or noninvasive, is followed by vestibular rehabilitation in an effort to speed the patient's vestibular compensation.

Many procedures have been designed for mechanical decompression of the endolymphatic space, including the Fick procedure, the Cody tack, cryosurgery, ultrasound, and otic-periotic shunt. The one procedure that seems to have best survived the test of time despite controversy, however, is the endolymphatic sac drainage/decompression procedure.[15] Since its description in 1927 by Portman[16] the efficacy of endolymphatic sac surgery in the treatment of Meniere's disease has been questioned. The low complication rate and nondestructive nature of endolymphatic sac surgery, as well as the ability to perform the procedure on an outpatient basis, make it an attractive option for patients with serviceable hearing and incapacitating vertigo. However, the natural history of Meniere's disease, specifically the spontaneous remission rate and the high placebo effect seen in Meniere's patients, has provoked many to question the effectiveness of endolymphatic sac procedures.

Reported long-term vertigo control rates with endolymphatic sac surgery vary from 100% to 46% based on the 1985 American Academy of Otolaryngology–Head and Neck Surgery (AAO-HNS) criteria.[17,18] In general, most studies report vertigo control rates approaching 80%.[19-22] These studies reported cure rates from endolymphatic sac surgery have been questioned, as spontaneous remission rates of vertigo in Meniere's disease have been reported to range from 30% to 71%.[23,24] Silverstein et al.[24] compared 50 patients who were candidates for surgery, but refused, with patients who underwent either endolymphatic sac surgery, vestibular nerve section, or labyrinthectomy. These investigators found that, at 2 years follow-up, 57% of patients who had not undergone surgery reported complete relief of vertigo, as compared with 40% of patients who had undergone sac surgery. Results at 7 years of follow-up showed about 70% relief in each group. By contrast, Filipo and Barbara[23] found that only 30% of their nonsurgical Meniere's disease patients reported disappearance of vertigo at 2 years of follow-up.

In addition to the spontaneous remission rate of Meniere's disease, placebo effects must be considered in this patient population. The Danish study on sham surgery performed a prospective randomized double-blind evaluation of the effects of a simple cortical mastoidectomy versus endolymphatic sac surgery with shunt placement in 30 patients with Meniere's disease refractory to medical management. These investigators found no difference between the groups postoperatively in levels of nausea or vomiting, dizziness, aural fullness, tinnitus, and hearing. In this study, 73% of the group receiving endolymphatic sac surgery reported benefit from the operation versus 67% of the sham group.[25] These patients have been followed now for more than 9 years without any change in their initial reported results.[26]

The results of the Danish sham study have been criticized by several groups, including independent statisticians.[27,28] Pillsbury et al.[27] analyzed the data reported in the Danish sham study and obtained different results. They noted significant differences between the sham groups and the endolymphatic sac surgery group with improved vertigo control rates, tinnitus levels, and low frequency hearing results for the group receiving sac surgery.

For obvious ethical reasons, repetition of the Danish study is not possible, but the effect of cortical mastoidectomy alone in controlling the vertigo of Meniere's disease has been evaluated. Kerr et al.[29] studied the outcome of 14 patients with incapacitating vertigo who underwent cortical mastoidectomy before planned vestibular nerve section and found that 57% had achieved complete control of vertigo with mastoidectomy alone. The observed benefits of mastoidectomy alone observed in Thomsen and Kerr's studies may relate to effects produced by surgery alone, such as disturbances in blood flow, shock to the inner ear, and/or inflammation. Thus, cortical mastoidectomy probably should not be referred to as sham or placebo surgery.

Despite the obvious conflicting beliefs concerning the benefits of endolymphatic sac surgery in Meniere's disease, most otologists routinely perform the procedure. The nondestructive nature of the surgery, low complication rate, minimal morbidity, and ability to perform the procedure as an outpatient are obvious advantages over labyrinthectomy or vestibular nerve section. For these reasons, and with a success rate approaching 80%, endolymphatic sac surgery remains a valuable option for treating the vertigo of Meniere's disease.

REFERENCES

Meyerhoff and Jordan—CHAPTER 48

1. Paparella MM. Methods of diagnosis and treatment of Meniere's disease. *Acta Otolarygol (Stockh)* 1991;485(suppl): 108–119
2. Morrison AW, Moffat DA, O'Connor AF. Clinical usefulness of electrocochleography in Meniere's disease: an analysis of dehydrating agents. *Otolaryngol Clin North Am* 1980;13: 703–722
3. Rubin W, Brookler KH. Dizziness: etiologic approach to management. New York: Thieme Medical Publishers; 1991
4. Hallpike CE, Cairns H. Observations on the pathology of Meniere's syndrome. *J Laryngol Otol* 1938;53:625–655
5. Blair RL. Medical management of vestibular dysfunction. *Otolaryngol Clin North Am* 1984;17:679–684
6. Furstenberg AC, Lashmet FH, Lathrop F. Meniere's symptom complex: medical treatment. *Ann Otol Rhinol Laryngol* 1934;43:1035–1046
7. Williams HL, Maher FT, Corbin KB, et al. Eriodictyol glycoside in the treatment of Meniere's disease. *Ann Otol Rhinol Laryngol* 1963;72:1082–1101
8. Mycek MI, Gertner SB, Perper MM, Harvey RA, Champe PC, eds. *Pharmacology*. Philadelphia: JB Lippincott; 1992
9. Fowler EP. Streptomycin treatment for vertigo. *Trans Am Acad Ophthalmol Otolaryngol* 1948;52:293–301
10. Graham MD, Sataloff RT, Kemink JL. Titration streptomycin therapy for bilateral Meniere's disease: a preliminary report. *Otolaryngol Head Neck Surg* 1984;92:440–447
11. Blakely BW. Clinical forum: a review of intratympanic therapy. *Am J Otol* 1997;18:520–526
12. Shea JJ, Norris CH. Streptomycin perfusion of the labyrinth. *Acta Otolaryngol (Stockh)* 1991;485(suppl):123–130
13. Pulec JL. The translabyrinthine section of the VIIIth nerve. *Otolaryngol Clin North Am* 1968;1:563–568

14. Belal A Jr, Linthicum FH, House WF. Middle fossa vestibular nerve section. *Am J Otol* 1979;1:72–79
15. Meyerhoff WL, Paparella MM. Meniere's disease and its various surgical therapies. *Otolaryngol Clin North Am* 1980;13: 767–773
16. Portman G. Vertigo, surgical treatment of opening the saccus endolymphaticus. *Arch Otolaryngol Head Neck Surg* 1927;6:309
17. Wright W, Hicks GW. Valved implants in endolymphatic sac surgery. *Am J Otol* 1987;8:307–312
18. Jackson CG, Dickens JR, Glasscock ME. Endolymphatic to mastoid shunt using the Denver Inner Ear shunt. *Otol Head Neck Surg* 1988;99:282–285
19. Huang TS, Lin CC. Endolymphatic sac ballooning surgery for Meniere's disease. *Am Otol Rhinol Laryngol* 1994;103:389–394
20. Kitahara M. Endolymphatic sac surgery for Meniere's disease: eighteen years experience with the Kitahara sac operation. *Am J Otol* 1987;8:283–286
21. Moffat DA. Endolymphatic sac surgery: analysis of 100 operations. *Clin Otolaryngol* 1994;19:261–266
22. Luetje CM. A critical comparison of results of endolymphatic subarachnoid shunt and endolymphatic sac incision operations. *Am J Otol* 1988;4:95–101
23. Filipo R, Barbara M. Natural course of Meniere's disease in surgically selected patients. *Ear Nose Throat J* 1994;73:254–257
24. Silverstein H, Smouha E, Jones R. Natural history vs. surgery for Meniere's disease. *Otolaryngol Head Neck Surg* 1989; 100:6–16
25. Thomsen J, Bretlau P, Tos M, et al. Placebo effect in surgery for Meniere's disease: a double blind, placebo-controlled study on endolymphatic sac shunt surgery. *Arch Otolaryngol* 1981; 107:271–277
26. Bretlau P, Thomsen J, Tos M, Johnsen NJ. Placebo effect in surgery for Meniere's disease: nine-year follow-up. *Am J Otol* 1989;10:259–261
27. Pillsbury HC, Arenberg IK, Ferraro J, Ackley RS. Endolymphatic sac surgery—the Danish sham surgery: an alternative analysis. *Otolaryngol Clinics North Am* 1983;16:123–127
28. Vaisrub N. Summary statement to "Placebo effect for Meniere's disease sac shunt surgery disputed." (Letter to the Editor.) *Arch Otolaryngol* 1981;107:774
29. Kerr AG, Toner JG, McKee GJ, Smyth GDL. Role and results of cortical mastoidectomy and endolymphatic sac surgery in Meniere's disease. *J Laryngol Otol* 1989;103: 1161–1166

17

The Intracanalicular Acoustic Neuroma

"We believe that patients with intracanalicular tumors who represent good candidates for treatment should be addressed surgically at the time of diagnosis. This is supported by the findings of the National Institutes of Health Consensus Development Conference in 1994: the ideal treatment of acoustic tumor is total surgical excision of the tumor in a single stage, with preservation of neurologic function."

Derald E. Brackmann

"During the past 10 years, the long-term safety and efficacy of stereotactic radiosurgery have established this technique as an important noninvasive first-line alternative to microsurgery. The absence of procedure-related mortality and morbidity and superior tumor control, hearing, and facial preservation rates, favor radiosurgery as the first management choice for patients with intracanalicular acoustic neuromas."

L. Dade Lunsford

"The role of the auditory brainstem response audiometry as a screening tool has been the subject of considerable discussion. For patients with intracanicular tumors, the sensitivity of ABR is highly suspect and the specificity poor. Many neurotologists (including the present author) are concerned about the low sensitivity and generally omit the ABR. Others counter that the ABR is widely available, less expensive, and likely to miss only small tumors that are not a threat to the patient."

Stephen G. Harner

The Intracanalicular Acoustic Neuroma

CHAPTER 49

Derald E. Brackmann, Robert M. Owens, and Jose N. Fayad

The management of acoustic tumors has become more complex through the years with the availability of multiple therapeutic options. Because of the relative limitations of early imaging techniques, most tumors were discovered only after they had grown to considerable size. During the 1970s, the development of computed tomograph (CT) air cisternography scanning permitted more accurate diagnosis of acoustic tumors. Advances in neuroradiology during the 1980s, specifically the advent of gadolinium-enhanced magnetic resonance imaging (MRI), led to earlier diagnosis of tumors. The use of MRI permits the detection of small intracanalicular tumors in patients with minimal early symptoms and represents the gold standard method for diagnosis. In addition, heightened clinical suspicion by otolaryngologists and primary care physicians attributable to an increased awareness of early symptoms has contributed to the earlier screening and eventual diagnosis of patients with tumors.

The increase in diagnosis of tumors at an early growth stage has led to controversy over management strategies. In 1994, the National Institutes of Health Consensus Development Conference determined that the treatment of patients with acoustic neuroma should be provided by an experienced multidisciplinary team and individualized with regard to tumor and patient characteristics.[1] The individualized approach is applicable, in particular, to the management of a patient with an intracanalicular tumor. The therapeutic options available in the management of these patients include surgery, stereotactic radiotherapy, and close observation with serial MRI. The discussion in this chapter assumes a unilateral tumor with normal hearing in the opposite ear.

Hearing Status of the Patient

Before discussing the therapeutic approaches to an intracanalicular acoustic neuroma, it is important to first consider that frequently these patients will possess near normal or at least "serviceable" hearing at the diagnosis. The presence of hearing in these patients directly impacts choices in all aspects of management. Controversy exists in defining exactly what constitutes serviceable hearing for determining candidacy for hearing preservation management approaches. The most commonly employed definitions include (1) a $\leq$50-dB average of the pure tones (PTA) at 500, 1, 2, and 3 kHz with a speech discrimination score (SDS) of $\geq$50%; or (2) a PTA of $\leq$30 dB and an SDS of $\geq$70%. Beyond these definitions, there have been a multitude of complex notions of serviceable hearing, including the presence of any measurable preoperative hearing. A true consensus on the definition of serviceable hearing has not been reached within the neurotologic and neurosurgical communities, and it is not the intention of this chapter to resolve this issue. However, it is important that individual clinicians managing patients with acoustic tumors develop a working definition of serviceable hearing in order to identify candidates for hearing preservation. For purposes of candidacy for hearing preservation surgery, we at the House Ear Clinic, in general, ascribe to the 50/50 rule.

Characteristics of Intracanalicular Acoustic Neuromas

An intracanalicular acoustic neuroma is $\leq$1 cm in length and appears rounded in the early stages. Upon filling the internal auditory canal (IAC), it assumes an oblong shape. At diagnosis, three variations are encountered, depending on the extent of involvement of the IAC: (1) medial IAC location near the porus acousticus, (2) lateral IAC involvement near the fundus, and (3) involvement of the entire IAC. True intracanalicular tumors involve only the IAC, although many tumors can be considered "primarily" intracanalicular with minimal cerebellopontine angle extension, and are readily accessible by surgical approaches to the IAC. It should be noted that whereas 90% of intracanalicular lesions are indeed acoustic neuromas, patients should be counseled regarding the possibility that a facial neuroma may be radiologically indistinguishable from an acoustic neuroma.[2] Alternative management schemes in the event of the presence of a facial neuroma should be discussed preoperatively with the patient.

Management Options

SURGICAL OPTIONS

The modern era of acoustic neuroma surgical management began during the early 1960s with the development of microsurgical techniques by Dr. William House. Before this, operative mortality rates approached 40%, and most patients experienced postoperative facial paralysis. With the advent of more technically advanced surgical procedures and intraoperative monitoring, the goals of acoustic neuroma surgery have evolved. Initially, the primary goal centered around decreasing operative mortality while providing total removal of the tumor mass. With technical advancements and increased knowledge of microsurgical anatomy, preservation of facial nerve function was emphasized. More recently, efforts have focused on preservation of serviceable hearing in appropriately selected patients. Three principal surgical approaches are appropriate for the removal of intracanalicular acoustic neuromas: the translabyrinthine approach, the middle fossa approach, and the retrosigmoid approach. Each of these approaches has certain advantages and disadvantages and can be considered to have different indications depending on individual patient and tumor characteristics.

PATIENTS WITH HEARING LOSS

In patients with a total loss of hearing or who do not meet criteria of candidacy for hearing preservation surgery, the translabyrinthine craniotomy (TLC) approach is selected. The procedure involves violation of the semicircular canals and vestibule, resulting in sacrifice of residual hearing. A major advantage of the TLC is that it provides a direct route to the internal auditory canal and cerebellopontine angle (CPA), while minimizing cerebellar retraction, thereby decreasing the incidence of postoperative ataxia.[3] This approach offers full exposure of the internal auditory canal, from the fundus laterally to the porus acousticus medially. It also provides direct access to the cerebellopontine angle in the event of CPA extension. The extent of the exposure gained by this approach ensures that any intracanalicular tumor may be addressed entirely under direct vision, facilitating total tumor removal and prevention of tumor recurrence. Recurrence rates after total translabyrinthine resection of acoustic neuroma are extremely low (<1%) despite the fact that most reports include data involving tumors of all sizes and level of CPA extension.[4] The level of exposure achieved also facilitates minimal traction on the facial nerve during tumor dissection, and facial nerve outcomes with this approach have historically been considered superior to other approaches. In patients with small tumors resected by the translabyrinthine approach, a House–Brackmann facial grade I or II was achieved in 92% of cases.[5]

PATIENTS WITH SERVICEABLE HEARING

Hearing preservation is possible by resecting intracanalicular tumors with either the middle fossa or retrosigmoid approaches. The decision to employ one of these approaches preferentially is largely dependent on the training of individual skull base surgeons. In many centers, neurotologists and neurosurgeons uniformly agree on using one approach primarily. Other skull base surgery teams tailor the decision of the approach to the precise location of the tumor within the IAC. Defining what constitutes serviceable hearing, and therefore candidacy for hearing preservation surgery, remains highly controversial. Similarly, controversy exists in reporting hearing outcomes of surgery performed to preserve hearing. These controversies contribute to the difficulty in analyzing and comparing the published rates of hearing preservation. Most investigators attempt to present postoperative results as hearing at or near preoperative levels as well as the presence of any measurable hearing. In 1995, the American Academy of Otolaryngology–Head and Neck Surgery Committee on Hearing and Equilibrium attempted to resolve this issue by establishing guidelines for reporting results of efforts to preserve hearing in the treatment of acoustic neuromas.[6]

We prefer the middle fossa approach to resect intracanalicular acoustic neuromas in patients with serviceable hearing in most cases. In our opinion, true intracanalicular tumors are best approached in this fashion, and we reserve the retrosigmoid approach for patients with serviceable hearing and tumors that involve the CPA with no extension to the fundus and minimal involvement of the porus acousticus. The middle fossa technique provides complete exposure to the contents of the internal auditory canal while eliminating any need for blind dissection.[7] Approaching the IAC superiorly avoids violation of the cochlea and semicircular canals, permitting the opportunity to preserve hearing. With full exposure of the facial and cochlear nerves at the fundus of the IAC, complete tumor removal in this region of the IAC is possible under direct vision. Furthermore, exposure of the fundus decreases the risk to the nerves and their intimate blood supply during tumor dissection, helping to preserve postoperative neurologic function. Using modifications to the original middle fossa approach, tumors that involve the entire IAC, those isolated to the lateral IAC, and tumors in the medial IAC with up to 2 cm of cerebellopontine angle extension can be readily removed.[8] A relative disadvantage of this approach is that dissection of tumor must be performed in close proximity to the facial nerve within the IAC. Tumor dissection can be more difficult in the event of a tumor arising from the inferior vestibular nerve. However, when the technique is performed in experienced hands and dissection is assisted by intraoperative facial nerve monitoring, facial nerve outcomes comparable to those achieved by the translabyrinthine approach can be attained.[5] In a recently published report of a large series of middle fossa removal of acoustic neuroma by the associates of the House Ear Clinic, facial function was preserved at a House–Brackmann grade of either I or II in 95% of patients with 1-year follow-up.[9] In other recent studies, facial nerve function of grades I and II are consistently noted in 90% or more patients postoperatively.[8,10,11] Gross preservation of the cochlear nerve is greatly facilitated by the IAC exposure provided by this approach. In addition, exposure of the cochlear nerve allows for real time intraoperative direct cochlear nerve monitoring, which is thought to aid in the dissection of tumor in close proximity to the cochlear nerve. In our most recent series, hearing was preserved to within 15 dB PTA and 15% SDS in 52% of patients, with measurable hearing preserved in 68% of all patients.[9] This series reported results not only of removal of intracanalicular tumors but also tumors with significant extension into the CPA. In a recent article published by Irving et al.,[12] hearing preservation rates of several series of both middle fossa and retrosigmoid cases were reclassified according to the AAO–HNS Committee on Hearing and Equilibrium guidelines. According to this reclassification, hearing was preserved by the middle fossa approach to a combined class A and B level (corresponding to a PTA of 50 dB and SDS of 50%) in 20 to 72% of cases in series with significant numbers of patients.[12] Complication rates associated with the approach are minimal. The incidence of cerebrospinal fluid (CSF) leak is consistently reported to be less than 10%, and leaks resolve with nonsurgical treatment in most cases. Meningitis is a rare complication, occurring in approximately 2% of cases. New cranial nerve deficits are essentially nonexistent postoperatively, as no direct manipulation of cranial nerves other than the facial and cochleovestibular nerves is required. The middle fossa approach obviates the need for cerebellar retraction, which reduces the risk of postoperative ataxia. Significant temporal lobe retraction is necessary with this approach, but complications attributed to temporal lobe retraction are not typically encountered. Additionally, operative and postoperative mortality is extremely rare, with no deaths reported in the majority of articles.

The retrosigmoid approach is routinely employed by many surgeons in attempts to preserve hearing while removing intracanalicular acoustic neuromas. With this technique, the tumor is approached posteriorly via a large suboccipital craniotomy with retraction of the cerebellum. By approaching tumors from this angle, tumor removal is possible without violating the cochlea or semicircular canals. Wide exposure of the cerebellopontine angle is achieved, and tumors of any size are approachable. A major limitation of the retrosigmoid approach is that tumors involving the fundus of the IAC are not readily accessible, and any attempt at tumor removal in the region of the fundus creates "blind dissection." The lack of a direct view of the contents of the lateral IAC creates a situation in which residual tumor may potentially be left intact near the fundus, and inadvertent trauma to the facial and/or cochlear nerves during tumor dissection may lead to increased rates of postoperative facial nerve weakness and loss of serviceable hearing.[13] For this reason, we limit our selection of the retrosigmoid approach to cases where the tumor is primarily located in the CPA, with essentially no involvement of the IAC. Actual data confirming an increase in recurrence of tumor with the approach is lacking, and it is unlikely that the rate of recurrence is significant if care is taken to select patients appropriately. The retrosigmoid approach allows a limited view of the facial nerve within the CPA. Rates of facial nerve function of grade I and II postoperatively are reported at 85 to 93% in appropriately selected patients with smaller tumors.[14-16] Drilling the posterior lip of the IAC and incising the dura of the canal facilitates enhanced exposure and decompression of the cochlear nerve. During this maneuver, great care must be taken to avoid violating the posterior semicircular canal. Reclassification of hearing results to the AAO–HNS guidelines in several recently published large series of retrosigmoid resection of tumors demonstrated a class A or B result in 11 to 50% of cases.[12] Although some surgeons feel that the incidence of CSF leak is increased with this approach, reported rates in the literature vary between 7% and 15%, with nonsurgical management effective in most cases. The incidence of postoperative meningitis and mortality is comparable to the middle fossa and translabyrinthine approaches. Postoperative headache recalcitrant to standard medical therapy, a rare finding in middle fossa patients, is reported after the retrosigmoid approach in 14 to 27% of patients and has been attributed to the necessary large suboccipital craniotomy or possibly irritative arachnoiditis resulting from intradural deposition of bone dust.[17,18]

STEREOTACTIC RADIOTHERAPY

Stereotactic radiotherapy refers to precise, mechanically directed, closed-skull destruction of an intracranial target by ionizing beams of radiation during a single treatment session.[19] This technique was first employed in the management of an acoustic neuroma in 1969 and was introduced in the United States in 1987 as an alternative to surgical removal of acoustic neuromas. Considerable advances have been achieved with the development of more advanced computerized methods of calculating both radiation dosage and targeting and the utilization of more sophisticated imaging techniques. Radiotherapy is performed by using either multisource cobalt-60 γ units or modified linear accelerators. The technique does not eliminate tumor, but appears to arrest tumor growth through cell death and tumor necrosis. Most radiation oncologists agree that this procedure should not be performed on patients with tumors >3 cm in size. A relative advantage of stereotactic radiotherapy over conventional surgery is that the procedure can be performed in an outpatient setting with local anesthesia and sedation. While some authors state that radiotherapy offers decreased cost as compared with surgery, surgeons argue that the long-term post-treatment imaging necessary with radiotherapy offsets initial costs associated with surgery and postoperative care. The ultimate goal of this procedure is "tumor control," which is the absence of tumor growth as detected by follow-up imaging studies. Rates of tumor control have been reported to be 70 to 98%, with variability in the length of follow-up.[20-23] Data demonstrating significant long-term control using consistent dosing protocols are lacking. Direct comparison of facial function and hearing outcomes is difficult due to differences in reporting guidelines and in radiation dosages between individual series. Facial nerve deficits may be transient or may occur late after therapy, and overall facial function outcomes of House–Brackmann grade I to II are reported to be anywhere from 62% to 92%.[20-22,24] A lack of consensus in reporting hearing outcomes creates difficulty in analyzing and comparing data on hearing preservation after stereotactic radiotherapy. As with facial neuropathy, hearing deterioration can be seen as a late sequela of treatment. Serviceable hearing in patients undergoing stereotactic radiotherapy is reported to exist over the long term

(>4 years) in 11 to 71% of patients.[23,25,26] A disadvantage of this procedure is post-treatment trigeminal nerve dysfunction, a condition that is extremely rare in patients undergoing surgery for small intracanalicular tumors. Reported rates of trigeminal nerve deficit vary from 19% to 59% of cases.[20-22,27] Thus, it is important to note that a certain percentage of patients undergoing radiotherapy are likely to develop combined facial and trigeminal neuropathies, with potentially serious ophthalmologic sequelae as a result. Permanent postirradiation hydrocephalus requiring shunt placement is reported to occur in 3 to 4% of cases, and malignant degeneration after intracranial radiation therapy has been documented in the literature.[28,29]

OBSERVATION WITH SERIAL IMAGING

Observation of patients with minimal symptoms and small acoustic neuromas has been advocated by some investigators, proposing that a more expectant attitude is an acceptable alternative to immediate treatment at the diagnosis.[30] The concept of observing patients is based on the premise that acoustic tumors demonstrate a slow growth rate, and that the potential mortality and morbidity associated with treatment justifies a wait-and-see policy. As a result of advances in the ability to manage tumors, this option has been reserved primarily for elderly patients, patients who represent poor candidates for treatment, and those who decline treatment. Attempts to accurately determine the average growth of acoustic neuromas have estimated the rate to be 0.11 to 3.2 cm/year as measured by serial MRI scanning.[31-34] Although some investigators advocate conservative management of tumors by citing low growth rates, the lack of visible tumor growth measured by imaging techniques does not necessarily imply that the tumor is quiescent. Microscopic growth of tumor cell undetectable by MRI may result in infiltration of intracanalicular nerves or their blood supply.[35] In fact, a recent study of the consequences of the wait-and-see policy demonstrated that 55% of patients who otherwise would have been considered candidates for hearing preservation surgery (by the "50/50" rule) lost serviceable hearing during the observation period.[33] In addition, serial imaging once or twice annually for many years may represent a considerable cost issue.

Conclusion

Modern technological advances have allowed clinicians to diagnose intracanalicular tumors at an early stage, often with patients exhibiting minimal or no symptoms. In parallel with gains in diagnostic capabilities, great advances have been achieved in the management of patients with acoustic neuroma. Indeed, the development of different management approaches has created most of the controversy in the management of small acoustic tumors.

In summary, we believe that patients with intracanalicular tumors who represent good candidates for treatment should be addressed surgically at the time of diagnosis. This is supported by the findings of the National Institutes of Health Consensus Development Conference in 1994: the ideal treatment of acoustic tumor is total surgical excision of the tumor in a single stage, with preservation of neurologic function. The translabyrinthine approach is used for all patients who are not candidates for attempts at hearing preservation. In patients with serviceable hearing, we prefer the middle fossa approach over the retrosigmoid approach. We believe this approach offers superior exposure to the contents of the entire internal auditory canal. A comparison of published series with significant numbers of patients and comparable methodology for reporting results suggests that the middle fossa approach provides better rates of hearing preservation. In addition, we believe that less postoperative morbidity is associated with the middle fossa approach. We restrict our usage of the retrosigmoid approach to a small subset of patients with serviceable hearing and tumors located primarily in the cerebellopontine angle that are too large to be resected with the middle fossa approach. In general, we do not advocate stereotactic radiotherapy as primary treatment for intracanalicular tumors in otherwise healthy patients. In fact, the majority of authors reporting results of stereotactic radiotherapy conclude that the procedure serves as an alternative to surgical treatment in patients who represent poor surgical candidates. Observation with serial imaging is appropriate for the elderly, for patients who otherwise are poor surgical candidates, or in special circumstances such as in patients with an intracanalicular tumor in the only hearing ear.

REFERENCES

Brackmann et al.—CHAPTER 49

1. National Institutes of Health Consensus Development Conference. Statement of acoustic neuroma. Arch Neurol 1994; 51:201–207
2. Lo WWM. Magnetic resonance imaging of vestibular schwannomas. In: *Techniques in Neurosurgery* Vol. 3, No. 2. Philadelphia: Lippincott-Raven Publishers;1997:95–108
3. Brackmann DE, Green JD. Translabyrinthine approach for acoustic tumor removal. *Otolaryngol Clin North Am* 1992; 25:311–329
4. Shelton C. Unilateral acoustic tumors: how often do they recur after translabyrinthine removal? *Laryngoscope* 1995;105: 958–966

5. Arriaga MA, Luxford WM, Berliner KI. Facial nerve function following middle fossa and translabyrinthine acoustic tumor surgery: a comparison. *Am J Otol* 1994;15:620–624
6. Committee on Hearing and Equilibrium. Committee on Hearing and Equilibrium guidelines for the evaluation of hearing preservation in acoustic neuroma (vestibular schwannoma). *Otolaryngol Head Neck Surg* 1995;113: 179–180
7. House WF, Shelton C. Middle fossa approach for acoustic tumor removal. *Otolaryngol Clin North Am* 1992;25: 347–359
8. Brackmann DE, House JR III, Hitselberger WE. Technical modifications to the middle fossa craniotomy approach in removal of acoustic neuromas. *Am J Otol* 1994;15: 614–619
9. Slattery WH, Brackmann DE, Hitselberger WE. Middle fossa approach for hearing preservation with acoustic neuromas. *Am J Otol* 1997;18:596–601
10. Gantz BJ, Harker LA, Parnes LS, McCabe BF. Middle fossa acoustic neuroma excision: results and complications. *Ann Otol Rhinol Laryngol* 1986;95:454–459
11. Dornhoffer JL, Helms J, Hoehmann DH. Hearing preservation in acoustic tumor surgery: results and prognostic factors. *Laryngoscope* 1995;105:184–187
12. Irving RM, Jackler RK, Pitts LH. Hearing preservation in patients undergoing vestibular schwannoma surgery: comparison of middle fossa and retrosigmoid approaches. *J Neurosurg* 1998;88:840–845
13. Domb GH, Chole RA. Anatomical studies of the posterior petrous apex with regard to hearing preservation in acoustic neuroma removal. *Laryngoscope* 1980;90:1769–1776
14. Cohen NL, Lewis WS, Ransohoff J. Hearing preservation in cerebellopontine angle tumor surgery: the NYU experience 1974–1991. *Am J Otol* 1993;14:423–433
15. Fischer G, Fischer C, Remond J. Hearing preservation in acoustic neurinoma surgery. *J Neurosurg* 1992;76: 910–917
16. Kemink JL, LaRouere MJ, Kileny PR, et al. Hearing preservation following suboccipital removal of acoustic neuromas. *Laryngoscope* 1990;100:597–602
17. Hanson MB, Glasscock ME III, Brandes JL, Jackson CG. Medical treatment of headache after suboccipital acoustic tumor removal. *Laryngoscope* 1998;108:1111–1114
18. Catalano PJ, Jacobowitz O, Post KD. Prevention of headache after retrosigmoid removal of acoustic tumors. *Am J Otol* 1996;17:904–908
19. Lunsford LD, Flickinger J, Lindner G, et al. Stereotactic radiosurgery of the brain using the first United States 201 cobalt-60 source gamma knife. *Neurosurgery* 1989;24: 151–159
20. Kondziolka D, Lunsford LD, McLaughlin MR, Flickinger JC. Long-term outcomes after radiosurgery for acoustic neuromas. *N Engl J Med* 1998;339:1426–1433
21. Pollock BE, Lunsford LD, Kondziolka D, et al. Outcome analysis of acoustic neuroma management: a comparison of microsurgery and stereotactic radiosurgery. *Neurosurgery* 1995; 36:215–229
22. Foote RL, Coffey RJ, Swanson JW, et al. Stereotactic radiosurgery using the gamma knife for acoustic neuromas. *Int J Radiat Oncol Biol Phys* 1995;32:1153–1160
23. Flickinger JC, Lunsford LD, Linskey ME, et al. Gamma knife radiosurgery for acoustic tumors: multivariate analysis of four year results. *Radiother Oncol* 1993;97:91–98
24. Noren G, Arndt J, Hindmarsh T. Stereotactic radiosurgery in cases of acoustic neurinoma: further experiences. *Neurosurgery* 1983;13:12–22
25. Forster DMC, Kemeny AA, Pathak A, Walton L. Radiosurgery: a minimally interventional alternative to microsurgery in the management of acoustice neuroma. *Br J Neurosurg* 1996;10:169–174
26. Ito K, Kurita H, Sugasawa K, et al. Neuro-otological findings after radiosurgery for acoustic neurinomas. *Arch Otolaryngol Head Neck Surg* 1996;122:1229–1233
27. Mendenhall WM, Friedman WA, Bova FJ. LINAC radiosurgery for acoustic schwannomas. *Int J Radiat Oncol Biol Phys* 1994;28:803–810
28. Ducatman BS, Scheithauer BW. Postirradiation neurofibrosarcoma. *Cancer* 1983;51:1028–1033
29. Lalwani A, Jackler RK, Gutin P. A lethal fibrosarcoma complicating radiation therapy for a benign glomus jugulare tumor. *Am J Otol* 1993;14:398–402
30. Cox GJ. Intracanalicular acoustic neuromas: a conservative approach. *Clin Otolaryngol* 1993;18:153–154
31. Nedzelski JM, Schessel DA, Pfleiderer A, et al. Conservative management of acoustic neuromas. *Otolaryngol Clin North Am* 1992;25:691–705
32. Deen HG, Ebersold MJ, Harner SG, et al. Conservative management of acoustic neuroma: an outcome study. *Neurosurgery* 1996;39:260–266
33. Charabi S, Thomsen J, Mantoni M, et al. Acoustic neuroma (vestibular schwannoma): growth and surgical and nonsurgical consequences of the wait-and-see policy. *Otolaryngol Head Neck Surg* 1995;113:5–14
34. Fucci MJ, Buchman CA, Brackmann DE, Berliner KI. Acoustic tumor growth: implications for treatment choices. *Am J Otol* 1999;20(4):495–499
35. Kartush JM, Brackmann DE. Acoustic neuroma update. *Otolarygol Clin North Am* 1996;29:377–392

The Intracanalicular Acoustic Neuroma

CHAPTER 50

Ajay Niranjan, L. Dade Lunsford, Douglas Kondziolka, and John C. Flickinger

Acoustic neuromas (vestibular schwannomas) arise in the vestibular portion of the eighth cranial nerve at the interface of its central neuroglial and peripheral Schwann cell components. After initial intracanalicular growth the tumor protrudes from the auditory canal into the cerebellopontine angle. The stage at which an acoustic tumor is detected is related to the nature of the symptoms and signs, the physician's alertness, and the availability of modern diagnostic imaging modalities. Toynbee[1] first described a primarily intracanalicular acoustic tumor in 1853. With the widespread availability of high-resolution magnetic resonance imaging (MRI) and sophisticated hearing tests, intracanalicular acoustic tumors are now diagnosed more easily. Purely intracanalicular neuromas differ from large cerebellopontine angle neuromas with regard to the effect of their growth. Asymptomatic tumors have also been discovered during imaging performed for other reasons. Because there is no consistent growth rate, there is no general consensus regarding the identification of candidates for therapeutic intervention. In general, management outcomes are better for smaller tumors, regardless of the strategy chosen. Owing to the small number of intracanalicular cases reported in most acoustic tumor series, it is difficult to define the exact rate of hearing preservation after intracanalicular acoustic tumor surgery.

Intracanalicular acoustic tumors as a separate entity have been addressed in relatively few reports.[2-5] In addition, there is wide variability in the criteria used to define hearing preservation. The criteria for preserved hearing in various series varies from as loose as any measurable hearing to as strict as having a pure-tone average (PTA) of ≤ 30 dB and a speech discrimination score of ≥ 70%. Terms like *measurable, valid, useful, usable, serviceable,* and *good hearing* are used to report post-operative hearing. A variety of classification systems have been used to document postoperative hearing. Although MRI has eliminated most diagnostic uncertainty, controversy still exists regarding the best management.

Background

Preservation of hearing has become the most challenging goal of intracanalicular acoustic tumor surgery. The reported hearing preservation after microsurgical excision of intracanalicular tumors varies from 12% to 82%.[2,5-10] In 1969, House and Hitselberger[6] first reported that they obtained functional hearing preservation in four out of five patients with intracanalicular tumors excised via the middle fossa approach. Ten years later, Brackmann[11] reported "some" hearing preservation in 5 out of 11 patients using this approach. Subsequently many surgeons further refined the middle fossa approach and reported better hearing preservation rates.[12] Both Silverstein et al.[9] and Jannetta et al.[13] used the retrosigmoid approach in order to achieve hearing preservation. Sterkers et al.[10] had a 66.7% hearing preservation rate using the retrosigmoid approach. Nadol et al.[14] reported a 50% useful hearing preservation rate but included patients with a speech discrimination score (SDS) as low as 15% and a speech reception threshold (SRT) of ≤ 70 dB in the useful hearing group. They also reported that 36% (5/14) had hearing preservation. Preserved hearing was defined as a change of < 15 dB in SRT and < 15% in SDS, as compared with preoperative levels.[14,15]

Samii et al.[5] recommended early surgery by the retrosigmoid approach in order to improve hearing preservation rates. In a review of 1000 acoustic tumors, Samii et al.[5] reported a 46% (17/37) hearing preservation rate in the subgroup of patients who had intracanalicular tumors. Samii et al.[5] advocated the Hannover classification, which included patients with PTA levels as poor as 80 dB and speech discrimination scores as low as 10%, in the preserved hearing group. Useful hearing preservation (defined as PTA ≤ 40 and SDS ≥ 70%) was noted to be 29%.[16] Haines et al.[2] reported an 82% (9/11) hearing preservation rate using both middle fossa (5/6) as well as retrosigmoid approaches (4/5), although in the next few patients hearing was not preserved so readily (personal communication). Irving et al.[7] compared hearing preservation rates (based on the 50/50 rule) using either a middle fossa or a retrosigmoid approach. They reported a 44% useful hearing preservation rate in the middle fossa group as compared with 12% in the retrosigmoid group. They concluded that the middle fossa approach has enhanced lateral exposure that facilitated lateral to medial dissection and promoted development of tumor arachnoid planes at the fundus. They hypothesized that this results in less traction on the distal cochlear nerve at its weakest point where it forms fine filaments in the modiolus and also less traction on the distal labyrinthine artery at its foraminal end.[7]

Most of the reported hearing preservation rates reflect immediate postoperative hearing status but do not document long-term hearing outcome at 1 or more years after surgery. Long-term follow-up of patients with preserved postoperative hearing showed delayed hearing loss in a significant number of patients.[17,18] Shelton et al.[18] reported further loss of preserved postoperative hearing in 56% of patients over a mean follow-up of 8 years.[18]

Facial nerve function has not been documented in most of the hearing preservation studies. Nadol et al.[14] observed postoperative facial paresis in 4 of 14 patients of smaller acoustic tumors that recovered in a year. Atlas et al.[19] described 3 patients with House–Brackmann grade II results and 2 with grade III results. Cohen and Ransohoff[20] reported a single intracanalicular tumor patient with preserved hearing; this patient had partial facial weakness with incomplete recovery. Irving et al.[7] noticed an increased incidence of transient facial nerve palsy after middle fossa surgery in the immediate postoperative phase.

Evolution of Radiosurgery

Lars Leksell coined the term *stereotactic radiosurgery* in 1951. He developed the technique for delivery of a single high dose of precisely focused radiation to achieve closed skull destruction of a small intracranial target. Acoustic tumor stereotactic radiosurgery using the Gamma knife unit was first performed by Leksell in 1969.[21] In a review of his 20 years' experience with treatment of acoustic neuromas by radiosurgery, Norén et al.[15] reported that more than 90% of patients had tumor growth control. The initial patient treated with the first North American 201-source Cobalt-60 Gamma knife unit at the University of Pittsburgh in 1987 had an acoustic neuroma.[22] Radiosurgery technique has evolved steadily during the past decade.[4,15,22-29] The results after radiosurgery of acoustic tumors have established it as an important minimally invasive alternative to microsurgery.[24,26,27] Pollock et al.[29] performed a retrospective matched cohort analysis of microsurgical and radiosurgical outcomes at the University of Pittsburgh and found radiosurgery as an effective and less costly management strategy. Ogunrinde et al.[3] described 10 patients with intracanalicular tumors managed by radiosurgery; no patient had a delayed facial or trigeminal neuropathy.

RADIOSURGICAL TECHNIQUE

Gamma knife radiosurgery begins with rigid fixation of an MRI-compatible Leksell stereotactic frame to the patient's head under local anesthetic infiltration and mild sedation. High-resolution-gadolinium enhanced T_1-weighted sagittal scout MRIs are obtained next, in order to localize the area of interest. To define the radiosurgery target volume, a multiplanar volume acquisition contrast-enhanced MRI (divided into 28 axial slices of 1-mm thickness) that covers the entire lesion and surrounding critical structures is performed. Planning is performed on axial images supplemented by coronal and sagittal reconstructed stereotactic images. A conformational plan is achieved using 1 to 6 isocenters of 4-mm beam diameter. After finalizing the plan, a maximum dose to the tumor margin is determined. The treatment isodose, maximum dose, and dose to the margin are jointly decided by a neurosurgeon, radiation oncologist and medical physicist after analysis of the hearing status of each patient. Since 1994, we have prescribed 13 Gy to the tumor margin in patients with serviceable hearing in an effort to preserve their hearing. Radiosurgery is performed with a 201-source cobalt-60 Leksell Gamma Knife (model U or B, Elekta Instruments, Atlanta, GA) by positioning the target serially at x-, y-, and z-coordinates of each isocenter. The stereotactic frame is removed immediately afterward, and the patients are discharged within the next 6 to 18 h.

UNIVERSITY OF PITTSBURGH EXPERIENCE

Between August 1987 and December 1997, 29 patients with intracanalicular acoustic tumors underwent stereotactic radiosurgery at our center. All patients were evaluated with high-resolution MRI or computed tomography (CT) scan and had clinical evaluation as well as audiology tests that included PTA and SDS. Hearing was graded using the Gardner-Robertson modification of the Silverstein and Norell classification, and facial nerve function was assessed according to the House–Brackmann grading system.[30,31] Serviceable hearing (class I and II) was defined as a PTA or SRT lower than 50 dB and an speech discrimination score better than 50%.

After radiosurgery, all patients had serial follow-up gadolinium-enhanced MRI scans, which were requested at 6-month intervals for 2 years. If there was no appreciable change in tumor size, subsequent MRIs were requested at 2-year intervals. All patients who had some preserved hearing were advised to obtain audiologic evaluation including PTA and SDS near the time of their MRI follow-up. No patient morbidity or mortality was observed. Tumor control, as documented by serial imaging, was achieved in all patients. Six of 29 patients showed clear-cut reduction in tumor volume in follow-up MRI. Three patients had minimal temporary enlargement followed by stabilization; loss of central contrast uptake was noted in two of these patients. Stable appearance without any evidence of further tumor growth was noted in 20 patients in a follow-up period ranging from 12 to 108 months. No patient in this series required subsequent surgical intervention.

A pre-radiosurgery Gardner–Robertson class was preserved in 49%, whereas testable hearing was present in 68% of patients (Fig. 50–1). Seventeen of 29 patients had serviceable hearing at radiosurgery. Audiologic follow-up was available on 15 of these 17 patients. Serviceable hearing was preserved in 73% (11/15) of patients at a mean follow-up of 33 months. Long-term follow-up showed serviceable hearing preservation in all 10 of

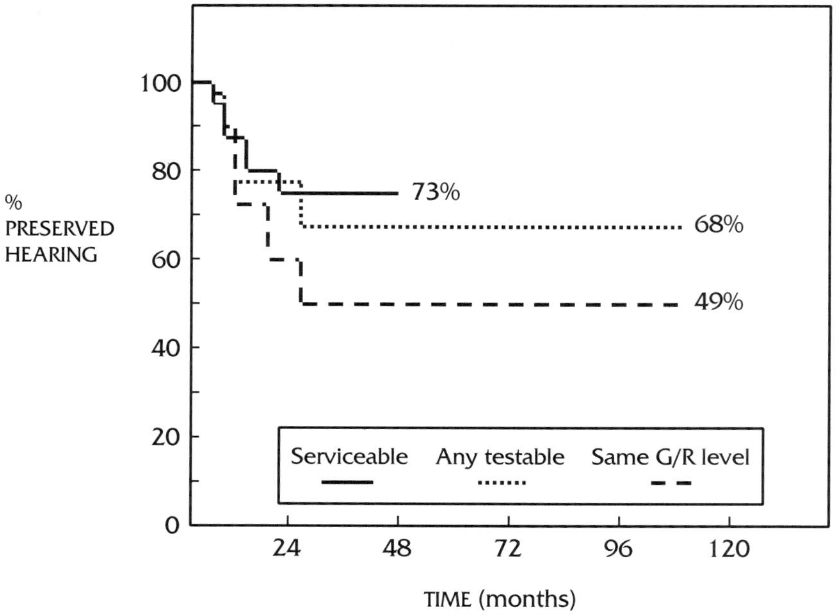

Figure 50–1 Graph showing preservation of serviceable, testable, and pre-radiosurgery hearing in the intracanalicular acoustic neuroma series at the University of Pittsburgh during the 10-year interval from 1987 to 1997.

10 patients (100%) treated with ≤14 Gy and in 1 of 5 patients (20%) treated with >14 Gy (Fig. 50–2). Five patients demonstrated significant improvement in hearing. No patient developed facial or trigeminal neuropathy. Seven of 13 patients with preoperative tinnitus continued to experience tinnitus in follow-up. Episodic vertigo continued in 3 of the 11 patients who presented with vertigo. No other perioperative complication occurred in any patient.

Our analysis suggests that the current technique (MRI-based conformal planning using exclusively 4-mm collimators and 13 to 14 Gy to the tumor margin) can achieve hearing preservation in almost all patients. The results of hearing preservation after stereotactic radiosurgery of intracanalicular tumors appear distinctly superior to results achieved after microsurgical excision even at centers of surgical excellence. Our current 100% preservation rates of facial and trigeminal

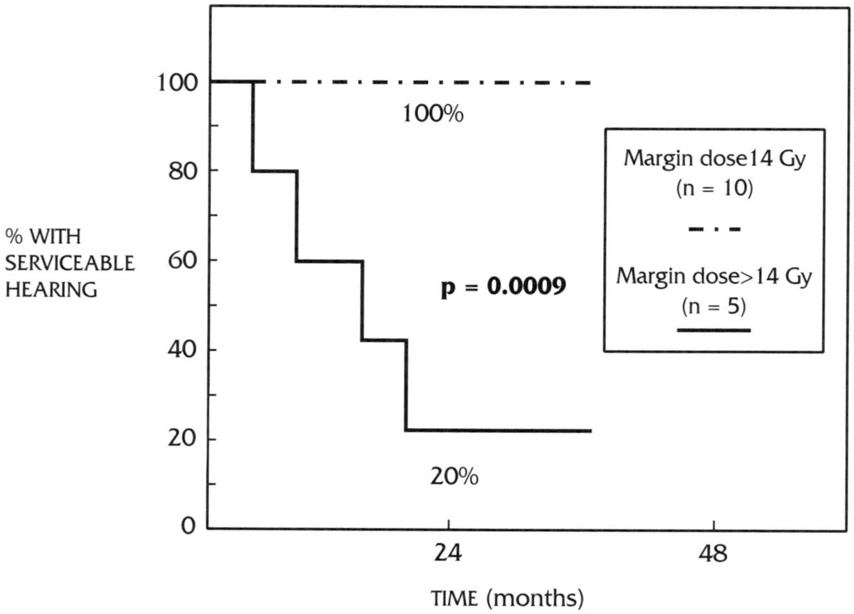

Figure 50–2 Graph showing preservation of serviceable hearing in the intracanalicular acoustic neuroma patients treated with ≤14 Gy versus >14 Gy to the tumor margin using the Gamma knife at the University of Pittsburgh.

nerve function are also superior to those reported after microsurgical excision of intracanalicular tumors. Hearing preservation is now the rule for such patients.

Possible Causes of Treatment-Related Hearing Loss

Mechanical damage to the axons or ischemia of the cochlea or auditory nerve may lead to immediate postoperative hearing loss during microsurgery. Stretch injury to the transitional Obersteiner–Redlich zone of the cochlear nerve has been suggested as the cause of hearing loss during tumor removal.[32] We did not observe immediate hearing loss in any patient after radiosurgery. If hearing impairment is noted, usually it is gradual. Early hearing loss after radiosurgery (within 3 months) is rare and may result from neural edema or demyelination.

Delayed hearing loss after microsurgery could result from the vascular or fibrotic changes or the development of endolymphatic hydrops after damage to the endolymphatic duct during surgery. The precise mechanism of delayed hearing loss after radiosurgery is still unclear. Perhaps delayed obliteration of microvessels or even direct radiation injury to the axons, in patients treated with higher radiosurgical doses, could account for hearing loss. Linskey et al.[26] hypothesized that length of the nerve irradiated predicts radiation injury to the nerve. The transitional Obersteiner–Redlich zone of the cochlear nerve may represent the most radiosensitive part of the cochlear nerve and may be responsible for hearing loss if a sufficiently high dose is given. The effect of radiation on normal microvessels supplying the cochlear nerve is still unclear. However, our experience suggests that doses of 13 or 14 Gy are well tolerated by auditory nerve and effectively prevent further tumor growth.[23,24] The conservation of hearing associated with the exclusive use of 4-mm collimator most likely is due to the sharp fall-off of the radiation field at the tumor margin. The 4-mm beam spares a substantial number of nerve fibers of the cochlear division which likely is compressed and pushed anteriorly by the tumor. A larger beam diameter not only covers the tumor but also encompasses most of the cochlear and facial nerve fibers within the 50% isodose volume, as the average diameter of normal internal auditory canal is only 4 mm (range 2 to 8 mm).[33]

Recommended Treatment Algorithm

Intracanalicular tumors usually present with acute or chronic hearing impairment, tinnitus, or imbalance. Most patients with acoustic tumors are not vertiginous because slow growth allows for gradual compensation by the central vestibular nuclei. The presence of vertigo may indicate compression of functioning vestibular nerve by an intracanalicular tumor before adequate compensation is established. Although a battery of tests have been described to diagnose acoustic tumors, MRI is the single most informative neurodiagnostic test. Gadolinium-enhanced T_1-weighted axial and coronal images provide excellent tumor delineation. The additional workup should include audiological testing to document pretreatment hearing status. In our view, PTA and SDS are necessary tests. The classification system proposed by Gardner and Robertson[30] appears quite useful for comparing hearing results.

All patients with newly diagnosed intracanalicular acoustic tumors should have a full explanation of the expected natural history of the tumor. The concepts of tumor growth control versus tumor removal should be discussed. All options, ranging from observation to microsurgery to radiosurgery, should be explained to patients (Fig. 50–3). Although serial observation may be a reasonable choice in selected elderly or asymptomatic pa-tients,[34] our experience indicates that more than 80% of tumors under observation grow within 4 years. Patients who are willing to accept tumor growth control coupled with enhanced hearing preservation rates should be offered radiosurgery as the treatment of choice. Those who elect microsurgery should be offered an approach best suited for hearing as well as facial preservation based on location of tumor in the internal auditory canal (medial or lateral) and the surgeon's experience. In general, patients with poor hearing undergo translabyrinthine removal, whereas patients with good hearing are operated on via the retrosigmoid approach or middle fossa approach. The goals of intracanalicular tumor management should be prevention of further tumor growth, and preservation of neurologic function. The treatment option should preserve serviceable hearing in those patients who have serviceable hearing at diagnosis. All patients at one point (during the early phase of tumor development) should be ideal candidates for hearing preservation.

Conclusion

Despite significant advances and improved results of microsurgical excision at centers of excellence, residual patient morbidity has not been eliminated. During the past 10 years, the long-term safety and efficacy of stereotactic radiosurgery have established this technique as an important noninvasive first-line alternative to microsurgery. The absence of procedure-related mortality and morbidity and superior tumor control, hearing, and facial preservation rates favor radiosurgery as the first management choice for patients with intracanalicular acoustic neuromas.

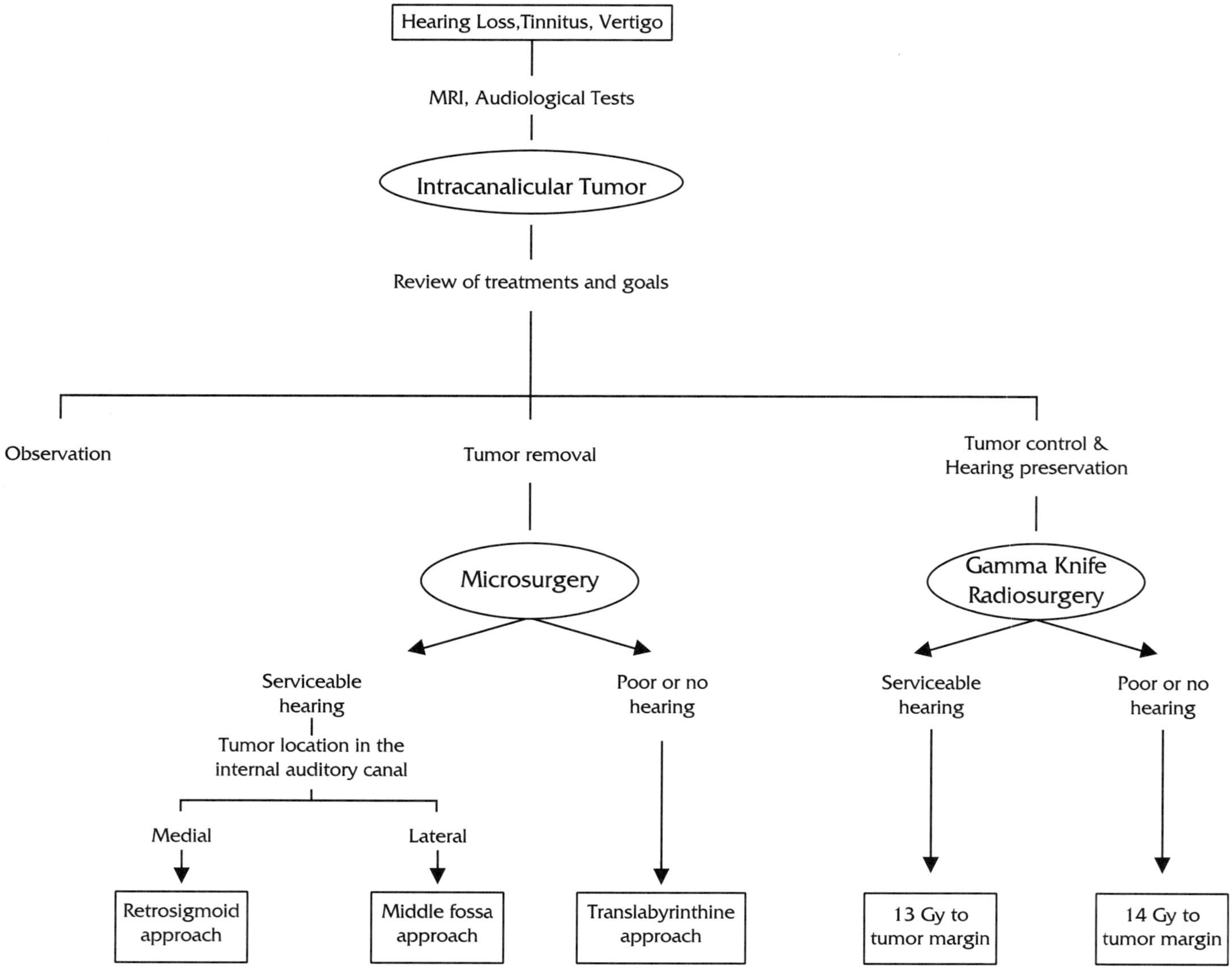

Figure 50–3 Management algorithm for intracanalicular acoustic tumors.

REFERENCES

1. Toynbee J. Neuroma of the auditory nerve. *Trans Pathol Soc Lond* 1853;4:259–260
2. Haines SJ, Levine SC. Intracanalicular acoustic neuroma: early surgery for preservation of hearing. *J Neurosurg* 1993;79:515–520
3. Kasantikul V, Netsky MG, Glasscock ME III. Intracanalicular neurilemmomas: clinicopathological study. *Ann Otol* 1980;89:29–32
4. Ogunrinde OK, Lunsford LD, Kondziolka D, et al. Cranial nerve preservation after radiosurgery for intracanalicular acoustic tumors. *Stereotact Funct Neurosurg* 1995;64(suppl 1):87–97
5. Samii M, Matthies C, Tatagiba M. Intracanalicular acoustic neuromas. *Neurosurgery* 1991;29:189–199
6. House WE, Hitselberger WE. The middle cranial fossa approach for removal of small acoustic tumor. *Acta Otolaryngol (Stockh)* 1969;67:413–427
7. Irving RM, Jackler RK, Pitts LH. Hearing preservation in patients undergoing vestibular schwannoma surgery: comparison of middle fossa and retrosigmoid approaches. *J Neurosurg* 1998;88:840–845
8. Nadol JB Jr, Levine R, Ojemann RG, et al. Preservation of hearing in surgical removal of acoustic neuromas of the internal

auditory canal and cerebello-pontine angle. *Laryngoscope* 1987; 97:1287–1294
9. Silverstein H, McDaniel AB, Norell H. Hearing preservation after acoustic neuroma surgery using intraoperative direct eighth nerve monitoring. *Am J Otol* 1985;(suppl):99–106
10. Sterkers JM, Sterkers O, Maudelonde C. Preservation of hearing by the retrosigmoid approach in acoustic neuroma surgery. *Adv Otorhinolaryngol* 1984;34:187–192
11. Brackmann DE. Acoustic neuroma surgery: otologic medical group results. In: Silverstein H, Norell H, eds. *Neurological Surgery for Ear*. Birmingham, AL: Aesculapus;1979:248–259
12. Dornhoffer JL, Helms J, Hoehmann DH. Hearing preservation in acoustic tumor surgery: results and prognostic factors. *Laryngoscope* 1995;105:184–187
13. Jannetta PJ, Moller AR, Moller MB. Technique of hearing preservation in small acoustic neuromas. *Ann Surg* 1984;200: 513–523
14. Nadol JB Jr, Chiong CM, Ojemann RG, et al. Preservation of hearing and facial nerve function in resection of acoustic neuroma. *Laryngoscope* 1992;102:1153–1158
15. Norén G, Greitz D, Hirsch A. Gamma knife radiosurgery in acoustic neurinoma. In: Steiner L, Lindquist C, Forester D, Backlund EO, eds. *Radiosurgery: Baseline and Trends*. New York: Raven Press;1992:141–148
16. Samii M, Matthies C. Management of 1000 vestibular schwannomas (acoustic neuromas): hearing function in 1000 tumor resections. *Neurosurgery* 1997;40:248–262
17. Palva T, Troupp H, Jauhiainer T. Hearing preservation in acoustic neuroma surgery. *Acta Otolaryngol* 1985;99:1–7
18. Shelton C, Hitselberg WE, House WE, Brackmann DE. Hearing preservation after acoustic tumor removal: long-term results. *Laryngoscope* 1990;100:115–119
19. Atlas MD, Harvey C, Fagan P. Acoustic neuroma hearing preservation surgery: five year follow-up results. In: Tos M, Thomsen J, eds. *Acoustic Neuroma*. New York: Kugler;1992: 681–687
20. Cohen NL, Ransohoff J. Hearing preservation—posterior fossa approach. *Otolaryngol Head Neck Surg* 1984;92: 176–185
21. Leksell L. Stereotactic radiosurgery. *J Neurol Neurosurg Psychiatry* 1983;46:797–803
22. Lunsford LD, Flickinger JC, Lindner G, Maitz A. Stereotactic radiosurgery of the brain using the first United States 201 cobalt-60 source gamma knife. *Neurosurgery* 1989;24: 151–159
23. Flickinger JC, Kondziolka D, Pollock BE, Lunsford LD. Evolution in technique for vestibular schwannoma radiosurgery and effect on outcome. *Int J Radiat Oncol Biol Phys* 1996; 36:275–280
24. Kondziolka D, Lunsford LD, Coffey RJ, Flickinger JC. Cranial nerve preservation after stereotactic radiosurgery of acoustic neurinomas. *Surg Forum* 1990;41:508–510
25. Kondziolka D, Lunsford LD, McLaughlin M, Flickinger JC. Long-term outcome after radiosurgery for acoustic neuromas. *N Engl J Med* 1998;339:1426–1433
26. Linskey ME, Flickinger JC, Lunsford LD. Cranial nerve length predicts the risk of delayed facial and trigeminal neuropathies after acoustic tumor stereotactic radiosurgery. *Int J Radiat Oncol Biol Phys* 1993;25:227–233
27. Lunsford LD, Kondziolka D, Flickinger JC. Stereotactic radiosurgery as an alternative to microsurgery for the treatment of acoustic neurinomas. *Clin Neurosurg* 1991;38:619–634
28. Lunsford LD, Kondziolka D, Flickinger JC. Acoustic neuroma management: evolution and revolution. In: Kondziolka D, ed. *Radiosurgery*. Vol 2. Basel: Karger;1998:1–7
29. Pollock BE, Lunsford LD, Kondziolka D, et al. Outcome analysis of acoustic neuroma management: a comparison of microsurgery and stereotactic radiosurgery. *Neurosurgery* 1995;36:215–229
30. Gardner G, Robertson JA, Tennessee M. Hearing preservation in unilateral acoustic neurinoma surgery. *Ann Otol Rhinol Laryngol* 1988;97:55–66
31. House JW, Brackmann DE. Facial nerve grading system. *Otolaryngol Head Neck Surg* 1985;93:146–147
32. Sekiya T, Moller AR. Cochlear nerve injuries caused by cerebello-pontine angle manipulations: an electrophysiological and morphological study in dogs. *J Neurosurg* 1987;67:144–249
33. Valvassori GE, Pierce RH. The normal internal auditory canal. *AJR* 1964;92:1232
34. Weit RJ, Zappia JJ, Hecht CS, et al. Conservative management of patients with small acoustic tumors. *Laryngoscope* 1995;105:795–800

The Intracanalicular Acoustic Neuroma

Stephen G. Harner

CHAPTER 51

Before 1960, the management of an intracanalicular acoustic neuroma was problematic. The tumor would have been almost impossible to diagnose, and microsurgical techniques and opening of the internal auditory canal were unknown. Beginning in the 1960s and continuing to the present, a number of events have made management of intracanalicular acoustic neuromas both interesting and exciting. The most significant events are the development of microsurgical techniques, the team approach, markedly improved imaging, and electrophysiologic monitoring.

Background

The acoustic neuroma arises from the vestibular nerve within the internal canal. The most likely point of origin is the juncture known as the glial–Schwann sheath junction. Theories have been proposed to explain this. One theory states that the vestibular nerve strikes the posterior portion of the internal auditory meatus and this trauma results in tumor formation. Other proposed theories such as genetic predisposition have not been substantiated. Regardless, the tumor begins within the canal and typically enlarges to fill the internal auditory canal before extending in the posterior cranial fossa. The length of the posterior wall of the internal auditory meatus is approximately 9 millimeters; therefore tumors classified as intracanalicular are ≤ 1.0 cm in length. In some surgical series, the intracanalicular portion of the acoustic neuroma is not included in the overall tumor size. Thus the measured tumor is only the portion in the posterior cranial fossa, and tumors within the internal auditory canal are grouped separately as intracanalicular. Other investigators include the intracanalicular portion; thus, a tumor that fills the internal auditory canal and that extends 1.5 cm into the posterior cranial fossa might be called a 1.5-cm tumor by the first group and a 2.5-cm tumor by the second group. I favor including the intracanalicular portion as part of the tumor.

The symptoms associated with an intracanalicular tumor are otologic.[1] The most common is unilateral hearing impairment. The hearing loss on audiometry is usually an asymmetric decrease in pure tones and some loss of speech discrimination. In addition, there is often a sense of sound distortion, which is disproportionate to the audiometric findings. Traditionally, the hearing loss has been thought to be primarily in the high frequencies, however the pure tones can assume any configuration, including a low tone loss, which resembles endolymphatic hydrops. A number of patients present with a sudden hearing loss.[2] These patients can be difficult to differentiate from idiopathic sudden hearing loss, particularly if the hearing then improves to normal or near-normal.

The second symptom of these tumors is unilateral tinnitus. Generally this is high pitched. When there is no clear-cut etiology for unilateral tinnitus, the symptom should be pursued. The third otologic symptom is dysequilibrium. Frequently the patient will remember unsteadiness in the past or describe some current persistent unsteadiness. Vertigo does occur but is rare. The other potential otologic symptom of an intracanalicular tumor is facial weakness. In a patient with an intracanalicular tumor and facial nerve paresis, a facial nerve neuroma should be the first consideration. Headache and diplopia are not associated with these tumors.

Physical findings are uncommon among patients with intracanalicular tumors. Potentially there could be nystagmus or facial weakness, but facial numbness, papilledema, and decreased corneal reflexes are not possible.

The important diagnostic tests are audiometry, vestibular testing, and imaging studies. Pure-tone audiometry, speech reception threshold, and speech discrimination are the most important initial tests. These tests are very sensitive and moderately specific. They confirm the patient's symptoms, define the degree of cochlear loss, and may suggest retrocochlear disease. Auditory brainstem response audiometry (ABR) can be useful among patients with mild asymmetry of the pure tones or a disproportionate decrease in the speech discrimination. As the hearing loss increases it becomes more prudent to use an imaging study. The role of the ABR audiometry as a screening tool has been the subject of considerable discussion.[3,4] For patients with intracanalicular tumors, the sensitivity of ABR is highly suspect and the specificity poor. Many neurotologists (including the present author) are concerned about the low sensitivity and generally omit the ABR. Others counter that the ABR is widely available, less expensive, and likely to miss only small tumors that are not a threat to the patient.

The role of vestibular testing as a diagnostic tool for intracanalicular tumors is limited. The sensitivity for use as a screening tool is marginal. When abnormal, this test might suggest the need to proceed with an imaging study. When normal, it does not exclude the need for further testing, thus like the ABR it is not sensitive or specific enough to play a major role in the evaluation of these patients.

The ultimate test is the imaging study. During the 1960s, imaging studies included plain radiographs and polytomography.

On occasion they would demonstrate enlargement of the internal auditory canal consistent with an expanding lesion. Unfortunately, this was not a definitive finding. Large tumors might cause no erosion; in addition, apparent erosion could be a normal variant. The most definitive test at that time was the posterior fossa myelogram, which depended on nonfilling of the internal auditory meatus to suggest an intracanalicular mass. Even for experienced radiologists this study was difficult to interpret. During the early 1970s, computed tomography (CT) first provided a positive image of the tumor. Unfortunately, the lesion had to be ≥2.5 cm to be visualized. CT with intravenous hypaque contrast allowed identification of most tumors that extended into the posterior cranial fossa. Intracanalicular tumors were still difficult to identify. The use of air contrast with CT permitted the definitive diagnosis of tumors within the internal canal. Initially the sensitivity of the magnetic resonance imaging (MRI) was equivalent to CT with hypaque. It could not regularly identify intracanalicular tumors. Gadolinium enhancement with MRI permitted identification of enhancing lesions within the internal auditory canal down to 2 mm. This increased sensitivity comes at a price. Lesions of ≥ 5 mm seem relatively easy to identify and diagnose. When the lesion is <5 mm, the enhancement is less specific and may represent inflammation rather than tumor. MRI with gadolineum has become the definitive imaging study. Recently there has been interest in a variation of MRI known as fast spin echo.[5-7] The major indications to look at this have been a reduction in cost and time. When a screening scan is desired, this has appeal. This study only looks at the cerebellopontine angle and does not use contrast material. The time to produce the image may be less, and it is definitely less costly. Unfortunately, it loses some of its sensitivity and is questionable in the smaller tumor. The complete MRI is clearly superior when looking for small tumors.

Discussion

The patient with an intracanalicular acoustic neuroma has three therapeutic options. The first is watchful waiting. An intracanalicular tumor usually causes well-defined otologic symptoms and poses no threat to life. For certain patients, observation is appropriate. The largest group would be those over the age of 65 or those with significant medical problems.[8] In addition, there are some patients who want to document growth of the tumor before they will submit to therapy. In these situations, a repeat MRI in 12 months is appropriate. Shorter waiting periods will not allow for definitive growth. Patients need to be aware that hearing preservation may be jeopardized with this choice. In theory the facial nerve preservation and postoperative function may lessen but that does not seem to be the case.

The second choice would be radiosurgery. The best-known technique would be the gamma knife.[9,10] As long as the tumor is limited to the internal canal, it seems inappropriate and unnecessary to treat with radiosurgery. This therapy should be reserved until the tumor extends beyond the internal auditory meatus. It should be used for patients who are older and/or who have significant medical problems. Concern has been expressed regarding the use of irradiation on a benign tumor, realizing that the tumor cannot be eradicated and over time there is potential for malignant degeneration.

The preferred option is surgical removal. The introduction of microsurgical techniques, electrophysiologic monitoring, and a team concept has vastly improved surgical results. In addition, surgery has the advantage of being definitive. Currently the surgical mortality should be less than 1%. The preservation of the facial nerve should occur in more than 95% of cases. Overall hearing preservation is around 50% with the retrosigmoid or middle fossa approach. Factors that influence hearing preservation include preoperative hearing levels, the presence of a wave V on the preoperative ABR, preservation of an ABR during surgery, and medial location of the tumor in the internal auditory canal. In the best cases, the hearing preservation is nearly 70%.[11] This is a major procedure and has the associated risks, including pain and disruption of lifestyle after surgery. However, most patients can return to full activity within 4 to 6 weeks. The tumor recurrence rate is low. Postoperative problems with headache, imbalance, facial weakness, and major hearing problems are infrequent.[12-15] A major concern for many patients who elect surgery is the choice of surgical approach.

The translabyrinthine approach is widely used and produces excellent results. Unfortunately, hearing will be uniformly sacrificed. In patients with less than serviceable hearing, this can be an appropriate choice. For the others, the retrosigmoid or middle fossa approach is preferred. Both produce excellent results when looking at tumor removal, facial nerve preservation and hearing preservation.[16] The middle fossa approach exposes the facial nerve to slightly higher risk. This results from the location of the facial nerve on top of the tumor and thus it is the first structure encountered when opening the internal auditory canal. Extension of the middle fossa procedure into the posterior fossa poses some difficulty. The middle fossa approach should not be used for patients aged 65 years or older because of concern regarding temporal lobe trauma.[17,18]

The retrosigmoid approach allows exposure for removal of these tumors. A potential problem has been that the lateral end of the canal is difficult to fully expose without opening the labyrinth. It appears that this area is also difficult to visualize by means of the middle fossa approach.[19] This does not hamper tumor removal, but it does jeopardize hearing preservation. The postoperative pain associated with this approach and persistent headache were believed to be significant, but studies do not seem to support this.[12,13] The most important factor in making a decision regarding surgical approach is the experience of the team and which approach the team feels most comfortable with. The results appear to be similar in experienced hands.

Conclusion

There are several conclusions that are based on this author's experience and on the observations of many surgeons who have shared experience in the literature and during informal discussions. First, an intracanalicular tumor poses no threat to the patient. Unless the lesion seen on MRI is ≥4 mm, the best choice is to recheck in 1 year. In patients over the age of 65, surgery is rarely indicated. The most significant exception is the patient with vertigo. Based on current knowledge, radiosurgery is never the best therapeutic option for intracanalicular tumors. When surgery is elected and hearing is present, the retrosigmoid or middle fossa approach is preferred. I prefer the retrosigmoid approach. When hearing is absent, the translabyrinthine approach is preferred. Electrophysiologic monitoring is useful but will not compensate for a lack of experience or skill. This surgery should be limited to those teams that perform one or more cerebellopontine angle procures per month.

REFERENCES

Harner—CHAPTER 51

1. Matthies C, Samii M. Management of 1000 vestibular schwannomas (acoustic neuromas): clinical presentation. *Neurosurgery* 1997;40:1–10
2. Weber PC, Zbar RI, Gantz BJ. Appropriateness of magnetic resonance imaging in sudden sensorineural hearing loss. *Otolaryngol Head Neck Surg* 1997;116:153–156
3. Zappia JJ, O'Connor CA, Wiet RJ, Dinces EA. Rethinking the use of auditory brainstem response in acoustic neuroma screening. *Laryngoscope* 1997;107:1388–1392
4. Ruchenstein MJ, Cueva RA, Morrison DH, Press G. A prospective study of ABR and MRI in the screening for vestibular schwannomas. *Am J Otol* 1996;17:317–320
5. Curtin HD. Rule out eighth nerve tumor: contrast-enhanced T1-weighted or high-resolution T2-weighted MR? *Am J Neuroradiol* 1997;18:1834–1838
6. Carrier DA, Arriaga MA. Cost-effective evaluation of asymmetric sensorineural hearing loss with focused magnetic resonance imaging. *Otolaryngol Head Neck Surg* 1997;116: 567–574
7. Allen RW, Harnsberger HR, Shelton C, et al. Low-cost high-resolution fast spin-echo MR of acoustic schwannoma: an alternative to enhanced conventional spin-echo MR. *Am J Neuroradiol* 1996;17:1205–1210
8. Glasscock ME III, Pappas DG Jr, Manolidis S, et al. Management of acoustic neuroma in the elderly population. *Am J Otol* 1997;18:236–241
9. Foote RL, Coffey RJ, Swanson JW, et al. Stereotactic radiosurgery using gamma knife for acoustic neuromas. *Int J Radiat Oncol Biol Phys* 1995;32:1153–1160
10. Pollock BE, Lunsford LD, Kondziolka D, et al. Outcome analysis of acoustic neuroma management: a comparison of microsurgery and stereotactic radiosurgery. *Neurosurgery* 1995;36:215–224
11. Slavit D, Harner SG, Harper CM Jr, Beatty CW. Auditory monitoring during acoustic tumor removal. *Arch Otolaryngol Head Neck Surg* 1991;117:1153–1157
12. Harner SG, Beatty CW, Ebersold MJ. Impact of cranioplasty on headache after acoustic neuroma removal. *Neurosurgery* 1995;36:1097–1099
13. Wiegand DA, Ojemann RG, Fickel V. Surgical treatment of acoustic neuroma (vestibular schwannoma) in the United States: report from the Acoustic Neuroma Registry. *Laryngoscope* 1996;10658–10666
14. van Leeuwen JP, Braspenning JC, Meijeer H, Cremers CW. Quality of life after acoustic neuroma surgery. *Ann Otol Rhinol Laryngol* 1996;105:423–430
15. Rigby PL, Shah SB, Jackler RK, et al. Acoustic neuroma surgery: outcome analysis of patient-perceived disability. *Am J Otol* 1997;18:427–435
16. Rowed DW, Nedzelski JM. Hearing preservation in the removal of intracanalicular acoustic neuromas via the retrosigmoid approach. *J Neurosurg* 1997;86:456–461
17. Slattery WH III, Brackmann DE, Hitselberger W. Middle fossa approach for hearing preservation with acoustic neuromas. *Am J Otol* 1997;18:596–601
18. Weber PC, Gantz BJ. Results and complications from acoustic neuroma excision via middle cranial fossa approach. *Am J Otol* 1996;17:669–675
19. Haberkamp TJ, Meyer GA, Fox M. Surgical exposure of the fundus of the internal auditory canal: anatomic limits of the middle fossa versus the retrosigmoid transcanal approach. *Laryngoscope* 1998;108:1190–1194

18

Temporal Bone Malignancies

"If the lesion is stage T3 or T4, the same protocol is offered as for T1 and T2, followed by removal of all positive and adjacent normal tissue in piecemeal fashion. If disease extends anteriorly into the glenoid fossa, the entire anatomic fossa is drilled out to the dura of the middle fossa, middle meningeal artery, and V3 as needed. The mandibular condyle, masseter, and pterygoid muscles may be removed."

Sam E. Kinney

"In a total temporal bone resection for stage T4 disease, the petrous carotid artery, sigmoid sinus, and involved dura are also resected en bloc. However, recent studies have shown that patients with such advanced disease succumb to it, regardless of therapy."

John P. Leonetti

"The advent of skull base surgery and free tissue transfers has extended the scope of surgery to include previously unresectable tumors, made surgery safer, decreased severe complication (CSF leaks, meningitis), and rendered the concept of piecemeal removal obsolete and indefensible."

Sebastian Arena

Temporal Bone Malignancies

Sam E. Kinney

CHAPTER 52

Malignancy of the temporal bone is a rare condition in otolaryngology–head and neck surgery. Conley[1] estimates that 1 in 3000 to 5000 patients with otologic disease will have a malignancy of the temporal bone. Manolidis et al.[2] reported from a referal otologic practice that 1 in 1167 new cases was an epithelial malignancy of the temporal bone.

The tumors can be divided into primary malignancies of the middle ear and mastoid and those with their origin from squamous epithelium or glandular tissue of the external auditory canal. The primary malignancies will be mentioned, with most of the discussion limited to malignancies with their origin in the external auditory canal.

The need to recognize and diagnose a malignancy early is not a controversial issue, but it must be included in this discussion. One of our obligations as otolaryngology–head and neck surgeons is to inform our colleagues in the primary care specialties to be suspicious of a possible malignancy. Infections of the external auditory canal are frequently treated in outpatient centers and primary care offices.

The usual course of treatment of external canal infections with either drops or wicks, or both, will result in resolution of pain and swelling within 5 to 7 days of treatment. Chronic infections may persist with some edema and discharge, but there is usually no pain.

In the elderly population, any external canal infection with persistent pain must be considered a possible malignancy. Any external canal infections with persistent bleeding, formation of granulation tissue, or lack of improvement with medical treatment, must be considered a possible malignancy. The lesion must be biopsied for histologic evaluation or referred to the otolaryngology–head and neck surgeon for biopsy.

Contemporary issues relative to temporal bone malignancy center on pretreatment evaluation, appropriate TNM staging, and designing appropriate treatment modalities. Recognizing that temporal bone malignancies are relatively rare, there are no large single-institution series.

Evaluation

The quality of high-resolution computed tomography (CT) scans has improved, resulting in a resolution that gives fine bone detail. Bone erosion by the tumor can readily be seen. However, when the CT scan shows abnormal soft tissue, the question of inflammation versus malignancy is not as certain. Arriaga et al.[3] presented a retrospective review of CT scans of patients with squamous cell carcinoma of the external auditory canal and temporal bone. T1 lesions have tumor limited to the external auditory meatus without bony erosion or soft tissue extension. T2 lesions would be limited to bone erosion of the external bony canal and <0.5-cm soft tissue extension. This category would include lesions extending through preformed pathways such as cartilaginous fissures of the bony cartilaginous junction of the external auditory meatus. T3 lesions would demonstrate full thickness erosion of the osseus external auditory meatus with <0.5 cm soft tissue involvement, tumor involving the middle ear mastoid, or facial nerve paralysis. T4 would be lesions eroding the cochlea, petrous apex, medial wall of the middle ear carotid canal, jugular foramen, or dura with >0.5 cm of soft tissue extension.

A careful clinical examination follows the histologic diagnosis of squamous cell carcinoma. The canal is evaluated for the location of the ulceration or granulation tissue. Evaluation of the tympanic membrane is important; however, it will not be possible to see the tympanic membrane in 50% of cases. Depth of disease in the canal can be helpful. Anterior lateral disease may extend into the glenoid fossa or the superficial lobe of the parotid gland. Anterior medial disease may extend into the deep lobe of the parotid gland. Posterior disease may spread to the postauricular lymph nodes.

A complete head and neck examination is accomplished, including cranial nerves, and the parotid, neck, and postauricular area. Imaging studies are performed. The thin-cut high-resolution CT scan is most important. The magnetic resonance imaging (MRI) scan may be helpful; however, false-positive soft tissue involvement such as brain extension may be seen. The CT scan is evaluated with the assistance of a temporal bone neuroradiologist. Careful attention is directed to the bone of the external auditory canal, the tympanic membrane, and the ossicles. Disease limited to these areas would be staged as T1 or T2, as noted by Arriaga et al.[3] There is no reliable sign to differentiate extension of disease through the tympanic membrane, and lateral ossicles as inflammatory granulation tissue or squamous cell carcinoma.

The structures of the medial wall of the middle ear, mastoid, dural plates, and otic capsule are evaluated. Disease in this area would be staged T3. The carotid canal, jugular bulb, foramen, and skull base are evaluated. Involvement of these structures would be staged T4.

The area of the glenoid fossa, the mandibular condyle, and the parotid gland is evaluated by CT scan and MRI scan. Consultations with colleagues in head and neck, neurotology, and neurosurgery are obtained as required. A treatment plan is outlined by the entire team.

Treatment

Treatment modalities presented in the literature have included radiotherapy alone, surgical resection, preoperative irradiation and surgery, surgery followed by radiotherapy, and occasional supplemental chemotherapy.

The ideal surgical approach to squamous cell carcinoma of the head and neck includes the external auditory canal and temporal bone in en bloc resection with the immediate adjacent tissues having the highest probability of lymphatic spread. The goal of surgical resection is to remove all tumor, as noted in the standard approach to squamous cell carcinoma of the head and neck, and to create the least amount of surgical morbidity and mortality with the best reasonable chance of 5-year or better survival. In some cases there may be a justification for a less than ideal surgical resection in order to provide relief of pain and a reasonable quality of life in the patient's last months to 1 year.

The literature during the past 40 years gives some insight into the ability to achieve the goals presented above. Boland[4] in 1963 presented the results of megavolt irradiation and felt that better than 50% of patients could be cured. This included T1 lesions as defined by Arriaga et al.[3] In 1975 Wang[5] reported about 50% cure rate of T1 lesions but believed that lesions beyond the external canal are not successful with radiotherapy alone. Wang and Doppke[6] reported on osteoradionecrosis of the temporal bone given postoperatively at doses of >6000 to 6500 rad.

Lewis[7] is credited by most investigators as presenting the best opportunity of en bloc resection of the temporal bone. He has also presented the largest series of cases in the literature. He advocated total en bloc resection of the temporal bone followed by radiotherapy. He had an overall 5-year survival rate of 28%. Arena[8] presented his modifications of the en bloc temporal bone resection, emphasizing the need for neurosurgical assistance to achieve total removal of the temporal bone. He noted that, in those cases in which the primary was not controlled, survival was less than 6 months.

Neely and Forrester,[9] in 1982, presented a temporal bone study to determine the feasibility of en bloc temporal bone resection, including the lateral wall of the bony carotid canal and jugular bone. These investigators noted the advisability of removing all pneumatized spaces when the tumor had invaded beyond the external canal. The ability to remove all of the air cell system without violation was remote.

Goodwin and Jesse,[10] in 1980, found that the survival rate for 35 patients with deep involvement of the squamous cell carcinoma was 28%. The reason for failure was incomplete resection of disease. Go et al.[11] presented the results of 16 cases of temporal bone resection noting that failures occurred because of incomplete resection of disease. There were positive margins on the surgical specimen.

Graham et al.[12] presented two cases of temporal bone resection, including the carotid artery. Sataloff et al.[13] presented an additional two patients with resection of the carotid artery and cranial nerves VI through XII and noted that there still was inadequate resection of the primary disease.

Willging and Pensak,[14] in 1991, presented their experience using temporal bone resection for squamous cell carcinoma of the temporal bone. These investigators emphasized early diagnosis and radical treatment. Imaging studies may be helpful in defining the extent of disease and limits of resection. They noted that inclusion of the petrous apex in an en bloc resection does not add to survival but significantly increases morbidity.

In 1987, Kinney and Wood[15-17] presented their experience of 30 cases of temporal bone malignancy. Based on the experience of Crabtree et al.[18] an external auditory canal resection, with further removal of all tumor as needed using frozen section margin control. Most patients were given full postoperative radiotherapy. The survival rate for external canal lesions, T1 of Arriaga et al.,[3] was 91%. T2 lesions survival rate was 72%. T3 and T4 lesions was 45%. As noted by Arena,[8] those cases not controlled died within 12 months.

The treatment algorithm for squamous cell carcinoma of the external auditory canal and temporal bone has evolved with some modifications. The high index of suspicion and early diagnosis remain the best prognostic tools in this disease.

Very limited lesions with low malignancy histology, such as verrucous carcinoma with no bone involvement, can be treated with a sleeve canal resection with or without split-thickness skin graft, depending on the size of the lesion. Radiotherapy is usually unnecessary during the postoperative period.

Recognizing the high incidence of tumor violation in the best designed en bloc temporal bone resection, this technique is not currently employed for primary treatment modality. Patients presenting with squamous cell carcinoma in an open mastoid cavity or who have undergone previous radiotherapy will be considered for attempted en bloc temporal bone resection.

Patients with T1 and T2 preoperative-stage lesions will be offered a lateral temporal bone resection with incontinuity removal of the superficial lobe of the parotid gland. If the lesion is anterior medial in the external canal, the deep lobe of the parotid gland may be removed. Level 2 and 3 lymph nodes are sampled for frozen-section evaluation to determine the need for formal radical neck dissection.

If the lesion is stage T3 or T4, the same protocol is offered as for T1 and T2, followed by removal of all positive and adjacent normal tissue in piecemeal fashion. If disease extends anteriorly into the glenoid fossa, the entire anatomic fossa is drilled out to the dura of the middle fossa, middle meningeal artery, and V3 as needed. The mandibular condyle, masseter, and pterygoid muscles may be removed.

The entire labyrinth, cochlea, facial nerve, and petrous apex may be removed. The entire mastoid middle fossa tegmen and posterior fossa dural plate may be resected. Dura is resected and grafted as needed. Squamous cell carcinoma rarely penetrates the dura but will track along the dura and must be resected.

The carotid artery can be removed from its bony canal and the external sheath stripped or carotid resection with bypass may be performed. Sacrifice of cranial nerves IX, X, and XI may be accomplished. All decisions are based on frozen-section control, often 20 to 30 samples in one case.

At present, all patients with CT evidence of bone involvement or histologic evidence of bone involvement, will be given full therapy postoperative radiotherapy. This is done in consultation with the radiation oncologist and will include the neck as considered necessary.

Recognizing the difficulties with late osteoradionecrosis of the temporal bone including bone death and cerebral spinal fluid leaks, the middle ear transformer is sacrificed in all cases for which irradiation will be given. This means that the operative field will be covered by vascularized soft tissue and skin. The original attempts to obliterate this site with sternocleidomastoid mastoid muscle have not been successful. The temporalis muscle with its anterior blood supply is useful for covering limited canal resections. Regional flaps or vascularized free flaps may be used particularly in those cases of auriculectomy and dural resection with grafts.

Appropriate cranial nerve rehabilitation to protect the eye, airway, and swallowing are also performed. Control of cerebrospinal fluid (CSF) and prevention of infection are concurrently employed.

Primary malignancies of the temporal bone are extremely rare. These would include rhabdomyosarcoma, aggressive middle ear adenoma, and adenocarcinoma of the endolymphatic sac. Current treatment of rhabdomyosarcoma consists of chemo-therapy and radiotherapy. Surgery is used only to reduce the bulk size of the tumor.

Aggressive middle ear adenoma[19] may be considered a form of adenocarcinoma or a benign papillary adenoma. The treatment is aggressive total removal of all tumor. It is advisable to plan a second-look operation about 1 year after the primary operation to ensure total removal.

Adenocarcinoma of the endolymphatic sac[20] is rare, and the diagnosis may not be apparent until the tumor has been violated. Aggressive total removal as advocated for T3 and T4 squamous cell carcinoma lesions of the external auditory canal followed by full-therapy irradiation would be given.

Conclusion

1. The most important prognostic factor in the treatment of malignancy of the temporal bone is early diagnosis. Any lesion of the external auditory canal not responding to medical treatment, with bleeding, forming granulation tissue, or persistent pain, must be biopsied.
2. An appropriate head and neck examination should also be performed, including cranial nerves and areas of potential lymphatic spread.
3. Imaging studies are performed, including high-resolution CT scans with bone algorithm and possible MRI scan. These studies are reviewed with the temporal bone neuroradiologist and other members of the treating team (i.e., head and neck surgeon, neurosurgeon, and neurotologist).
4. The tumor is staged according to the TNM classification of Arriaga et al.[3] The literature and experience will show that there often will be intraoperative findings that will change the TNM classification.
5. T1 and T2 lesions will be treated with a lateral temporal bone resection in continuity with superficial lobe of the parotid gland, possible resection of the deep lobe of the parotid gland, sampling of level 2 and 3 neck nodes, and neck dissection as needed. The area will be covered with vascularized tissue and skin, sacrificing the middle ear transformer. Postoperative full-therapy irradiation will be given.
6. T3 and T4 lesions will begin with the lateral temporal bone resection, followed by piecemeal removal of all tumor and adjacent normal structures based on frozen-section control. Parotidectomy and neck evaluation will be as with T1 and T2 lesions. Those T1 and T2 lesions that experience violation of tumor by the resection, will be treated as a T3 or T4 lesion. The surgical field will be covered by vascularized tissue and skin. Appropriate steps to protect the exposed eye, airway, and swallowing will be taken. Full-therapy postoperative irradiation will be given.
7. Cases of squamous cell carcinoma in a previous mastoid cavity, or when radiotherapy has been given with persistence, will be treated with attempted en bloc resection based on the imaging studies. This approach may be used for palliation in those patients with severe pain.

REFERENCES

Kinney—CHAPTER 52

1. Conley J. Cancer of the middle ear. *Ann Otol Rhinol Laryngol* 1965;74:555–572
2. Manolidis S, Pappas D, Von Doersten P, et al. Temporal bone and lateral skull base malignancy: experience and results with 81 patients. *Am J Otol* 1998;19:S1–S15
3. Arriaga M, Curtin H, Takahashi H, et al. Staging proposal for external auditory meatus carcinoma based on preoperative clinical examination and computed tomography findings. *Ann Otol Rhinol Laryngol* 1990;90:714–721
4. Boland J. The management of carcinoma of the middle ear. *Radiology* 1963;80:285
5. Wang CL. Radiation therapy in the management of carcinoma of the external canal, middle ear, or mastoid. *Radiology* 1975;116:713–715

6. Wang CL, Doppke K. Osteoradionecrosis of the temporal bone—considerations of nominal standard dose. *Int J Radiat Oncol Biol Phys* 1976;1:881–883
7. Lewis JS. Surgical management of tumors of the middle ear and mastoid. *J Laryngol Otol* 1983;97:299–311
8. Arena S. Tumor surgery of the temporal bone. *Laryngoscope* 1974;84:615–670
9. Neely JG, Forrester M. Anatomic considerations of the medial cuts in subtotal temporal bone resection. *Otolaryngol Head Neck Surg* 1982;90:641–645
10. Goodwin WJ, Jesse RH. Malignant neoplasms of the external auditory canal and temporal bone. *Arch Otolaryngol* 1980;106:675–679
11. Go KG, Annyas AA, Vermey A, et al. Evaluation of results of temporal bone resection. *Acta Neurochir* 1991;110:110–115
12. Graham MD, Sataloff RT, Kemink JL, et al. Total en bloc resection of the temporal bone and carotid artery for maligant tumors of the ear and temporal bone. *Laryngoscope* 1984;94: 528–533
13. Sataloff RT, Myers DL, Lowry LD, et al. Total temporal bone resection for squamous cell carcinoma. *Otolaryngol Head Neck Surg* 1987;96:4–14
14. Willging JP, Pensak ML. Temporal bone resection. *Ear Nose Throat J* 1991;70:612–617
15. Kinney SE, Wood BG. Malignancies of the external ear canal and temporal bone: surgical techniques and results. *Laryngoscope* 1987;97:158–164
16. Kinney SE, Wood BG. Surgical treatment of skull base malignancy. *Otolaryngol Head Neck Surg* 1984;92:94–99
17. Kinney SE. Squamous cell carcinoma of the external auditory canal. *Am J Otol* 1989;10:111–116
18. Crabtree JA, Britton BH, Pierce MK. Carcinoma of the external auditory canal. *Laryngoscope* 1976;86:405–415
19. Batsakis JG. Adenomatous tumors of the middle ear. *Ann Otol Rhinol Laryngol* 1989;98:749–752
20. Li JC, Brackmann DE, Lo WWM, Carberry JN, House JW. The reclassification of aggressive adenomatous mastoid neoplasms as endolymphatic sac tumors. *Laryngoscope* 1993;103:1342–1348

Temporal Bone Malignancies

Sam J. Marzo and John P. Leonetti

CHAPTER 53

The human temporal bone occupies the inferolateral skull base. Although osseous, it also possesses an epithelialized ear canal, mastoid, and middle ear, as well as other foramina and canals. Cranial nerves VII to IX, the carotid artery, and the sigmoid sinus all traverse the temporal bone. Almost every type of tissue, from cartilaginous to glandular, can be found within it. Athough any of these structures can give rise to a malignancy, most temporal bone cancers arise from the external auditory canal, and of these, squamous cell carcinoma (SCCA) is the most common.[1] Table 53–1 lists a classification of temporal bone malignancies.

It is often difficult to determine the tissue of origin in patients with temporal bone malignancy. Patients with a biopsy-proven ear canal SCCA and an otherwise normal head and neck examination most likely have primary SCCA of the temporal bone. Patients with a prior history of head and neck SCCA who present with a lesion in the temporal bone may have metastatic disease. A diligent search for other evidence of metastases should be sought before embarking on surgical therapy. This might include a contrast computed tomography (CT) scan of the head, neck, and chest. Uncommon lesions such as adenocarcinoma may require a search for metastatic disease, including a thorough breast examination with or without mammography, and a contrast CT scan of the chest, abdomen, and pelvis. Primary tumors metastatic to the temporal bone include carcinoma of the breast, lung, stomach, prostate, and kidney. Of these, most are from the breast.[2] This chapter focuses primarily on the management of SCCA of the temporal bone. Principles apply to other isolated less common lesions as well, with the exception of pediatric rhabdomyosarcoma, which is treated with limited surgical resection, chemotherapy, and radiotherapy.[3]

TABLE 53–1
Differential Diagnosis of Temporal Bone Malignancies

Origin	Type
Ear canal	Squamous cell carcinoma Basal cell carcinoma Adenoid cystic carcinoma Ceruminal gland adenocarcinoma Malignant melanoma Kaposi's sarcoma
Middle ear	Squamous cell carcinoma Adenocarcinoma Rhabdomyosarcoma Malignant lymphoma Plasmacytoma
Metastatic	Breast carcinoma Squamous cell carcinoma from other head and neck site Pulmonary adenocarcinoma Malignant melanoma Renal cell carcinoma Prostate adenocarcinoma Thyroid papillary adenocarcinoma

SOURCE: Wenig B, ed. *Pathology of the Head and Neck*. New York: McGraw-Hill; 1990.

Epidemiology

The incidence of squamous cell carcinoma of the temporal bone is approximately six cases per million in the general population, with most patients more than 50 years of age.[4] The main risk factor is a long, often two or more decade history of chronic suppurative otitis media.[5] Other potential inciting factors include chronic dermatitis,[6] cholesteatoma,[7] history of employment as a radium dial painter,[8] and intracranial irradiation.[9]

Clinical and Radiographic Examination

The most common presenting symptom is otalgia; the most common presenting sign is a mass in the external auditory canal.[10] Other clinical manifestations are detailed in Table 53–2. Binocular microscopic otoscopy, a complete head, neck, and cranial nerve examination, and audiometry are then performed. Since SCCA of the temporal bone routinely invades bone and soft tissues within and near the temporal bone, most patients should ideally undergo CT of the temporal bone as well as magnetic resonance imaging (MRI) of the head and neck.

Although no consensus has been reached on the ideal staging system for SCCA of the temporal bone, one of the better systems is from the University of Pittsburgh[11] and is summarized as follows: T1, tumor limited to the external auditory meatus without bone or soft tissue extension; T2, tumor with

TABLE 53–2
Clinical Manifestations of Patients with Squamous Cell Carcinoma of the Temporal Bone

Symptoms:	
	Otalgia
	Hearing loss
	Headache
	Facial numbness
	Hoarseness
	Dysphagia
Signs:	
	EAC mass
	Bloody otorrhea
	Facial nerve paralysis
	Other cranial nerve deficits
	Parotid and/or cervical mass
	Temporal mass

SOURCE: Leonetti JP, Smith PG, Kletzker R, Izquierdo R. Invasion patterns of advanced temporal bone malignancies. *Am J Otol* 1996;17: 438–442.

limited bone and soft tissue extension; T3, full-thickness external auditory meatus erosion, middle ear or mastoid extension, and facial nerve paralysis; and T4, tumor eroding cochlea, carotid canal, jugular foramen, dura, petrous apex, or extensive (>0.5 cm) soft tissue extension. Nodal and metastatic disease is staged according to the American Joint Committee System. Most pa-tients present with stage T3 and T4 lesions. T1 and T2 lesions have cure rates of 50 to 70%, whereas T3 and T4 lesions have a 35% cure rate.[12]

Treatment

Modern skull base surgery has expanded our capability of resecting temporal bone malignancies. However, the ability to resect structures such as the petrous carotid artery can cause significant morbidity without increasing surgical cure rates. Small surgical series and lack of a universal staging system further cloud this issue. Pensak et al.[13] believe contraindications to surgical resection include invasion of any of the following structures: the cavernous sinus, the carotid artery, the infratemporal fossa, and the paraspinous musculature. All patients in their series of 46 individuals with squamous cell carcinoma of the temporal bone with such invasion died within 3 years despite surgery and postoperative radiotherapy. Although some investigators have found preoperative staging to be highly accurate,[11] the senior author of this chapter has found that CT and MRI scanning underestimated involvement of the mastoid mucosa, tegmen tympani, middle fossa dura, middle ear mucosa, and carotid canal.[10] Furthermore, all such patients had a very high incidence of local recurrence.

The technique of temporal bone resection has been described previously.[14-16] Partial temporal bone resection is performed for tumors located within the external auditory canal, stage T1 and T2. Through a postauricular approach with appropriate canal incisions to obtain negative margins, a complete mastoidectomy with an extended facial recess is performed. Dissection continues anteriorly through the root of the zygoma. The incudostapedial joint is sectioned and the incus removed. Bone anterior to the vertical facial nerve and medial to the tympanic anulus is removed. The vertical segment of the facial nerve is followed into the stylomastoid foramen. A parotidectomy and cervical lymphadenectomy is performed. The entire specimen is retracted superiorly and a final chisel cut lateral to the styloid process liberates the specimen. After negative margins confirmed on frozed section, the cavity is filled with an abdominal fat graft, and the ear canal is closed on itself or with a skin graft.

A subtotal temporal bone resection is performed for tumors involving the middle ear and mastoid, stage T3. The entire pinna may have to be included with the specimen. A parotidectomy and cervical lyphadenectomy is performed. The entire temporal bone lateral to the internal auditory canal and carotid artery is resected. The wound is closed, using either a trapezius flap or a rectus abdominus free tissue transfer.

In a total temporal bone resection for stage T4 disease, the petrous carotid artery, sigmoid sinus, and involved dura are also resected en bloc. However, recent studies have shown that patients with such advanced disease succumb to it, regardless of therapy. Manolidis et al.[17] had 6 patients, Pensak et al.[13] had 3 patients, and Leonetti et al.[10] had 9 patients. All 18 of these patients had T4 disease and expired within 3 to 5 years after surgery and radiotherapy.

Adjuvant therapy after surgery for temporal bone SCCA should include radiotherapy. Chemotherapy has only been shown to be effective for rhabdomyosarcoma.[3] Total radiotherapy dosages are usually 60 Gy, with the limiting structures the optic nerve and brain.[18] Most failures after radiotherapy occur at the basicranium, in either the surgical bed or a contiguous site.[19]

Postoperative complications can include hematoma, infection, stroke, cerebrospinal fluid (CSF) leakage, cranial nerve deficits, and deep venous thrombosis. Trapezius pedicle flaps and rectus abdominus free flaps have shown promise in defect reconstruction. With appropriate wound closure, many CSF leaks can be controlled with short-term lumbar drainage.[20] Immediate primary thyroplasty has shown promise in improving immediate voice and swallowing results when the vagus nerve has to be resected. In short, aside from a cerebrovascular accident after carotid resection, most postoperative complications can be adequately managed.

REFERENCES

1. Lederman M. Malignant tumors of the ear. *J Laryngol Otol* 1965;79:79–85
2. Feinmesser R, Libson Y, Uziely B, Gay I. Metastatic carcinoma to the temporal bone. *Am J Otol* 1986;7:119
3. Wiatrak BJ, Pensak ML. Rhabdomyosarcoma of the ear and temporal bone. *Laryngoscope* 1989;99:1188
4. Lodge WP, Jones HM, Smith ME. Malignant tumors of the temporal bone. *Arch Otolaryngol* 1995;61:535–541
5. Conley J. Cancer of the middle ear. *Ann Otol Rhinol Laryngol* 1965;74:555–572
6. Conley J, Schuller DE. Malignancies of the ear. *Laryngoscope* 1976;86:1147–1163
7. Coachman EH. Squamous cell carcinoma secondary to cholesteatoma. *Arch Otolaryngol* 1951;54:187
8. Beal DD, Lindsay JR, Ward P. Radiation-induced carcinoma of the mastoid. *Arch Otolaryngol* 1965;81:9–16
9. Ruben RJ, Thaler SU, Holzer N. Radiation induced carcinoma of the temporal bone. *Laryngoscope* 87;1977: 1613-1621
10. Leonetti JP, Smith PG, Kletzker R, Izquierdo R. Invasion patterns of advanced temporal bone malignancies. *Am J Otol* 1996;17:438–442
11. Arriaga M, Curtin H, Hirsch BE, et al. Staging proposal for external auditory meatus carcinoma based on preoperative clinical examination and CT findings. *Ann Otol Rhinol Laryngol* 1990;99:714–721
12. Lewis JS. Temporal bone resection—review of 100 cases. *Arch Otolaryngol* 1975;101:23–25
13. Pensak ML, Gleich LL, Gluckman JL, Shumrick KA. Temporal bone carcinoma: contemporary perspectives in the skull base surgical era. *Laryngoscope* 1996;106:1234–1237
14. Graham MD, Sataloff RT, Kemik JL, et al. Total en bloc resection of the temporal bone and carotid artery for malignant tumors of the ear and temporal bone. *Laryngoscope* 1984; 94:528–533
15. Sataloff RT, Myers DL, Lowry LD, Spiegel JR. Total temporal bone resection for squamous cell carcinoma. *Otolaryngol Head Neck Surg* 1987;96:4–14
16. Kinney SE, Wood BG. Malignancies of the external ear canal and temporal bone: surgical techniques and results. *Laryngoscope* 1987;97:158–163
17. Manolidis S, Papas D, VonDoersten P, Jackson CG, Glasscock ME 3rd. Temporal bone and lateral skull base malignancy: experience and results with 81 patients. *Am J Otol* 1988;19:S1–S15
18. Marks J, Wong J. The risk of cerebral radionecrosis in relation to dose, time and fractionation. *Prog Exp Tumor Res* 1985;29: 210–218
19. Paulino AC, Marks JE, Leonetti JP. Postoperative irradiation of patients with malignant tumors of the skull base. *Laryngoscope* 1996;106:880–883
20. Jackson CG, Netterville JL, Glasscock ME, et al. Defect reconstruction and cerebrospinal fluid management in neurotologic skull base tumors with intracranial extension. *Laryngoscope* 1992;102:1205–1213
21. Wenig B, ed. *Pathology of the Head and Neck*. New York: McGraw-Hill; 1990

Temporal Bone Malignancies

Sebastian Arena

CHAPTER 54

The diagnosis and management of malignancies of the temporal bone remain an area that presents a severe challenge to the otolaryngologist. The complex anatomy of the temporal bone and surrounding neurovascular structures mandates that any surgeon who undertakes a formidable procedure such as temporal bone tumor resection have an intimate knowledge of the galaxy of anatomic details of this area. Familiarity with patterns of invasion of these malignancies is a prerequisite. Advanced imaging with computed tomography (CT) and magnetic resonance imaging (MRI) has greatly enhanced preoperative evaluation and surgical planning, but there is still no uniformly accepted staging system for these tumors.

The most viable systems of staging are reviewed. Advances in skull base surgery have extended the boundaries of surgery, made surgery safer, and decreased the mortality, but have they really decreased the morbidity of multiple cranial nerve palsies? Have the cure rates improved? Free tissue transfers have significantly reduced cerebrospinal fluid (CSF) leaks and ascending meningitis and have helped make postoperative radiation better tolerated.

Primary malignancies of the temporal bone are rare.[1] Squamous cell carcinoma (SCC; also abbreviated SCCA) is the predominant primary carcinoma arising from the external canal and middle ear.[2] Adenoid cystic carcinoma is the next most common, although its incidence is far below that of SCC.[3] Papillary tumors of the temporal bone (also classified as adenomas or adenocarcinomas) are thought to arise from the endolymphatic sac.[4,5] The temporal bone can be secondarily invaded by cancer of the pinna, parotid, and temporomandibular joint (TMJ). Although rare, the temporal bone can be the focus of metastasis from distant sites (e.g., breast, lung, kidney, thyroid, larynx), that are thought to be hematogenous to the petrous apex.[6] In children, rabdomyosarcoma is the most frequent somatic tumor and carries a poor prognosis, although combined therapy (surgery, radiotherapy, and chemotherapy) has improved the outlook. Early diagnosis, which is difficult, is essential to a favorable outcome.

Diagnosis

The diagnosis of SCC of the external canal and middle ear is often made late in the disease because of long-standing suppurative disease. By the time the diagnosis is made, the tumor may have involved the carotid canal, dura, facial nerve, and extended into the temporomandibular (TMJ) or pterygoids. It is important in assessment of these patients to be familiar with the behavior patterns of these tumors. Leonette et al.[3] described five patterns of invasion as determined by CT and MRI findings correlated with operative and pathologic findings. They described anterior, inferior, medial, superior, and posterior extension. In other words, extension occurs in all directions, including natural pathways such as the fissures of Santorini.[3]

CT is essential for staging. MRI is helpful in determining soft tissue invasion including dural involvement and pterygoid involvement. Curtin et al.[7] have proposed what has become known as the Pittsburgh Staging System for SSC of the temporal bone. In their system, T1 is a tumor limited to the external canal with no bone erosion, T2 includes erosion of the bony canal, T3 tumor involves middle ear and/or mastoid, and T4 is a tumor involving petrous apex, carotid canal, jugular, foramen, and soft tissue involvement. In my view, this system of staging is the best yet proposed but still is not entirely satisfactory. Further staging refinements will require that subclassifications of staging include dural and skull base involvement, as suggested by Clark et al.[8] inasmuch as anterior extension carries a better prognosis than medial and posterior extension and should be identified in the staging system. I suggest modifying the Pittsburgh Staging System to include Clark's subdivision of extratemporal spread. Curtin's T4 would become a T4a, T4b would include intracranial involvement of dura, brain, and cranial nerves.

Management

In 1954, Parsons and Lewis[9] reported their landmark paper on en bloc subtotal resection of the temporal bone and introduced the present day concept for management of the temporal bone malignancies. Conley and Novack,[1,4] in 1960, described an operation for malignancies limited to the external canal, with preservation of the facial nerve. Before this, piecemeal removal followed by radiation was advocated with poor 5-year survival rates.[10] With the advent of skull base surgery, many previously unresectable tumors have become amenable to en bloc surgical extirpations. In addition, free tissue transfers have decreased wound complications and made postoperative radiotherapy more feasible. Before the introduction of free tissue transfers, the temporal bone defect was dressed with only a split-thickness skin graft. This precluded resection of dura and would on occasion result in CSF leaks and ascending meningitis.

Treatment of SCC of the external canal is determined by accurate preoperative clinical, CT, and MRI staging of this disease. Complete surgical resection followed by radiation yields the highest cure rate, and incomplete surgical removal almost certainly will result in death or recurrence within a few years.[11]

In T1 SCC (limited to the ear canal without bone involvement), the lateral temporal bone resection as described by Conley and Novack[4] with preservation of the facial nerve is the treatment of choice. I always include the parotid gland (in a retrograde dissection of the facial nerve) as part of the specimen because of possible migration of tumor through the fissures of Santorini. Postoperative radiotherapy in stage 1 disease is determined by the final pathologic findings. For stages 2 and 3, a subtotal temporal bone resection, as described by Parsons and Lewis,[9] is the treatment of choice, followed by radiation. The technique for subtotal temporal bone resection has been described extensively by many investigators; it is not be described here, except to state that the medial osteotomies are directed just lateral to the petrous ICA and medial to the arcuate eminence.[9,12]

For T4a and T4b, a total en bloc resection is necessary along with a neck dissection including the soft tissues, dura, and the ICA, if necessary. Sekhar et al.[13] use a saphenous vein interposition graft to reconstruct the petrous ICA. Malata et al.[14] describe their techniques for total enbloc resection with preservation of the ICA. This procedure invariably results in multiple cranial nerve palsies and their sequelae. Curtin and Som[15] have described the air cell system in the petrous apex and other anatomic feature of the petrous apex with which surgeons should be familiar. Total temporal bone resection will invariably result in CSF leaks and STSG are not adequate to reconstruct the defect. Various myocutaneous flaps and local muscle flaps have been used, but large defects are ideally reconstructed with free tissue transfers because they are free of reach limitation. The rectus abdominus flap is the ideal flap to use because the patient does not have to be repositioned, its bulk obliterates the cavity, and the rectus sheath can be used for dural repair, avoiding CSF leaks and ascending meningitis.[14] Temporal bone resection and free flap reconstruction require the skills of the ablationist, the neurosurgeons, and a microvascular surgeon, not to mention the skills of a neurosurgical anesthesiologist.

Postop radiotherapy is mandatory but is of no benefit if the tumor has not been completely resected.[11] Facial reanimation is accomplished by either a cable graft or a hypoglossal facial crossover. However, the latter is not indicated when a total temporal bone resection is done and IX and X nerve paralysis are anticipated, because a XII nerve palsy would further complicate the swallowing function. However, in subtotal temporal bone resection, a hypoglossal to facial nerve neurarraphy serves well. Some do not recommend a neck dissection because of the low incidence of metastasis (10 to 15%). However, a suprahyoid dissection affords good exposure and access for recipient vessels for free tissue transfer. I subscribe to this approach because a suprahyoid dissection takes very little time and gives excellent exposure.

The operative and perioperative mortality has decreased markedly from 10% in 1954 to less than 5%, but the morbidity associated with cranial nerve palsies has not decreased. Free tissue transfers have significantly decreased the morbidity due to CSF leaks and meningitis.[14]

Cure rate reports by many investigators range from 28% to 50%.[17] These are difficult to interpret because of differences in histology, sites of origin, and staging systems in addition to different surgical approaches (including piecemeal removal as advocated by Kinney and Wood),[16] and the use of postoperative radiotherapy. The small number of cases in each report study is statistically insignificant.

Conclusion

1. A uniform staging system is mandatory before an accurate analysis of treatment modalities can be made.
2. The best staging system at present is that presented by Curtin et al.[7] in 1990 with the modification by Clark et al.[8] to subdivide Curtin's T4 to reflect the difference in prognosis between anterior soft tissue extension and posterior and medial extension into dura and brain.
3. Different histologic malignancies and sites of origin should be differentiated when cure rates and survival rates are calculated inasmuch as different tumors have different biologic patterns of behavior.
4. Technological advances in imaging have enhanced adequate evaluation of the extent of disease and more realistic preoperative planning.
5. The advent of skull base surgery and free tissue transfers has extended the scope of surgery to include previously unresectable tumors, made surgery safer, decreased severe complication (CSF leaks, meningitis), and has rendered the concept of piecemeal removal obsolete and indefensible.
6. Postoperative radiotherapy is mandatory after temporal bone resection, but it is beneficial for local control only if the tumor has been totally resected with clear margins.
7. Forty-four years ago, Parsons and Lewis[9] presented their landmark contribution on subtotal temporal bone resections. Since then, many advances in surgery have extended our surgical ability to perform this surgery more safely.

It is my opinion we have reached the pinnacle of our surgical ability in treating carcinoma of the temporal bone and must now devote our energies to adjunctive modalities either after or in conjunction with surgery. Temporal bone resection is the cornerstone in the treatment of malignancies of the temporal bone.

REFERENCES

Arena—CHAPTER 54

1. Conley JJ.Cancer of the middle ear and temporal bone. *NY State J Med* 1994;9:1575–1579
2. Conley JJ, Schuller K. Malignancies of the ear. *Laryngoscope* 1976;86:1147–1163
3. Leonette JP, Izquierdo R, Kletzer R, Smith PG. Invasion patterns of advanced temporal bone malignancies. *Am J Otol* 1996;17:438–442
4. Conley, JJ, Novack AJ. The surgical treatment of tumors of the ear and temporal bone. *Arc Otolaryngol* 1960;71:635–652
5. Graham MD, Kemink JL, McGillicuddy JE, et al. Total en bloc resection of the temporal bone and carotid artery for malignant tumors of the ear. *Laryngoscope* 1984,94: 528–533
6. Steel PM. Epithelial tumors of the external meatus and middle ear. *Otology*. Vo. 3. *Scott-Brown's Otolaryngology*. 5th Ed. Oxford: Butterworth–Heinemann; 1987:534–545
7. Curtin HD, Hirsch B, Takahashi H, Kamerer DB. Staging proposal for external auditory meatus carcinoma based on preoperative clinical examination and computed tomography findings. *Ann Otolaryngol Rhinol Laryngol* 1990;99:714–721
8. Clark LJ, Morgan DA, Narula AA, Bradley PJ. Squamous cell carcinoma of the temporal bone: a revised staging. *J Laryngol Otol* 1991;105:346–348
9. Parsons H, Lewis JS. Subtotal resection of the temporal bone for malignancies of the middle ear. *Cancer* 1954;7:995–1001
10. Ward GE, Lock WE, Lawrence W. Radical operation for carcinoma of the external canal and middle ear. *Am J Surg* 1951, 82:169–178
11. Zreski LA, Johnson JT, Myers EN. Squamous cell carcinoma with positive margins; surgery and postoperative irradiation. *Arch Otolaryngol* 1986,112:863–866
12. Arena S. Tumor surgery of the temporal bone. *Laryngoscope* 1974,84:645–670
13. Sekhar LN, Pomeranz S, Janecka IP, et al. Temporal bone neoplasms, a report on twenty surgically treated cases. *J Neurosurg* 1992,76:578–587
14. Malata CM, Cooter RD, Towns GM, Batchelor GG. Petrosectomies for invasive tumors: surgery and reconstruction. *Br J Plast Surg* 1996;49:370–378
15. Curtin HD, Som PM. The petrous apex. *Otolaryngol Clin North Am* 1995;28:473–496
16. Kinney SE, Wood BG. Malignancies of the external ear canal and temporal bone: surgical techniques and results. *Laryngoscope* 1987;97:158–164
17. Goodwin WJ, Jesse RH. Malignant neoplasms of the external canal and temporal bone. *Arch Otolaryngol* 1980;106:675–679

19

Perilymph Fistulae

"In about 50% of patients with bilateral PLFs, the PLFs will close in the second ear during the period of bed rest after surgery on the first ear. In the event that both ears require tympanotomy, we recommend a minimum 3-month interval between operations."

F. Owen Black

"A sensitive and specific marker of perilymph would greatly facilitate identification of PLF. Attempts to find a marker using colorimetric markers such as fluorescein have not been successful. Chemical markers specific for CSF (β-2-transferrin) have also not proven reliable as an indicator of perilymph in clinical studies."

Richard R Gacek

"The existence of microfissures or patent tracts in the fissula ante fenestra have been postulated as sources for the perilymph fistula by various investigators. The precise pathophysiologic mechanism has not been described, obviously lending concern to the actual existence of this disorder."

John F. Kveton

Perilymph Fistulae*

F. Owen Black, Susan C. Pesznecker, and Joan St. Jean

CHAPTER 55

A perilymph fistula (PLF) is defined as an abnormal connection between the perilymphatic fluid spaces of the inner ear and the air spaces of the middle ear. As a result of the abnormal connection, perilymph fluid may leak and/or ambient pressure changes may be transmitted between the two spaces. Most PLFs occur at or near the oval and/or round windows. Physiologic alterations associated with PLFs result in significant morbidity and disability and profound lifestyle changes. In some cases, PLFs may also result in serious or life-threatening complications, including hearing loss, loss of vestibular function, and meningitis, respectively.

The controversy regarding PLF diagnosis arises in part from the adherence to the belief that PLFs are a diagnosis of exclusion. PLFs have been confirmed histopathologically in blinded prospective studies, establishing the pathologic "gold standard" for PLF diagnosis.[1,2] Unfortunately, this standard for pathologic diagnosis cannot be used in the clinical setting for obvious reasons. However, chronic or persistent combinations of dysequilibrium, headache, adult-onset motion sickness (motion-related nausea and vomiting), and neurocognitive disruption, particularly when exacerbated by exertion or physical activity, are classic symptoms of a PLF in one or both ears, until proved otherwise. Contrary to popular belief, only about one-half of traumatic PLF patients have an objective hearing loss. Hearing loss is usually a complication of PLF, not a primary result of otic capsule compromise.

Background

PLFs were first recognized as a result of pathologic causes, such as tumors or virulent middle ear or mastoid infections. PLFs were later documented as a complication of otic capsule erosion by cholesteatomas, usually at the lateral extent of the horizontal canal.[3,4]

Traumatic PLFs have been recognized clinically for more than 100 years.[5] PLFs were later identified in military personnel exposed to sudden decompression or blasts and in scuba divers, who presented with sudden hearing loss from round window rupture.[6-14] Barotrauma is a well-documented cause of PLFs.[13,15-17] Conditions associated with sudden or dramatic changes in ambient air pressure can rupture the oval or round window via extreme implosive forces.[18-20] Certain types of acoustic trauma may also cause PLFs. We have confirmed reports of PLFs in patients exposed to explosions or to sudden or catastrophically loud sound.[21]

With the advent of stapedectomy, PLFs were implicated as a complication of stapes surgical procedures,[22-24] particularly if Gelfoam was used as the graft or if polyethylene tubing was used as a prosthesis.[25,26]

In 1971, Goodhill[27] advanced the theory of implosive and explosive mechanisms for traumatic PLFs. According to Goodhill, an explosive PLF occurs when a sudden increase in the cerebrospinal fluid (CSF) pressure that ruptures the oval or round window due to increased intracranial pressure is transmitted to the perilymphatic fluid space. An implosive event occurs when sufficient external (ambient) pressures were applied to the tympanic membrane or entered the middle ear through the eustachian tube, driving the stapes into the inner ear and causing rupture of the oval or round window, or both.

G.A. Fee, an astute Canadian otolaryngologist,[28] was among the first to identify trauma as a cause of PLFs[5,29-35] in patients suspected of having Meniere's disease. The most likely mechanism of PLFs after blunt body or head trauma is a transient dramatic increase in intracranial pressure, as proposed by Goodhill's explosive theory.[27] The head trauma need not be severe. Whiplash injury has been linked to PLFs.[36] Goodhill's explanations probably account for PLFs occurring in association with whiplash trauma to the neck, and without direct head blow.[36]

A more recent example of implosive PLF formation is airbag deployment trauma. According to Ferber-Viart et al.,[37] airbags may reach peak volume in 50 ms after impact, inflating at a speed of 156 mph, and with an opening force equivalent to a shotgun blast. Traumatic injury to head, neck, upper body, and face in association with airbag deployment has been well documented.[38-40] These reports suggest that PLFs from airbag injury are likely to increase.

The patient with spontaneous or idiopathic PLF exhibits signs, symptoms, and findings fully consistent with PLFs but that lack correlation to a specific cause.[41-45] In reality, spontaneous PLFs probably do not exist per se but are more likely a reflection of the inability to correctly identify a causative event.

Anatomic variants have been associated with PLFs,[46,47] including patent fissula ante fenestrae,[1,2,48,49] large patent cochlear aqueducts,[50,51] the Mondini deformity,[52,53] and oval window microfissures.[2,54,55] In some cases, anatomic variants may show familial tendency.[56] Congenital PLFs have been described by many clinicians;[47,56-59] in some cases, congenital PLFs appear to have anatomic and/or familial links.

* This work was supported in part by National Institutes of Health grant RO 1 DC00204, NASA grant NAGW-3799, and a grant from the Legacy Portland Hospitals Research Advisory Committee.

Within the modern otologic community, great diversity exists with regard to the identification and management of PLFs. A detailed review is beyond the scope of this chapter. The following discussion summarizes our methods and approaches in dealing with some of the purported controversies associated with the care of the PLF patient.

Discussion

CLASSIFICATION OF PLFs

A myriad of different etiologies for PLFs have been described in the literature. To simplify this discussion, we suggest a global classification of PLF etiology: (1) pathologic (e.g., cholesteatoma, infection/erosion, tumors); (2) traumatic (e.g., acoustic, blast or barotrauma, surgical complication); and (3) spontaneous (idiopathic) (Table 55–1).

We have encountered a wide array of interesting causes of PLFs, including PLFs that resulted from prolonged vomiting after exposure to toxic fumes, PLFs in a young weightlifter, PLFs developing during labor and delivery, and PLFs that occurred after a frozen 24-lb turkey fell from a freezer on a patient's head. In our experience, trauma to the head and neck is by far the most common cause of PLFs. However, our experience is heavily weighted toward trauma patients. There are two level I regional trauma centers in our metropolitan area, one of which is located within our hospital system.

TABLE 55–1
Classification of Perilymphatic Fistula

Pathologic
Congenital
Cholesteatomas
Neoplasms (particularly tumors of the mastoid or skull base)
Middle ear infections
Mastoid infections
Stapedectomy and stapedotomy
Traumatic
Implosive
Barotrauma
SCUBA diving
Rapid descent in aircraft
Acoustic trauma (e.g., exposure to loud noise or explosions)
Explosive
Head and neck trauma (including whiplash)
Airbag trauma
Conditions associated with sudden or sustained increases in intracranial or intrathoracic pressure (e.g., heavy lifting, protracted or violent vomiting, childbirth, obstructive sleep apnea)
Spontaneous or unknown causes
Anatomic variants? (e.g., persistent aqueduct patentency or congenital defects?)

CLINICAL PRESENTATION

Our experience confirms the observation by Healy et al.[60, 61] that dysequilibrium is the most common presenting symptom of PLF[62] (Fig. 55–1). The typical PLF patient has disabling difficulty with gait and imbalance; the patient "cruises," touching or holding onto walls or furniture, subconsciously attempting to increase proprioceptive input. The PLF patient is constantly spatially disoriented and often is visually dependent. In addition to constant or persistent balance difficulties, physical exertion, especially lifting or straining, will exacerbate or initiate symptoms.

Low-pressure headache, similar or identical to the headache associated with a persistent CSF leak after a spinal tap, is also a primary complaint in patients with active PLFs.[62] The typical PLF headache is unilateral and almost always present on the side of the active PLF. In the case of bilateral PLFs, the pain is often worse on the most active side. The PLF headache is severe, sometimes throbbing, and often accompanied by hypersensitivity to light and sound. Headaches persist as long as PLFs are active; when the PLFs are closed surgically or with bed rest, the headaches resolve immediately, similar to the resolution of symptoms after successful blood patching of postspinal tap CSF leaks. Because headache is not a standard part of most otologic questionnaires and interview forms, and many PLF patients have significant short-term memory impairment and are poor or incomplete historians, this important symptom may be missed if not specifically sought.

Adult-onset motion sickness, or exacerbation of previously existing motion sickness, occurs in virtually 100% of PLF patients. Successful closure of PLFs resulted in either immediate improvement in, or cessation of, motion sickness symptoms in 100% of adult PLF patients ($n = 31$).[63] The combined problems associated with motion sickness and with exertional exacerbation of symptoms are extremely disabling to PLF patients, often resulting in loss of mobility, loss of employment, inability to complete normal activities of daily living (ADLs), and even self-imposed reclusive behavior. Often there is comorbid (secondary) psychopathology, including anxiety, depression, and panic-type behavior, especially in undiagnosed patients. These symptoms, and the patient's attempts to control or avoid them, often lead to misdiagnosis as primary mental or neurologic disorders.

Neurocognitive dysfunction is a well-documented and frequent complaint in patients with PLFs[64, 65] (also K.R. Erickson, personal communication, 1989). It is commonly manifested by short-term memory impairment, multitasking problems, difficulties sorting and/or prioritizing tasks and information, and sometimes vague dyslexic disturbances with reading, writing, or difficulty tracking written words. A few patients also have speech difficulties, or dysphasic-mimicking problems with word recall. Cognitive dysfunction increases the patient's sense of frustration and greatly complicates problems with ADL, schooling, and employment.

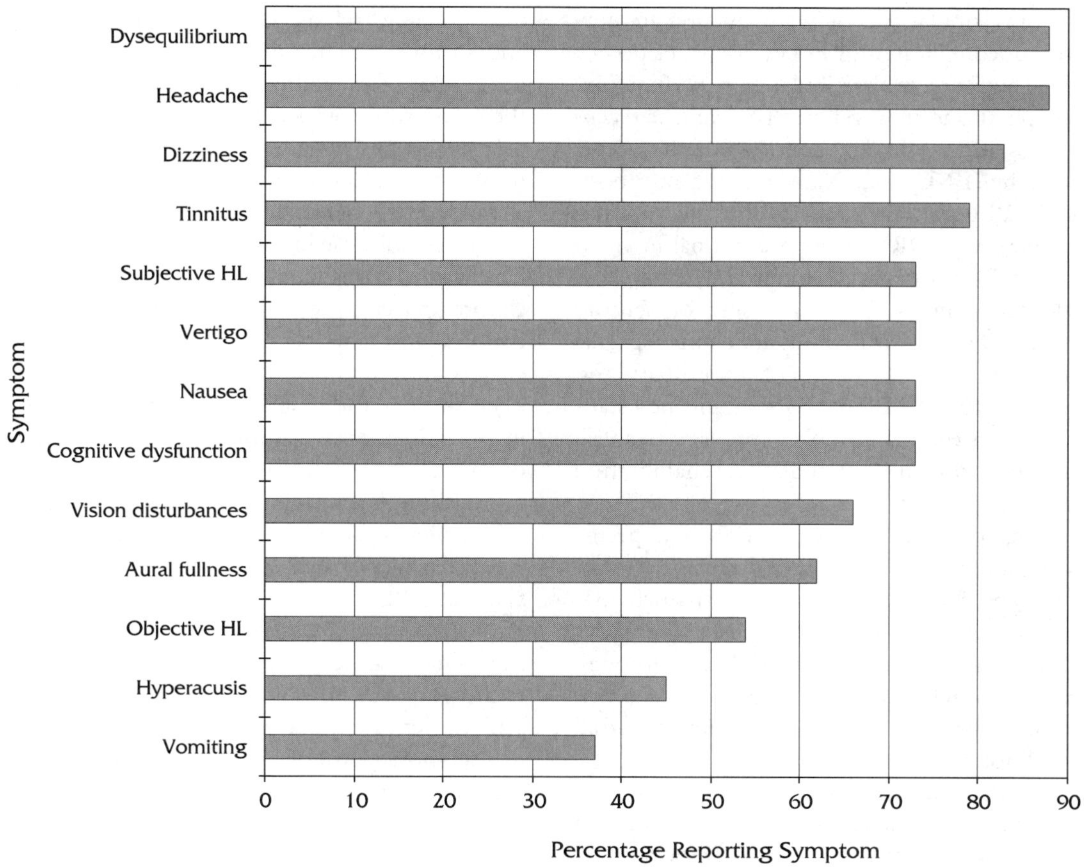

Figure 55–1 Presenting symptoms of perilymphatic fistula.

Hearing loss is not present in all patients with a PLF.[66] In our practice, objective hearing loss occurs in about 55% of patients with post-traumatic PLF[62] and in about 25% of all patients with PLFs. However, a much higher percentage of PLF patients will complain of subjective hearing loss/fluctuation, or of other auditory symptoms, including tinnitus, aural fullness/pressure, hyperacusis, and aural discomfort. It is obvious that subjective hearing loss and other auditory dysfunction is more common than our ability to document the PLF patient's consistent complaint of compromised auditory function.[67, 68] Objective hearing loss is therefore not an absolute criterion for PLF diagnosis, as is widely believed.

Acute-onset hearing loss in a PLF patient requires emergent care. If the hearing loss does not rapidly improve with restricted physical activity, surgical exploration for identification and PLF closure should be offered the patient.

DIAGNOSIS

The diagnosis of PLF can be established only at tympanotomy. Although imperfect, the clinical gold standard for PLF diagnosis remains visual inspection for perilymph leakage into the middle ear at tympanotomy. Unfortunately, this method is subjective, and two competent surgeons inspecting the same visual field may come to two different conclusions regarding the absence or presence of a perilymph leak. This is especially true if one of the surgeons is viewing the field from a monocular side arm or with any other monocular instrument such as an endoscope.

Even if a clinical fistula test[69-72] is positive, the results are not diagnostic of PLF because any anatomic or pathologic condition permitting transfer of middle inner ear or intracranial pressure changes to stimulate vestibular receptors will result in a positive fistula test based on external canal pressure changes as the stimulus. Examples include otic capsule softening from lues, Paget's disease, or labyrinthine fibrosis.[73] Conversely, a negative PLF test does not rule out a PLF because external auditory canal pressures may not be transmitted to the inner ear receptors (e.g., with ossicular discontinuities). It is also possible that persons with a loss or absence of vestibular hair cell function in the affected ear will yield negative responses (objective and subjective) to conventional fistula tests. Reduced ability of the vestibular hair cells to respond to stimulation must be considered (established) when interpreting negative fistula test results. Although the only generally accepted way that a PLF can be confirmed is identification of perilymphatic leakage at tympanotomy, failure to observe a PLF leak at tympanotomy does not rule out a PLF because otic capsule integrity can be compromised without perilymph fluid leak.

Standard tests of vestibular and auditory function are normal in patients with uncomplicated PLFs because PLFs do not directly cause loss of auditory and vestibular hair cell function. It is only when complications of persistent PLFs damage receptors that hearing loss and vestibular function deficits occur. Electronystagmography (ENG) may or may not show a positional nystagmus in PLF patients, and caloric and rotation (vestibulo-ocular reflex, or VOR) testing are normal in virtually all uncomplicated PLF patients. Computed dynamic posturography (CDP) often shows abnormal results on sensory organization testing (SOTs); these findings are neither specific for, nor diagnostic of, PLFs. However, the auditory and vestibular functional status of PLF patients should be established by objective tests as early as possible in order to establish a baseline and in order to plan treatment and rehabilitation based on quantitative data.

Hearing loss complicating PLFs does not present a specific pure-tone threshold pattern or configuration, but most are sensorineural in type. Some clinicians have used electrocochleography (ECoG) to assist in the diagnosis of PLFs;[74,75] we have not found ECoGs to be useful for diagnosis of PLFs, although we do employ ECoG to help identify a secondary endolymphatic hydrops, which is probably the most frequent comorbid (complicating) condition accompanying PLFs.

Strohm[5] was among the first to observe that PLFs may arise many years after the initial traumatic event. Strohm reported a case of a PLF that became symptomatic more than 30 years later in the second ear of a patient with a traumatic PLF. The clinical dictums regarding the close temporal relationship between the traumatic event and onset of symptoms must therefore be regarded with circumspection in patients with traumatic PLF.

BILATERALITY

In our experience, PLFs resulting from pathologic causes are almost always unilateral, whereas those from trauma are more likely to be bilateral. In our practice, at least 50% of patients with PLFs caused by trauma have bilateral fistulas.[62]

CONSERVATIVE TREATMENT

In the absence of complications, such as sensorineural hearing loss, treatment of active, uncomplicated PLFs should always begin with conservative treatment. About 85% of patients will improve with 6 weeks of bed rest.[62] The goal of bed rest is to minimize movement across the defect causing PLF. This immobilization technique is accomplished by minimizing changes in intracranial, intrathoracic, and/or intra-abdominal pressure and is analogous to the principles of wound healing employed by all successful surgeons.

Patients placed on bed rest are instructed to recline on bed or couch with their head at or above 30 to 45 degrees elevation at all times (including during sleep) and are allowed up only for meals, and bathroom/bathing privileges. Patients are given a list of pressure-related activities to avoid, which include bending, straining, yelling, drinking liquids through a soda straw, and so forth.[76] They may not work, perform house or yard chores, care for children, run errands, attend school, or leave the house while on bed rest. They are given a vitamin–mineral preparation and encouraged to eat a well-balanced diet and to drink 6 to 8 glasses of water each day. Stool softeners are used as needed to avoid constipation.

PLFs will close in approximately 80 to 85% of patients who have followed this regimen for 4 to 6 weeks. The likelihood of closure is inversely related to time elapsed from PLF onset; those patients with new PLFs are much more likely to obtain good closure from bed rest than are the patients whose PLFs have been present for months, or years. For successful management of PLF, early diagnosis is a critical factor for satisfactory outcome.

Although this regimen may seem strict and prolonged, our results in using it have been very good, with a high rate of return to work or ADL.[62] Most of our patients have post-traumatic PLFs, and most have come to us months or years after the development of PLFs, usually as a tertiary referral. Many have undergone less strict attempts at conservative treatment with poor results. Typically, the PLF patient will self-restrict physical activities that cause symptoms, resulting in a temporary seal of PLFs with middle ear mucosa. Because middle ear mucosa contains little or no collagen, resumption of physical activity typically results in rupture of the mucosal seal and recurrence of PLF symptoms. The more often this sequence is repeated, the more likely that complications will develop.

A critical aspect of bed rest treatment is the patient's psychosocial support system. Patients cannot complete the demanding regimen of strict bed rest without a great deal of external assistance. Before beginning this treatment, we counsel the patients and their family, making sure that they understand and are fully able and ready to commit to a lengthy and treatment plan, with a proper support network.

Maximum healing occurs within 12 months of closure; if characteristic of connective tissue in other sites, the PLF heals with approximately 80% of its original tensile strength. (Note that the round window membrane in the human is only 0.3 mm thick.[77]) After a successful course of PLFs with bed rest, patients are allowed to gradually and incrementally increase their activities through a progression of six stages.[76] Activities that are likely to cause recurrence (e.g., airplane flight) are restricted for at least 1 year after PLF closure. Successfully treated PLF patients are instructed never to fly if they have an upper respiratory infection or if they have poor eustachian tube function (i.e., cannot clear their ears when exposed to altitude or barometric pressure changes).

TRANSTYMPANIC GENTAMICIN ABLATION

Transtympanic administration of drugs, especially ototoxic preparations, should be avoided in PLF patients. While ototoxic ablation of inner ear hair cells might improve or relieve

PLF-related symptoms in patients with unilateral PLFs and a normal opposite ear, ablation of inner ear hair cells does not address the mechanical problem of the open fistula or otic capsule defect. The instillation of ototoxic agents into the middle ear of the PLF patient is associated with a greater risk of ototoxic hearing loss and destruction of vestibular hair cells than would occur in a nonfistulous ear. The treatment also leaves the fistula open, placing the patient at risk of potentially serious complications (see below). For these reasons, we believe that treating the symptoms of active PLF with transtympanic ototoxic agents is inappropriate.

SURGICAL TREATMENT

An inherent problem in the surgical repair of PLFs is the difficulty of getting graft tissue to heal securely to bone (the bony otic capsule), especially in the environs of a middle ear system, which is in constant motion. Modifications of technique in surgically treating PLFs have been aimed at solving these problems.[62]

We favor a post-auricular areolar tissue graft[78] because, if placed into the oval and round window niches as very small pieces, areolar tissue conforms by capillary action to the underlying denuded bone. We use multiple small pledgets of postauricular areolar graft material, rather than a single large graft, which tends to quickly migrate or contract out of the oval or round window niche as healing commences. We use an argon laser to prepare the graft bed. Removing the mucoperiosteum is an essential prerequisite for optimal grafting of the oval and round window PLF. The graft can be further buttressed by congealing the graft in layers with an out-of-focus laser to weld the graft as the tissue pledgets are mounded up to fill the oval and round windows.

We strongly advise use of autologous cryoprecipitated fibrinogen adhesive.[62] We have reduced our recurrence rate from about 25% to less than 8% using this technique combined with laser preparation (vaporization of the mucoperiosteum) of the graft site.[62]

Traumatic PLFs may be associated with stapes fractures and/or stapes footplate subluxations. In our experience, an oval window PLF complicated by a stapes footplate fracture (or a displaced stapes) will not close until a stapedectomy is performed and a prosthesis is placed over a tissue graft. However, if footplate fragments are not displaced, it is advisable to attempt closure of the PLF without stapedectomy.

Patients are admitted the morning of surgery and are discharged the next day. Before discharge, patients are evaluated by a trained physical therapist for safe ambulation, and are instructed on a bed rest regimen (see the previous section, Conservative Treatment) for 4 to 6 weeks. Stool softeners are prescribed, and antiemetics used as needed. External auditory canal packing is removed 7 to 10 days postoperatively by a caregiver.

In about 50% of patients with bilateral PLFs, the PLFs will close in the second ear during the period of bed rest after surgery on the first ear. In the event that both ears require tympanotomy, we recommend a minimum 3-month interval between operations.

TREATMENT FAILURES

In our experience, PLF treatment failures almost always result from one of three reasons: (1) failure to recognize a PLF in the contralateral ear, (2) failure to recognize a comorbid condition, and (3) failure of the patient to follow recommended postoperative regimens.

COMORBIDITY

Secondary Endolymphatic Hydrops

The most common complication of chronic, persistent, or recurrent PLFs is secondary endolymphatic hydrops (SEH). This condition can occur acutely, especially after traumatic PLFs, but more typically occurs after repeated openings of the PLF. ECoG is often positive (SP/AP ratio > 0.4)[79-81] in many, if not most patients with spontaneously fluctuating symptoms in addition to or superimposed on the classic PLF symptom pattern outlined above. The occurrence of SEH in association with PLFs is the primary reason that PLFs are often misdiagnosed as Meniere's disease.[82]

Symptomatic patterns in PLF and Meniere's patients are very different.[83] PLF symptoms consist of nearly continuous dysequilibrium, headache, motion sickness, cognitive dysfunction, and subjective auditory symptoms, all of which are exacerbated by exertion and activity. Conversely, Meniere's disease is characterized by unprovoked sudden, violent, and spontaneous episodes of vertigo, vomiting, tinnitus, and hearing loss, with symptom-free and often lengthy periods between attacks.

Most cases of post-traumatic SEH tend to improve with time, especially after successful PLF closure and a great many resolve completely within 1 to 2 years of the causative accident. In the interim, conservative treatments (e.g., after a hydrops dietary regimen, judicious use of diuretics, and mild vestibular suppression with a titrated daily dose of 75 to 150 mg of meclizine hydrochloride) may help make the patient more comfortable until the SEH resolves. The hydrops dietary regimen is aimed at maintaining a consistent (osmotically constant) intake of foods, fluids, and solutes throughout the day and from day to day. Although a low intake of all substances that might affect fluid or volume status (e.g., salt, sugar, caffeine, alcohol) is desired, the most important consideration is even dietary (osmotically constant) intake, thus avoiding irregular and unexpected shifts in the body's intracellular fluid compartment.

Benign Paroxysmal Positional Nystagmus and Vertigo

Benign paroxysmal positional nystagmus and vertigo are commonly seen in patients with traumatic PLFs. In addition to reporting symptoms related to exertional activity characteristic of PLFs, the PLF patient who also reports transient episodes of vertigo in association with specific (pitch plane) head movements, or who awakens with rotary vertigo after turning onto either ear, may be describing post-traumatic benign paroxysmal positional nystagmus and vertigo.

The diagnosis and treatment of comorbid benign paroxysmal nystagmus and vertigo in a patient with active PLFs can be challenging. Performing the Hallpike maneuver in a PLF patient may be contraindicated, as the sudden intracranial pressure increase during Hallpike maneuvers can precipitate severe PLF-induced symptoms and may also cause or worsen a sensorineural hearing loss. For the same reasons, canalith repositioning (CRP) maneuvers[84] must be performed with caution in the PLF patient with active benign paroxysmal nystagmus and vertigo. Vigorous positioning activities associated with physical therapy, including the Semont maneuver[85,86] should be avoided in PLF patients. Although benign paroxysmal nystagmus and vertigo is certainly uncomfortable and distressing, the active PLFs pose risks of hearing loss and meningitis and should therefore be treated (closed) before proceeding with treatment of benign paroxysmal nystagmus and vertigo. Ideally, we recommend that CPR be delayed 1 year after PLF closure or as long as possible after PLF closure. If CRP maneuvers are planned in the patient with suspected PLFs in one or both ears, the patient should be fully informed of the alternatives, risks (especially hearing loss) and benefits before the procedure is performed.

In our experience, most post-traumatic benign paroxysmal nystagmus and vertigo cases will resolve spontaneously within 1 year of the causative injury, which may obviate the need for active treatment. Conversely, a comorbid benign paroxysmal nystagmus and vertigo that does not resolve may become more of a problem after PLF treatment, as the positional symptoms arising from benign paroxysmal nystagmus and vertigo will typically exacerbate during bed rest and activity restriction. Mild oral vestibular suppressive drugs (e.g., Meclizine) may help reduce the severity of positional vertigo in the short term, and vestibular protocol physical therapy (with PLF precautions) may be useful, once PLFs are closed.

Obstructive Sleep Apnea

Patients with obstructive sleep apnea (OSA) have a much higher rate of PLF recurrence and/or treatment failure. The increased intracranial pressure gradient created as the patient attempts to inspire against the pharyngeal obstruction apparently causes rerupture of incompletely healed PLFs, in a manner analogous to the rerupture of inguinal hernias in patients with exertion, chronic cough, or constipation. We now believe OSA to be a major cause of recurrent PLFs and postoperative failures, and question whether OSA might also be an unrecognized cause of spontaneous PLFs. If history or physical findings suggest the presence of OSA (or any sleep disorder) in patients with suspected or confirmed PLFs, they are referred for laboratory sleep studies. Treatment of the OSA must be successfully completed before attempts to manage PLFs are begun.

COMPLICATIONS OF PLFs

Curiously, PLF-related complications are rarely, if ever, discussed in the literature. In addition to the comorbid conditions discussed above, there are three significant complications of PLFs: Hearing loss, vestibular function loss, and meningitis.

Hearing loss is a complication of a PLF and should never be regarded as either a primary consequence or inevitable result of PLF. Hearing loss complicating PLFs is a true otologic emergency. Sensorineural hearing loss indicates hair cell damage and/or death, whereas a conductive or mixed loss (often seen in cases of post-traumatic PLF) indicates a superimposed middle ear component. Probability of improvement in SNHL after PLF closure is 50/50 at best,[62] and the likelihood of improvement diminishes rapidly with time.

Once SNHL occurs, it must be treated aggressively. In our experience, the best chance of improving or regaining SNHL thresholds is to begin treatment within 48 to 72 h of the loss. In our practice, sudden SNHL is treated with an ABCS approach consisting of activity restriction, bed rest, carbogen, and surgery.[76]

Carbogen, a mixture of 95% oxygen and 5% carbon dioxide, has proved an effective treatment in many cases of sudden, emergent SNHL related to PLFs.[87-89] The patient is admitted to the hospital, placed on strict bed rest with head elevated, and given carbogen inhalations for 15 min of every hour, around the clock. Treatment is continued for a minimum of 48 h. Serial audiograms are performed and treatment may be continued for an additional 1 to 2 days if hearing is recovering. In our experience, carbogen treatment has often restored sudden SNHL and obviated the need for emergent tympanotomy and PLF repair.

Loss of vestibular function is relatively uncommon in PLFs. The likelihood of vestibular damage is higher in persons with pathologic PLFs or removal of a fractured or unstable stapes. Once vestibular function is lost, it is usually not regained.

Meningitis is an infrequent but potentially life-threatening complication of PLFs.[41, 90-93] The abnormal opening between the sterile inner ear and an infected middle ear potentially allows bacteria and viruses to enter the inner ear space. Since perilymph is continuous with the CSF, invading organisms can infect the CSF, meninges, and brain, causing meningitis and cerebritis. Because meningitis and cerebritis are life-threatening,[94] PLFs from any cause should be closed, through either conservative or surgical means, without delay. Patients with active PLFs should also be instructed to seek medical treatment immediately if they develop symptoms or signs of an upper respiratory or middle ear infection.

Conclusion

There is an extensive literature on PLFs. Substantial data and confirmed observations in the peer-reviewed literature have already addressed topics considered controversial by some members of the otologic community. The clinical presentation of PLFs is clear, the various treatment options available have been well described, and the recent prospective histopathologic confirmation of PLFs has established a gold standard for diagnosis.[1,2,48]

It is the responsibility of otologists to become familiar with the extensive PLF literature. Scholarly discourse should be encouraged so that we may better care for patients whose lives and livelihood have been devastated by PLFs.

REFERENCES

Black et al.—CHAPTER 55

1. Kohut RI, Hinojosa R, Budetti JA. Perilymphatic fistula: a histopathologic study. *Ann Otol Rhinol Laryngol* 1986;95: 466–471
2. Kohut RI, Hinojosa R, Ryu JH. Perilymphatic fistula: a single blind histopathological study. *Adv Otol Rhinol Laryngol* 1988;42:148–152
3. Dawes JD, Watson RT. Labyrinthine fistulae. *J Laryngol Otol* 1978;92(2):83–98
4. Sheehy JL, Brackmann DE. Cholesteatoma surgery: management of the labyrinthine fistula—a report of 97 cases. *Laryngoscope* 1979;89:78–87
5. Strohm M. Traumatic lesions of the round window membrane and perilymphatic fistulae. *Adv Otolol Rhinol Laryngol* 1986; 35:177–247
6. Parell GJ, Paige GD. Inner ear barotrauma in SCUBA divers. *Arch Otolaryngol Head Neck Surg* 1993;119:455–457
7. Edmonds C. Hearing loss with frequent diving (deaf divers). *Undersea Biomed Res* 1985;12:315–319
8. Molvaer OI, Natrud E. Ear damage due to diving. *Acta Otolaryngol (Stockh)* 1979;360(suppl):187–189
9. Caruso VG, Winkelmann PE, Correia MJ, et al. Otologic and otoneurologic injuries in divers: clinical studies on nine commercial and two sport divers. *Laryngoscope* 1977;4:508–521
10. Farmer JC. Diving injuries of the inner ear. *Ann Otol Rhinol Laryngol* 1977;86(suppl 36):1–20
11. Edmonds C, Freeman P, Tonkin J. Fistula of the round window in diving. *Trans Am Acad Ophthalmol Otolaryngol* 1974;78:444–447
12. Lundgren CEG. Alternobaric vertigo—a diving hazard. *BMJ* 1965;2:511–513
13. Head PW. Vertigo and barotrauma. In: Dix MR, Hood JD, eds. *Vertigo*. Bath, Avon, England: John Wiley & Sons Ltd; 1984:199–214
14. McNicoll WD. Traumatic perforation of the tympanic membrane with associated rupture of the round window membrane. *J Laryngol* 1978;92:895–903
15. Whinney DJD, Parikh AA, Brookes GB. Barotraumatic fracture of the stapes footplate. *Am J Otol* 1996;17:697–699
16. Miyazawa T, Ueda H, Yanagita N. Eustachian tube function and middle ear barotrauma associated with extremes in atmospheric pressure. *Ann Otol Rhinol Laryngol* 1996;105:887–892
17. Freeman P, Tonkin J, Edmonds C. Rupture of the round window membrane in inner ear barotrauma. *Arch Otolaryngol* 1974;99:437–442
18. Bruins WR. Blast injuries of the ear as a result of the Peterborough lorry explosion: 22 March 1989. *J Laryngol Otol* 1991;105:890–895
19. Konrádsson KS, Carloborg BR, Farmer JC. Pressure gradients affecting the labyrinth during hypobaric pressure. Experimental study. *Ann Otol Rhinol Laryngol* 1997;106:495–502
20. Beuerlein M, Nelson RN, Welling B. Inner and midde ear hyperbaric oxygen-induced barotrauma. *Laryngoscope* 1997; 107:1350–1356
21. Guyot JP. Acoustic trauma caused by the telephone. *Otorhinolaryngology* 1988;50:313–318
22. Schuknecht HF, Reisser C. The morphologic basis for perilymphatic gushers and oozers. *Adv Otol Rhinol Laryngol* 1988;39:1–12
23. Schepens YM, Schepens P. Complications which may be encountered in surgery for otospongiosis. *Acta Otol Rhinol Laryngol Belg* 1977;31:5–36
24. Glasscock ME. The stapes gusher. *Arch Otolaryngol* 1973; 98:82–91
25. Hemenway WG, Hildyard VH, Black FO. Post stapedectomy perilymph fistulas in the Rocky Mountain area: the importance of nystagmography and audiometry in diagnosis and early tympanotomy in prognosis. *Laryngoscope* 1968;78:1687–1715
26. House HP. The fistula problem in otosclerosis surgery. *Laryngoscope* 1967:1410–1426
27. Goodhill V. Sudden deafness and round window rupture. *Laryngoscope* 1971;81:1462–1474
28. Fee GA. Traumatic perilymphatic fistulas. *Arch Otolaryngol* 1969;88:43–46
29. Glasscock ME, McKennan KX, Levine SC. Persistent traumatic perilymph fistulas. *Laryngoscope* 1987;97:860–863
30. Goodhill V. Traumatic fistulae. *J Laryngol Otol* 1980;94: 123–128
31. Sidi J, Tovi F. Traumatic labyrinthine fistulas. *Isr J Med Sci* 1979;15:156–158
32. Lehrer JF, Rubin RC, Poole DC, et al. Perilymphatic fistula—a definitive and curable cause of vertigo following head trauma. *West J Med* 1984;141:57–61
33. Hemenway WG, Black FO, Grimm RJ, Pesznecker SC. Traumatic perilymph fistula. In: Claussen CF, Kirtane MV, eds. *Vertigo, Nausea, Tinnitus, and Hypoacusis Due to Head and Neck Trauma. Proceedings of the Seventh Scientific Meeting of the Neurotological and Equilibriometric Society*. Amsterdam: Elsevier; 1991:167–170
34. Healy GB. Hearing loss and vertigo secondary to head injury. *N Engl J Med* 1982;306:1029–1031
35. Healy GB, Friedman JM, Strong MS. Vestibular and auditory findings of perilymphatic fistula: a review of 40 cases. *Trans Am Acad Ophthalmol Otolaryngol* 1976;82:44–49
36. Chester JB. Whiplash, postural control, and the inner ear. *Spine* 1991;16:716–720
37. Ferber–Viart C, Postec F, Duclaux R, Dubreuil C. Perilymphatic fistula following airbag trauma. (Letter to the Editor.) *Laryngoscope* 1998;108:1255–1257
38. Huelke DF, Moore JL, Compton TW, Samuels J, Levine RS. Upper extremity injuries related to airbags deployments. *J Trauma* 1995;4:482–488

39. Thomas P, Bradford MO. The nature and source of the head injuries sustained by restrained front-seat car occupants in frontal collisions. *Accident Anal Prev* 1995;4:561–570
40. Duma SM, Kress TA, Porta DJ, et al. Airbag-induced eye injuries: a report of 25 cases. *J Trauma* 1996;41:114–119
41. Facer GW, Farrell KH, Cody DT. Spontaneous perilymph fistula. *Mayo Clin Proc* 1973;48:203–206
42. Althaus SR. Spontaneous and traumatic perilymph fistulas. *Laryngoscope* 1977;87:364–371
43. Shea JJ III. The myth of spontaneous perilymph fistula. *Otolaryngol Head Neck Surg* 1992;107:613–616
44. Cole GG. Validity of spontaneous perilymphatic fistula. *Am J Otol* 1995;16:815–819
45. Meyerhoff WL. Spontaneous perilymphatic fistula: myth or fact. *Am J Otol* 1993;14:478–481
46. Sando I, Takahara T, Ogawa A. Congenital anomalies of the inner ear. *Ann Otol Rhinol Laryngol* 1984;93:110–117
47. Reilly JS. Congenital perilymphatic fistula: a prospective study in infants and children. *Laryngoscope* 1989;99:393–397
48. Kohut RI, Hinojosa R, Ryu JH. The histologic characteristics of the core of the fissula ante fenestram. *Acta Otolaryngol (Stockh)* 1991;481(suppl):158–162
49. Dawes JD, Pearman K, Kochilas X. Patent fissula ante fenestram. *J Laryngol Otol* 1983;97:357–360
50. Jackler RK, Hwang PH. Enlargement of the cochlear aqueduct: fact or fiction? *Otolaryngol Head Neck Surg* 1993; 109:14–25
51. Griffith AJ, Arts HA, Downs C, et al. Familial large vestibular aqueduct syndrome. *Laryngoscope* 1996;106:960–965
52. Illum P. The Mondini type of cochlear malformation. *Arch Otolaryngol* 1972;96:305–311
53. Schuknecht HF. Mondini dysplasia: a clinical and pathological study. *Ann Otol Rhinol Laryngol* 1980;89(suppl 65):3–23
54. Kamerer DB, Sando I, Hirsch BE, Takagi A. Perilymph fistula resulting from microfissures. *Am J Otol* 1987;8:489–494
55. Harada T, Sando I, Myers EN. Microfissure in the oval window area. *Ann Otol Rhinol Laryngol* 1981;90:174–180
56. Weider DJ, Musiek FE. Bilateral congenital oval window microfistulae in a mother and son. *Laryngoscope* 1984;94: 1455–1458
57. Bluestone CD. Otitis media and congenital perilymphatic fistula as a cause of sensorineural hearing loss in children. *Pediatr Infect Dis J* 1988;7:141–145
58. Crook JP. Congenital fistula in the stapedial footplate. *South Med J* 1967;60:1168–1170
59. Guindi GM. Congenital labyrintho-tympanic fistula—a recently recognized entity in children. *J Laryngol Otol* 1981; 10:1:67–71
60. Healy GB, Friedman JM, DiTroia J. Ataxia and hearing loss secondary to perilymphatic fistula. *Pediatrics* 1978;61:238–241
61. Healy GB, Strong MS, Sampogna D. Ataxia, vertigo, and hearing loss. *Arch Otolaryngol* 1991;100:130–135
62. Black FO, Pesznecker SC, Norton TL, et al. Surgical management of perilymph fistulas: a new technique. *Arch Otolaryngol Head Neck Surg* 1991;117:641–648
63. Black FO, Pesznecker SC. Surgical management of motion sickness in perilymph fistula patients. In: Twentieth Meeting of the International Barany Society. Würzburg, Germany; 1998
64. Grimm RJ, Hemenway WG, LeBray PR, Black FO. The perilymph fistula syndrome defined in mild head trauma. *Acta Otolaryngol* 1989;464(suppl):5–40
65. Erickson KR, DeWeese M, Simons A. A specific syndrome of memory impairment in patients with vestibular disorder: selective acquisition and retrieval deficits. International Conference: Perilymph fistula—a common cause of dizziness and dysequilibrium? September 6, 1990;Portland, Oregon. *Am J Otol* 1990:887–891
66. Kohut RI, Waldorf RA, Haenel JL, Thompson JN. Minute perilymph fistulas: vertigo and Hennebert's sign without hearing loss. *Ann Otol Rhinol Laryngol* 1979;88:153–159
67. Simmons FB. Fluid dynamics in sudden sensorineural hearing loss. *Otolaryngol Clin North Am* 1978;11:55–61
68. Simmons FB. Perilymph fistula: some diagnostic problems. *Adv Otol Rhinol Laryngol* 1982;28:68–72
69. Daspit CP, Churchill D, Linthicum FH. Diagnosis of perilymph fistula using ENG and impedance. *Laryngoscope* 1980; 90:217–223
70. Causse JR, Causse JB, Bel J. Tympanometry and fistula test. *Audiology* 1983;22:451–462
71. Black FO, Lilly DJ, Nashner LM, Peterka RJ, Pesznecker SC. Quantitative diagnostic test for perilymph fistula. *Otolaryngol Head Neck Surg* 1987;96:125–134
72. Black FO, Lilly DJ, Peterka RJ, et al. The dynamic posturographic pressure test for the presumptive diagnosis of perilymph fistulas. *Neurol Clin* 1990;8:361–374
73. Nadol JB Jr. Positive Hennebert's sign in Meniere's disease. *Arch Otolaryngol* 1977;103:524–530
74. Arenberg IK, Ackley RS, Ferraro JA, Muchnik C. ECoG results in perilymphatic fistula: clinical and experimental studies. *Otolaryngol Head Neck Surg* 1988;99:435–443
75. Campbell KCM, Savage MM, Harker LA. Electrocochleography in the presence and absence of perilymphatic fistula. *Ann Otol Rhinol Laryngol* 1992;101:403–407
76. Black FO, Pesznecker SC. Perilymphatic fistula. The method of F. Owen Black. In: Gates GA, ed. *Current Therapy in Otolaryngology Head and Neck Surgery.* 6th Ed. St. Louis, MO: CV Mosby; 1998:71–78
77. Nomura Y. *Otologic Significance of the Round Window.* Munich: Karger-Basel; 1984
78. Seltzer S, McCabe BF. Perilymph fistula: the Iowa experience. *Laryngoscope* 1986;94:37–49
79. Coats AC. The summating potential and Meniere's disease. Summating potential amplitude in Meniere's and non-Meniere's ears. *Arch Otolaryngol Head Neck Surg* 1979;107: 199–208
80. Coats AC. Electronystagmography. In: Bradford LJ, ed. *Physiological Measures of the Audio-vestibular System.* San Diego, CA: Academic Press, 1975:37–83
81. Coats A. On electrocochleographic electrode design. *J Acoust Soc Am* 1974;56:708–711

82. Arenberg IK, May M, Stroud MH. Perilymphatic fistula: an unusual cause of Meniere's syndrome in a prepubertal child. *Laryngoscope* 1974;84:243–246
83. Black FO. Vertigo: the method of F. Owen Black, M.D., F.A.C.S. In: Decker BC, ed. *Current Therapy in Otolaryngology–Head and Neck Surgery.* 1990:59–65
84. Epley JM. The canalith repositioning procedure: for management of benign paroxysmal positional vertigo. *Otolaryngology Head Neck Surg* 1992;107:399–404
85. Semont A. Curing the BPPV with a liberatory maneuver. In: *Annual Meeting of the Barany Society*, Marseille, France; 1987
86. Serafini G, Palmieri AMR, Simoncelli C. Benign paroxysmal positional vertigo of posterior semicircular canal: results in 160 cases treated with Semont's maneuver. *Ann Otol Rhinol Laryngol* 1996;105:770–775
87. Fisch U, Murata K, Hossli G. Measurement of oxygen tension in human perilymph. *Acta Otolaryngol* 1981;81:278–282
88. Nagahara K, Fisch U, Yagi N. Perilymph oxygenation in sudden and progressive sensorineural hearing loss. *Acta Otolaryngol (Stockh)* 1983;96:57–68
89. Fisch U. Management of sudden deafness. *Otolaryngol Head Neck Surg* 1983;91:3–8
90. Bhansali SA. Perilymph fistula. *Ear Nose Throat J* 1989; 68:11–27
91. Bennett RJ. On subarachnoid–tympanic fistulae: a report of two cases of the rare indirect type. *J Laryngol Otol* 1966;80: 1242–1252
92. Lingam S, Singh A. Recurrent meningitis due to labyrinthine fistula. *J Neurol Neurosurg Psychiatry* 1982;45:1168–1176
93. Grewal DS, Hiranandani NL, Pusalkar AG. Traumatic perilymph fistulae of the round and oval windows. *J Laryngol Otol* 1983;97:1149–1155
94. Schuknecht HF. *Pathology of the Ear.* 2nd Ed. Philadelphia: Lea & Febiger; 1993

Perilymph Fistulae

CHAPTER 56

Richard R. Gacek

Since the description by Fee[1] of perilymphatic fistula (PLF) to the middle ear space, there has been an explosion in the number of reports describing PLF. It is likely that PLF has been used to explain clinical cases of unexplained sensorineural hearing or vertigo, or both. The diagnostic criteria of PLF are not clearly defined and surgical exploration has been used as the principal approach to diagnosis as well as management. A major impediment to recognition of perilymph in the oval or round window niches (RWN) is the presence of tissue fluid produced by middle ear mucosa that reaccumulates when aspirated. An additional misconception responsible for reported round window membrane fistulae is the assumption that a fenestrated membrane, which often covers the entrance to the RWN, represents the RWM. Removal of the bony overhang of the RWN is necessary for exposure of the RWM. It is not surprising that PLF is overdiagnosed and overtreated. This has formed the basis for controversy regarding the issue of diagnosis, recognition, and treatment of PLF.

A perilymphatic fistula (PLF) may be defined as a communication of the perilymphatic space to the middle ear space. The volume of perilymph in the labyrinth is normally small, as it is derived as a transudate of the vasculature in the spiral ligament and, to a limited degree, the cerebrospinal fluid (CSF) space through the cochlear aqueduct. Therefore, perilymph loss in a PLF is small and reaccumulates slowly. A large volume of fluid from a fistula in the oval or round windows (surgical or traumatic) represents the flow of CSF through a congenital defect in the labyrinth that allows the subarachnoid space to communicate with the perilymphatic space. This form of CSF otorrhea will not be considered in this discussion of PLF, as its presence is easily recognized by its copious flow, and treatment is noncontroversial. The PLF, which has attracted considerable controversy, is represented by a defect either in the ligamentous or bony structures of the oval or round windows in a normal labyrinth. It should also be pointed out that fistulization of the bony labyrinth (cochlea and semicircular canals) from chronic middle ear inflammation, particularly cholesteatoma, does not include communication into the perilymphatic compartment. The inflammatory response to bone erosion from cholesteatoma creates fibrosis of the endosteal membrane and variable degrees of labyrinthitis rather than a defect permitting perilymph loss. Issues of diagnosis and recognition of PLF at surgery form the main areas of disagreement.

Vast clinical experience is based on the signs and symptoms that result from a humanmade fistula in the oval window. This derives from the stapedectomy or stapedotomy procedure where either a large or small fenestra is fashioned in a fixed footplate and sealed with a tissue prosthesis to reconstruct a sound transmission mechanism. Although the fenestra with PLF in this procedure is of short duration, as it is sealed with tissue and the healing response of the labyrinth and the middle ear, poststapedectomy symptoms reflect a controlled PLF. Both vestibular and auditory symptoms follow stapedectomy with the vestibular symptoms consisting of dizziness and dysequilibrium, occasionally accompanied by spontaneous nystagmus being the most troublesome. Auditory system effects appear as elevated bone conduction thresholds with some decrease in speech discrimination, which may require one or several weeks to return to normal levels. It is for this reason that the usual post stapedectomy auditory examination is obtained at 4 to 5 weeks. Animal research[2] has demonstrated rapid healing of a defect in the oval window by regeneration of the endosteal membrane within 24 to 48 h, followed by regeneration of middle ear mucous membrane. This reparative response is more rapid with a small fenestra than with a large (total stapedectomy) fistula.

Clinical experience with the end result of an unhealed PLF comes from our experience with direct trauma to the tympanic membrane and ossicular chain as a result of the introduction of an instrument (toothpick, hairpin) into the external ear canal. When such an injury is accompanied by vestibular symptoms, it is axiomatic that immediate surgical exploration and removal of a subluxed or fractured stapes footplate with soft tissue seal of the PLF be performed.[3,4] If such repair is not performed the PLF leads to irreversible sensorineural hearing loss with eventual resolution of vestibular symptoms as a result of central vestibular compensation. Early surgical repair of the oval window fistula insures recovery of auditory and vestibular deficits. Thus, surgical repair of PLF is capable of reversing the labyrinthine deficits caused by PLF.

Round window membrane ruptures can be produced in the laboratory animal (cat) by increasing subarachnoid pressure.[5] However, the cochlear aqueduct is short and wide in the cat but is long, narrow, and filled with periotic duct tissue in humans. Therefore, this pathway usually will not permit transmitted CSF pressure in humans as in the laboratory animal, at least in the majority of temporal bones. Furthermore, the RWM is very thin with a reduced lamina propria in the laboratory animal (cat, guinea pig, chinchilla),[6] whereas the human RWM has a thick lamina propria that will resist disruption by increased pressure.[7]

Animal research has demonstrated that cochlear potentials do not change[8,9] after RWM ruptures. Furthermore, RWM breaks, no matter how large, undergo spontaneous healing in 7 to 10 days.[8] However, when such RWM ruptures are accompanied by intracochlear membrane breaks (Reissner's membrane, basilar membrane) there is a significant sensorineural hearing loss or change in cochlear potentials.[10,11]

These clinical and experimental observations indicate that a serous labyrinthitis occurs in PLF. The definition of serous labyrinthitis rests on the reversibility of auditory and vestibular dysfunction, implying that if function does not recover, a more advanced stage of labyrinthitis has been reached. Therefore, if the PLF does not heal either spontaneously or by repair, the serous labyrinthitis may progress to a serofibrinous labyrinthitis with irreversible loss of auditory and vestibular function. If the PLF is repaired while the stage of inflammation is serous, recovery of the function and reversibility of auditory and vestibular symptoms will occur.[12] The time period beyond which repair will not prevent irreversible loss of function is unknown but probably has a duration of 1 to 2 weeks. This suggested time period is based on clinical experience with treatment of post-stapedectomy granuloma. Most ears with the granuloma removed within 2 weeks recover function completely, whereas those removed later than 2 weeks, or not at all, are associated with severe sensorineural hearing loss.

The main controversy centers around the diagnosis and management of PLF. In my opinion, history is an extremely important diagnostic criterion for spontaneous PLF. A traumatic event, either direct or indirect, to the tympanic membrane and ossicular chain must precede the onset of symptoms. This may occur after severe barotrauma, in which the patient feels sudden pressure change as a result of rapid ascent or descent. A similar force can be created in head injury without TB fracture, where a concussive force is delivered to the labyrinth and ossicular chain. The presence of auditory and vestibular symptoms after such an event may represent the diagnostic manifestations of PLF. These should be demonstrated with auditory and vestibular tests that include pneumatic otoscopy to exhibit a possible fistula.[13-15]

Marked displacement of the ossicular chain is more likely to produce a tear in the ligamentous structures of the oval window than the RWM because of the shearing force between the footplate and the margin of the oval window. This may produce disruption of the stapediovestibular ligament and the creation of PLF. This author has identified four PLFs in the oval window out of 20 surgically explored cases over a 25-year period. No PLFs were identified in the RWM. A higher incidence of PLF in the oval window than in the round window has also been reported by Singleton et al.[13] It is possible that the thicker RWM in close proximity to a channel (cochlear aqueduct), which may decompress the pressure within the perilymphatic compartment, is at least partially responsible for the infrequency of disruption at this area. Adequate exposure is necessary to precisely identify a tear in the RWM. Because the RWM is usually obscured by the bony overhang of the round window niche, exposure requires drilling off the overhang after the removal of the mucosal fold that is frequently draped over the aperture of the round window niche. This mucosal fold often has a small fenestra which may be mistaken for an RWM defect. This mucosal curtain may assume various positions in the RW niche that simulate the RWM.

When the criteria for diagnosis of PLF are fulfilled, a conservative management is recommended initially. The following criteria are sufficient to support a diagnosis of PLF: (1) a history of trauma (barotrauma or head trauma), (2) sensorineural hearing loss and dysequilibrium, and (3) dissimilarity to other known labyrinth disorders. The presence of a positive fistula test is additional supporting evidence. Conservative management consists of a period of bed rest with head elevation for a period of 7 to 10 days to provide an opportunity for spontaneous healing of the defect by the endosteal membrane of the vestibular wall as well as the middle ear mucosa. Procedures that reduce subarachnoid pressure and possibly perilymphatic pressure are encouraged to assist healing. Should there be no improvement or should auditory or vestibular symptoms worsen, surgical exploration for PLF is indicated.

Exploration of the middle ear for PLF should be performed under local anesthesia with light sedation. Local rather than general anesthesia reduces the incidence of bleeding and fluid accumulation from manipulation of the middle ear mucosa. It also allows the patient to respond with a Valsalva maneuver when requested to enhance perilymph leakage. Complete control of bleeding is necessary before examination of the middle ear space is performed. Adequate exposure of the oval and round windows may require curettage of the posterior and superior ear canal wall. Both labyrinthine windows should be examined without manipulation of a mucosal surface since this maneuver may induce a serous transudate that can simulate perilymph. A sensitive and specific marker of perilymph would greatly facilitate identification of PLF. Attempts to find a marker using colorimetric markers such as fluorescein have not been successful. Chemical markers specific for CSF (β-2-transferrin) have also not proven reliable as an indicator of perilymph in clinical studies.[16] A recent report[17] described detection of human apolipo-protein D using chemo- luminescent Western blot assay in human perilymph taken at surgery. A 75% positive identification rate for perilymph and no false-positive results among 15 controls (middle ear fluid) were recorded. Further confirmation of the use of such protein fractions specific for perilymph will aid the diagnosis of PLF.

A No. 24 aspirator tip is carefully used to examine the margins of the oval window with and without displacement of the ossicular chain. If no fluid accumulation is seen, the patient is asked to perform Valsalva maneuvers at least twice to determine whether an enhancement of subarachnoid pressure will produce perilymph flow. If the oval window examination is negative, the round window niche is examined initially without instrumentation following a Valsalva maneuver and ossicular manipulation. If no fluid has accumulated, the bony overhang of the round window niche is carefully removed with a microdrill to expose and examine the RWM while depressing the ossicular chain. If this examination is also negative, tissue augmentation of the membrane is not performed. I believe that repair in the absence of any visible evidence of PLF confuses the evaluation of the effectiveness of the procedure. A fistula small enough to escape detection by the preceding method of examination should have healed spontaneously.

If fluid has been detected in either of the labyrinthine windows, the precise location of the defect is revealed by use of a No. 24 aspirator and is prepared to receive a tissue graft by removal of mucosal membrane from adjacent bony surfaces. Small (1-mm) adipose tissue grafts are secured in place with gelfoam pledgets. The patient's activity postoperatively should be restricted for at least 1 week to 10 days to aid adequate fibrous healing of the PLF. Auditory function should be evaluated in 6 to 8 weeks postoperatively and at later periods if incomplete recovery is seen initially.

A reasonable statement of PLF incidence is that they do occur but are infrequent. The survey conducted by Hughes et al.[18] of 167 surgeons of the American Otologic Society indicated that most (60%) performed three or fewer explorations for PLF per year. The average number of explorations for the group was less than five per year. The number of confirmed PLF was even smaller. If the diagnosis of PLF is based on strict criteria and surgical exploration carried out only after a conservative therapeutic trial has been offered, the number of confirmed PLFs will be very small.

REFERENCES

Gacek—CHAPTER 56

1. Fee GA. Traumatic perilymphatic fistulas. *Arch Otolaryngol* 1968;88:477–480
2. Hohmann A. Inner ear reactions to stapes surgery (animal experiments). In: Schunecht HF, ed. *Otosclerosis.* Boston: Little, Brown; 1962:305–317
3. Silverstein H. Penetrating wounds of the tympanic membrane and ossicular chain. *Trans Am Acad Ophthalmol Otolaryngol* 1973;77:125–135
4. Emmett JR, Shea JJ. Traumatic perilymph fistula. *Laryngoscope* 1980;90:1513–1520
5. Harker L, Norante JD, Ryu JH. Experimental rupture of the round window membrane. *Trans Am Acad Ophthalmol Otolaryngol* 1974;78:448–452
6. Richardson T, Ishiyama E, Keels E. Submicroscopic studies of the round window membrane. *Acta Otolaryngol* 1971;71:9–21
7. Kawabata I, Paparella M. Fine structures of the round window membrane. *Ann Otol Rhinol Laryngol* 1971;80:13–26
8. Simmons FB, Burton RD, Beatty D. Round window injury: auditory, behavioral and electrophysiological consequences in the cat. *Trans Am Acad Ophthalmol Otolaryngol* 1962;66:715
9. Weisskopf A, Murphy JT, Merzenich MM. Genesis of the round window rupture syndrome: some experimental observations. *Laryngoscope* 1978;88:389–397
10. Oshiro EM, Shelton C, Lusted HS. Role of perilymphatic fistula in sudden hearing loss: an animal model. *Ann Otol Rhinol Laryngol* 1989;98:491–495
11. Simmons FB. The double-membrane break syndrome in sudden hearing loss. *Laryngoscope* 1979;89:59–66
12. Arragg F, Paparella M. Traumatic fracture of the stapes. *Laryngoscope* 1964;74:1329
13. Singleton GT, Post KN, Karlan MS, Bock DG. Perilymph fistulas: diagnostic criteria and therapy. *Ann Otol Rhinol Laryngol* 1978;87:797–803
14. Simmons FB. Perilymph fistula: some diagnostic problems. *Adv Otorhinolaryngol* 1982;18:68–72
15. Love JT, Waguespack RD. Perilymphatic fistulas. *Laryngoscope* 1981;91:1118–1128
16. Buckman CA, Luxford WM, Hirsch BE, et al. Beta-2-transferrin assay in the identification of perilymph. In: *Abstracts of the One hundred thirty-first Meeting of the American Otologic Society*; May 9–10, 1998
17. Telian SA, Disher MJ, Sun Q, Andrews PC. Biochemical markers for identification of human perilymph. In: *Abstracts of the One hundred thirty-first Meeting, of the American Otologic Society;* May 9–10, 1998
18. Hughes GB, Sismanis A, House J. Is there consensus in perilymph fistula management? *Otolaryngol Head Neck Surg* 1990; 102:111–117

Perilymph Fistulae

CHAPTER 57

John F. Kveton

The diagnosis of perilymph fistula continues to be elusive, spawning both extremes of overdiagnosis and underdiagnosis. In this situation, the otolaryngologist is confronted with the possibility of becoming either a charlatan for overdiagnosing, and therefore overoperating on patients, or a therapeutic nihilist, and so failing to eliminate inner ear symptoms in one of the rare instances in which surgical intervention can remedy sensorineural impairment. The question of whether such a condition even exists has been raised by some investigators.[1,2] By contrast, Goodhill's[3] original descriptions of the pathophysiology of perilymphatic fistula and my personal experience with elimination of symptoms after surgical repair of obvious perilymph leaks would indicate that this condition does in fact exist. This chapter reviews my understanding of this entity and outlines my approach to arriving at the diagnosis and management of patients who present with the appropriate symptoms.

Pathophysiology

Perilymph fistula refers to a pathologic condition in which there is a persistent communication between the inner ear and the middle ear. Perilymph fistula implies that there is an egress of perilymph, either constantly or intermittently from the inner ear, and it is this loss of perilymph from the inner ear that produces symptoms. The precise effect of this change in the volume of perilymph is not understood. Temporary loss of perilymph occurs often in stapedectomy with little or no permanent effect on inner ear function. Chronic perilymphatic leak, as seen in fistulization of the labyrinth by cholesteatoma, can result in permanent auditory and vestibular dysfunction. Although not proved, the chronic loss of fluid from the perilymphatic space should lead to expansion of the endolymphatic spaces, producing a condition similar to endolymphatic hydrops. This most likely explains the reason that the symptoms of perilymph fistula and endolymphatic hydrops are at times indistinguishable.

The mechanisms for the development of perilymph fistula are credited to Goodhill.[3] He described both implosive and explosive causes. Implosive fistulae occur when a force is exerted on the oval and round windows through the middle ear. This might involve severe excursion of the tympanic membrane or ossicular chain, such as in acoustic trauma, or by direct positive pressure on the oval and round windows due to severe change in middle ear pressure as in a sudden decompression syndrome (scuba diving). The explosive mechanism occurs by transmission of a sudden increase in intracranial pressure to the inner ear. This occurs primarily through the cochlear aqueduct, theoretically, when the aqueduct is abnormally patent, but it also can occur through the internal auditory canal in congenital anomalies such as Mondini dysplasias. This increase in intracranial pressure can occur as a result of head trauma, coughing, or any type of straining activity. The existence of microfissures or patent tracts in the fissula ante fenestra have been postulated as sources for the perilymph fistula by various investigators. The precise pathophysiologic mechanism has not been described, obviously lending concern to the actual existence of this disorder.

Perilymph fistulae are either traumatic, iatrogenic, idiopathic, or congenital. Trauma may be blunt, such as a head injury with a temporal bone fracture, barotrauma, increased intracranial pressure; acoustic, as occurs with a blast injury; or penetrating, as in ossicular fracture due to foreign body injury. Iatrogenic causes of perilymph fistula most commonly occur after stapedectomy but may occur in any case of inadvertent ossicular disruption. Idiopathic, or spontaneous, perilymph fistulae occur in cases in which no identifiable preceding condition can be recognized. Congenital malformations such as Mondini dysplasias carry a high risk of perilymph fistulae because of the more extensive communication with intracranial cerebrospinal (CSF) pressure due to the foreshortened patent internal auditory canals that often open directly into the otic capsule.

Signs and Symptoms

As with most disorders of the inner ear, hearing loss, tinnitus, fullness, and vestibular symptoms are all possible symptoms of perilymph fistula.[4] Obtaining a careful history with attention to onset, duration, and frequency of symptoms, in addition to an understanding of events antecedent to the development of the symptoms and other associated symptoms, will lead in most instances to the appropriate diagnosis.

HEARING LOSS

The hearing loss associated with perilymph fistula varies according to the mechanism that produced the fistula. In the majority of cases the onset of hearing loss is sudden, and can be correlated with a particular event (e.g., head trauma, a sneeze, explosion, foreign body). Hearing loss may be complete, but it is usually partial. The sudden hearing loss is often associated with vertigo at the time of the incident. Tinnitus commonly occurs around the time of the hearing loss as well. There may be partial or complete recovery of hearing days after the inciting event. If the fistula becomes chronic, the hearing loss may fluctuate or progressively deteriorate over time. A positive diagnosis can be made if fluctuation or progressive deterioration can be correlated with activities that increase intracranial pressure.

Progressive or fluctuating hearing loss without a sudden onset is more likely to occur in idiopathic or congenital perilymph fistula. In these cases, a pre-existing hearing loss worsens with symptoms of tinnitus and vertigo during the hearing loss. This is usually the first indication that a perilymph fistula may be the etiology of the hearing loss.

TINNITUS AND AURAL FULLNESS

Tinnitus and aural fullness are vague symptoms that should not be used alone to make the diagnosis of perilymph fistula. In perilymph fistula tinnitus usually occurs with hearing loss or may increase during instances of increased intracranial pressure without any further hearing loss occurring. A sense of fullness in the involved ear can often be elicited from patients as beginning after the initial precipitating event. Aural fullness without other symptoms such as hearing loss or vertigo are nonspecific in the diagnosis of perilymph fistula.

VERTIGO

The abrupt onset of vertigo after direct ear trauma such as a foreign body penetration into the ear canal should immediately prompt the diagnosis of perilymph fistula. Unfortunately such instances are rare, and more commonly, consideration of the diagnosis of perilymphatic fistula in patients with vertigo symptoms is more nonspecific. Attention to the nature of the vestibular symptoms along with onset, duration, frequency, and associated symptoms is helpful in establishing the differential diagnosis. Vertigo caused by a traumatic perilymph fistula occurs at the time of the injury and is abrupt and violent. Vertigo can last from minutes to hours and is often accompanied by nausea and vomiting. If the fistula closes, the usual recovery from the vestibular insult occurs over the next 6 to 8 weeks. Persistent vestibular symptoms after this time should alert the clinician to the possibility of a persistent or intermittent fistula. In most cases, the recurrent vertigo will not be as severe in duration as the initial injury. The vertigo is abrupt with a strong sense of rotation and at times falling, but usually lasts minutes with less severe vegetative symptoms. Vertigo attacks are often triggered by increased intracranial pressure and may be associated with hearing loss, tinnitus, or aural fullness. Positional vertigo to the side of the lesion is an interesting and unexplainable phenomenon that can occur with persistent perilymph fistula. This positional vertigo is not associated with increases of intracranial pressure and seems to develop as a chronic condition after the initial injury.

In addition to vertigo, the whole array of vestibular symptoms associated with varying degrees of vestibular compensation after an acute vestibular injury may be present in perilymph fistula. It is into this diagnostic miasma that some otologists fall, becoming charlatans at worst, and zealots at best, in over-diagnosing perilymphatic fistula in these chronic symptoms. Integral to entertaining the diagnosis of perilymph fistula in patients with these symptoms is an antecedent history of some type of trauma. Fluctuation or worsening of the symptoms with changes in intracranial pressure may also be confirmatory. Chronic lightheadedness or spatial disorientation alone are too vague to be used solely to entertain the diagnosis of perilymph fistula. Dysequilibrium that persists after severe vertigo, especially if associated with progressive hearing loss and tinnitus, may be caused by a perilymph fistula. Chronic nausea is at times a predominant symptom associated with such dysequilibrium.

SIGNS

Physical examination is generally of little help in making the diagnosis of perilymph fistula. Spontaneous nystagmus is rarely seen, and if identified, is nondiagnostic. The fistula test is routinely noted as means to diagnose a fistula, but correlation of a positive fistula test with identification of an actual fistula at surgical exploration ranges from 24 to 77%.[4,5] A positive fistula test itself is somewhat variable, in that there can be an objective result (i.e., induced nystagmus) or a subjective result (i.e., induced sense of vertigo or dysequilibirum without nystagmus). Enhancements of the fistula test with impedance testing and electrooculographic recordings[6] or determining changes in body sway using dynamic posturography[7] have not been uniformly adopted. Other signs of vestibular abnormalities, such as abnormal Romberg testing, are nonspecific for perilymph fistula.

Diagnostic Testing

To complicate matters further, there is neither an auditory or vestibular function test that will confirm the diagnosis of perilymph fistula. Although the simplest test in the diagnostic battery, the audiogram provides the most consistent information to consider the diagnosis of perilymph fistula. The hearing loss is usually a sloping high-frequency sensorineural hearing loss with impaired speech discrimination. Progressive sensorineural hearing loss with or without deterioration of speech discrimination is a finding that should bring perilymph fistula to the forefront of the differential diagnosis. Electrocochleography has not been shown to enhance the ability to confirm the diagnosis, as a positive finding of the summation potential/action potential ratio of ≥ 0.5 was identified in 52% of patients with confirmed perilymph leaks.[8]

Vestibular function tests are of little value in making the diagnosis of perilymph fistula. As in endolymphatic hydrops, the degree of damage to the vestibular system will vary depending on the time course of the disease when the testing is performed. In a recent fistula, as in early endolymphatic hydrops, caloric testing will be normal; in an advanced stage of the disease, a caloric weakness will be present. Similarly, rotational vestibular testing will be normal in early stages and the 5 to 6 pattern of vestibular dysfunction noted on dynamic platform posturography will only be present in advanced stages of the disorder.

Diagnosis

A method to arrive precisely at the diagnosis of perilymph fistula remains impossible. As in many inner ear conditions, we have been hampered by a lack of pathologic data because the condition is not lethal and so timely pathologic examination of the inner ear is impossible. This situation is not dissimilar to most inner ear disorders and forces the otolaryngologist to integrate and interpret all data (history, physical examination, and diagnostic tests) to position perilymph fistula high in the differential diagnosis for the condition. If the diagnosis of perilymph fistula is entertained, surgical exploration of the oval and round windows is the only way to confirm the diagnosis. Controversy abounds, even in this realm of intraoperative identification of a perilymph leak. Fluid in the oval or round window niches has been attributed to pooling of residual local anesthetics,[9] and perilymph labeling, especially with fluorescein, has yielded mixed results.[10] Moreover, the number of negative explorations associated with improvement of symptoms raises the question of the placebo effect versus closure of intermittent perilymph leaks that simply are not active at the time of surgical exploration.

Management

Acute perilymphatic fistulae caused by nonpenetrating trauma or idiopathic etiologies should be first managed conservatively with bed rest and avoidance of any increase in intracranial pressure. If symptoms do not improve, or even worsen during this time, surgical exploration should be considered.

Once the decision has been made to explore the middle ear for a perilymph fistula, a routine should be followed to minimize the possibility for inaccurate diagnosis. Injection of topical anesthetics should be kept to a minimum to avoid pooling of anesthetic fluids in the window niches. Once the tympanomeatal flap has been raised, the round window niche should be gently suctioned and briefly examined. The entire oval window niche must be visualized, which usually requires curettage of the scutum. Using microsuction and high-power magnification, both the oval and round windows should be inspected with the patient in the Trendelenburg position, while the anesthetist performs a Valsalva maneuver. Gentle manipulation of the ossicular chain should also be done while visualizing both window niches. If the stapedial footplate is fractured, a total stapedectomy should be performed. More commonly, the perilymph leak is around the annular ligament of the footplate or in the round window niche. In such cases, the mucosa around the windows should be escarified with a micropick and a piece of soft tissue placed over the region. In the round window niche, a plug of fibrofatty tissue works well to obliterate the niche and directly contact the round window membrane. The oval window niche is best managed by using a thin piece of perichondrium cut in a pants-leg fashion, to cover the annular ligament of the footplate completely, overlapping only at the posterior margin of the footplate. This type of repair is performed, even if no perilymph leak has been identified at surgery. It is my philosophy that if I have entertained this diagnosis so seriously that I have advised the patient to undergo an operative procedure, I seal both windows in the event that this is an intermittent fistula.

Epilogue

It should be apparent that the diagnosis of perilymph fistula relies for the most part on the clinical acumen of the otolaryngologist. It is the art, rather than the science, of medicine that takes precedence. As in many inner ear conditions, a diagnosis is made with no precise documentation as to the accuracy of that diagnosis. How many cases of viral labyrinthitis are misdiagnosed? How many procedures are performed for Meniere's disease for which a pathologic diagnosis is never made? The clinician must entertain the diagnosis of perilymph fistula, keeping in mind that it is an unusual event. Careful attention must be paid to antecedent history of trauma or a congenital anomaly, mindful that spontaneous fistulae are rare or possibly nonexistent.

REFERENCES

1. Schuknecht HF. Myths in neurotology. *Am J Otol* 1992; 13:124–126
2. House JW, Morris MS, Kramer SJ, Shasky GL, Coggan BB, Putter JS. Perilymphatic fistula: surgical experience in the United States. *Otolaryngol Head Neck Surg* 1991;104: 239–243
3. Goodhill V. Leaking labyrinth lesions, deafness, tinnitus, and dizziness. *Ann Otol Rhinol Laryngol* 1981;90:99–106
4. Seltzer S, McCabe BF. Perilymph fistula: the Iowa experience. *Laryngoscope* 1986;96:37–49
5. Podosin L, Fradis M, Ben-David J, Berger SI, Feiglin H. Perilymphatic fistula—the value of diagnostic tests. *J Laryngol Otol* 1994;108:560–563
6. Vartiainen E, Nuutinen J, Karjalainen S, Nykanen K. Perilymph fistula—a diagnostic dilemma. *J Laryngol Otol* 1991; 105:270–273
7. Black FO, Lilly DJ, Nashner LM, Peterka RJ, Peznecker SC. Quantitative diagnostic test for perilymph fistula. *Otolaryngol Head Neck Surg* 1987;96:125–134
8. Arenberg IK, Ackley RS, Ferraro JA, Muchnik C. ECoG results in perilymphatic fistula: clinical and experimental studies. *Otolaryngol Head Neck Surg* 1988;99:435–443
9. Arenberg IK, Wu CM. Fluorescein as an easy, low-cost, indirect, or reverse intraoperative marker to rule out perilymph versus local injection. *Am J Otol* 1996;17:259–262
10. Poe DS, Gadre AK, Rebeiz EE, Pankratov MM. Intravenous fluoroscein for detection of perilymphatic fistulae. *Am J Otol* 1993;14:51–55

20

Fistulae in Head and Neck Surgery

"A wound infection is always present when a fistula occurs, due to contamination of the wound by saliva. Perioperative antibiotics should always be used when mucosa is entered, since their use has long been proven effective in decreasing the incidence of wound infection when the pharynx is entered."

Paul A. Levine

"In our institution, the rate of postlaryngectomy pharyngocutaneous fistulae and its association with age, gender, preoperative radiation, TNM staging, and a number of other clinical and therapeutic parameters, was investigated. The overall fistula rate was 22% and no association was found between any of the above clinical or treatment parameters and the likelihood of developing a fistula."

Patrick J. Gullane

"In our experience, prior full-course radiotherapy (>5000 cGy) and brachytherapy have a detrimental effect on wound healing and are considered a risk of compromised healing and fistulization."

Clarence T. Sasaki

Fistulae in Head and Neck Surgery

CHAPTER 58

Richard Gallagher and Paul A. Levine

One of the most frustrating complications of surgery of the upper aerodigestive tract is the development of a salivary fistula, which results in a prolonged hospitalization and morbidity. The patient's recovery, rehabilitation of swallowing, speech, and adjuvant treatment are delayed, and the fistulae may predispose to serious complications, such as great vessel rupture or mediastinitis.

A fistula may develop as a consequence of any operation where the mucosa of the upper aerodigestive tract is approached by a neck incision and is entered, whether planned or iatrogenic. Saliva leaks through the line of mucosal closure and appears at an external skin incision line. The challenge for the surgeon then becomes thoughtful management of the problem to achieve wound healing, while avoiding significant complications. This chapter presents our thoughts and philosophy regarding the prevention and management of salivary fistulae.

Background

Salivary fistulae are most commonly associated with major oncologic resections of the upper aerodigestive tract, but can occur when resecting benign disease, such as the closure for the resection of a Zenker's diverticulum. All salivary fistulae, whether pharyngocutaneous or orocutaneous, present similar management problems. The best time to manage a fistula is by prevention at the primary operation.[1] Operative technique that avoids excessive tissue destruction is the first step, along with ensuring that the mucosal suture line be watertight. For the mucosal suture, interrupted Vicryl (polyglactic acid) or silk sutures are used. After total laryngectomy, closure of mucosa is achieved using an inverting suture of polyglactic acid which maintains integrity during wound repair. Soylu et al.[2] showed a statistically significant reduction in the incidence of pharyngocutaneous fistula when this suture was used for closure (8.6%) compared with catgut (24%).

At the completion of mucosal closure in total laryngectomy and laryngopharyngectomy, a test of the integrity of the closure is performed by filling the neopharynx with saline, noting leaks, and repairing them with additional sutures for closure. It makes sense that a saline leak at the time of operation will produce a salivary leak postoperatively. Tension on the suture line should be minimized, and a two- to three-layer closure can usually be achieved by closing the fascial and muscle layers overlying the repair. In the case of a total laryngectomy, at least a two-layer repair is favored (i.e., submucosa and pharyngobasilar fascia). When enough constrictor muscle is present on one side, it can be used to bolster the line of closure by securing it across the suture line but not providing pharyngeal constriction. This provides an additional layer of closure without reuniting the inferior constrictor and narrowing the neopharynx, affecting swallowing and tracheoesophageal puncture speech. The larger the tumor and the resection, the greater the potential for tension on the mucosal closure.[3] Several authors have demonstrated an increased incidence of fistula as the amount of mucosa resected increases, particularly in pyriform sinus cancers.[4-6] Closure in these cases results in increased tension on the suture line as well as increased intraluminal pressure. To avoid these problems, a vascularized flap may be necessary to provide an adequately sized neopharynx.

The choice of flap depends on the available resources and surgical capabilities. Whether using a pectoralis major myocutaneous flap, radial forearm flap, or jejunal free flap, it is imperative that the flap is inset securely. In the oral cavity, when a flap is inset adjoining the mandible, additional support can be provided by anchoring the flap to any remaining teeth or to the mandible itself, if the patient is edentulous, to provide flap support and reduce suture line tension. When a modified radical or radical neck dissection has been performed in conjunction with a pharyngeal resection, coverage of the carotid artery by a dermal graft or sternomastoid or levator scapulae muscle should be considered as a prophylactic maneuver to reduce the risk of carotid blow-out in the event of a fistula developing.[7] Suction drainage is used to minimize fluid beneath the skin flaps and control the spread of saliva if a fistula develops.[8] The drains should not be placed on the mucosal closure lines but should lie in close proximity.

The type of neck incision used is important. Trifurcations should be avoided, since these points have the poorest blood supply, predisposing to wound breakdown. If a fistula develops, it will appear at these sites.[4,9] If necessary, the modified Schobinger incision places the trifurcation along the anterior trapezius border, away from the carotid artery. The use of apron incisions or McFee incisions is our preference to avoid this problem.

A wound infection is always present when a fistula occurs, due to contamination of the wound by saliva. Perioperative antibiotics should always be used when mucosa is entered, since their use has long been proven effective in decreasing the incidence of wound infection when the pharynx is entered.[10,11]

The nutritional status of the patient affects all major surgery, with starvation, trauma, sepsis, and malignancy all resulting in a catabolic state.[12] In these situations, wound healing may be impaired and patients are predisposed to the development of complications such as fistulae. Although a precise methodology for quantifying malnutrition is not available, any history of significant weight loss with a patient who appears cachectic on physical exam, with a low albumin and pre-albumin, makes it peremptory to consider hyperalimentation, even before surgery, to minimize postoperative complications. In addition, thyroid-stimulating hormone (TSH) should be checked to evaluate for hypothyroidism, which is especially important for salvage surgery following radical radiotherapy.

Several authors have found that low postoperative hemoglobin is associated with the development of fistulae,[5,13,14] although few have offered an explanation for this finding. Frederickson and Haight[15] suggest that the decrease in blood volume, which is reflected by the lowered hemoglobin, results in lowered wound oxygen tension, which has been shown to increase bacterial colonization of wounds and slow the rate of healing.

The impact of radiotherapy as a cause of fistula formation is still a topic of considerable debate. Radiotherapy is known to result in endothelial fibrosis with reduced tissue blood supply.[16] McCombe and Jones[17] demonstrated an incidence of fistulae of 39% in salvage laryngectomy and only 4% in the group having laryngectomy as the primary treatment, though others have been unable to demonstrate a statistical difference between the rate of fistulae in irradiated and nonirradiated patients.[7,13,18]

There is no common system for classifying salivary fistulae, and most authors divide them into small, medium, and large.[3,19,20] Small and medium fistulae generally heal with local wound care.[4,5,20] The exception to this is medium-size fistulae in an irradiated wound, which will usually require surgical intervention.[19] Large fistulae with loss of skin will always require surgical repair with a flap.[3] The timing of closure is also debated. Most investigators recommend waiting 4 to 6 weeks, a time when the wound will be clean and granulating.[14,20,21] Earlier repair or intervention is mandatory when the carotid artery is exposed,[3,22] if not for wound closure, at least for carotid protection. Small fistulae are usually packed with ribbon gauze. Dedo et al.[23] recommended soaking in povidone-iodine, while Cummings[24] has used 0.25% acetic acid. Both substances will clean the wound and promote granulation tissue.

Stell and Cooney[21] conceptualized surgical closure of fistulae into three types, and all require closure by two epithelial surfaces.

Type 1 Both tissue surfaces provided locally.
Type 2 One tissue surface provided locally and one provided from a distance.
Type 3 Both surfaces provided from a distance.

All successful closure depends on using healthy, well-vascularized tissue. Historically, the deltopectoral flap was used most often for repair of medium and large fistulae[3,19] and, although still an option, myocutaneous flaps have become more popular for fistula repair due to the large amount of tissue provided with a reliable blood supply that does not need to be delayed.[22,24-26] Free flaps are always an option for repair.[27]

Discussion

A salivary fistula may occur at any time following surgery but most commonly is detected 5 to 10 days postoperatively, though they may occur later in patients who have undergone prior irradiation.[18] A late-developing fistula, one that occurs 3 to 4 weeks after surgery, or a few months after complete healing, is considered persistent or an indication of recurrent malignancy until proven otherwise. The patient will develop a low-grade fever 3 to 4 days postoperatively, which will occur a few days before significant induration of the wound is noted, and no other etiology of the elevated temperature is noted. Typically, the wound skin becomes inflamed, and the most dependent fistula drainage point becomes edematous and red. It is prudent to open an area along the suture line to permit drainage of purulent material. This controlled drainage should be made to divert saliva away from the carotid artery. Opening the wound limits the spread of saliva and infected material beneath the skin flaps. Cultures should be sent, even though the results most often exhibit mixed oral flora. Irrigation of the wound with half-strength hydrogen peroxide and packing with plain gauze soaked in 1% povidone-iodine is performed 4 times per day.

Hyperalimentation, most commonly via nasogastric or gastrostomy tube, is peremptory to assist in providing a caloric load of about 2000 calories/day.

If the suction drains are still in place when a fistula occurs, the drain volumes increase and the character of the drainage changes. Saliva is usually obvious, but the drainage may be frankly purulent, with a volume within the range of 50 to 100 ml/day. If the increased drainage, ≥150 ml, is on the left side, a chylous fistula is easily ruled out by placing cream down the feeding tube and observing the drainage at 1 h when it will become obviously milky. Although primarily on the left, a chyle leak may occur on the right by the transection of accessory thoracic ducts. It is best to control the fistula drainage with suction, if necessary, to create a mature fistula tract. This allows the skin flaps to heal to the deep neck tissue and avoids the potential problem of necrosis of a large amount of skin, which exposes underlying structures. It is hoped that, as the fistula heals, granulation tissue will stimulate closure and healing will be exhibited by a reduction in fistula fluid volume.

High-dose intravenous (IV) antibiotics are used until the wound is clean and the drainage clear. Once frankly purulent drainage has ceased and the wound is clean, antibiotics can be given enterally until the fistula is healed, or can potentially be discontinued.

The local management of the fistula depends on its site and size. Fistulae related to the great vessels and the laryngectomy stoma have the highest morbidity. If the skin flaps are intact, the fistula can be managed conservatively with irrigation and packing, since the underlying tissue will not be exposed to the added drying effect of air exposure. In the case of a high-volume fistula, the fistula should be directed medial to the great vessels.[3,28] This is done by incising directly over the pharyngeal defect, which is then sutured to the overlying skin. Pressure dressings or suction drains are used to permit healing of the surrounding skin flaps. The resulting mature fistula will require secondary closure with a flap when the wound is clean and granulating.

More problematic is the case of significant tissue necrosis, leaving a large soft tissue defect. In these cases, the wound should be irrigated and dressed regularly to prevent drying and excoriation of the tissues. Necrotic material may be debrided in the operating room and, if the carotid artery is exposed, tissue coverage is required. The choices are a dermal graft or the rotation and suturing of the sternomastoid or levator scapulae muscle over the vessel to the prevertebral fascia. Preferably, these defensive maneuvers would have been performed at surgery. A further option is the early application of a pectoralis major myocutaneous flap. Because a "good" flap will not heal to "bad" tissue, the wound may have to be temporized with defensive maneuvers until it is clean and granulating. Depending on the size of the defect, split skin grafts may need to be applied to the muscle.

In total laryngectomy and laryngopharyngectomy patients, the fistula will often be small, but troublesome, because it is sited directly above the laryngectomy stoma. Left unattended, this can result in continued wound breakdown and severe aspiration. They are best dealt with by insertion of a cuffed tracheotomy tube and placement of a suction catheter to detour the saliva, or a salivary bypass tube inserted endoscopically and packing placed through the fistula. We traditionally wait 2 weeks after the complete closure of the fistula before feeding by mouth, and do not normally perform a barium swallow before oral intake.

In general, our policy is to create a clean granulating fistula wound by local wound care and observation. The patient is supported nutritionally, and any systemic disorders such as diabetes or hypothyroidism are controlled. Small fistulae, in our experience, will close over several weeks. Larger fistulae with significant loss of skin and mucosa are closed with usage of myocutaneous or free flap, after a 4- to 6-week wound cleaning and healing period.

Conclusion

Salivary fistulae are a troubling complication in surgery of the upper aerodigestive tract. Their prevention is based on sound surgical technique and decision making. Attention to mucosal closure without tension and great vessel protection are the most important factors. If a fistula occurs, the initial management is conservative and supportive unless the carotid artery or jugular vein is exposed. Nutrition should be maximized and hypothyroidism and diabetes corrected. Saliva should be diverted away from the great vessels and protection of the carotid artery provided (Fig. 58–1). If the fistula fails to close after a 4- to 6-week period, surgical closure will be required. The main principle is to close both mucosal and skin defects with well-vascularized tissue, as a single procedure.

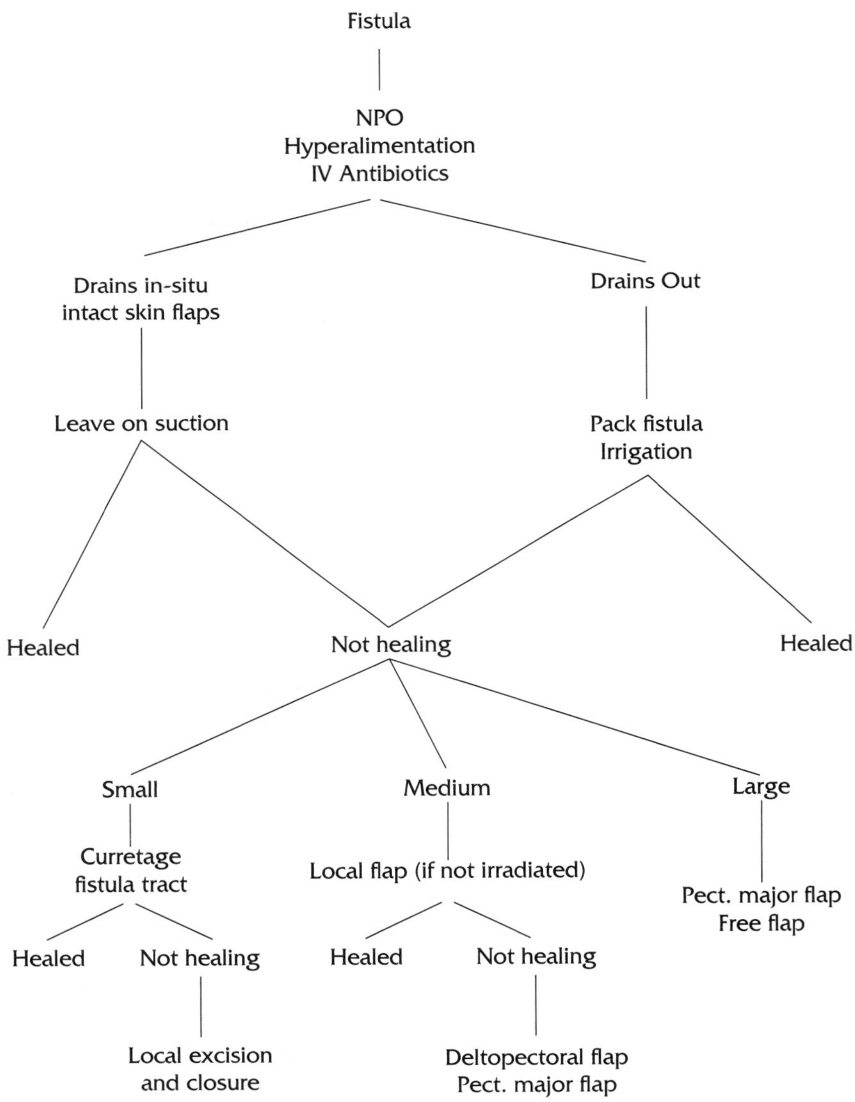

Figure 58–1 Algorithm of treatment choices (options) for postoperative salivary fistulae.

REFERENCES

Gallagher and Levine—CHAPTER 58

1. Cantrell R. Pharyngeal fistula: prevention and treatment. *Laryngoscope* 1978;88:1204–1208
2. Soylu I, Kiroglu M, Aydogan B, et al. Pharyngocutaneous fistula following laryngectomy. *Head Neck* 1998;20:22–25
3. Myers E. The management of pharyngocutaneous fistula. *Arch Otolaryngol* 1972;95:10–17
4. Dedo D, Alonso W, Ogura J. Incidence, predisposing factors and outcome of pharyngocutaneous fistulas complicating head and neck cancer surgery. *Ann Otol Rhinol Laryngol* 1975; 84:833–840
5. Mendelsohn M, Bridger G. Pharyngocutaneous fistulae following laryngectomy. *Aust NZ J Surg* 1985;55:177–179
6. Boyce S, Meyers A. Oral feeding after total laryngectomy. *Head Neck* 1989;11:269–273
7. Thawley S. Complications of combined radiotherapy and surgery for carcinoma of the larynx and inferior hypopharynx. *Laryngoscope* 1981;91;677–700
8. Bastian R, Park A. Suction drain management of salivary fistulas. *Laryngoscope* 1995;105:1337–1341
9. Freeland A, Rogers J. The vascular supply of the cervical skin with reference to incision planning. *Laryngoscope* 1975;85:714–724
10. Burke J. The effective period of preventative antibiotic action in experimental incisions and dermal lesions. *Surgery* 1961;50: 161–168
11. Newman RK, Weiland FL, Johnson JT, et al. Salivary scan after major ablative head and neck surgery with prediction of postoperative fistulization. *Ann Otol Rhinol Laryngol* 1983;92:366
12. Hill G. Surgical metabolism and nutrition. In: Marshall V, Ludbrook J, eds. *Clinical Science for Surgeons*. Boston: Butterworths; 1988:103–121
13. Lavelle R, Maw A. The aetiology of post-laryngectomy pharyngo-cutaneous fistulae. *J Laryngol Otol* 1972:785–793
14. Wei W, Lam K, Wong J, Ong G. Pharyngocutaneous fistula complicating total laryngectomy. *Aust NZ J Surg* 1980;50: 366–369
15. Frederickson J, Haight J. Prevention of pharyngeal fistulae. In: Snow JB, ed. *Controversy in Otolaryngology*. Philadelphia, PA: WB Saunders; 1980:371–378
16. Walter J, Israel M. *General Pathology*. 6th Ed. New York: Churchill Livingstone; 1987:117–129
17. McCombe A, Jones A. Radiotherapy and complications of laryngectomy. *J Laryngol Otol* 1993;107:130–132
18. Cummings C, Johnson J, Chung C, Sageman R. Complications of laryngectomy and neck dissection following planned preoperative radiotherapy. *Ann Otol Rhinol Laryngol* 1977; 86:745–750
19. Maw A, Lavelle R. The management of post-operative pharyngo-cutaneous pharyngeal fistulae. *J Laryngol Otol* 1972; 86:795–805
20. Papazoglou G, Doundoulakis G, Terzakis G, Dokianakis G. Pharyngocutaneous fistula after total laryngectomy: incidence, cause, and treatment. *Ann Otol Rhinol Laryngol* 1994;103: 801–805
21. Stell P, Cooney T. Management of fistulae of the head and neck after radical surgery. *J Laryngol Otol* 1974:819–834
22. Cohen M, Marschall M, Greager J. Early, aggressive management of postoperative oropharyngocutaneous fistulas. *Plast Reconstr Surg* 1992;89:56–61
23. Dedo D, Alonso W, Ogura J. Povidone-iodine: an adjunct in the treatment of wound infections, dehiscences, and fistulas in head and neck surgery. *Trans Am Acad Ophthalmol Otolaryngol* 1977;84:68–74
24. Cummings C. Complications of surgery of the larynx. In: Eisele D, ed. *Complications in Head and Neck Surgery*. St Louis, MO: CV Mosby; 1993:333–343
25. Zbar R, Funk G, McCulloch T, et al. Pectoralis major myofascial flap: a valuable tool in contemporary head and neck reconstruction. *Head Neck* 1997;19:412–418
26. Rubin J. Repair of post-laryngectomy pharyngeal fistulae. *J Laryngol Otol* 1989;103:302–305
27. Stell P, Maisels D. Closure of pharyngocutaneous fistulae. In: Ballantyne J, Harrison D, eds. *Rob and Smith's Operative Surgery*. Boston: Butterworths; 1986:448–458
28. Gall A, Sessions D, Ogura J. Complications following surgery for cancer of the larynx and hypopharynx. *Cancer* 1977;39: 624–631

Fistulae in Head and Neck Surgery

CHAPTER 59

Aongus J. Curran and Patrick J. Gullane

Fistula formation after head and neck surgery is a serious complication as it leads to prolonged hospitalization and increased patient morbidity. The overall reported incidence varies considerably in the literature, although generally one-third of people who undergo major ablative surgery for oral, pharyngeal, hypopharyngeal, and laryngeal cancers will develop a fistula.[1,2] Despite this frequency, there is considerable debate among surgeons as to the most important risk factors and how best to prevent fistula formation. Any factor that impairs wound healing, such as poor nutritional status and preoperative radiotherapy, is likely to contribute to the formation of a fistula.[3,4] Synchronous neck dissection, low postoperative hemoglobin, type of pharyngeal closure (T versus linear), and residual disease are other factors that may predispose to this complication.[5,6] Technical factors, such as gentle atraumatic handling of the soft tissues, achieving a watertight anastomosis, ensuring complete hemostasis, and using closed suction drains to eliminate dead space, are key factors in its prevention. In our institution, the rate of postlaryngectomy pharyngocutaneous fistulae and its association with age, gender, preoperative radiation, TNM staging, and a number of other clinical and therapeutic parameters, was investigated.[7] The overall fistula rate was 22% and no association was found between any of the above clinical or treatment parameters and the likelihood of developing a fistula. The development of a fistula post head and neck surgery remains a common and poorly understood problem. This chapter focuses on the main types of fistulae and how they are best managed.

Pharyngocutaneous Fistula

Pharyngocutaneous fistulae usually follows oncologic resection of oropharyngeal, hypopharyngeal, or laryngeal tumors. Once this occurs, saliva pours into the neck and this may lead to skin breakdown, flap necrosis, vessel exposure, and/or rupture. Initially erythema and tenderness in the lower neck incision or skin flap are present, which leads to the development of a fistula. There may be an associated pyrexia and leukocytosis. The extent of the fistula will become apparent over a number of days and is primarily dependent on the degree of mucosal separation at the site of closure. With massive fistulae, the entire neck skin may slough, exposing major neural and vascular structures.

Management

This may be conservative or surgical and is dictated by size and location of the fistula. Small fistulas often heal spontaneously with meticulous wound care, consisting of antiseptic dressings, minimal debridement, and antibiotics. The patient is fed by nasogastric/gastrostomy tube or parenterally with careful monitoring of nutritional and biochemical status. With this form of management, most fistulae heal by secondary intention. Every attempt is made to divert the flow of saliva medial to the carotid artery, usually with the aid of a carefully placed Penrose drain and to minimize tracheal aspiration. Oral feeding is commenced once the integrity of the upper aerodigestive tract is ensured by contrast medium or Methylene Blue dye swallow. Small fistulae may take up to 1 month or more to close by such a conservative approach.

Massive fistulas are associated with extensive overlying skin loss and mucosal dehiscence. Initial management consists of controlled exteriorization after surgical debridement. Residual or recurrent disease must be considered a possibility when a large fistula fails to close by secondary intention. The conservative measures described above for smaller fistulae also apply to this group of patients; once clean/fresh granulation tissue appears, the wound is usually ready for closure. The exception is the patient with major vessel exposure where urgent cover with vascularized tissue is needed to prevent carotid artery or internal jugular vein blow-out. Local, pedicled, and free flaps may be employed to cover exposed vascular structures. The most commonly used flaps are pectoralis major myocutaneous and free radial forearm flaps for this purpose. The goal is to ensure that mucosal continuity is maintained and adequate skin cover is established. One flap may suffice to provide skin cover when enough local tissue is available to close the mucosal defect. Occasionally, extensive loss of mucosa combined with skin may require two flaps. A free radial forearm flap is a good choice to ensure mucosal continuity is maintained and a pectoralis major myocutaneous flap provides bulk to cover vital vascular structures and skin cover. Various flaps may be utilized alone or in combination, and this will depend on the surgeon's preference and previous experience.

Orocutaneous Fistula

Cancer of the oral cavity accounts for approximately 30% of head and neck carcinomas. Surgical intervention ranges from simple excision with minimal morbidity to composite resection with significant attendant complications. When large resections are necessary and mandibulotomy is required for access, a fistula may ensue. Currently as mandibular osteotomy has become the preferred method of access for the majority of large oral cavity and oropharyngeal tumours, this complication is not infrequent.[8,9] Previous investigators have attempted to identify factors that may predispose to mandibulotomy sepsis and fistula formation, although no consensus has been reached as to the precise cause. Preoperative irradiation and type of fixation (wire or plate) does not appear to influence the incidence of sepsis, although most studies have been retrospective in nature.[10,11] A failure to achieve a watertight mucosal closure adjacent to the mandibulotomy site, even when using a free flap to reconstruct the defect, is an important factor. Patients who undergo step osteotomy as opposed to linear cuts and those who have a marginal mandibulectomy in combination with the resection are not at an increased risk of infection.

Generally, the management of this complication is similar in principal to that of pharyngocutaneous fistulae. Small fistulae respond to conservative measures with meticulous wound care and antibiotic therapy. Early recognition and intervention are key to the successful management of this complication. Diverting the flow of saliva away from the great vessels and keeping skin flaps viable will result in spontaneous healing of most fistulae. Placement of a Savory tube into the pharynx may be useful to direct saliva away from the neck. Necrotic tissue must be carefully excised, and appropriate antibiotic therapy is guided by culture and sensitivity. Larger fistulae and those extending over the carotid artery require vascularized tissue flaps to avoid carotid artery or jugular vein blowout. When plate exposure is contributing to persistence of the fistula, removal of the plate and reconstruction with an appropriate flap are necessary.

Chylous Fistula

Chylous fistulae occur in approximately 2% of neck dissections and mostly on the left side (75% of cases).[12] Chyle is composed of the products of fat digestion (chylomicrons), and therefore persistent loss can lead to significant electrolyte disturbance, impaired wound healing, and nutritional imbalance. Intraoperatively, a leak may be recognized by the presence of a clear/milky fluid collection in the lower neck or by a greasy feel to the surgical gloves.

A suspected leak should be confirmed by placing the patient in the Trendelenburg position and asking the anaesthesiologist to apply continuous positive airway pressure (i.e., Valsalva). This increases the flow of chyle by raising the venous and lymphatic pressures. Ligation of the thinned walled thoracic duct in isolation is not recommended, and it is better to include the surrounding tissue with the duct using a nonabsorbable suture. The scalene muscle can be included with this suture ligature. Many leaks are not treated adequately when noticed intraoperatively; attention at this stage will reduce the incidence of fistula formation. Surgical glues and sclerosing agents such as tetracycline have been used with some reported success.[12]

The presence of fluid with a milky appearance or continuous fluid from the neck drains once feeding begins is likely to be due to a chylous fistula. An intense inflammatory response due to chyle may cause flap compromise or loss of the overlying skin. When in doubt, the presence of triglycerides in this fluid confirm the diagnosis. The goal of management is to optimize the patient's nutritional status and reduce the volume of chyle production.

Management

A low output leak can usually be managed with aspiration, a pressure dressing, and dietary manipulation. The patient should have nasogastric feeding discontinued and a medium chain triglyceride diet or a compound such as Vivonex (98% fat-free solution) commenced. Collaboration with a dietitian and careful monitoring of electrolytes are also necessary.

Failure of the above regimen or in the presence of a high output leak (>500 ml/day) for 3 days or longer despite conservative management, warrants surgical intervention. A neck reexploration on the 4th or 5th postoperative day is the best approach in this setting.[13] Feeding the patient 100 to 200 ml of cream 1 to 3 h preoperatively will improve the changes of identifying the leak at the time of reexploration. Placing the patient in the Trendelenburg position with the use of continuous positive pressure also helps in localization. Also, the application of a sclerosing agent such as tetracycline after ligating the duct may also be beneficial at this stage.[13] Close suction drainage is used, and the patient is managed postoperatively with a medium chain triglyceride diet and careful electrolytic monitoring. A thoracoscopic ligation of the thoracic duct is an effective method of controlling a leak if neck reexploration fails or in the rare clinical situation of a chylothorax.[14]

Conclusion

In summary, fistula formation after head and neck surgery is common, with uncertainty regarding predisposing factors. Because of the retrospective nature of previous studies, this controversy is bound to continue. This chapter attempts to address factors important in the prevention of this problem and to detail how best to manage a fistula once it develops. It is important to realize that clinically the fistula may range from a tiny opening to a wide-open pharyngeal cavity in size; this can represent a considerable challenge to the surgeon. In most cases, conservative treatment is appropriate initially. Successful closure of the larger fistula is possible in most instances, although considerable technical skill and planning are necessary to achieve this goal.

REFERENCES

Curran and Gullane—CHAPTER 59

1. Dedo DD, Alonso WA, Ogura JH. Incidence and predisposing factors and outcome of pharyngocutaneous fistulas. *Ann Otol Rhino Laryngol* 1975;84:833–838
2. Lavell RJ, Maw AR. The etiology of post-laryngectomy pharyngocutaneous fistulae. *J Laryngol Otol* 1972,86: 785–793

3. Havas TE, Gullane PJ. Prevention of complications in head and neck surgery. A self-instructional package. American Academy of Otolaryngology–Head and Neck Surgery Foundation. Alexandria, VA; 1987
4. Giordano AM, Adams GL. Pharyngocutaneous fistula after laryngeal surgery. *Otolaryngol Head Neck Surg* 1984;92: 19–23
5. Gullane PJ, Jabbour JN, Conley JJ, et al. Correlation of pharyngeal fistulization with pre-operative radiotherapy, reduced serum albumin and dietary obstruction. *Otolaryngol Head Neck Surg* 1979;87:311–317
6. Hooley R, Levin H, Flores TC, et al. Predicting post-operative head and neck complications using nutritional assessment: the prognostic nutritional index. *Arch Otolaryngol* 1983;107: 725–729
7. Parikh SR, Irish JC, Curran AJ, et al. Pharyngocutaneous fistulae in laryngectomy patients: the Toronto Hospital experience. *Otolaryngol* 1998;27:3:136–140
8. MacGregor IA, McDonald DG. Mandibular osteotomy in the surgical approach to the oral cavity. *Head Neck Surg* 1983,5: 457–462
9. Spir RH, Gerold F0, Shah JP, et al. Mandibulotomy approach to oropharyngeal tumours. *Am J Surg* 1985;150:466–469
10. Davidson J, Freeman J, Gullane P, et al. Mandibulotomy and radical radiotherapy: compatible or not? *J Otolaryngol* 1988; 17:279–281
11. McCann K, Irish J, Gullane P, et al. Complications associated with rigid fixation of the mandibulotomies. *J Otolaryngol* 1994;23(3):210–215
12. Kassel RN, Havas TE, Gullane PJ. The use of topical tetracycline in the management of persistent chylous fistula. *J Otolaryngol* 1987:16:174–178
13. Crumley RL, Smith JD. Postoperative chylous fistula prevention and management. *Laryngoscope* 1976,86:804–813
14. Kent RB, Pinson TW. Thorascopic ligation of the thoracic duct. *Surg Endosc* 1993;7:52–55

Fistulae in Head and Neck Surgery

CHAPTER 60

Clarence T. Sasaki, James Alex, and Sanchayeeta Mitra

A head and neck fistula typically refers to an unplanned postoperative communication between the upper aerodigestive tract and skin. Although this term may also refer to other types of fistulae, such as a tracheal fistula or chylous fistula, this chapter focuses primarily on pharyngocutaneous fistulae. Postoperative fistula formation remains a challenging problem that can be managed only with understanding of causative factors, diagnosis, methods of prevention, and treatment options.

Background

All patients undergoing surgery of the upper aerodigestive tract are at risk of pharyngocutaneous fistula, even in the hands of the most technically competent surgeons. The first laryngectomy carried out by Billroth in 1873 was complicated by a large pharyngocutaneous fistula and eventual death. The current incidence of pharyngocutaneous fistula after laryngectomy varies widely in the literature. Giordano et al.[1] report an average fistulization rate of 17%, whereas Weissler[2] ranged from 9% to 21%, and Papazoglou et al.[3] note an incidence varying between 2 and 66%.

Causative Factors

Several factors are thought to cause or predispose to fistula formation. They are most easily classified into local and systemic factors with several subdivisions in each group. Because preventing a fistula is much less costly and morbid than treating one, identifying and minimizing these risks helps promote uncomplicated wound healing and prevents fistula formation.

LOCAL FACTORS

The most significant factor in fistula formation is an associated wound infection. The oral cavity, pharynx, and larynx are clean contaminated surgical sites, exposed not only to saliva, but also to tracheal, pulmonary, and regurgitant gastric secretions. Kirchner at al.[4] have shown bacterial counts in saliva of irradiated subjects to be as high as 10^5/ml. Others have shown decreased fistula rates when dental prophylaxis precedes tumor resection. As shown by Weber et al.,[5] wound infection rates are 30 to 80% without antibiotic prophylaxis and decrease to about 5 to 30% with appropriate antibiotic administration. Modern surgical techniques and preoperative administration of prophylactic antibiotics have been critical factors in preventing wound infections and fistula formation in head and neck surgery.

Gastroesophageal reflux has been identified as an important factor in many inflammatory and neoplastic disorders of the aerodigestive tract. Although no definitive studies have shown a correlation between reflux and fistulization, Seikaly and Park[6] showed a decreased rate of fistulae formation in patients treated with a postoperative antireflux regimen. We routinely maintain intravenous H_2 blocking agents until gastric feeding can be started via tube feeds.

The effect of preoperative radiation therapy on fistula formation remains controversial. Studies reported by Dedo et al.,[7] Mendelsohn et al.[8] and others report that preoperative radiation predisposes to fistula formation by damaging tissue, decreasing vascular perfusion, and delaying healing. However, other studies, including Thawley[9] and, more recently, Fradis et al.[10] and Soylu et al.,[11] concluded that radiation does not correlate with the likelihood of fistulization. Studies of patients undergoing brachytherapy show wound complication rates ranging from 10% to 50% in patients undergoing either brachytherapy as part of their initial cancer treatment or combined surgery–brachytherapy for salvage. In our experience, prior full-course radiotherapy (>5000 cGy) and brachytherapy have a detrimental effect on wound healing and are considered risk factors for compromised healing and fistulization. As a general practice, a trial of oral intake that might routinely take place on postoperative day 7 is deferred until postoperative day 10 in the previously irradiated or implanted patient.

Another well-established cause of fistula formation is tight wound closure that places undue tension on the suture line. Advanced T3 and T4 tumors have a higher incidence of fistula formation, due primarily to the added resection of the pharyngeal wall and consequent tighter closure. Similarly, pharyngocutaneous fistulae are more common with total laryngectomy or partial laryngopharyngectomy than with supraglottic resection due to extension of the resection to include the pyriform area. Although the extent of oncologic resection is not within the reconstructive surgeon's control, reconstructive efforts should strive to minimize tight closure. If the pharyngeal closure is tight enough to impair the outflow of the swallowed bolus, saliva will follow the path of least resistance and may leak through the suture line during swallowing. Similarly, distal anastomotic stricture in gastric pullup may lead to outflow resistance and cause backup of secretions. The problem of tense closure can be managed by recruiting additional tissue for closure of the pharyngeal mucosa over a nasogastric tube. As shown by Horowitz and Sasaki,[11] upper esophageal sphincter myotomy at total laryngectomy significantly decreases peak pharyngeal pressures, minimizing proximal fistulization through the suture line. Clayman and Weber[12] report a 20% fistula rate with gastric pullup reconstruction of circumferential hypopharyngeal defects, with a rate of only 2% with free jejunal transfer—a difference they attribute to decreased tension of closure with free jejunal transfer giving less concern about tethering. At our institution, laryngopharyngoesophagectomy with gastric transposition is more commonly performed than free jejunal transfer, with a fistulization rate of 3%.

The last local predisposing factor in the development of pharyngocutaneous fistula is residual gross or microscopic tumor at the surgical site or resection margins. Residual tumor disrupts the healing process, leads to wound infection, and results in early dehiscence and fistula formation. Fistulae that occur within 1 to 2 weeks postoperatively frequently reflect problems relating to systemic and local factors in wound healing. Those occurring about 2 to 3 weeks postoperatively may also be due to these same factors, however, persistent cancer should also be considered, particularly if the fistula persists despite appropriate management.

SYSTEMIC FACTORS

In addition to the local factors reviewed previously, there are several systemic considerations that impact on a patient's ability to heal. Many of these systemic factors are related directly to the risk factors that predispose to head and neck cancer itself: heavy alcohol use and smoking. Patients who continue to smoke until surgery often not only suffer from compromised pulmonary status but are at increased risk of wound breakdown due to poor distal vascular perfusion caused by a direct nicotine effect.

Similarly, patients with a history of alcohol abuse are at an increased risk for poor wound healing due to nutritional depletion. For patients who continue to drink actively up to the time of surgery, delirium tremens also poses a concern. The signs of delirium tremens usually begin approximately 48 to 72 h postoperatively and may be life-threatening if unattended promptly. In addition to cardiopulmonary compromise, significant concern is maintained for the physical disruption of the wound by an agitated thrashing patient, particularly in the setting of a tight closure or underlying free flap.

Most head and neck cancer patients present with some degree of malnutrition. Poor oral intake due to mechanical obstruction, and/or chronic alcoholism is common. In this situation, properly diagnosing malnutrition and restoring the patient to a positive nitrogen balance becomes critical.

Other systemic conditions, such as cardiopulmonary compromise, diabetes mellitus, chronic steroid use, hypothyroidism, or other conditions leading to immune system deficiency should also be addressed in the preoperative evaluation and followed closely postoperatively.

Prevention and Optimization

Identifying and minimizing the factors that predispose to fistula formation helps improve the chance of successful wound healing. Since most fistulae are associated with a wound infection, appropriate antibiotic coverage is essential. Studies by Johnson et al. and more recently by Weber et al.[5] show a marked decrease in wound infection rates with appropriate antibiotic administration. For maximum efficacy, one dose should be given preoperatively so that antibiotics are in the circulation before the skin incision is made. The spectrum of coverage should include oral anaerobes as well as aerobic gram-positive and negative bacteria, including *Staphylococcus aureus*. We favor the standard combination of cefazolin and metronidazole, and reserve clindamycin for patients with penicillin allergy. Although ampicillin with sulbactam and single coverage with cefuroxime (second-generation cephalosporin) or cefotaxime (third-generation cephalosporin) have been found effective, we do not routinely use them in uncomplicated cases. A short 48-h postoperative course of parenteral prophylaxis is sufficient in routine cases and minimizes the risk of bacterial resistance, superinfection, and antibiotic-associated colitis. Clindamycin mouth rinses have been shown by Kirchner and Sasaki to reduce levels of both aerobic and anaerobic bacteria significantly and are usually started on postoperative day 1 in patients who have undergone oral cavity procedures.

Patients with a recent history of alcohol abuse should receive postoperative thiamine, folate, and vitamin B_{12} supplementation. For patients who continue to drink actively up to the time of operation, aggressive delirium tremens prophylaxis should be initiated. We typically administer benzodiazepines, either as a standing dose or as needed, depending on the patient's preoperative level of alcohol consumption.

Initial preoperative assessment of nutritional status includes weight (loss of >10% ideal body wt is significant), albumin, and protein levels. Patients with poor nutrition can undergo counseling about adequate vitamin supplementation and the use of high-protein or high-calorie nutritional supplements. For patients who are significantly malnourished or dehydrated, we place a nasogastric tube preoperatively and commence tube feedings. We do not routinely employ preoperative gastrostomy tube placement, except for those patients in whom we anticipate prolonged aspiration or postoperative dysphagia. Postoperative nutritional status is monitored with weight gain and serum prealbumin levels, which are thought to be a more sensitive indicator of nutritional status than albumin alone.

Cardiopulmonary status should be maximized with maintenance of hematocrit ideally above 30%. Although the selective use of perioperative blood transfusions and beta blockers for cardioprotective effect are advocated by some surgeons, they remain an area of debate. In patients with free flaps, vasoconstrictive agents should be avoided. In addition, the threshold for transfusion is kept much higher (hematocrit approximately 25%), primarily given concern for increasing viscosity of blood. Diabetes should be followed closely with tight perioperative control of blood sugar levels and with awareness maintained of the correlation with vascular disease which may impact on flap survival and wound healing. Pulmonary status should be evaluated fully with pulmonary function tests and preoperative arterial blood-gas levels in patients for whom there is concern about persistent postoperative aspiration or chronic ventilator requirement. Subclinical hypothyroidism may be associated with poor wound healing; however, we do not routinely obtain thyroid function tests preoperatively unless the patient has symptoms of hypothyroidism or a history of radiotherapy to the head and neck. Patients with chronic steroid use are started on preoperative vitamin A supplementation to aid in wound healing, as shown in studies by Hunt et al.[13] Finally, some consideration should be given to the patient's age. Although elderly patients undergoing major resection have complication rates similar to those of younger patients, they suffer from more severe medical conditions thus increasing the hazards of any operation.

In all patients, careful handling of tissues and thoughtful planning of skin incisions are important for adequate wound healing. They are particularly important in patients who have previously been irradiated. Care should be taken to preserve the vascular supply to the skin flap and to design the flap closure away from the carotid artery or underlying mucosal closure. Linear incisions paralleling major vessels should be avoided, and may be accomplished with an inverted Y-incision or modifications of the apron flap. Incisions in previously operated patients should use prior skin incisions to prevent devascularization of skin islands.

Meticulous hemostasis is needed and suction drains should be placed to diminish dead space, promote apposition of tissue, and decrease hematoma formation, all of which promote uncomplicated healing. Ideally, the drains should be placed away from an unprotected carotid artery. We usually leave drains on high wall suction until the output is <30 ml over 24 h. Continued assessment of drain function and drainage quality (serosanguinous, bloody, chylous) should be performed to assist in determining the appropriateness of drain removal.

In patients who have undergone previous irradiation or brachytherapy, coverage of underlying vessels or microvascular anastomosis with vascularized soft tissue should be considered. To protect the exposed and radiated carotid artery, vascularized muscle flaps from the levator scapulae, digastric and mylohyoid muscles, or prevertebral fascia can be used for local coverage. Dermal grafts can also be used; however, no definitive improvement in fistulization rates have been seen with their use. Local muscle flaps, such as the sternocleidomastoid, or muscle flaps from areas distant to the radiated fields, such as the pectoralis myocutaneous and trapezius muscle flaps, can also be transposed to cover the carotid artery and support the pharyngeal closure. The pectoralis myocutaneous flap, in particular, has become the workhorse flap in head and neck surgery, largely because it is rapidly harvested and easily transposed into most defects. In addition it provides excellent coverage for vascular structures, protects the pharyngeal closure, replaces lost epithelial lining or compromised neck skin, and provides well-vascularized tissue coverage.

Planned Fistula

In patients with local and systemic risk factors at high risk of spontaneous fistula formation, the deliberate construction of a planned pharyngocutaneous fistula may be considered. A controlled pharyngostoma can be helpful in protecting the suture line and skin flaps in wounds that have undergone previous radiation or are under tight tension. A controlled fistula may be made by placing a large passive drain from the phayrnx to the skin, or with a midline controlled pharyngostoma along the pharynx or tongue base . Salivary flow is then temporarily channeled along the path of least resistance and directed away from major vessels or underlying microvascular anastomosis until definitive reconstruction is possible.

Diagnosis

Early diagnosis of postoperative fistula is imperative to prevent excessive breakdown or spillage along the wound. Fistulae that occur within approximately 1 week postoperatively generally reflect factors relating to poor wound healing, while those occurring within approximately 2 to 3 weeks may reflect persistent cancer. The intraoral and neck suture lines should be examined carefully for evidence of nonhealing. Erythema, firmness, or tenderness of the skin flaps may indicate early infection or hematoma formation. Temperature spikes, leukocytosis, and oral or wound malodor may also be an early sign of fistula formation.

With these signs and symptoms, the suture line should be opened under sterile conditions in the area of greatest erythema and swelling. It is essential that the wound be opened as far away from the carotid artery, tracheostoma, and underlying microvascular anastomosis as possible. Gentle palpation will usually confirm the diagnosis of a localized infection. The presence of a fistula may be detected by visualization of saliva or palpation of a tract. A swallow test with Methylene Blue dye and gauze packing of the wound site can confirm the diagnosis if needed.

Treatment

Upon detection of a fistula, initial management is to gently open the wound as previously described and to palpate carefully for the extent of infection. Identification of the relationship to vascular structures, microvascular anastomoses, and the trachea can be attempted with conservative, careful exploration of the wound. A cuffed tracheotomy tube should be placed in the stoma to prevent aspiration of infected secretions, and the patient made NPO. Nutritional support can ideally be provided by tube feeds, although parenteral nutrition may be used if enteral feeding is not possible. Cultures of wound drainage should be obtained, with empiric intravenous broad spectrum antibiotics (covering anaerobes and gram-negative organisms) started while awaiting culture and sensitivity results.

After the initial standard management, therapy includes both conservative medical management and different levels of surgical management. The appropriate choice of treatment depends on the size and location of the fistula, prior radiation status, and general medical condition. Generally, in patients with no history of radiotherapy, fistulas under <2 cm close spontaneously within 2 to 4 weeks with proper wound care. Moist gauze packings of the fistula tract are applied 3 times each day. The infected tract is packed with gauze soaked in betadine solution or 0.5% acetic acid. As the infection appears to clear, dressing changes should continue with Dakins gauze to stimulate granulation tissue. When granulation tissue appears, packing may be continued with saline soaked strips alone. Oral 0.5% acetic acid solutions, shown to be bacteriostatic, may also be administered (as swish and swallow) to acidify the upper digestive tract. Sharp debridement of overlying necrotic debris and fibrinous exudate should also be performed at least once a day, with care to avoid underlying structures. In otherwise healthy, nonradiated patients, the fistula tract should improve within 2 to 4 weeks of treatment, and persistence of the tract should raise suspicion for residual tumor or distal outflow obstruction.

For patients with a small fistula who have received prior radiotherapy, similar conservative measures are started with the understanding that wound healing is delayed. If the fistula tract lies over vascular structures or a microvascular anastomosis, more aggressive treatment is warranted. Although some investigators recommend immediate return to the operating room, we usually attempt conservative measures for several days. If the wound appears to be infected, debridement and packing are continued to allow for a noninfected bed of granulation tissue should flap reconstruction be necessary. If the tract is unchanged, appears to have worsened after a few days of conservative treatment, or if there is increasing concern for the underlying vessels or anastomosis, the patient is returned to the operating room, the fistula site is opened, and the extent of infection evaluated with gentle blunt dissection. Copious irrigation with warm bacitracin solution is performed after removal of purulent debris and necrotic tissue. Excessive manipulation of the wound is avoided to minimize injury to underlying structures. If the infection appears relatively contained and does not involve vascular structures, a pharyngostome can be created by placement of a passive drain (Penrose, suction drain tubing without application of suction), thus diverting the salivary stream away from the vessels. If the infection is widespread or the skin and vessels tenuous, vascularized tissue should be brought into the wound to hasten healing and to provide protection for the underlying vasculature. Local flaps may be used for coverage if nonirradiated. If the surgical field has been irradiated or epithelial lining is required, the use of the pectoralis myocutaneous flap is a popular choice. First, necrotic edges and nonviable tissue should be removed from the recipient site, and then the pectoralis muscle brought into contact with underlying mucosa and sutured to surrounding tissue. The muscle flap provides a barrier between the vessels and the fistula site. A passive drain should be placed over the muscle flap and advanced over several days, allowing the fistula to close slowly.

Larger pharyngocutaneous fistulae are usually associated with prior radiotherapy and/or a more compromised host. Often there is significant loss of neck skin and wide exposure of underlying structures. The first priority in this type of fistula is protection of the carotid artery and prevention of carotid rupture. If the defect appears infected or is so extensive that local vascularized muscle transfer may not be large enough to provide definitive closure, conservative measures should begin with betadine gauze packing, changed 3 times per day, and debridement twice daily. Adequate nutrition, optimization of cardiopulmonary status, correction of hypothyroidism, and management of any other correctable systemic conditions should also be addressed during this time. Conservative treatment for 1 to 2 weeks usually results in significant decrease in the size of the fistula. Although controversial, hyperbaric oxygen appears to improve wound healing and may be considered for those patients who seem unimproved with other conservative measures. Advocates believe hyperbaric oxygen promotes angiogenesis and helps healing by improving wound oxygenation. Patients who are at risk for carotid artery hemorrhage are followed closely in the hospital. Infected wounds are debrided and packed until gross resolution of infection or a tissue bacterial count of $>10^5$ colony-forming units (CFU)/g is reached. At this time, the bacterial count is felt to be low enough to attempt definitive closure.

In choosing a reconstructive method, the patient's general condition, the extent of the defect, and the availability of vessels in the neck for possible microvascular anastomosis should be considered. Many surgical methods of repair have been reported, but the principles of providing both an internal and external lining remain constant. The pectoralis myocutaneous flap remains an excellent option. It is a sturdy, well-vascularized source of tissue for support and protection of the repair site. The negative features about the flap include its large and bulky size which may put tension on the suture line or cause it to unfurl away from the wound site. In patients who can tolerate a longer procedure or for those patients in whom a pectoralis flap failed or is unavailable, radial forearm free flaps provide another option. This flap can be constructed either alone, providing both the internal pharyngeal and external skin lining, or in conjunction with a myofascial flap to provide the external lining. Other alternatives include the latissimus dorsi free or pedicled flap, in which the skin paddle replaces the internal pharyngeal lining, with skin graft coverage of the external muscle. This flap provides a large amount of coverage; however, it may be excessively thick and bulky. Other reports in the literature include removal of the fistula site and repair with free jejunal transfer or gastric pullup. These operations have higher potential morbidity, but offer the benefit of not requiring a tubular suture line as with a forearm flap.

REFERENCES

Sasaki et al.—CHAPTER 60

1. Giordano AM, Cohen J, Adams GL. Pharyngocutaneous fistula after laryngeal surgery: the role of barium swallow. *Otolaryngol Head Neck Surg* 1984;92(1):19–23
2. Weissler MC. Management of complications resulting from laryngeal cancer treatment. *Otolaryngol Clin North Am* 1997; 30:269–278
3. Papazoglou G, Doundoulakis G, Terzakis G, et al. Pharyngocutaneous fistula after total laryngectomy: incidence, cause, and treatment. *Ann Otol Rhinol Laryngol* 1994;103:801–805
4. Kirchner JC, Edberg SC, Sasaki CT. The use of topical oral antibiotics in head and neck prophylaxis: is it justified? *Laryngoscope* 1988;98:26–29
5. Weber RS, Read I, Frankenthaler R, et al. Ampicillin-sulbactam vs clindamycin in head and neck oncologic surgery. *Arch Otolaryngol Head Neck Surg* 1992;118:1159–1163
6. Seikaly H, Park P. Gastroesophageal reflux prophylaxis decreases the incidence of pharyngocutaneous fistula after total laryngectomy. *Laryngoscope* 1995;105(11):1220–1222
7. Dedo DD, Alonso WA, Ogura JH. Incidence, predisposing factors and outcomes of pharyngocutaneous fistulas complicating head and neck cancer surgery. *Ann Otol Rhinol Laryngol* 1975;84:833–840
8. Mendelsohn MS, Bridger GP. Pharyngocutaneous fistulae following laryngectomy. *Aust NZ J Surg* 1985;55(2): 177–179
9. Thawley SE. Complications of combined radiation therapy and surgery for carcinoma of the larynx and inferior hypopharynx. *Laryngoscope* 1981;91:677–700
10. Fradis M, Podoshin L, Ben David J. Post-laryngectomy pharyngocutaneous fistula—a still unresolved problem. *J Laryngol Otol* 1995;109:221–224
11. Horowitz JB, Sasaki CT. The effect of cricopharyngeus myotomy on postlaryngectomy pharyngeal contraction pressures. *Laryngoscope* 1993;103:138–140
11. Soylu L, Kiroglu M, Aydogan B, et al. Pharyngocutaneous fistula following laryngectomy. *Head Neck* 1998;20(1): 22–25
12. Clayman GL, Weber RS. Pharyngocutaneous fistula. In: Gates GA, ed. Current therapy in otolaryngology–head and neck surgery. St Louis: Mosby; 1994
13. Hunt TK, Ehrlich HP, Garcia JA, et al. Effect of vitamin A on reversing the inhibitory effect of cortisone on healing of open wounds in animals and man. *Ann Surg* 1969;170: 633–641

SUGGESTED READINGS

Sasaki et al.—CHAPTER 60

Freeland AP, Rogers JH. The vascular supply of the cervical skin with reference to incision planning. *Laryngoscope* 1975;85:714–725

Girod DA, McCulloch TM, Tsue TT, Weymuller EA. Risk factors for complications in clean-contaminated head and neck surgical procedures. *Head Neck* 1995;17:7–13

Johnson J, Bloomer WD. Effect of prior radiotherapy on post surgical wound infection. *Head Neck* 1989;11:132–136

Johnson JT, Myers EN, Thearle PB, et al. Antimicrobial prophylaxis for contaminated head and neck surgery. *Laryngoscope* 1984; 94:46–51

Murakami Y, Ikari T, Haraguchi S, et al. Repair of salivary fistula after reconstruction of pharyngoesophagus. *Arch Otol Head Neck* 1998;114:770–774

Nemiroff PM, Lungu AL. The influence of hyperbaric oxygen and irradiation on vascularity in skin flaps. *Surg Forum* 1987; 38:565

Peat BG, Boyd JB, Gullane PJ. Massive pharyngocutaneous fistula: salvage with two-layer flap closure. *Ann Plast Surg* 1992;29:153–156

Redleaf MI, Bauer CA. Topical antiseptic mouthwash in oncological surgery of the oral cavity and oropharynx. *J Laryngol Otol* 1994;108:973–979

Sasaki CT, Salzer SJ, Cahow E, et al. Laryngopharyngoesophagectomy for advanced hypopharyngeal and esophageal squamous cell carcinoma: the Yale experience. *Laryngoscope* 1995;105:160–163

Sasaki CT, Gardiner LJ, Kirchner JC. The split muscle flap in pharyngeal closure after laryngectomy—"how I do it." *Laryngoscope* 1983;93:821–822

Weber RS, Callender DL. Antibiotic prophylaxis in clean-contaminated head and neck oncologic surgery. *Ann Otol Rhinol Laryngol* 1992;102:16–20

Zbar RIS, Funk GF, McCulloch TM, Graham SM, Hoffman HT. The pectoralis major myofascial flap: a valuable tool in contemporary head and neck reconstruction. *Head Neck* 1997;19: 412–418

21

Assessment and Management of the Unknown Primary with Neck Disease

"Suspicious areas of mucosa (e.g., leukoplakia, erythroplasia, or mucosal irregularities seen on prior physical examination or on imaging studies) should be biopsied. If no such lesions are seen, random biopsies should be performed on mucosal sites with the known highest probability of harboring a tumor (i.e., nasopharynx, tonsil, tongue base, pyriform sinus.)"

J. Oliver Donegan

"The routine use of CT or MRI for the purpose of attempting to identify a primary site responsible for the cervical metastasis, however, is controversial. Some consider the routine use of either of these studies as unnecessary; others regard them as indispensable."

Robert P. Zitsch III

"The potential to improve management of patients with an unknown primary SCC metastatic to the neck through administration of adjuvant chemotherapy is attractive. However, there are currently no strong data to support the use of chemotherapy in this setting."

Henry T. Hoffman

Assessment and Management of the Unknown Primary with Neck Disease

CHAPTER 61

J. Oliver Donegan

Metastatic disease in cervical lymph nodes may be the initial manifestation of cancer. Most of these patients will have an apparent primary at presentation. However despite the most exhaustive search, approximately 5 to 10% of these tumors remain undetected at the primary site.[1-3]

Each year, an estimated 40,000 patients with a new unknown primary tumor present in the United States.[4] Most (>85%) are adenocarcinomas. In the head and neck, approximately 60% of such occult primaries represent squamous cell carcinoma. Thirty percent are adenocarcinomas and the remainder are tumors originating in the thyroid gland, melanoma of the skin and mucosa, and poorly differentiated carcinoma.

If the metastases are from a squamous cell carcinoma, the primary is found in the head and neck region in the majority of cases.[1] Metastatic adenocarcinoma most often originates in a primary tumor below the clavicles, such as in the lung, the gastrointestinal (GI) tract, the genito-urinary (GU) tract, breast, and pancreas. However, a small number of these adenocarcinomas may originate in the head and neck from the salivary glands, paranasal sinuses, and the nasal cavity.

Metastases to the cervical lymph nodes as an initial presenting event from tumors below the clavicles are quite uncommon, representing only approximately 4% of such cases. Only 1.5% of lung tumors, for example, will present in such a manner.[1]

Lymph nodes in zone 2 of the neck are the most common sites of metastases from an unknown primary, representing approximately 60 to 70% of cases. A significant proportion of supraclavicular lymph nodes represent metastatic adenocarcinoma and the majority of these tumors originate below the clavicles. Of known primary lesions metastatic to supraclavicular lymph nodes, approximately 20% only originate in the head and neck.

Several aspects of the assessment and management of patients with occult primary tumors have generated controversy and debate over the years. These issues include (1) the role of radiologic studies in identifying the primary lesion and assessment of cervical adenopathy; (2) the possible adverse effects of early open neck biopsy; (3) the value of tonsillectomy in identifying the primary lesion; (4) the question of branchiogenic carcinoma as a possible diagnosis; (5) the role of surgery, radiation, and chemotherapy in the management of these patients; (6) the advantages and disadvantages of treating the likely mucosal sites of the primary lesion; and (7) the value of random or directed biopsies at time of endoscopy.

The successful treatment of the metastatic neck disease and prevention of the primary tumor growth are the keys to patient survival. The management of a patient with an unknown primary carcinoma with metastatic disease in the neck remains a challenge to the head and neck surgeon and others including radiation therapists and oncologists involved in the management of these patients. However with appropriate evaluation and treatment, many of these patients have an excellent prognosis. Those patients with squamous cell carcinoma most of whom likely have primaries in the head and neck, can expect a favorable response to treatment especially if the nodal disease is limited. By contrast, patients with adenocarcinoma, most of which originate below the clavicles, generally have a very poor prognosis.

Evaluation of Patient

It is important that every effort be made to locate the primary tumor. If found, the primary can be adequately and appropriately treated and the patient's prognosis therefore better assessed. In addition, locating the primary lesion may avoid extensive mucosal radiation and therefore avoid the often severe adverse effects of wide-field mucosal irradiation. These adverse effects include severe xerostomia, dental caries, laryngeal edema, osteoradionecrosis of the mandible, laryngeal chondritis, persistent pain, dysphagia due to submucosal fibrosis of the pharynx, hypothyroidism, hypopituitarism, and aspiration.[5-8]

Most patients with head and neck cancer have squamous cell carcinoma arising from mucosal surfaces of the head and neck. Most of these patients are more than 40 years of age with a 4 or 5 to 1 male/female ratio. The vast majority of these patients relate a history of tobacco use, usually cigarette smoking, and many have a history of alcohol abuse. A patient presenting with a mass in the neck that is nontender and enlarging and who matches the above profile, should be regarded as having cancer until proven otherwise. An orderly stepwise approach should be taken in evaluating these patients. Most physicians treating these patients agree that open biopsy of the neck mass should be delayed until later stages of evaluation.

A careful history may elicit symptoms of pain in the oral cavity, the oropharynx, or hypopharyngeal areas, possibly with referred otalgia. Symptoms of hoarseness, dysphagia, odynophagia, or hemoptysis, or the awareness of a mass or ulcer in the oral cavity or the oropharynx, may alert the physician to the possible site of a primary tumor. One should inquire about symptoms such as weight loss, fever or night sweats, abdominal pain, melena, diarrhea, and hematuria. The patient should be questioned about history of thyroid or skin cancer or other tumors, including tumors below the clavicles (i.e., in the GI tract, lung, or GU tract). For example, renal cell carcinoma may metastasize to the head and neck 10 to 15 years or more after the initial diagnosis.

A detailed examination of the head and neck should follow. The number and location of lymph nodes in the neck are then assessed. Contralateral neck disease should not be overlooked. The site of lymph node involvement may suggest the location of the primary tumor.[8,9]

Primary Cancer Sites Based on Neck Node Location

The primary cancer sites based on neck node location are as follows:

Level 1. submandibular/submental: lips, buccal mucosa, anterior nasal cavity, soft tissues of the cheek, oral cavity
Level 2. upper jugular: oral cavity, oropharynx, nasopharynx, supraglottic larynx, hypopharynx
Level 3. mid jugular: larynx, hypopharynx, thyroid
Level 4. lower jugular: larynx, thyroid, esophagus, lung, upper GI tract
Level 5. posterior triangle of neck: nasopharynx, thyroid, cervical esophagus

When assessing cervical adenopathy, one should also note the size of the lymph nodes, mobility or possible fixation of these lymph nodes to the skull base, prevertebral muscles, or carotid artery. The neck is staged according to the American Joint Committee on Cancer Clinical Nodal Staging Guidelines (1988).

The skin of the head and neck including the scalp should be assessed, as squamous cell carcinoma or melanoma may metastasize to cervical lymph nodes. The major salivary glands should also be examined. A cranial nerve examination is undertaken.

The oral cavity and the oropharynx are next examined. The patient is requested to remove dentures if these are present. Particular attention is paid to the posterior floor of the mouth and the adjacent tongue and tonsillar fossae as tumors in these areas can be easily missed on a cursory examination. Palpation of the oral cavity and oropharynx should be included in the assessment as some tumors are often palpable before being readily visualized. The ears are evaluated for the possible presence of a middle ear effusion which may be an early finding in cancer of the nasopharynx.

Flexible fiberoptic evaluation of the nasal cavities, the nasopharynx, larynx, and hypopharynx is the next step in the patient's evaluation. Indirect laryngoscopy and nasopharyngoscopy remain a valuable technique for examination but many physicians simply find the fiberoptic instruments permit a more thorough and detailed evaluation in most patients. The nasal mucosa is prepared by spraying with a topical anesthetic/vasoconstrictor mix. The nasal mucosa is then carefully evaluated, followed by evaluation of the nasopharynx.

The fiberoptic instrument is now advanced and the hypopharynx and larynx examined. The mobility of the vocal cords should be assessed and during phonation, the depths of the pyriform sinuses and the postcricoid regions may be visualized. The subglottis may be seen during this part of the examination. The tongue base and vallecula should be evaluated and again during phonation, the deeper region of the vallecula including the lingual surface of the epiglottis are usually well seen. The majority of the mucosal surfaces of the larynx, the hypopharynx, and tongue base can thus be thoroughly evaluated. Note should be made of areas of mucosal leukoplakia, erythroplasia, asymmetry, or friability with easy bleeding, as these areas may harbor neoplastic change. Pooling of secretions in the pyriform sinus may also be a clue to the presence of a tumor in the hypopharynx.

In many patients, the primary carcinoma will be identified following such a thorough examination in an office setting. However, if a primary lesion remains undetected at this point, the patient should undergo a further orderly evaluation to include fine needle aspiration of the neck mass, imaging studies, and endoscopy under anesthesia. An open biopsy of the neck mass is best avoided until the rest of the evaluation has been completed.

A recommendation for delaying an open biopsy of the neck mass has been axiomatic in head and neck surgery for many years. McGuirt and McCabe[10] demonstrated an increased incidence of wound necrosis, regional recurrence, and distant metastatic disease in patients who had a nodal biopsy before a full diagnosis and definitive treatment with neck dissection. Other investigators have shared this concern.[3,11] However, a subsequent study by Robbins and others, did not corroborate these findings.[12-18] Robbins et al.[12] concluded that an open biopsy does not signify a poor prognosis provided adequate therapy is subsequently given. Mack et al.[13] concluded, based on their data and on a review of the pertinent literature, that excisional biopsy of a solitary neck node does not have a detrimental effect on neck control or distant metastatic rate as long as the next step in treatment includes radiation therapy. Ellis et al.[14] concluded that the potential adverse effect of violating the neck before definitive treatment cannot be demonstrated if radiation therapy is the next step in the patient's management. McGuirt's results might be explained by the fact that open biopsy may spread cancer cells into tissues not removed by classic radical neck dissection, but these cells are often sterilized by adequate doses of radiotherapy. However, as many of these patients with neck masses will be diagnosed as having squamous cell carcinoma, an ongoing search for the primary should be undertaken before open biopsy, so that both the primary and neck can receive definitive treatment. It is recommended that an open biopsy take place at the conclusion of the full evaluation.

A fine-needle aspiration biopsy (FNAB) of the neck mass may now be undertaken. A 22-gauge needle and 10 cc syringe are used to obtain the aspirate. Several passes with the needle through different portions of the neck node should be accomplished in order to obtain an adequate sample. If an adequate sample is obtained, and if squamous cell carcinoma is present in the lymph node, there is an approximately 95 to 98% chance of establishing this diagnosis correctly.[7] If such a diagnosis is established, the search for the primary tumor should proceed with imaging studies, and endoscopy of the upper aerodigestive tract under anesthesia. The fine-needle aspirate may establish the presence of other malignancies, such as thyroid carcinoma, lymphoma, or adenocarcinoma, in which case the search may be directed to the appropriate regions. Fine-needle aspiration may often establish the histologic diagnosis at this stage. There is no evidence that fine-needle aspiration causes tumor seeding of the needle tract, an increased rate of metastases, or other adverse effects.

If the fine-needle aspirate demonstrates squamous cell carcinoma, the nasopharynx is one possible site of the primary tumor. There is a strong association between carcinoma of the nasopharynx and the Epstein-Barr virus (EBV). High titers of the EBV may be detected in patients with nasopharyngeal carcinoma on serologic testing. The presence of EBV genomes may be detected in cells from the neck aspirate using the polymerase chain reaction (PCR).[19] These findings may point to the nasopharynx as the possible site of the primary.

Imaging Studies

There are physicians who believe that radiologic studies of these patients have a minor role to play in the evaluation.[20,21] However, most believe that radiologic evaluation should be undertaken and may yield valuable information.[22,23] The purpose of pursuing radiologic evaluation is twofold: (1) to assess the extent of nodal disease in the ipsilateral neck and the possible presence of disease in the contralateral neck. Lymph nodes in the retropharyngeal area and the paratrachial region may also be assessed as these are often difficult to detect on clinical examination, (2) possible detection of the primary tumor. Radiologic studies should precede endoscopy and mucosal biopsies. Such studies undertaken after biopsy may be more difficult to interpret because of edema and inflammation at the biopsy sites. Before endoscopy, these studies may alert the physician to mucosal abnormalities that may harbor the primary tumor.

Computed tomography (CT) scanning is the recommended study for evaluation of nodal disease in the neck.[24,25] This modality will assist in delineating the presence of single versus multiple lymph nodes, the presence of contralateral lymph nodes, and the possible extranodal extension of disease. Tumor involvement of the carotid artery, the skull base, and the prevertebral musculature may also be detected. Mancuso and others[24-26] have defined the criteria for the diagnosis of tumor-bearing lymph nodes and also for the possible extranodal extension of disease. The CT criteria for suspecting metastatic disease in lymph nodes includes the following: (1) diameter of the lymph node >15 mm, (2) grouping of three or more 8- to 15-mm lymph nodes, (3) central decreased density of a lymph node, and (4) poorly defined mass in a lymph node-bearing area.

The CT criteria for possible extranodal extension of disease include (1) ill-defined margins around abnormal lymph nodes, (2) edema or thickening of adjacent fat and muscle, (3) loss of facial planes between a mass and adjacent structures such as the carotid sheath.

Magnetic resonance imaging (MRI) scans may also play a valuable role in assessing neck disease and possible location of the primary tumor.[24,25] However, MRI scans have been shown to be less accurate than CT scans in demonstrating the presence of central necrosis in metastatic lymph nodes and in detecting the presence of extracapsular spread of disease. MRI appears to be superior to CT in detecting more subtle mucosal changes possibly due to neoplastic change. The consensus of opinion favors CT over MRI in evaluating these patients and, certainly, CT has been proved more cost effective. In a study by Mendenhall et al.[22] CT and/or MRI correctly identified the primary site in 50% of patients evaluated who had no suggestive findings on physical examination.

The involvement of the carotid artery system by tumor can be quite difficult to ascertain. Van den Brekel et al.[24] noted that tumor encircling a blood vessel more than 270 degrees on CT or MRI scans or tumor that is immobile from the vessel using sonopalpation [palpation with ultrasound] indicates involvement of the vessel wall. Angiography does not appear to enhance findings obtained from CT or MRI studies of vessel involvement.

The role of positron emission tomography (PET) in the evaluation of these patients has recently been reported.[22,27] PET uses 18-F-labeled-floro-2-D-glucose (FDg) to assess the rate of glucose turnover in malignant cells. In limited studies to date, PET has shown promising results in detecting occult primaries and assessing lymph nodes for the presence of metastatic disease. However, this technique remains in the investigational stage for these purposes and its availability is limited due to cost factors.

Thallium-201 Spect scans have also been evaluated in the management of these patients. In a report by Valdes Olmos et al.,[28] the primary site was successfully detected in five of six patients using this technique. This technology may complement the role of CT and/or MRI in the detection of primary tumors. Ultrasound has been reported to be a valuable adjunct to palpation in the detection of lymph node metastases in the neck.[24]

A chest radiograph should be obtained prior to endoscopy. Other radiologic studies are usually not undertaken at this point but may be indicated in certain circumstances. If there is increased concern regarding distant metastases, for example in patients with very extensive neck disease, a CT scan of the chest and the abdomen and a bone scan should be undertaken. If adenocarcinoma has been demonstrated on the fine needle aspirate, these studies should also be undertaken, and an upper and lower GI series may also be indicated. Radiologic evaluation of the sinuses may also be appropriate if no other site for a primary adenocarcinoma has been discovered. If thyroid carcinoma is detected on needle aspiration, then appropriate evaluation of the thyroid, including a thyroid scan is indicated.

Endoscopy

The final step in evaluating the patient is to perform endoscopy of the upper aerodigestive tract under general anesthesia. This examination consists of inspection and palpation of the oral cavity and the oropharynx, direct laryngoscopy, bronchoscopy, esophagoscopy, and nasopharyngoscopy. Suspicious areas of mucosa (e.g., leukoplakia, erythroplasia, or mucosal irregularities seen on prior physical examination or on imaging studies) should be biopsied. If no such lesions are seen, random biopsies should be performed on mucosal sites with the known highest probability of harboring a tumor (i.e., nasopharynx, tonsil, tongue base, pyriform sinus).[7,23] The use of toluidine blue has not proved effective in identifying possible early mucosal carcinoma.[20] If the primary lesion has not been found on physical examination or on radiologic studies, most lesions detected at endoscopy are found in the tonsil or tongue base (80%).[22]

The issue of performing an ipsilateral tonsillectomy during this evaluation has been controversial.[20] However, there is growing evidence that such a procedure should be done, as a tumor located in the depths of the tonsil may be missed on a simple biopsy. In a report by Righi and Sofferman[29] 6 of 19 patients had occult carcinoma in an ipsilateral tonsil which was diagnosed only by examination of the whole tonsil. Microscopy demonstrated that all six tonsils had extensive areas of normal squamous epithelium overlying the malignancies suggesting that simple random biopsies might well have missed the lesion. CT scanning, inspection, and palpation showed no evidence of disease in all of these six patients. There are other reports in the literature supporting such a recommendation.[22,30]

The combination of CT, MRI scanning, and endoscopy with directed biopsies will demonstrate the presence of approximately 20% of occult tumors.[7]

The issue of carcinoma in a branchial cleft cyst may arise in a situation where a cystic neck mass is found to contain squamous cell carcinoma and no obvious primary lesion is found despite appropriate evaluation.[1,31] This concept of carcinoma in a branchial cleft cyst was first reported by Von Volkmann in 1882.[32] Since then, there has been ongoing controversy regarding this issue. Most authorities believe that if this lesion occurs at all, it is very rare indeed.[1] Guidelines for establishing such a diagnosis were outlined by Martin, Morfit, and Ehrlich in 1950:[33] (1) cervical tumor occurs along a line from the tragus extending along the anterior border of the sternocleidomastoid muscle to the clavicle, (2) histology should demonstrate branchial vertigia, (3) no primary lesion is found after 5 years of follow-up, and (4) there is histologic evidence of cancer developing in the wall of an epithelium-lined cyst.

Treatment

The challenge facing the head and neck surgeon and others dealing with these patients with an occult primary includes not only appropriate evaluation but also maximizing the chance of survival while minimizing the morbidity of treatment. The goals of treatment include control of the ipsilateral neck, the contralateral neck, and control of disease at the mucosal primary site.

If the primary tumor remains occult following the above evaluation, then management should proceed as follows. If there is any doubt regarding the histologic diagnosis based on fine needle aspirate, the patient is taken back to the operating room and an open biopsy of the neck mass is performed. If possible, an excisional biopsy rather than an incisional biopsy should be carried out. If lymphoma is diagnosed, no further surgery is indicated and the patient is referred for appropriate treatment. If thyroid carcinoma is identified, further workup of the thyroid is undertaken. If adenocarcinoma is found on biopsy of the neck node, the patient is further evaluated for evidence of a primary adenocarcinoma and the possibility of metastatic disease at other sites. In patients with adenocarcinoma, a nodal biopsy is necessary to attempt to establish the primary tumor site (e.g., signet ring cells suggest a stomach primary). Other immunocytochemistry studies may point to the GI tract, the breast, or the thyroid. If the primary adenocarcinoma remains occult following a very thorough evaluation and if no other metastatic disease is found a neck dissection is performed and postoperative radiation is delivered to the neck.[4] If, as so often happens, there is evidence of widespread metastatic disease, the patient should be referred for possible chemotherapy; there is no indication to operate on the neck in such a situation.

If malignant melanoma is encountered on open neck biopsy, the primary site should be sought in the head and neck, including the scalp and mucosal surfaces. If the primary is not found, it is appropriate to proceed with a radical neck dissection if a search for other metastatic disease is negative. The value of postoperative radiotherapy to the neck in this setting remains controversial. Radiation appears to enhance local control, but not long-term survival.[34] There are optimistic reports that chemotherapy and therapy with interferon may also benefit some of these patients with metastatic malignant melanoma.[35]

If open neck biopsy reveals squamous cell carcinoma, then further management is based on the stage of the neck disease and the treating physician's philosophy regarding management of the possible mucosal primary site. The management of these patients has been quite controversial and review of the literature reveals varying and often confusing results. Treatment options, however, can be summarized as follows: (1) biopsy of the neck (N1), neck dissection, no treatment to the possible primary mucosal sites; (2) biopsy neck (excisional, N1) radiation to the ipsilateral neck and possible primary sites; (3) biopsy neck (excisional, N1), radiation to both necks and possible primary sites; (4) biopsy neck (N2–N3), neck dissection, radiation to both necks and primary mucosal sites; and (5) biopsy neck mass (neck unresectable) radiation to both necks, primary sites with or without concurrent or sequential chemotherapy.

The issue of irradiation to the possible primary mucosal sites in these patients has been very contentious. Many physicians take the view that withholding irradiation to the primary mucosal sites is reasonable. This approach would allow for careful follow-up of the patient following initial treatment and if a primary tumor is subsequently detected, it is then treated appropriately. The rationale for this approach is based on reports in the literature that would suggest that the rate of appearance of the mucosal primary is not affected by withholding radiation to the mucosa, and the patient's outcome is not adversely affected by this management. In addition, this approach avoids the often severe side effects of wide-field mucosal irradiation. DeSanto and Neel[36] at the Mayo Clinic reported on 15 such patients treated with neck dissection only. No primary tumor developed in any of these patients during a follow-up period ranging from 3 to 13 years. Coster et al.[37] updated the Mayo Clinic experience, and subsequently analyzed a series of 24 patients with unilateral cervical node metastases from squamous cell carcinoma of unknown origin. These patients were treated with neck dissection only. A primary tumor subsequently developed in only one, or 4%, of these patients. The 5-year overall survival rate was 60%. Based on this series and a literature review, these investigators state there is no convincing evidence that RT to the mucosa lowers the rate of primary tumor development.

However, other authorities report evidence that radiotherapy to the mucosal primary sites significantly reduces the subsequent appearance of the primary tumor. These same workers also report an adverse effect on survival if the primary tumor develops. In Reddy and Marks's series, the incidence of occult primary appearance was 44% in those patients who did not receive radiation therapy to the primary mucosal sites.[38] In those patients who received radiation to the possible primary mucosal sites, the incidence of subsequent occult primary appearance was 8%. In this series, the 5-year disease-free survival was 20% for those patents in whom a primary appeared versus 54% in those patients who never developed a primary tumor. In a recent report by Colletier et al.,[39] the M.D. Anderson experience for patients treated with surgery and postop radiation therapy for metastatic squamous cell carcinoma to cervical lymph nodes from an unknown primary is updated. This series reports a 6.5% incidence of subsequent appearance of tumor at the primary mucosal sites. In a report by Batani et al.,[40] a 4% incidence of primary mucosal occurrence after prophylactic RT to the mucosa was reported. This author cites a 20 to 40% incidence of primary mucosal occurrence in those patients who did not receive radiation to the mucosal sites. In a review of other series, the reported incidence of occurrence of the primary after radiation ranges within 6 to 16%.[17,18,41,42] In other series, in which patients were not treated with radiation to the mucosa, the reported incidence of subsequent primary appearance ranges within 0 to 40%.[18,38,43] Overall, the consensus would appear to favor radiotherapy to the mucosa, but this view must be balanced against the frequently severe complications of wide-field mucosal radiation. The approach to management of the neck is based on the stage of the nodal disease. Contralateral nodal disease increases with increasing nodal stage.

There is continuing controversy over the management of the N1 neck.[20,21] Many physicians adhere to the view that surgery (neck dissection) should always play a role in the management of the N1 neck. However, there is now convincing evidence that neck dissection alone or excisional biopsy of the neck node followed by radiotherapy may be sufficient to control patients at this stage. Parsons et al.[15] studied a group of patients in whom there was no gross residual disease after excisional biopsy and who were treated with radiation only. The absolute 5-year disease-free survival for this group was 79%, and the rate of neck disease control was 96%. Mendenhall et al.[44] noted that in patients with a single node in the neck less than 3 cm in size, the neck disease control rate was the same in those patients treated with radiation only versus those treated with radiation and neck dissection. These same investigators noted that as the size and number of lymph nodes increased, there was a higher rate of neck control for those patients treated with combined surgery and radiation versus those treated with radiation only. Mack et al.[13] noted comparable results. In this series, 38 patients underwent radiotherapy to the neck following excisional biopsy of a solitary metastatic nodule. The reported incidence of control of neck disease at 5 years was 95%. In Reddy's series, patients treated with excisional biopsy followed by radiotherapy for N1 neck disease were evaluated.[38] All patients in this series treated in this manner had control of disease in the ipsilateral neck. This author also concluded that bilateral neck and mucosal irradiation lowers the incidence of contralateral metastatic disease when compared with radiotherapy to the ipsilateral neck only. The control rate in the contralateral neck for those patients who received radiation to both necks was 86%, as compared with 56% for patients receiving radiation to the ipsilateral neck only.

These studies emphasize that excisional, and not incisional, biopsy should be performed on the single node if radiotherapy only is used to treat the neck. If there is obvious residual disease in the neck after biopsy, or if multiple nodes are found or if there is evidence of extracapsular extension of disease, the neck should be treated with a combination of neck dissection and postoperative radiotherapy. If excision biopsy and radiotherapy are used to treat the N1 neck, the possible primary mucosal sites and both necks may be treated.

By contrast, there is more general agreement that advanced neck disease should be treated with a combination of neck dissection and postoperative irradiation.[39,44-48] Patients with N2 and N3 disease should undergo a neck dissection followed by radiotherapy to both necks and the likely primary mucosal sites. The type of neck dissection used under these circumstances has also been controversial. The traditional approach has been a radical neck dissection with excision of the sternocleidomastoid muscle, the internal jugular vein and the 11th cranial nerve. However, in carefully selected patients, it may be appropriate to perform a modified neck dissection allowing preservation of the 11th cranial nerve and therefore improved shoulder function postoperatively. This modification can be carried out as long as tumor-bearing lymph nodes are not detected along the course of the 11th nerve in the neck or at the skull base. Selective neck dissections are best reserved for management of patients with an N0 neck.[49-52]

In more advanced neck disease where there is fixation to nonresectable structures (i.e., the skull base), radiation has been the management of choice. In more recent years, the combination of radiation and chemotherapy has shown promising results in the management of patients with advanced head and neck cancer. The most promising results have been achieved to date with concomitant multiagent chemotherapy and radiation, with the radiation frequently administered in a hyperfractionated manner.[41,53,54] Further studies are needed to assess the role of these modalities, but certainly results to date are encouraging. Treatment of these patients should include radiation therapy to both necks and to the primary mucosal sites. If residual potentially resectable disease remains in the neck following treatment, it is reasonable to perform a neck dissection. This will achieve significant control of disease in the neck in many of these patients.[53]

After treatment, all patients should be examined at regular intervals. Recurrence in the neck or at the primary site if detected early, may be amenable to salvage surgery and/or radiotherapy. Those patients with squamous cell carcinoma are also at significant risk of the development of a second primary lesion. If a primary lesion does subsequently develop, many of these do so during the first 24 months after treatment.

Prognosis

Several factors impact on the outcome of these patients. These issues include histology, the location and number of lymph nodes in the neck, the presence or absence of extracapsular spread of disease, and the treatment decision. Preventing the development of the primary tumor appears to enhance prognosis.

Adenocarcinoma has a generally very poor prognosis. Lee et al.[4] studied a group of 223 patients with metastatic adenocarcinoma to the neck from an occult primary. The supraclavicular fossa was the presenting site of involvement in 77% of these patients. Only 14% presented with nodes in the upper neck, classified in this study as above the cricoid cartilage; 84% of these patients also had metastatic disease outside the head and neck region. Treatment of these patients involved combinations of neck dissection, radiotherapy, and chemotherapy. There was a 90% mortality at 5 years. The mean survival was 17 months. Patients in this group with unilateral neck disease and with nodes confined above the cricoid cartilage had a slightly increased survival rate.

Patients with squamous cell carcinoma, in general, have a better prognosis than those with adenocarcinoma. The overall survival at 5 years for these patients is approximately 50%.[38,39] Again, however, supraclavicular nodes with squamous cell carcinoma have a very poor prognosis, with approximately 15% surviving only 3 to 5 years.[7] Patients with lymph nodes confined to the upper neck and those without extracapsular spread of disease have a better prognosis.

N1 nodal disease has a very favorable prognosis whether treated with surgery alone, with excisional biopsy and radiation therapy, or with neck dissection and radiation. Five-year disease specific survival rates for this group of patients ranges from 70% to 90%.[13,15,38,44] Early open nodal biopsy does not appear to compromise prognosis as long as radiation is included in subsequent treatment. Patients with N2 to N3 nodal disease do not fare as well. Five-year disease-specific survival rates reported for these patients range from 30% to 60%.[37,44-46]

The rate of distant metastases increases with nodal stage. In Colletier's study, the patients with multiple nodes had a rate of 23% versus 8% in those who presented with a single node in the neck.

For those patients with advanced disease, the prognosis has improved in recent years with the use of hyperfractionated irradiation and concurrent chemotherapy. In Brizels' study, 122 patients with advanced head and neck cancer were treated with hyperfractionated RT with or without concurrent chemotherapy.[53] Most of these patients had unresectable disease. The 3-year overall survival rate was 55% in the combined therapy group and 34% in the hyperfractionation radiotherapy group. The rate of local regional control of disease at 3 years was 70% in the combined treatment group versus 44% in the radiotherapy-only group. This study supports an increasing role for chemotherapy in the management of patients with advanced or unresectable disease. Other series also report encouraging results.[54]

Conclusion

Patients presenting with metastatic disease in the neck from an occult primary tumor remain a diagnostic and therapeutic challenge. However, many patients presenting with squamous cell carcinoma, especially those with early stage disease, may be offered effective treatment with the prospect of a favorable outcome. It is essential that a thorough evaluation be undertaken before definitive therapy. Careful physical examination, imaging studies, and endoscopy with biopsies will detect the primary tumor in 90% of patients presenting with a node in the neck. The outcome for patients with advanced disease may be improving with the advent of hyperfractionated radiation and concurrent chemotherapy.

REFERENCES

Donegan—CHAPTER 61

1. Batsakis JG. Metastatic neoplasms to and from the head and neck. In: *Tumors of the Head and Neck.* 2nd Ed. Baltimore: Williams & Wilkins;1979:40–251
2. Nguyen C, Shenouda G, Black MJ, et al. Metastatic squamous cell carcinoma to cervical lymph nodes from unknown primary mucosal sites. *Head Neck* 1994;16:58–63
3. Jones AS, Cook JA, Phillips DE, Roland NR. Squamous carcinoma presenting as an enlarged cervical lymph node. *Cancer* 1993;72:1756–1761
4. Lee NK, Byers RM, Abbruzzese JL, Wolf P. Metastatic adenocarcinoma to the neck from an unknown primary source. *Am J Surg* 1991;162:306–309
5. Freeman D, Mendenhall WM, Parsons JT, Million RR. Unknown primary squamous cell carcinoma of the head and neck: is mucosal irradiation necessary? *Int J Radiat Oncol Biol Phys* 1992;23:889–890
6. Collins SL. Controversies in management of cancer of the neck. In: Thawley SE, Panje WR, Batsakis JG, Lindberg RD, eds. *Comprehensive Management of Head and Neck Tumors.* 2nd Ed. Philadelphia: WB Saunders, 1998:1479–1562
7. Metastatic cancer of occult origin to cervical lymph nodes. In: Gluckman JL, ed. *Renewal of Certification Study Guide in Otolaryngology Head and Neck Surgery.* Dubuque, IA: Kendall/Hunt; 1998:447–453
8. Strasnick B, Moore DM, Abemayor E, et al. Occult primary tumors: the management of isolated sub-mandibular lymph node metastases. *Arch Otolaryngol Head Neck Surg* 1990; 116:173–176
9. Lindberg R. Distribution of lymph node metastases from squamous cell carcinoma of the upper respiratory and digestive tracts. *Cancer* 1972;29:1446–1449
10. McGuirt FW, McCabe BF. Significance of node biopsy before definitive treatment of cervical metastatic carcinoma. *Laryngoscope* 1978;88:594–597
11. Kleid S, Millar MS. The case against open neck biopsy. *Aust N Z J Surg* 1993;63:678–681
12. Robbins KT, Cole R, Marvel J, et al. The violated neck: cervical node biopsy prior to definitive treatment. *Otolaryngol Head Neck Surg* 1986;94:605–610
13. Mack Y, Parsons JT, Mendenhall WM, et al. Squamous cell carcinoma of the head and neck: management after excisional biopsy of a solitary metastatic neck node. *Int J Radiat Oncol Biol Phys* 1993;25:619–622
14. Ellis ER, Mendenhall WM, Rao PV, et al. Incisional or excisional neck node biopsy before definitive radiotherapy, alone or followed by neck dissection. *Head Neck* 1991;13:177–183
15. Parsons JT, Million RR, Cassisi NJ. The influence of excisional or incisional biopsy of metastatic neck nodes on the management of head and neck cancer. *Int J Radiat Oncol Biol Phys* 1985;11:1447–1454
16. Razack MS, Sako K, Marchetta FC. Influence of initial neck node biopsy on the incidence of recurrence in the neck and survival in patients who subsequently underwent curative resectional surgery. *J Surg Oncol* 1977;9:347–353
17. Silverman CL, Marks JD, Lee F, Ogura JH. Treatment of epidermoid and undifferentiated carcinomas from occult primaries presenting in cervical lymph nodes. *Laryngoscope* 1983;93:645–648
18. Jesse RH, Perez CA. Cervical lymph node metastasis: unknown primary cancer. *Cancer* 1973;31:854–859
19. Walter MA, Menarguez-Palanca J, Peiper SC. Epstein-Barr virus detection in neck metastases by polymerase chain reaction. *Laryngoscope* 1992;102:481–485
20. Gluckman JL, Robbins KT, Fried MP. Cervical metastatic squamous carcinoma of unknown or occult primary source. *Head Neck* 1990;12:440–443
21. Johnson J. Cervical metastases. In: Gluckman J, Gullane P, Johnson J, eds. *Practical Approach to Head and Neck Tumors.* New York: Raven Press;1994:47–63
22. Mendenhall WM, Mancuso AA, Parsons JT, et al. Diagnostic evaluation of squamous cell carcinoma metastatic to cervical lymph nodes from an unknown head and neck primary site. *Head Neck* 1998;20:739–752
23. Otto PM, Otto RA. Metastatic cervical lymph nodes with occult primary carcinomas. *Curr Opin Otolaryngol Head Neck Surg* 1998;6:102–105
24. Van den Brekel MWM, Castelijns JA, Snow GB. Diagnostic evaluation of the neck. *Otolaryngol Clin North Am* 1998;31: 601–620
25. Madison MT, Remley KB, Latchaw RE, Mitchell SL. Radiologic diagnosis and staging of head and neck squamous cell carcinoma. *Otolaryngol Clin North Am* 1998;31: 727–754
26. Mancuso AA, Harnsberger HR, Muraki AS. Computed Tomography of cervical and retropharyngeal lymph nodes: normal anatomy, variants of normal, and applications in staging head and neck cancer. *Radiology* 1983;148:715–723
27. Paulus P, Sambon A, Vivegnis D, et al. ^{18}FDG-PET for the assessment of primary head and neck tumors: clinical, computed Tomography and histopathological correlation in 38 patients. *Laryngoscope* 1998;108:1578–1583
28. Valdes Olmos RA, Balm AJ, Hilgers FJ. Thallium-201 Spect in the diagnosis of head and neck cancer. *J Neul Med* 1997;38:873–879
29. Righi PD, Sofferman RA. Screening unilateral tonsillectomy in the unknown primary. *Laryngoscope* 1995;105:548–550

30. McQuone SJ, Eisele DW, Lee J, Westra WH, Koch WM. Occult tonsillar carcinoma in the unknown primary. *Laryngoscope* 1998;108:1605–1610
31. Singh B, Balwally AN, Sundaram K, Har-el G, Krgin B. Branchial cleft cyst carcinoma: myth or reality. *Ann Otol Rhinol Laryngol* 1998;107:519–524
32. Von Volkmann R. Das Tiefe Branchiogege Halskarcinom. *2 Entralbl Chir* 1882;9:49–63
33. Martin H, Morfit HM, Ehrlich H. The case of branchiogenic cancer [malignant Brachioma]. *Ann Surg* 1950;132:867–887
34. Storper IS, Lee SP, Abemayor E, Juillard G. The role of radiation therapy in the treatment of head and neck cutaneous melanoma. *Am J Otolaryngol* 1993;14:426–431
35. Kirkwood JM, Strawderman MH, Ernstoff MS, Smith TJ, Borden EC, Blum RH. Interferon alfa-2B adjuvent therapy of high risk resected cutaneous melanoma: the Eastern Cooperative Oncology Group Trial EST 1684. *J Clin Oncol* 1998;14:7–17
36. DeSanto LW, Neel HB. Squamous cell carcinoma metastasis to the neck from an unknown primary. *Otolaryngol Clin N Am* 1985;18:505–513
37. Coster JR, Foote RL, Olsen KD, Jacks M, Schaid DJ, DeSanto LW. Cervical node metastasis of squamous cell carcinoma of unknown origin: indications for withholding radiation therapy. *Int J Radiat Oncol Biol Phys* 1992;23:743–749
38. Reddy SP, Marks JE. Metastatic carcinoma in the cervical lymph nodes from an unknown primary site: results of bilateral neck plus mucosal irradiation vs. ipsilateral neck irradiation. *Int J Radiat Oncol Biol Phys* 1997;37:797–802
39. Colletier PJ, Garden AS, Morrison WH, Goepfert H, Geara F, Angk K. Postoperative radiation for squamous cell carcinoma metastatic to cervical lymph nodes from an unknown primary site: outcomes and patterns of failure. *Head Neck* 1998;20: 674–681
40. Batani JP, Rodriquez J, Jaulerry C, Brugere J, Ghossein NA. Treatment of metastatic neck nodes secondary to an occult epidermoid carcinoma of the head and neck. *Laryngoscope* 1987;97:1080–1084
41. deBraud F, Heilbrun LK, Ahmed K, et al. Metastatic squamous cell carcinoma of an unknown primary localized to the neck. *Cancer* 1989;64:510–515
42. Harper CS, Mendenhall WM, Parsons JT, Stringer SP, Cassisi NJ, Million RR. Cancer in neck nodes with unknown primary site: role of mucosal radiotherapy. *Head Neck* 1990;12: 463–469
43. Wang RC, Goepfert H, Barber AE, Wolf P. Unknown primary squamous cell carcinoma metastatic to the neck. *Arch Otolaryngol Head Neck Surg* 1990;116:1388–1393
44. Mendenhall WM, Million RR, Cassisi NJ. Squamous cell carcinoma of the head and neck treated with radiation therapy: the role of neck dissection for clinically positive neck nodes. *Int J Radiat Oncol Biol Phys* 1986;12:733–740
45. Davidson BJ, Spiro RH, Patel S, Patel K, Shah JP. Cervical metastases of occult origin: the impact of combined modality therapy. *Am J Surg* 1994;168:395–399
46. Maillard E, Housset M, Brunel P, et al. Postoperative radiation therapy for cervical lymph node metastases from an occult squamous cell carcinoma. *Laryngoscope* 1992;102:884–889
47. Spiro RH, DeRose G, Strong EW. Cervical node metastasis of occult origin. *Am J Surg* 1983;146:299–304
48. Rice DH, Spiro RH. Metastatic carcinoma of neck primary unknown: current concepts in head and neck cancer. *Am Cancer Soc* 1989;127–133
49. Johnson JT. Neck dissection. *Arch Otolaryngol Head Neck Surg* 1998;124:1044–1045
50. Johnson JT. Selective neck dissection in patients with squamous cell carcinoma of the upper respiratory and digestive tracts. *Arch Otolaryngol Head Neck Surg* 1998;124:353
51. Clayman GL, Frank DK. Selective neck dissection of anatomically appropriate levels is as efficacious as modified radical neck dissection for elective treatment of clinically negative neck in patients with squamous cell carcinoma of the upper respiratory and digestive tracts. *Arch Otolaryngol Head Neck Surg* 1998;124:348–352
52. Myers EN, Fagan JJ. Treatment of the N+ neck in squamous cell carcinoma of the upper aerodigestive tract. *Otolaryngol Clin N Am* 1998;31:671–686
53. Brizel DM, Albers ME, Fisher SR, et al. Hyper-fractionated irradiation with or without concurrent chemotherapy for locally advanced head and neck cancer. *N Engl J Med* 1998; 338:1798–1998
54. Weissler MC. Combined chemotherapy and radiation therapy for advanced squamous cell cancer of the head and neck. *Current Opinion Otolaryngol Head Neck Surg* 1998;6: 120–123

Assessment and Management of the Unknown Primary with Neck Disease

CHAPTER 62

Robert P. Zitsch III and Russell B. Smith

Cancer in the head and neck region commonly manifests in an otherwise asymptomatic patient as metastatic disease to the cervical lymph nodes. In most cases, a complete history and physical examination are sufficient to ascertain the primary site of origin of the metastatic disease. The primary lesion is found to be in the head and neck region at least 70% of the time.[1,2] Occasionally, however, the primary lesion responsible for the cervical metastasis is found to have originated at a site remote from the head and neck, and therefore, metastatic neck disease often represents a distant metastasis from this primary site.

Among those patients with head and neck cancer presenting with cervical lymph node metastases, a primary lesion may sometimes fail to be identified despite a thorough diagnostic evaluation. This is reported to occur in approximately 5% of all patients presenting with cervical lymph node metastases, and the term occult primary or unknown primary has been commonly used to describe this clinical situation.[1] The diagnosis of metastatic cancer to the neck from an occult primary requires histologic or cytologic evidence of malignancy in a cervical lymph node as well as the failure to identify the primary site of origin after a systematic, comprehensive search. Thyroid cancers and lymphomas are excluded from this definition. Traditionally, this search has implied a complete history, a thorough physical examination of the upper aerodigestive tract, and multiple endoscopic examinations (direct laryngoscopy, esophagoscopy, bronchoscopy, nasopharyngoscopy) under anesthesia, usually with random or directed biopsies.

There are several controversial issues regarding both the assessment and the treatment of patients with cervical metastases from an unknown primary site. In the realm of assessment, controversy arises over which of the diagnostic studies should be routinely done in order to find the primary site. Imaging studies such as computed tomography (CT), magnetic resonance imaging (MRI), positron emission tomography (PET), and 2-[fluorine-18]-2-deoxy-D-glucose single photon emission computed tomography (FDG-SPECT) for surveillance of potential primary sites are central to any assessment controversy.[3] In addition, the role of serologic Epstein-Barr viral (EBV) tests or EBV genomic DNA assays in patients with cervical lymph node metastases from an occult primary is also uncertain.[4] Furthermore, the routine use of random aerodigestive tract biopsies and routine ipsilateral tonsillectomy in the diagnostic workup has been recommended by some and rejected by others.[3,5]

New technology that has been found to be useful in the assessment of head and neck cancer patients has not always generated controversy. Rigid and flexible endoscopes, generally regarded as indispensable for conducting a thorough examination of the pharynx and larynx today, have been an obvious improvement over the traditional indirect examination methods, particularly for the nasopharynx.

As with most head and neck cancer patients in general, both radiotherapy and surgery have important roles for patients having metastatic cervical disease with an occult primary. Some disagreement exists about whether single-modality treatment, particularly surgery, should be used for earlier-stage disease. The routine practice of irradiating potential primary mucosal sites has also been challenged. Finally, a role for chemotherapy in this group of patients has been suggested.

Discussion

HISTOPATHOLOGIC DIAGNOSIS

The histopathologic type of metastatic cervical lymphadenopathy for which a primary cannot be identified is squamous cell carcinoma in about 80% of the cases.[2] The remainder are adenocarcinomas, melanomas, undifferentiated carcinomas, and small cell carcinomas.[6] The diagnosis can usually be reliably established in most cases with a fine-needle aspiration biopsy (FNAB), particularly with metastatic squamous cell carcinoma. Certain instances in which the aspiration biopsy is indeterminate or suggestive of lymphoma require an open cervical lymph node biopsy.

The histopathology of the metastasis provides information that can aid in the search for a primary site and that is used for appropriate management decisions. Adenocarcinoma in low cervical lymph nodes only is strongly suggestive of an infraclavicular primary lesion. In such cases, further exhaustive evaluation of the upper aerodigestive tract is not warranted. The diagnostic evaluation would shift to focus on the organs being the most likely sources of the metastasis. The potential primary sites in decreasing order of frequency for an infraclavicular adenocarcinoma are lung, gastrointestinal tract, breast, pancreas, prostate, and ovary. Adenocarcinoma from an infraclavicular site manifesting as cervical adenopathy represents distant metastatic disease and, as might be expected, has a very poor prognosis.[7] By contrast, metastatic adenocarcinomas presenting in the upper neck often arise from salivary tissue in the major or minor salivary glands. Metastatic differentiated or medullary thyroid carcinoma must be considered for adenocarcinoma metastatic to cervical lymph nodes in any location. Immunohistochemical stains specific for these malignancies are useful in establishing a diagnosis. Obviously, histopathologic findings consistent with melanoma require a systematic evaluation of all cutaneous sites, as well as a thorough aerodigestive tract examination to rule out a rare mucosal primary. Finally, small cell or undifferentiated carcinoma may elude detection if evaluation of the salivary glands and paranasal sinuses is omitted from the routine evaluation of the aerodigestive tract and the potential infraclavicular sites.

EVALUATION

Cancer manifesting as cervical lymphadenopathy will be discovered in the upper aerodigestive tract in about 70% of cases.[1] Obviously, the evaluation for the primary should initially focus on this region until other diagnostic information suggests the primary is elsewhere. Specific historic information should be gathered for every patient who has an undiagnosed neck mass suspected to be malignant. Features such as absence of tenderness and progressive enlargement, particularly in a patient with a history of tobacco use or excessive alcohol use, are associated with a higher probability of malignancy. Further questioning about hoarseness, dysphagia, odynophagia, epistaxis, or nasal obstruction may help identify a head and neck primary site. A history of prior malignancy, including skin cancer of the head and neck or removal of pigmented lesions, should be noted. A history of prior head and neck radiation exposure should be elicited. A system review should investigate any gastrointestinal, pulmonary, or constitutional symptoms that may allude to the primary site.

The evaluation continues with a physical examination that focuses on the head and neck region. This examination should always include palpation of the oral cavity and oropharynx as well as direct endoscopic examination of the nasopharynx, larynx, and hypopharynx. Any area found to be unusual or abnormal should be biopsied.

The location in the neck of a mass confirmed to be a metastatic cervical node can guide the evaluation, as certain nodal groups will primarily drain specific areas in the head and neck. Obviously, this information is only useful when the cervical disease is very localized or solitary. Adenopathy in the submental region often corresponds to a primary lesion of the nose, the lips, or the anterior nasal cavity. Submandibular adenopathy is usually secondary to a primary site in the oral cavity, whereas intraparotid nodal enlargement is common for lip, nasal vestibule, face, and scalp cancers.[8] Upper and middle posterior cervical metastases usually originate from nasopharyngeal carcinomas. A supraclavicular metastasis will usually arise from an infraclavicular primary site, although thyroid cancer or cervical esophageal cancer is sometimes manifested in this manner.

Various diagnostic imaging studies are available, any one of which may, in some instances, provide useful information about the extent of the cancer. In every case, the chest radiograph should be obtained to assess for either primary or metastatic disease of the lungs. In some cases, patients having advanced neck disease should have a CT scan or an MRI to help gauge the extent of the metastatic neck disease in order to provide the most effective treatment. Also, these studies may be used to evaluate for distant metastases in cases of advanced cervical disease.

The routine use of CT or MRI for the purpose of attempting to identify a primary site responsible for the cervical metastasis, however, is controversial.[9] Some consider the routine use of either of these studies as unnecessary; others regard them as indispensable. Many of those who favor these imaging studies on a routine basis consider MRI or CT as potentially able to identify an occult primary site, as well as to identify suspicious areas needing careful endoscopic examination and biopsy. A recent retrospective study attempted to ascertain the role of these studies in the context of the evaluation of the occult primary tumor with cervical metastases.[3] These investigators found that either CT or MRI correctly identified the primary site in 50% of patients who had no abnormal findings on physical examination. Whether one or the other of these two studies is better able to identify a primary lesion was not addressed in this study and has not yet been determined. However, for cases in which nasopharyngeal carcinoma is suspected to be the primary site, it has been suggested that because early lesions can be seen more readily on MRI, it is the preferred imaging study for this site.[10]

When MRI or CT is used to assist with the identification of an occult primary site, the images should evaluate the paranasal sinuses and salivary gland regions for abnormalities that are indicative of a source of the metastasis. This is particularly important for adenocarcinoma that has metastasized to upper cervical lymph nodes.

Recently, the FDG-SPECT or PET scan has been found a useful diagnostic imaging study for differentiating malignancy from normal tissue. This property has led to studies investigating its role in detecting the primary site producing metastatic cancer to the cervical lymph nodes. One study using FDG-SPECT as a diagnostic tool to identify a primary site in patients with metastatic squamous cell carcinoma to the cervical lymph nodes from an unknown primary demonstrated a positive scan in 20 of 24 patients. Of the 20 patients with the positive scans, only 7 had a primary cancer site found, and only 1 of those 7 were otherwise without findings suggestive of the primary.[3] In four patients with a negative scan, two were found to have tumor. It was concluded that the value of this study for the purpose of discovering an occult primary lesion is very modest. At this time, the routine use of this study in patients with cervical metastases from an occult primary cannot be justified, and its role remains undefined.

A close association of the EBV and nasopharyngeal carcinoma has resulted in the widespread use of EBV antibody titers as post-treatment markers for cancer at this site.[11] This has led to the use of EBV assays for diagnostic purposes in patients having metastatic squamous cell carcinoma to the cervical lymph nodes for which the primary site is unknown, but suspected to be the nasopharynx.[10,12] Fu[10] suggests that for patients with poorly differentiated or undifferentiated metastatic carcinomas, the identification of the EBV genome in the cervical metastasis of a patient also having elevated IgA antiviral capsid antigen is strongly suggestive of a nasopharyngeal primary. However, it has been shown that the presence of EBV genomic DNA in metastatic lymph nodes alone is predictive of the presence of nasopharyngeal carcinoma.[13] Testing a metastatic node for EBV DNA or obtaining EBV immunoglobulin titers is a reasonable approach that should be considered for any case of metastatic poorly differentiated or undifferentiated carcinoma of cervical lymph nodes, particularly if upper deep cervical or posterior cervical nodes are involved.

The usual and preferred manner of diagnosis for a cervical mass with a nonrevealing history and physical examination is FNAB. This can be done relatively early in the diagnostic evaluation of such cases, even at the initial visit, if a complete history and examination are normal. The diagnostic accuracy and ability to yield a diagnosis for this test are high. If a single attempt fails to provide diagnostic information, it should be repeated, or a core needle biopsy should be considered.

Only after a repeated needle biopsy fails to establish a diagnosis should an open biopsy procedure be contemplated. Open biopsy is also often necessary for cases in which FNAB shows a probable lymphoma or an epithelial malignancy of uncertain type. If open biopsy is done, frozen section examination should be performed to determine whether the biopsied tissue should be processed for a lymphoma evaluation or for an infectious disease etiology.

In the past, the usual approach to open biopsy of a suspicious neck mass by head and neck oncologists involved the performance of an immediate complete neck dissection if the biopsy confirmed a metastatic squamous cell carcinoma. Failing to do a neck dissection or being unprepared to perform this operation at the time of an open biopsy showed metastatic carcinoma was regarded as very poor and risky patient management. Some recent studies, however, suggest that if an open biopsy of a metastatic squamous cell carcinoma is subsequently followed by adequate treatment with either radiotherapy or surgery, but not necessarily immediate neck dissection, the outcome is not compromised.[14,15] One study reported a 5-year disease-specific survival of 95% among patients whose treatment included excisional biopsy.[16] Nevertheless, open biopsy remains the least preferred way to establish a diagnosis in a patient with metastatic carcinoma presenting with a cervical mass.

The remaining part of the diagnostic evaluation that is generally regarded as indispensable for a patient presenting with a metastatic carcinoma from an occult primary is the endoscopic examination under anesthesia. This usually includes careful palpation of the oral cavity and oropharynx, with particular attention given to the base of tongue and palatine tonsils, as well as direct laryngoscopy, pharyngoscopy, esophagoscopy, and bronchoscopy. Any abnormal or suspicious areas should be biopsied. The yield of primary site identification for panendoscopy after an unrevealing history and physical examination is 24 to 44%.[3]

Of a more controversial nature is the value of random biopsies taken from head and neck mucosal sites when the endoscopic examination is normal. One approach is to biopsy the sites where the occult primary is statistically most likely to be located.[9] These would be the nasopharynx, the base of tongue, the ipsilateral palatine tonsil, and the ipsilateral pyriform sinus. Another approach is to select biopsy sites on the basis of the location of the involved lymph nodes.[9] The rationale for this approach is that head and neck cancer will metastasize in a relatively predictable fashion to the cervical lymph nodes and that the location of an occult primary lesion can be inferred by the location of the nodal metastasis. Finally, biopsy sites can be selected on the basis of suspicious areas identified on CT or MRI scans. In addition to random biopsies, bronchial washings have been recommended.[12]

The value of routine ipsilateral tonsillectomy to identify the source of a metastatic squamous cell carcinoma has been debated.[3,9] One small retrospective review concluded that ipsilateral tonsillectomy was the only reliable screening technique to rule out an occult tonsil carcinoma.[17] This conclusion was made on the basis of a case series; no comparison was made to other methods of detection, such as palpation under anesthesia or tonsil biopsy. By contrast, a larger review by Mendenhall et al.[3] concluded that the diagnostic value of routine ipsilateral tonsillectomy was uncertain.

TREATMENT

Several reasonable treatment options are available for metastatic cancer to the cervical lymph nodes for which no primary lesion is found. The most appropriate treament choices, however, are dependent on the specific pathology of the neck disease and on the stage of the metastatic disease. The usual treatment modalities selected for curative treatment in these cases are surgery or radiotherapy, or both. The goals for treatment are to control the known neck disease and to prevent eventual clinical manifestation of any occult disease in the neck or at the occult primary site.

Patients with metastatic poorly differentiated squamous cell carcinoma or undifferentiated carcinoma that is suspected to originate from the Waldeyer's ring area, often on the basis of suggestive anti-EBV antibody titers or the presence of EBV DNA, should receive definitive radiotherapy to the cervical lymph nodes and the pharyngeal lymphoid tissue. Surgical management with a cervical lymphadenectomy is used in these cases when the metastatic cervical disease persists after completion of radiotherapy or if it recurs. Whether adjuvant chemotherapy, using the regimen found to improve survival for nasopharyngeal carcinoma in a recent intergroup phase III trial, should be used in this subgroup of patients is uncertain. At the very least, however, its use should be considered in those having compelling evidence for an occult nasopharyngeal primary lesion.

All other cases of metastatic squamous cell carcinoma from an occult primary should be managed according to the extent (stage) of the cervical disease. For those patients having N1 cervical disease, definitive radiotherapy alone and cervical lymphadenectomy alone have been regarded as equally effective treatments.[10,18] Combination therapy for this stage of disease may not be justified.[18] When irradiation alone is chosen, the potential mucosal primary sites are also often included in the radiation fields, as irradiation of the neck alone may compromise the subsequent use of radiation to a primary lesion that may manifest at a later time.[10] Surgery alone, usually as a comprehensive cervical lymphadenectomy, is also reasonable and effective for N1 disease with an occult primary site, with 3-year disease-free survival rates of 67% reported by Jesse et al.[18] The treatment that is ultimately selected in this situation is dependent on other patient factors, such as age, health, reliability for follow-up, and individual preference.

Cases of more advanced neck disease are not normally treated using a single therapeutic modality but rather with surgery and radiotherapy.[19] The only possible exception would be a case of N2b neck disease, in which only two metastatic nodes at a single level are found, each <3 cm in size and with no evidence of extracapsular spread. Surgery alone might be considered in such a case.

One large review showed improved neck control with combination therapy over single-modality treatment for patients with advanced neck disease (N2 or N3).[19] This improved control, however, did not translate into improved survival, presumably because of significant development of distant metastases and second primary tumors in this group of patients. Cervical lymphadenectomy in this stage of neck disease should be a complete dissection as a minimum. Functional modifications can be considered when oncologically feasible. Regardless of the stage of the neck disease, postoperative radiotherapy should be used for any case exhibiting extracapsular extension, perineural or vascular invasion, or known residual disease.[10]

Another debatable aspect of the management of patients presenting with regionally metastatic squamous cell carcinoma from an occult primary site is the value of prophylactic irradiation of the potential head and neck mucosal sites. To date, no randomized trial to evaluate such treatment has been published; recommendations must be made on the basis of retrospective reviews. In one review, an attempt was made to assess the value of mucosal radiotherapy in cases of metastatic squamous cell carcinoma from an unknown primary by comparing the rates of subsequent primary lesions developing in patients treated for occult primary lesions with those treated for known primary lesions.[20] It was concluded that since the mucosal failure rates were equivalent in the two groups, elective radiotherapy of the mucosa is highly effective. Consequently, they recommend the elective irradiation of the nasopharynx, the oropharynx, the hypopharynx, and the supraglottic larynx. Others have also recommended the routine use of mucosal irradiation in order to reduce the incidence of eventual primary site identification.[21,22] These three series had eventual failures at head and neck mucosal sites after elective mucosal radiotherapy ranging from 4% to 12%, as compared with 20 to 40% mucosal failures among historic controls.[20-22] Unfortunately, no study to date has demonstrated improved survival with elective mucosal irradiation in patients with cervical metastases from an occult primary.

Others do not recommend routine mucosal radiation, but rather use it selectively for only those cases for which radiotherapy is otherwise indicated for control of metastatic neck disease.[16,19] The Memorial Sloan-Kettering group will electively irradiate only the hypopharyngeal and oropharyngeal mucosa, excluding the nasopharynx in cases in which the cervical metastases are not consistent with a nasopharyngeal primary.[19] By limiting wide-field mucosal radiation, significant morbidity in the form of xerostomia can be avoided. In addition, the modality would be available for future use should a head and neck primary eventually manifest.[19]

Adenocarcinoma manifesting in upper cervical lymph nodes for a primary that cannot be found often arises from the major or minor salivary glands. If an exhaustive evaluation including CT or MRI fails to disclose the primary site, a complete cervical lymphadenectomy should be done. This should always include the submandibular gland and, in cases of nodal pathology adjacent to the parotid gland, a parotidectomy may be justified. No clear indications for radiotherapy exist in this subset of patients, although it should be considered for multiple positive lymph node metastases or extracapsular spread of tumor.

Adenocarcinoma of lower cervical nodes with an occult primary is usually a manifestation of distant metastatic disease from an infraclavicular primary site, although it must be ascertained that the metastasis is not from the thyroid gland. Having excluded the latter, excisional biopsy is all that should be undertaken. The prognosis in this situation is poor, despite treatment attempts using chemotherapy and radiotherapy.[7,12] Metastatic melanoma for which no primary site can be identified is treated with a complete (usually radical or modified radical) neck dissection after the prospect of distant metastasis is eliminated.

The precise role, if any, of chemotherapy in the treatment of metastatic carcinoma to cervical lymph nodes for which no primary has been found is unclear. This is not unlike the uncertainty of the role of chemotherapy for head and neck cancer, in general, for which a clear role has been identified only for organ preservation for known primary sites such as larynx and hypopharynx and as an effective adjuvant therapy for nasopharyngeal carcinoma.

Two studies have attempted to address the question of the role of chemotherapy for patients with metastatic squamous cell carcinoma for which no primary was identified. One of these, a retrospective review, showed improved survival for patients with N3 disease who received chemotherapy as part of their treatment as compared to those who were treated with surgery and/or radiotherapy alone.[23] All patients treated with chemotherapy received cisplatin. Another nonrandomized phase II trial of patients with metastatic squamous cell carcinoma from an unknown primary, showed durable responses with 58% showing no evidence of recurrence after three cycles of induction chemotherapy using cisplatin and 5-fluorouracil (5-FU).[24]

As no randomized trials using chemotherapy have been conducted, or will unlikely be conducted, in this group of patients, the value of adjuvant chemotherapy for metastatic carcinoma with unknown primary will probably have to be established by extrapolating from other adjuvant chemotherapy head and neck trials. One current phase III intergroup trial is evaluating the benefit of adding cisplatin to surgical resection and radiotherapy for patients at high risk of recurrence. This includes patients with advanced neck disease and patients having extracapsular spread of their nodal metastatic disease. Should chemotherapy be found to improve survival among patients with high-risk neck disease, this treatment would likely be given consideration for those having occult primary disease as well.

OUTCOME

Recent series of patients treated for cervical lymph node metastasis from an occult primary site show disease-specific survivals at 5 years of 60 to 74%, with overall survival of 35 to 60%.[16,19,22] These, and other studies, have confirmed that neck control and survival are determined by the extent of the neck disease, including the N stage, node fixation, extracapsular spread, and the number of involved nodes.[10,16,19,21,22] Five-year survival rates by N stage are reported at 60 to 62% for N1, 40 to 50% for N2, and 19 to 38% for N3 groups.[19,21]

Whether survival is influenced by the eventual manifestation of the primary site above the clavicle remains uncertain. Primary lesions will eventually manifest in about 16% of patients treated for cervical metastasis from an occult primary, with nearly 50% of these presenting within the first 2 years.[25] Significantly more primaries manifest in patients who have not received radiotherapy as part of their management (27% vs 6% with radiation).[25] A review conducted at M.D. Anderson Hospital failed to show any effect of an eventual primary site discovery on survival or neck control at 5 years compared with those whose primary site remained occult.[25] The same conclusion has been reached by others.[2,10]

Not all would agree with this conclusion, however. Several reviews provide some evidence to support the view that the ultimate discovery of a primary lesion above the clavicles is associated with a worse prognosis than if the occult primary site remained undetected.[18,26] Jesse et al.[18] stated that the 3-year survival was 31% for those patients manifesting a primary site above the clavicles, compared to 58% for those who did not manifest one. However, their findings of complete failure to control disease among patients whose primaries developed below the clavicles are consistent with other studies.

Conclusion

Cancer in the head and neck commonly presents as a cervical lymph node metastasis. A thorough, systematic evaluation will allow the primary site to be identified in most cases. When no primary site is found, endoscopic examination under anesthesia with biopsy, radiography, and other ancillary tests are used to help identify the primary site. A high-resolution imaging study such as CT or MRI is often of value in the identification of primary site among patients without any abnormal history or physical findings other than the neck mass. The selection of biopsy sites should be based, in part, on suspicious areas on imaging studies and the location of the metastatic lymph nodes.

If a primary site is not discovered despite an extensive evaluation, and if an infraclavicular primary site is not suspected, treatment is directed at the cervical disease and potential primary sites. Limited and early neck disease is often treated with a single therapeutic modality, either radiotherapy or cervical lymphadenectomy. Prophylactic treatment to potential primary sites is often not delivered in these cases of limited disease when surgical management is used. Survival is primarily determined by the extent of the cervical metastasis, with 5-year survivals averaging better than 50% among patients with the most limited cervical disease.

REFERENCES

Zitsch III and Smith—CHAPTER 62

1. Richard JM, Micheau C. Malignant cervical adenopathies from carcinomas of unknown origin. *Tumori* 1977;63:249–258
2. Barrie JR, Knapper WH, Strong EW. Cervical nodal metastases of unknown origin. *Am J Surg* 1970;120:466–470
3. Mendenhall WM, Mancuso AA, Parsons JT, et al. Diagnostic evaluation of squamous cell carcinoma metastatic to cervical lymph nodes from an unknown head and neck primary site. *Head Neck* 1998;20:739–744
4. Walter MA, Menarguez-Palanca J, Peiper SC. Epstein-Barr virus detection in neck metastases by polymerase chain reaction. *Laryngoscope* 1992;102:481–485
5. Righi PD, Sofferman RA. Screening unilateral tonsillectomy in the unknown primary. *Laryngoscope* 1995;105:548–550
6. Davidson BJ, Spiro RH, Patel S, et al. Cervical metastases of occult origin: the impact of combined modality therapy. *Am J Surg* 1994;168:395–399
7. Templer J, Perry MC, Davis WE. Metastatic cervical adenocarcinoma from an unknown primary tumor: treatment dilemma. *Arch Otolaryngol* 1981;107:45–47
8. Strasnick B, Moore DM, Abeymayor E, et al. Occult primary tumors: the management of isolated submandibular lymph node metastases. *Arch Otolaryngol Head Neck Surg* 1990;116:173–176
9. Gluckman JL, Robbins KT, Fried MP. Cervical metastatic squamous cell carcinoma of unknown or occult primary source. *Head Neck* 1990;12:440–443

10. Fu KK. Neck node management from unknown primary. *Front Radiat Ther Oncol* 1994;28:66–78
11. Pearson GR, Weiland LH, Neel HB III, et al. Application of Epstein-Barr virus serology to the diagnosis of North American nasopharyngeal carcinoma. *Cancer* 1983;51:260–268
12. Harwick RD. Cervical metastases from an occult primary site. *Semin Surg Oncol* 1991;7:2–8
13. Macdonald MR, Freeman JL, Hui MF, et al. Role of Epstein-Barr virus in fine-needle aspirates of metastatic neck nodes in the diagnosis of nasopharyngeal carcinoma. *Head Neck* 1995;17:487–493
14. Robbins KT, Cole R, Marvel J, et al. The violated neck: cervical node biopsy prior to definitive treatment. *Otolaryngol Head Neck Surg* 1986;94:605–610
15. Ellis ER, Mendenhall WM, Rao PV, et al. Incisional or excisional neck node biopsy before definitive radiotherapy, alone or followed by neck dissection. *Head Neck* 1991;13:177–183
16. Colletier PJ, Garden AS, Morrison WH, et al. Postoperative radiation for squamous cell carcinoma metastatic to cervical lymph nodes from an unknown primary site: outcomes and patterns of failure. *Head Neck* 1998;20:674–681
17. Righi PD, Sofferman RA. Screening unilateral tonsillectomy in the unknown primary. *Laryngoscope* 1995;105:548–550
18. Jesse RH, Perez CA, Fletcher GH. Cervical node metastasis: unknown primary cancer. *Cancer* 1973;31:854–859
19. Davidson BJ, Spiro RH, Patel S, et al. Cervical metastases of occult origin: the impact of combined modality therapy. *Am J Surg* 1994;168:395–399
20. Harper CS, Mendenhall WM, Parsons JT, et al. Cancer in the neck nodes with unknown primary site: role of mucosal radiotherapy. *Head Neck* 1990;12:463–469
21. Maulard C, Housset M, Brunel P, et al. Postoperative radiation therapy for cervical lymph node metastases from an occult squamous cell carcinoma. *Laryngoscope* 1992;102:884–890
22. Bataini JP, Rodriguez J, Jaulerry C, et al. Treatment of metastatic neck nodes secondary to an occult epidermoid carcinoma of the head and neck. *Laryngoscope* 1987;97:1080–1084
23. De Braud F, Heilbrun LK, Ahmed K, et al. Metastatic squamous cell carcinoma of an unknown primary localized to the neck—advantages of an aggressive treatment. *Cancer* 1989;64:510–515
24. Jeremic B, Zivic DJ, Matovic M, Marinkovic J. Cisplatin and 5–fluorouracil as induction chemotherapy followed by radiation therapy in metastatic squamous cell carcinoma of an unknown primary tumor localized in the neck. A phase II study. *J Chemother* 1993;5:262–265
25. Wang RC, Goepfert H, Barber A, Wolf PF. Squamous cell carcinoma metastatic to the neck from an unknown primary site. In: Larson DL, Ballantyne AJ, Guillamondegu OM, eds. *Cancer in the Neck: Evaluation and Treatment.* New York: Macmillan;1986:183–192
26. Talmi YP, Wolf GT, Hazuka M, Krause CJ. Unknown primary of the head and neck. *J Laryngol Otol* 1996;110:353–356

Assessment and Management of the Unknown Primary with Neck Disease

CHAPTER 63

David J. Arnold and Henry T. Hoffman

Patients with cancer of the upper aerodigestive tract (UADT) commonly present to their primary caregivers with a mass in the neck. It is important that an appropriate evaluation be undertaken to include a search for the primary tumor from which the cervical metastasis developed. It is the inability to find the source that has led to the concept of the unknown primary. However, the meaning of unknown primary has a great deal to do with the extent of the treating physician's ability to search for this often elusive lesion. The staging of the tumor is TX when complete evaluation has not been accomplished. This is changed to T0 if a complete evaluation has not revealed the primary tumor.[1] Frequently, surgical excision of a neck mass is carried out to secure a diagnosis after a course or two of antibiotics has failed to cause resolution without consideration of a neoplastic cause for the mass. Several deleterious effects can arise from this course of treatment if the disease process proves to be malignant. Violation of the fascial planes of the deep neck may give a decreased rate of control in the neck when compared to formal neck dissection, especially if radiotherapy is not employed. Perhaps more distressing is the potential for the primary lesion to go undiagnosed until local symptoms prompt further investigation. It was this very situation that prompted warnings from Martin as early as 1961 when he wrote, "excisional or incisional lymph node biopsy should be used only as a last resort and then preferably by the surgeon who accepts responsibility for the treatment himself if the diagnosis eventually proves to be cancer."[2]

The pivotal question that lies at the heart of this subject is: How should the head and neck surgeon approach a patient with a neck mass? This process begins with establishing a diagnosis. The evaluation includes a physical examination, a careful history, radiologic studies, histologic studies, and often examination under anesthesia.

A thorough history and physical examination includes specific questioning regarding exposure to potentially carcinogenic agents such as ethanol and tobacco products. A complete exam is carried out to visualize all visible surfaces of the UADT possible during an office examination. This exploration includes an exam with a flexible fiberoptic nasopharyngoscope to evaluate otherwise difficult to visualize areas such as the fossae of Rosenmueller and the pyriform sinuses. A modified Valsalva maneuver may be performed with the fiberoptic laryngoscope in place to maximally expose the hypopharynx.

In most patients in whom the cervical mass is suspected to be malignant, the primary site will be apparent on physical exam in the office setting. When the primary is not visible, additional effort is necessarily spent to search for the source of the neck metastasis. Identification of the primary site at the time treatment has begun has been shown to improve ultimate rates of disease control.[3] Several tools are available to help with this search.

Histologic evaluation of the neck mass is best first approached with fine needle aspiration biopsy (FNAB). This technique has been shown to be both sensitive and specific for detecting many of the common histologic entities responsible for head and neck neoplasms.[4] Accuracy approaching 100% has been described in diagnosing squamous cell carcinoma (SCC).[4] This technique is easily carried out in the office and for this reason the histology of the cervical disease is usually known by the time the patient is evaluated under anesthesia. It is our practice to attempt histologic diagnosis in patients with a neck mass on the day of their first presentation. In most cases involving neoplasm, SCC will be the histologic class of cancer. There are other entities that can present as masses in the neck. These include tumors of thyroid or salivary gland origin, lymphoma, benign masses, and rare tumors such as sarcoma. If FNAB does not suggest carcinoma, open biopsy may be required to make a diagnosis. The remainder of this discussion focuses on SCC presumed to be metastatic to the neck.

A new dimension was added to this diagnostic scheme during the 1970s with the advent of computed tomographic (CT) scanning. This modality has continued to evolve with advancements in computer software and now is capable of providing the clinician with images with quite good resolution. This three-dimensional imaging technique, as well as the techniques of magnetic resonance imaging (MRI) and positron emission tomography (PET) scanning, extends the evaluation beyond that accomplished through physical inspection of mucosal surfaces.[5,6] As early as 1983, Muraki et al.[7] were convinced that CT evaluation "should be used as part of the routine evaluation of patients with this clinical problem (unknown primary)." This group was able to find a primary site in four cases among 17 patients who had been previously evaluated with a negative endoscopic examination under anesthesia. We routinely obtain a CT for all patients with a neck mass thought to be neoplastic in origin. The information gained from contrast-enhanced CT scan from skull base to clavicles often provides crucial information beyond that gained by physical examination, especially for patients with short or bulky necks with difficult physical examinations. Continuous refinement of additional imaging techniques has given rise to new modalities such as MRI and PET scanning that hold future promise in helping to find an unknown primary. Great effort is now under way to explore physiochemically based imaging that can differentiate normal and malignant tissue.

In contrast to CT and MRI, PET scanning capitalizes on the different physiochemical properties of tumor and nontumor cells.[8] Imaging is possible because tumor cells have been shown to have increased glycolysis (compared with normal cells) as monitored by PET using ^{18}F-labeled 2-deoxy-D-glucose. Work done by Braams et al. has shown this modality to have approximately 30% sensitivity for detecting an unknown primary as we have defined above.[8] It is still difficult to recommend PET scanning as the standard of care in the search for an unknown primary because of its low sensitivity.

MRI scanning has allowed greater resolution for evaluating soft tissue structures than does CT. As a result, MRI is most useful when there is question of whether a soft tissue structure is fluid trapped in a paranasal sinus or a solid anatomically abnormal tissue mass as often presents a dilemma when evaluating anomalies of the paranasal sinuses. Additionally, resolution afforded by MRI is unsurpassed when evaluating intracranial structures for metastatic involvement because MRI is able to show subtle differences between similar soft tissues that are not discernible with CT.

Molecular genetics has received attention as a potential tool in the evaluation of patients with a cervical metastasis. This approach has found greatest application through the association between Epstein-Barr virus (EBV) and nasopharyngeal carcinoma. Macdonald et al.[9] have identified a clear association between polymerase chain reaction (PCR)-amplified sequences of EBV in FNAB samples of cervical metastatic disease and presence of nasopharyngeal carcinoma. This test is limited by the fact that a positive result only proves exposure to EBV. Many more patients have been exposed to EBV than actually have nasopharyngeal carcinoma. Until specificity can be improved, this assay will have an unacceptably high false-positive rate. It does, however, hold promise as an interesting diagnostic tool.

An extension of physical examination is endoscopy under anesthesia. The combination of laryngoscopy, bronchoscopy, esophagoscopy, nasopharyngoscopy with biopsies directed at any mucosal abnormalities is needed. In the absence of identifiable tumor, directed biopsies to likely sites of occult disease such as base of tongue, pyriform sinus, larynx, and tonsils are needed to reveal an occult primary. Questions have arisen as to whether it is necessary to remove the entire tonsil as a means of biopsy.

Tonsillectomy has been advocated by many as a part of the search for a primary of the UADT. Lapeyre and collegues showed that 26% of 87 patients with cervical metastases of unknown primary proved to have a lesion of origin in the tonsil. The author asserts that this intervention (tonsillectomy) saved this 26% of his group of patients from the morbidity of receiving radiation to the larynx and nasopharynx and further supports this intervention by demonstrating significant cases of appearance of a previously unknown primary tumors of the tonsil in formerly radiated fields. They also state that "tonsillectomy never induced specific complications" (in his group of patients).[10] Mendenhall et al.[11] showed similar rates of discovery (35%) in their series of patients (n = 34) undergoing tonsillectomy in search of a primary. They point out that their patients received tonsillectomies only when physical exam or radiographic studies indicated the tonsil as a primary site. Righi and Sofferman[12] echo this experience in their group of 19 patients, 32% of whom proved to have occult primary tumors in their tonsils.

We agree that tonsillectomy, although not completely without complications, is worthwhile for patients not at increased risk of bleeding. Moreover, we believe that removing the entire tonsil will demonstrate lesions that can be overlooked by noncomprehensive tonsil biopsies. A strong argument for bilateral tonsillectomy exists in avoiding a confusing physical examination secondary to oropharyngeal asymmetry for future examiners. This procedure is likely to demonstrate a site of primary in a significant number of patients. The capacity to narrow treatment fields when a primary tumor is found helps decrease morbidity. Patients with a tonsil primary that has been treated appropriately have significantly better prognoses than do patients whose primaries remain unknown.[3,7] For these reasons, it is our practice to perform bilateral tonsillectomy as part of our routine directed biopsies in the search for an occult primary.

We believe that only after an extensive search that reveals no primary lesion can a neck metastasis be said to have no primary and therefore be staged as T0 rather than TX.[1] Several theories exist to explain this phenomenon. The simplest proposes that a primary tumor does exist and is not found. Others propose that a primary lesion did exist but was eliminated by the immunologic defense mechanisms. Still other investigators suggest that epithelial cells lining a congenital cyst can convert to malignant cells that present as cervical carcinoma without an apparent primary source. Although there is no definite pathophysiologic mechanism to explain the occult primary there is a general consensus that epithelial malignancy does not arise de novo in the neck.

The standard of care at our institutions for patients in whom the primary remains occult is most often neck dissection performed at the diagnostic endoscopy with biopsies directed at high-risk sites as outlined above, followed by radiotherapy. If no primary is found at endoscopy, it is safe to assume that the primary (if present) is a T1 at most and, as such, is amenable to treatment with radiation as a single modality. The field of the radiation is designed to encompass all potential mucosal sites of the primary tumor, usually including naso-, oro-, and hypopharynx as well as larynx and both sides of the neck. There is controversy concerning several aspects of this routine.

Coster et al.[13] take issue with the assertion that all patients with unknown primary sites should receive radiation after neck dissection. They make the point that some of these patients will have disease originating from below the clavicles and that irradiation of wide mucosal fields will only increase the morbidity for these people. They also state that approximately one-half of the tumors eventually identified as potential head and neck primaries present more than 5 years after the original and must be considered second primaries. As such, these patients would not benefit from prior radiotherapy, and they would have one less treatment option if a new lesion is diagnosed in the field of previous radiation. This group does agree that N2 or higher disease and histologic evidence of extracapsular spread or lymphoepithelioma are indications for postoperative radiotherapy both to the neck and to potential sites of the primary tumor.[13] The experience of Mohit-Tabatabai and colleagues[14] mirrors these findings. These workers found 8 of 35 patients treated with radiation had primaries arise at a later date in field (although it is not clear how far out from treatment). The numbers of patients in these studies are too small to propose definite conclusions. However, we feel that the decision to withhold radiation in the face of unknown primary disease can only be made with a much greater experience and should not be routinely advised on the basis of the available data.

There is strong support for bilateral technique (as opposed to treating only the neck with obvious neoplastic disease) when using radiotherapy to treat cervical metastases from an unknown primary. Reddy and Marks[15] demonstrated significantly lower rates of subclinical metastasis in the contralateral neck (higher rates of control) when both sides of the neck were irradiated. Our groups support this practice not only because it promises better locoregional control, but also because it does not add significant morbidity as compared with an ipsilateral technique.

The potential to improve management of patients with an unknown primary SCC metastatic to the neck through administration of adjuvant chemotherapy is attractive. However, there are currently no strong data to support the use of chemotherapy in this setting. Khansur et al.[16] prospectively showed a 53% response rate in patients with occult primary disease and cervical metastasis treated with a combination of cisplatinum and 5-fluorouracil (5-FU). Similarly, DeBraud et al.[17] showed that the addition of either of these agents to a regimen of surgery and XRT seemed to improve outcome. Tabatabai and his group[14] also support the idea that adjuvant chemotherapy holds much promise in improving survival in patients with cervical SCC of unknown primary. No survival advantage has been demonstrated with any of these regimens and further study is needed before acceptable regimens can be adopted. At this time, the role of chemotherapy is limited to palliative treatment, as an adjuvant to radiotherapy in the treatment of nasopharyngeal cancer, and as part of controlled clinical trials. The use of chemotherapy in other situations is strongly discouraged.

It is common for practitioners in a tertiary referral center to see patients with neck metastasis from an unknown primary who have already received treatment. Most commonly the patient has undergone open biopsy of the neck mass and it is at this point that the histologic diagnosis is made. Mack et al.[18] have claimed that there is no detriment to outcome in patients with cervical disease diagnosed by open biopsy whose primary tumor has remained occult after an extensive search as outlined above as long as radiotherapy is given as the next step in treatment after the biopsy. Others support this idea.[19-22] Many times, there has not been significant search for a site of primary, and it is then incumbent on the treating physician to undertake this search. There is often concern that the scar resulting from the incisional biopsy may be seeded with tumor. It is our practice to excise this scar if it can be included in an incision for the definitive neck dissection and to have it remain attached to the neck dissection specimen. Parsons et al.[20] have discussed the management dilemma of patients diagnosed with cervical carcinoma of unknown primary by open biopsy. They point out that the initial biopsy and possible hematoma have the potential to spread tumor cells outside of the normal fascial planes in a manner that is impossible to predict. They believe that an operation to eradicate these malignant cells is difficult to design and that in this situation radiation therapy should be the next step in treatment. These investigators suggest that radiotherapy to both sides of the neck is preferred, in the belief that open biopsy of the neck can alter patterns of lymph flow significantly enough to change normal patterns of metastasis.

Appropriate management of the majority of patients with SCC metastatic to the neck from an unknown primary (T0, N+) results in control of locoregional disease. Outcome has been shown to be linked to several identifiable factors. Survival decreases as tumor stage increases. Extracapsular spread in cervical metastatic nodal disease portends a worse outcome both in terms of local control and overall survival. It is prudent to follow these patients frequently, as they are likely to demonstrate a mucosal neoplasm over time. Some have advocated the practice of close observation with fiberoptic endoscopy in an office setting during the course of radiotherapy. These clinicians believe that radiation tumoritis will often make the primary site visually obvious and allow a planned excision. It is hoped that work in areas such as adjuvant chemotherapy will hold promise for improved outcomes, especially with advanced-stage tumors, in the near future.

REFERENCES

Arnold and Hoffman—CHAPTER 63

1. American Joint Committee on Cancer. *Cancer Staging Manual.* 5th Ed. Philadelphia: Lippincott-Raven; 1997
2. Martin H. Untimely lymph node biopsy. *Am J Surg* 1961; 102:17–18
3. Marcal-Vega VA, Cardenes H, Perez CA, et al. Cervical metastases from unknown primaries: radiotherapeutic management and appearance of subsequent primaries. *Int J Radiat Oncol Biol Phys* 1990;19:919–928

4. Shaha A, Webber C, and Marti J. Fine-needle aspiration in the diagnosis of cervical lymphadenopathy. *Am J Surg* 1986;152: 420–423
5. Mancuso AA, Hanafee WN. Elusive head and neck carcinomas beneath intact mucosa. *Laryngoscope* 1983;93:133–139
6. Schaefer SD, Merkel M, Diehl J, Maravilla K, Anderson R. Computed tomographic assessment of squamous cell carcinoma of oral and pharyngeal cavities. *Arch Otolaryngol* 1982; 108:688–692
7. Muraki AS, Mancuso AA, Harnsberger HR. Metastatic cervical adenopathy from tumors of unknown origin: the role of CT. *Radiology* 1984;152:749–753
8. Braams JW, Pruim J, Kole AC, et al. Detection of unknown primary head and neck tumors by positron emission tomography. *Int J Oral Maxillofac Surg* 1997;26:112–115
9. Macdonald MR, Freeman JL, Hui MF, et al. Role of Epstein-Barr Virus in fine-needle aspirates of metastatic neck nodes in the diagnosis of nasopharyngeal carcinoma. *Head Neck* 1995; 487–493
10. Lapeyre M, Malissard L, Peiffert D, et al. Cervical lymph node metastasis from an unknown primary: is a tonsillectomy necessary? *Int J Radiat Oncol Biol Phys* 1997;39:291–296
11. Mendenhall WM, Mancuso AA, Parsons JT, Stringer SP, Cassisi NJ. *Head Neck* 1998;20:739–744
12. Righi PD, Sofferman RA. Screening unilateral tonsillectomy in the unknown primary. *Laryngoscope* 1995;105:548–550
13. Coster JR, Foote RL, Olsen KD, Jack SM, Schaid DJ, DeSanto LW. Cervical nodal metastasis of squamous cell carcinoma of unknown origin: indications for withholding radiation therapy. *Int J Radiat Oncol Biol Phys* 1992;23:741–749
14. Mohit-Tabatabai MA, Dasmahapatra KS, Rush Jr. BF, Ohanian M. Management of squamous cell carcinoma of unknown origin in cervical lymph nodes. *Am Surg* 1986;52(3):152–154
15. Reddy SP, Marks JE. Metastatic carcinoma in the cervical lymph nodes from an unknown primary site: results of bilateral neck plus mucosal radiation vs. ipsilateral neck irradiation. *Int J Radiat Oncol Biol Phys* 1997;37:797–802
16. Khansur T, Allred C, Little D, Anand V. Cisplatin and 5-Fluorouracil for metastatic squamous cell carcinoma from unknown primary. *Cancer Invest* 1995;13(3):263–266
17. DeBraud F, Heilburn LK, Ahmed K, et al. Metastatic squamous cell carcinoma with unknown primary localized to the neck. *Cancer* 1989;64:510–515
18. Mack Y, Parsons JT, Mendenhall WM, Stringer SP, Cassisi NJ, Million RR. Squamous cell carcinoma of the head and neck: management after excisional biopsy of a solitary metastatic neck node. *Int J Radiat Oncol Biol Phys* 1993;25:619–622
19. Ellis ER, Mendenhall WM, Rao PV, et al. Incisional or excisional neck-node biopsy before definitive radiotherapy, alone or followed by neck dissection. *Head Neck* 1991;13:177–183
20. Parsons JT, Million RR, Cassisi NJ. The influence of excisional or incisional biopsy of metastatic neck nodes on the management of head and neck cancer. *Int J Radiat Oncol Biol Phys* 1985;11:1447–1454
21. Robbins KT, Cole R, Marvel J, Fields R, Wolf P, Goepfert H. The violated neck: cervical node biopsy prior to definitive treatment. *Otolaryngol Head Neck Surg* 1986;94:605–610
22. Wang RC, Goepfert H, Barber AE, Wolf P. Unknown primary squamous cell carcinoma metastatic to the neck. *Arch Otol Head Neck Surg* 1990;116:1388–1393

22

The Parotid Neoplasm

"A few experts feel rather strongly that the routine use of CT or MRI is not cost-effective and that it should not be recommended, even though they concede that useful information can be obtained from these studies in certain situations. They believe that the use of CT or MRI should be restricted to patients with recurrent neoplasms, high suspicion of malignancy, very large neoplasms, suspected parapharyngeal space involvement, suspected carotid artery involvement, or any other finding that introduces the possibility of inoperability."

Byron J. Bailey

"Functioning facial nerves are retained in the presence of any grade malignancy, including nerve encasement by tumor."

Marshall Strome

"There is universal agreement in the literature that a neck dissection is indicated when there is clinical evidence of metastatic disease from the parotid gland to the cervical lymph nodes. However, the surgical management of the clinically negative neck (N0) remains controversial. Both the indications and type of elective neck dissection are not well defined in the literature."

James Y. Suen

The Parotid Neoplasm

Byron J. Bailey

CHAPTER 64

Parotid neoplasms are quite diverse in terms of their histology and biologic behavior. As a group, they represent about 2% of all head and neck neoplasms, and parotid gland tumors account for 70 to 80% of all neoplasms of the salivary glands. Parotid neoplasms are usually benign (80% for adults), and the most common benign neoplasm is the pleomorphic adenoma (about 85%) in adults, whereas hemangiomas and lymphangiomas are the most common neoplasms in children. Malignant tumors are divided into low-grade and high-grade neoplasms. The low-grade category comprises (1) low-grade mucoepidermoid, (2) low-grade adenocarcinoma, (3) acinic cell carcinoma, (4) basal cell adenocarcinoma, and (5) terminal duct adenocarcinoma. The high-grade group includes intermediate and high-grade mucoepidermoid, (2) adenoid cystic, (3) carcinoma ex pleomorphic adenoma, (4) adenocarcinoma, (5) undifferentiated carcinoma, (6) salivary duct carcinoma, and (7) dedifferentiated acinic cell carcinoma.

The controversies that arise concerning the diagnosis and management of salivary gland neoplasms reflect the necessity to achieve an accurate pathologic diagnosis in order to initiate the proper therapy. In most circumstances, the surgeon will not have definitive diagnostic information until the surgical specimen has undergone permanent section analysis by the surgical pathologist. In this situation, we are pushed to the limit to outline a treatment course most likely to preserve facial nerve function, prevent tumor recurrence, and deal appropriately with a broad range of tumor aggressiveness.

The controversies dealt within this section are: (1) the role of fine-needle aspiration biopsy, (2) imaging parotid neoplasms, (3) selecting the proper surgical procedure, and (4) the role of radiotherapy.

Fine-Needle Aspiration Biopsy

Our understanding of salivary gland neoplasms has undergone considerable change over the past three decades and newer methods of tissue sampling and tissue processing have improved the ease and accuracy of diagnosis and have therefore helped us select more appropriate therapy. Fine-needle aspiration biopsy (FNAB) is still viewed by many as controversial, in terms of its value in the diagnosis and management of salivary gland neoplasms. A recent Scandinavian study[1] provides a typical report of the findings of 218 patients whose FNAB was confirmed histologically after surgical excision. The benign lesions were diagnosed accurately with 76% sensitivity and 83% specificity. FNAB was not as helpful with malignant lesions, and only 26 of 47 FNAB samples were considered malignant (sensitivity = 55%), whereas there were 11 false-positive diagnoses for malignancy (92% specificity). Misdiagnosis resulted in a delay of therapy in some patients because of reliance on the FNAB report by physicians who did not understand the limitations of that study. FNAB accuracy is higher when the surgical pathologist is experienced in interpreting these results. It is common to find reports of approximately 85% accuracy for detecting malignant tumors, 80% accuracy for detecting benign lesions, and 90% accuracy for diagnosing pleomorphic adenoma. It is clear that FNAB can provide useful information that has value in planning therapy, but it should not be the sole basis for management decisions. It has been performed in large series of patients without major complications and, when it is used routinely, it is found to shorten the time required for diagnosis. One of the important benefits of FNAB is the opportunity to avoid unnecessary operative risk for patients who have benign parotid neoplasms but who are very poor candidates for surgery because of other general medical conditions.

Some surgeons have not found good support for the routine use of FNAB and have emphasized the low accuracy of this study in diagnosing malignant parotid neoplasms. They believe that FNAB should be considered only as a screening examination in view of the fact that pathologists generally have much greater difficulty reaching a definitive diagnosis with salivary gland tumors, even when they are given a large tissue specimen. They emphasize that superficial lobe parotidectomy should be considered the gold standard for diagnosis and that this procedure is essentially an excisional biopsy for diagnosis.[2]

Clearly, FNAB is not as useful in salivary gland neoplasia as it has been for squamous cell carcinoma and thyroid neoplasia, and the report cannot be relied on as definitive. The clinical value of FNAB is a function of the experience of the cytopathologist; it must be combined with the impression gained from other studies as well as the history and physical examination.[3]

At this point, some experts advocate the routine use of FNAB in evaluating all parotid neoplasms, emphasizing the diagnostic accuracy, rapidity, patient convenience, and cost-effectiveness of this study and feel that it is probably the single most important piece of information to be obtained.[4,5] Other experts advocate the use of FNAB only for three specific indications: (1) for patients who are poor surgical risks, (2) for patients with a history of previous malignancy/metastasis, and (3) for patients in whom it is difficult to determine whether the lesion is neoplastic or inflammatory.[6]

IMAGING STUDIES

The options available for the imaging of parotid neoplasms include plain films, sialography, ultrasound, computed tomography (CT), magnetic resonance imaging (MRI), and positron emission tomography (PET) scanning. Considerations of cost-effectiveness have placed increasing pressure on physicians to pursue imaging studies that are most likely to be useful on the basis of the presumed pathology after careful history and physical examination. It appears that CT scanning is the most widely accepted and routine form of imaging for parotid neoplasms[3,7] because it permits assessment of the entire parotid gland, the parapharyngeal space, the mandible, the skull base, and the mastoid region.

Some radiologists disagree with this approach and believe that the MRI gives more valuable information because it is more sensitive than CT for soft tissue lesions.[8-12]

A few experts feel rather strongly that the routine use of CT or MRI is not cost-effective and that it should not be recommended, even though they concede that useful information can be obtained from these studies in certain situations. They believe that the use of CT or MRI should be restricted to patients with recurrent neoplasms, high suspicion of malignancy, very large neoplasms, suspected parapharyngeal space involvement, suspected carotid artery involvement, or any other finding that introduces the possibility of inoperability.[13]

Parotid neoplasms in children are a special case, even though they are uncommon. We know that about 50% of these neoplasms in infants will be hemangiomas and that they usually present within the first few months of life. The CT scan is not helpful in this diagnostic situation. The first attempt at imaging should be to obtain plain films, as these will sometimes show calcifications that will strongly suggest that the tumor is a hemangioma. If the plain films are negative and there is a need for diagnostic precision, the use of technetium 99–labeled red blood cells can provide nearly 100% specificity for diagnosing hemangioma if the imaging demonstrates poor activity in the profusion phase with gradual uptake in the early pool images and increased uptake in the delayed scan.[14]

In my experience, the controversy is usually a moot point, as patients usually present in our office carrying a CT scan under their arm at the time of our initial contact. Once this controversy has been resolved, it will be important to educate primary care physicians concerning the most appropriate imaging studies to be requested.

Operative Procedure of Choice

The treatment of choice for salivary gland neoplasms is surgical excision. In the United States, it is generally agreed that superficial parotidectomy consisting of the identification and preservation of the facial nerve and removal of the portion of the gland superficial to the nerve is both diagnostic and curative for most parotid gland neoplasms.

French surgeons[15] recommend a procedure called total conservative parotidectomy with facial nerve preservation for the most common parotid neoplasm, benign pleomorphic adenoma. On the basis of their experience with 256 patients, their analysis showed pleomorphic adenoma to involve the deep lobe of the gland in17% of patients and both the superficial and deep lobe in 32%. They conclude that a superficial parotidectomy would have been inadequate in almost one-half of this large series of patients. The procedure carried a rather high complication rate in terms of temporary facial paresis (65%) and permanent facial paresis (4%). These surgeons noted postoperative Frey syndrome in two-thirds of their patients. Using this procedure, they observed only one recurrent pleomorphic adenoma in the entire series.

Role of Radiotherapy for Malignant and Recurrent Parotid Neoplasms

In recent years radiotherapy has been added to surgical excision in a variety of situations. Some have proposed its use as adjuvant therapy for all malignancies, for all pleomorphic adenomas, for recurrent pleomorphic adenomas only, for malignancy metastatic to the parotid gland, and for those occasions in which there is known spillage of pleomorphic adenoma cells during the course of a superficial parotidectomy.

Radiotherapy is recommended widely as an adjuvant modality after surgical excision of malignant neoplasm. It is used for patients with adenoid cystic carcinoma because of its effectiveness in controlling perineural invasion.[13] Studies have shown the results of combined therapy to be superior to surgery alone.[16,17] The observed success with adenoid cystic carcinoma has prompted the recommendation for surgery plus radiotherapy for all malignant salivary gland tumors except for T1 or T2 N0 disease with low-grade histology and clear margins.[18] A large Scandinavian study[19] reported that the change from surgery alone to surgery plus radiotherapy resulted in increased facial nerve preservation and a significantly higher rate of local control. Studies have shown that the addition of radiotherapy has reduced the local recurrence rate by 50% in some clinical reports. Truelson[3] recommends the addition of radiotherapy to surgical excision for patients with advanced tumors, high-grade malignancy (squamous cell carcinoma, undifferentiated carcinoma, malignant mixed tumors, and high grade mucoepidermoid carcinoma) as well as for patients with recurrent tumors or suspected residual tumor cells.

The value of radiotherapy as a routine adjuvant for pleomorphic adenoma is unclear. A study from Norway[20] reported that in a series of 238 patients with follow-up averaging 18 years, there was an overall recurrence rate of pleomorphic adenoma of 2.5%. The recurrence rate increased to 8% when there was a known rupture of the tumor capsule. Buchman et al.[21] concluded that the addition of radiotherapy is extremely important when the surgical pathologist reports inadequate resection margins on the tumor specimen. These investigators observed recurrence in 36% of patients who were not irradiated and no recurrence in the group of patients receiving postoperative radiotherapy. He also recommends postoperative radiotherapy for those patients who have undergone enucleation as the initial surgical procedure and after all patients undergoing surgical excision of recurrent pleomorphic adenoma.

Conclusion

We have followed a general plan for the routine evaluation and management of an adult patient who presents with a parotid mass, as illustrated in the algorithm depicted in Figure 64–1. For further information on this subject, the reader is referred to two recently published, concise and excellent sources.[22,23]

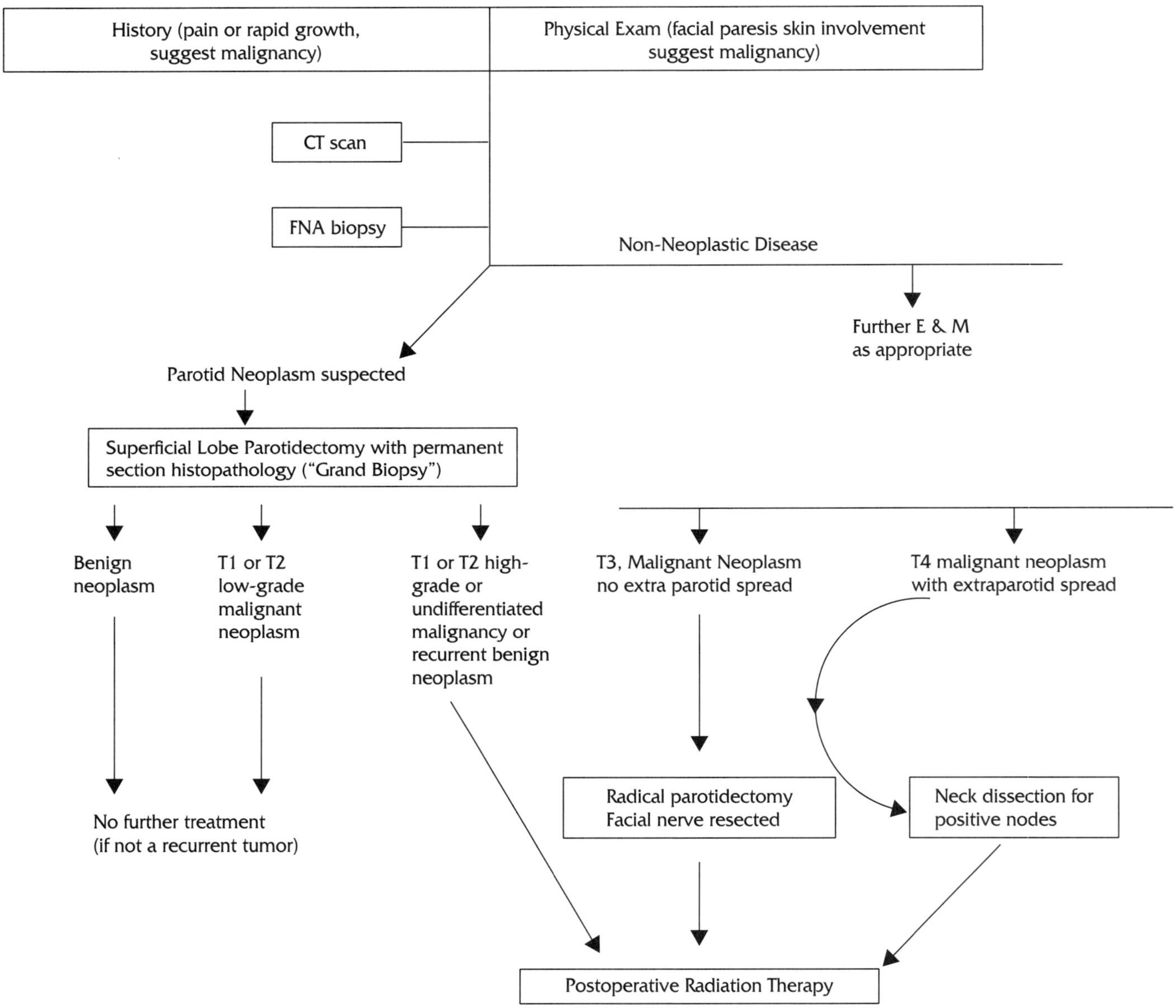

Figure 64–1 Routine pathway for evalutation and management of a parotid mass in an adult patient.

REFERENCES

Bailey—CHAPTER 64

1. Atula T, Grenman R, Laippala P, Klemi PJ. Fine-needle aspiration biopsy in the diagnosis of parotid gland lesions: evaluation of 438 biopsies. *Diagn Cytopathol* 1996;15:185
2. Boles R. Needle biopsy of salivary gland tumors. In: Snow JB Jr, ed. *Controversy in Otolaryngology.* Philadelphia: WB Saunders; 1980:87–91
3. Truelson JM. Controversies in salivary gland disease. In: Bailey BJ, ed. *Head and Neck Surgery—Otolaryngology.* 2nd Ed. Philadelphia: Lippincott-Raven; 1998:851–857
4. Johns ME. Parotid mass. In: Holt GR, Mattox DE, Gates GA, eds. *Decision Making in Otolaryngology.* BC Decker; 1984:92–93
5. McGuirt WF, Keyes JW Jr, Greven KM, et al. Preoperative identification of benign versus malignant parotid masses: a comparative study including positron emission tomography. *Laryngoscope* 1995;105:579
6. Weber RS, Eisele DW, El–Naggar A, et al. Contemporary classification of salivary gland tumors: fine needle aspiration cytology (FNA). In: Gluckman JL, ed. *Renewal of Certification Study Guide in Otolaryngology—Head and Neck Surgery.* Kendall/Hunt; 1998:548
7. Becker T. Salivary gland imaging. In: Bailey BJ, ed. *Head and Neck Surgery—Otolaryngology.* 2nd Ed. Philadelphia: Lippincott-Raven; 1998:541–559
8. Barsotti JB, Westesson PL, Coniglio JU. Superiority of magnetic resonance over computed tomography for imaging parotid tumor. *Ann Otol Rhinol Laryngol* 1994;103:737–740
9. Som PM, Shugar JMA, Sacher M, et al. Benign and malignant parotid pleomorphic adenomas: CT and MR studies. *J Comput Assist Tomogr* 1988;12:65–69
10. Mees K, Vogl T, Kellermann O. Magnetic resonance tomography in tumors of the salivary glands—a diagnostic advantage? *Laryngol Rhinol Otol (Stuttg)* 1988;67:355–361
11. Mirich DR, McArdle CB, Kulkarli MV. Benign pleomorphic adenomas of the salivary gland. Surface coil MR imaging versus CT. *J Comput Assist Tomogr* 1987;11:620–623
12. Teresi LM, Lufkin RB, Wortham DG, et al. Parotid masses: MR imaging. *Radiology* 1987;163:405–409
13. Eisele DW, Johns ME. Salivary gland neoplasms. In: Bailey BJ, ed. *Head and Neck Surgery—Otolaryngology.* 2nd Ed. Philadelphia: Lippincott-Raven; 1998:1485–1508
14. Liu KKW, Lam WWM. Parotid hemangioma in infancy: diagnosis with technetium 99m–labeled red blood cell pool imaging. *Otolaryngol Head Neck Surg* 1995;112:780–781
15. Laccourreye H, Laccourreye O, Cauchois R, et al. Total conservative parotidectomy for primary benign pleomorphic adenoma of the parotid gland: a 25-year experience with 229 patients. *Laryngoscope* 1994;104:1487–1494
16. Garden AS, Weber RS, Morrison WG, et al. The influence of positive margins and nerve invasion in adenoid cystic carcinoma of the head and neck treated with surgery and radiation. *Int J Radiat Oncol Biol Phys* 1995;32:619
17. Miglianico L, Eschwege F, Marandas P, et al. Cervicofacial adenoid cystic carcinoma: study of 102 cases: influence of radiation therapy. *Int J Radiat Oncol Biol Phys* 1987;13:673–678
18. North CA, Lee DJ, Piantadosi S, et al. Carcinoma of the major salivary glands treated by surgery or surgery plus postoperative radiotherapy. *Int J Radiat Oncol Biol Phys* 1990;18:1319
19. Pedersen D, Overgaard J, Sogaard H, et al. Malignant parotid tumors in 110 consecutive patients: treatment results and prognosis. *Laryngoscope* 1992;102:1064–1069
20. Natvig K, Soberg R. Relationship of intraoperative rupture of pleomorphic adenomas to recurrence: an 11–25-year follow-up study. *Head Neck* 1994;16:213–217
21. Buchman C, Stringer SP, Mendenhall WM, et al. Pleomorphic adenoma: effect of tumor spill in inadequate resection of tumor recurrence. *Laryngoscope* 1994;104:1231–1234
22. Adams GL. Malignant tumors of the parotid gland. In: Gates GA, ed. *Current Therapy in Otolaryngology—Head and Neck Surgery.* 6th Ed. St Louis, MO: CV Mosby; 1998:228–234
23. Medina JE, Byers RM, Maves MD, et al. *Clinical Practice Guidelines for Diagnosis and Management of Cancer of the Head and Neck (Parotid).* American Society for Head and Neck Surgery and The Society of Head and Neck Surgeons; 1996:65–67

The Parotid Neoplasm

Marshall Strome

CHAPTER 65

Given the remarkable advances during the last decade in our understanding of tumor biology, intracellular ultrastructural aberrations, imaging, radiotherapy delivery, and the synergism of radiotherapy with chemotherapeutic agents, it is remarkable that management controversies facing otolaryngologists 30 years ago remain today for parotid neoplasia. Some issues defy ready resolution in part because prospective data of statistical import are and have been difficult to acquire. It is the rarity and multiplicity of these malignancies that makes the former so. Further, in some instances, accuracy would require a 20-year follow-up period, because of growth characteristics and long intervals before recurrences are identified.

Given the complexities of the diagnosis and management of malignant parotid tumors, differences of opinion are both understandable and inevitable. Questions legitimately disputed are the efficacy and indications for fine-needle aspiration biopsy (FNAB), imaging technology, nerve monitoring, frozen section, surgical extent, facial nerve sacrifice, the use of radiotherapy, and chemotherapy. Classic articles are reviewed in virtually all book chapters and recent articles, with some presenting raw data for reader interpretation, others suggesting a format for management. My approach is to define the issues, followed by a personal philosophy based on an extensive experience with parotid neoplasia.

General Truisms

Malignant parotid neoplasms represent 1 to 3% of carcinomas of the head and neck. Recurrence of these malignancies is often synonymous with future therapeutic failure. Identifying the covariables suggestive of aggressive behavior and recurrence could alter initial therapeutic planning. Tumor stage, including extension, facial nerve involvement, and histologic grading are the most significant prognostic indicators.[1] Integrating the aforementioned into a realistic therapeutic plan is still best accomplished by case individualization, with decision making reflecting significant physician experience. Some points as to data acquisition and interpretation follow. The realities of cost containment are reflected in the management strategies proposed but are not further specified.

MRI and CT

Magnetic resonance imaging (MRI) and computed tomography (CT) are sophisticated techniques, each with independent strengths. However, rarely do these procedures alter the decision to perform surgery. Their relative value is in evaluating the extent of larger tumors, and associated nodal status and in differentiating deep lobe neoplasms from primary parapharyngeal space lesions.[2] Although some controversy exists as to which provides the most meaningful data, MRI in most situations appears to have some advantages. For soft tissue definition, resolution is generally superior. Further, some neoplasms have identifying characteristics noted on MRI studies. Warthin's tumors, for example, are well marginated and heterogeneous, whereas pleomorphic adenomas are homogeneous and smoothly marginated. Differences in signal intensity have been noted for low- and high-grade malignancies. If bone and/or skull base definition is needed, CT can be added as an adjunct to MRI. It should be stated that there is no longer a need for radionuclide imaging or sialography in the management of parotid neoplasms.

For the isolated easily palpable parotid mass, preoperative imaging is not a necessity. Imaging studies are beneficial preoperatively in defining the extent of larger infiltrative tumors. MRI is the initial imaging modality of choice.

Fine-Needle Aspiration Biopsy

Three alternatives are present when considering FNAB. First, the choice not to use FNAB as a diagnostic technique rests with the premise that it will not alter management. Second, proponents of routine use want to have as much information as possible available preoperatively for counseling patients, often with reference to facial nerve management. Third, selective use of FNAB depending on the situation, which would appear to have the most merit. Any advantage conferred by having FNAB data depends entirely upon the accuracy of the information obtained. The latter unquestionably is experience driven, both in performing the procedure itself and in the interpretation thereof. It is acknowledged that FNAB is better at identifying and classifying benign lesions. Today, in 93% of cases, it is possible to differentiate benign from malignant. However, it is clearly more difficult to classify the malignant group with this technique.[3] The difficult question as to the value of FNAB is whether it alters decision making. Further, with a small but acknowledged false-positive rate, should a more aggressive surgical procedure be performed based primarily on FNAB data? The answer is, selectively, yes. For example, squamous cell carcinoma should be readily identifiable on FNAB. Mucoepidermoid tumors can often be identified as well. Appropriate preoperative counseling could then be given, with intraoperative frozen-section confirmation leading to an appropriate surgical procedure. It is interesting, however, that a recent survey of 34 head and neck surgeons found that FNAB data did not alter decision making for a discrete parotid mass.[3] In such a setting, patient and physician comfort with the clinical preoperative information gleaned from the history and physical examination will be the final arbiter as to the value of FNA for the isolated parotid mass.

I find FNAB efficacious when lymphadenopathy is suspected, (e.g., inflammation, benign lymphoepithelial disease, sarcoid, or lupus erythematosus). It has merit if lymphoma is a consideration and also for the elderly in whom confirmation of a benign neoplasm might affect surgical decision making. FNAB is beneficial in identifying recurrent neoplasia, benign or malignant.

In summary, as a technique, FNAB has stood the test of time, spanning several decades. It has some value in tumor identification without evidence of tumor seeding and has very limited morbidity. It is better in separating benign from malignant pathology than determining specific malignant histologic characteristics.

Frozen Section

More than any of the other available diagnostic techniques, the way in which frozen section is used will determine its value. Some malignancies (e.g., squamous cell carcinoma) will be diagnosed with nearly 100% accuracy. Further definition for problematic lesions will depend in great measure on the experience of the pathologist and the surgeon. Implicit is a discussion with the pathologist at the time of frozen section of intraoperative tumor patterns. Clinical cues in T3 or T4 tumors (e.g., tumor interface with the facial nerve, discussed further under Facial Nerve) and pattern of extension (e.g., skin proximity) can reasonably infer malignancy in many instances. If the interpretation on frozen section is malignant and a benign neoplasm is subsequently diagnosed on permanent section, it is only problematic if inappropriately radical surgery is the endpoint. This is where surgical judgment plays such an important role.

Although a thorough knowledge of the recent literature can augment judgment, there is no substitute in this setting for experience. Wheelis and Yarington,[4] reporting on 256 frozen section results, noted a 5% error in benign to malignant and four instances of incorrectly diagnosing cancer. Error rates as high as 25% have been reported on frozen section. However, in an isolated study, Hillel and Fee[5] reported no misdiagnoses of malignancy on frozen section. If the important details as iterated above are considered, a problematic error on frozen section should not occur. Problematic again refers to inappropriately aggressive surgery (e.g., sacrifice of the facial nerve, muscle, or bone). If malignancy is diagnosed on frozen section with clinical correlation for T2 or greater staging, a total parotidectomy should be performed with sampling of adjacent lymph nodes. A normally functioning facial nerve, irrespective of tumor encasement, should not be removed. This prudent approach based on frozen section will almost uniformly serve the patient well. If there ever is a question that cannot be resolved with certainty, waiting for permanent sections and then returning, should it be necessary for more extensive surgery, is the only reasonable approach.

Facial Nerve

MONITORING

Monitoring of the facial nerve was introduced with the hope of decreasing the acknowledged incidence of paresis 20 to 25% or paralysis 3 to 5%. Comparative studies have not supported the theory.[6] For the relative neophyte, for deep lobe tumors with potentially displaced nerves, and for recurrences, monitoring may have merit. In other settings, the use of nerve integrity monitors is optional.

CLINICAL OPERATIVE CONCEPTS

Adherence characteristics to the facial nerve at the tumor interface can in most instances clinically separate benign from malignant pathology. The adherent facial nerve branches readily elevate in the presence of benign neoplasms. Inflammatory masses may not separate easily, but there is usually more associated bleeding than in similarly adherent malignant neoplasms.

Functioning facial nerves are retained in the presence of any grade malignancy, including nerve encasement by tumor. The nerve is meticulously separated from tumor circumferentially if necessary using the operative microscope. Although the latter is clearly controversial, all advanced grade malignancy will require adjunct radiotherapy. There are no confirmatory data to suggest leaving microscopic disease on nerve increases local recurrence when postoperative radiation therapy is administered.[7] Although there is initial paresis uniformly in most such instances, there is a return to full facial nerve function if such is present preoperatively. With this approach, there is an obvious decrease in morbidity.

The facial nerve is resected when function is impaired preoperatively. In such cases, frozen section is performed on the cut nerve endings, both proximal and distal, to obtain negative margins when feasible. Immediate nerve grafting is performed when tumor-free margins are obtained, as postoperative radiotherapy does not adversely affect graft reinnervation. If a facial nerve is positive at the first genu, further resection has no survival advantage and an intracranial resection has significantly increased morbidity. In the latter setting, the facial nerve is not grafted.

Radiotherapy

The mindset of many based on historical percepts is that radiotherapy has limited efficacy in the management of parotid malignancies. Even recently published data have suggested that adjunctive radiotherapy did not favorably affect prognosis related to recurrence.[1] Retrospective studies are clearly of concern. Vastly improved imaging, dose sequencing, planning, and delivery systems during the past 5 years make older studies of questionable significance. Current wisdom suggests that, in the appropriate setting, radiotherapy does, in fact, reduce the rate of local recurrence.[8] Further, for recurrent or inoperable malignant neoplasms, with or without prior irradiation, a neutron-based regimen has documented efficacy.[9] Under these circumstances, neutrons have an approximately threefold improvement in survival at 2 years as compared with daily photon sequences. Acknowledged comorbidities have arisen years after neutron therapy, but recent improvements in planning and dosimetry should decrease these late sequelae. Photon sequencing remains controversial, but efficacy could reasonably be expected in epithelial-based malignancies. I currently recommend suggesting postoperative radiotherapy for all stage 3 and 4 malignant tumors. The inclusion of T2 tumors is dependent on histologic grade. For small high-grade malignancies with extension or adherence to the facial nerve, postoperative radiotherapy is individualized as decided by our tumor board.

More problematic is defining the role of radiotherapy for recurrent pleomorphic adenoma. Radiotherapy has been shown to decrease recurrence when administered after limited local excision with or without tumor spill and after surgery for recurrences. This led to a period of use for multifocal recurrence after reoperation. However, this form of management for initially benign disease is far from innocuous. Complications, including xerostomia, osteoradionecrosis, and fibrosis, are recognized. Further, after a 20-year therapeutic interval, the incidence of carcinoma is increased if radiotherapy was used. A recent review of 126 cases of recurrent pleomorphic adenoma makes the case for surgery as the treatment modality of choice.[10] In this study, the average time of follow-up was 14.5 years. Interestingly, tumor recurrence was 32.5% after the first reoperation, 7.1% after the second operation, and 1.6% after the third. If excision of the biopsy site accompanied a parotidectomy shortly after local excision had been performed, no tumor recurred. Importantly, after all procedures, total paralysis occurred in 5.5% and partial paralysis in 13.5% of cases. In my practice, I manage recurrent pleomorphic adenoma with repeated extirpation until such an option no longer exists, which is rare.

Chemotherapy

Efficacy, albeit limited, has been suggested using Adriamycin, cisplatin, and 5-fluorouracil (5-FU). For squamous cell-based malignancies, the traditional cisplatin/5-FU combination may have merit. Further, synchronous postsurgical cisplatin, 5-FU, and radiotherapy on protocol in a small number of high-grade advanced-stage mucoepidermoid carcinomas under my care has shown efficacy (no recurrence) at more than 3 years. Longer follow-up and combined trials will define utility in time.

Neck Management

There can be no argument as to the need for nodal removal in the clinically positive neck. For the N0 neck, tumor size and/or stage, histology (squamous cell carcinoma), grading (high-grade mucoepidermoid carcinoma), and facial nerve paralysis (60 to 77%) suggest occult metastasis. For the latter group, ultrasound may identify adenopathy in the clinically N0 neck and subsequent ultrasound-guided FNAB of identified adenopathy would provide additional meaningful data. If the FNAB was positive, this would obviously lend support for lymphadenectomy. If there is no clinical evidence preoperatively of nodal spread in these high-risk pathologies, I sample readily identifiable level I and intraparotid nodes. If frozen section is negative, no further nodal removal is performed. If positive, levels I to III are cleared, with the lowest nodes in level III submitted for frozen section. The latter algorithm would appear to decrease morbidity, while maximizing efficacy.

Having proposed the latter, to my knowledge, no data are available confirming that removal of microscopic disease confers a survival advantage in aggressive parotid neoplasms, as virtually all are managed with postoperative radiotherapy. However, the approach espoused provides prognostic information potentially identifying and clearing microscopic disease. Although unsubstantiated, it is my bias that removal of microscopic disease could confer a survival advantage with little or no associated morbidity.

Low-grade malignancies of <4 cm in size in most instances require no neck nodal sampling. Intraparotid nodes >1 cm, if identified, are submitted for frozen section at surgery, as low-grade tumors infrequently will be found to have intraparotid nodal spread requiring then and only then a total parotidectomy.

Surgery and Adjunctive Therapy

Surgery remains the cornerstone of management for primary parotid malignancies. The extent of resection is TNM grounded. For stage I tumors, <4 cm, low grade, and located in the superficial lobe, a superficial parotidectomy is the procedure of choice. The deep lobe is also removed if it is the primary site, if involved via tumor extension or if microscopic intraparotid nodes are detected intraoperatively. In rare occasions, otherwise histologically low-grade malignancies (e.g., mucoepidermoid carcinoma) are associated with microscopic intraglandular nodal extension. These tumors are biologically and clinically more significant. Intraglandular nodal spread because of lymphatic patterns mandates a total parotidectomy. If more than one node is identified, even in the face of low-grade pathology, a supraomohyoid selective neck dissection would be performed. If the neck were positive in the presence of a low histologic grade, radiotherapy would be suggested. If negative, even with intraparotid spread for a low-grade malignancy, radiotherapy would not be considered. Again, as a routine, unless identified preoperatively or suggested above, the neck nodes are not addressed surgically for low-grade stage I parotid malignancies. High grade T1 lesions are managed with total parotidectomy. The facial nerve is preserved unless clinically involved. A neck dissection is not performed unless positive nodes are detected preoperatively (e.g., palpation, imaging, ultrasound-guided aspiration) or intraoperatively with selective nodal sampling of suspicious intraparotid and level I nodes.

For stage II or greater without nodal involvement, the resection is tailored to provide a reasonable margin encompassing areas of local extension. Bone and/or muscle are to be included as indicated. All functioning branches of the facial nerve are preserved whenever possible. If more than one branch is found to supply a given anatomic area, only then is a functional tumor encased branch removed. Neck dissection is performed if positive nodes are encountered at surgery or if the preoperative evaluation infers such. Juxtaposed nodal sampling is routine. Postoperative radiotherapy is essential. If positive nodes are encountered with any T stage, obviously some form of neck dissection is indicated. Nodal size and or number will determine the magnitude of the neck dissection performed. As a general rule, two levels below the lowest identified node are cleared. Nodal status has no direct bearing on the management of the facial nerve.

Any neck nodal involvement in conjunction with a high-grade primary tumor should raise consideration of postoperative chemotherapy. When applicable, this should only be given as part of a planned protocol such that efficacy can be determined. The rationale for the latter is grounded in the knowledge that extended surgical resections correlate with substantively increased recurrence rates.

The precepts put forward are the synthesis of more than two decades of experience with parotid neoplasia. Albeit conservative, this approach provides a needed balance between quality of life, cost, and survival.

REFERENCES

1. Calearo C, Storchi OF, Pastore A, et al. Parotid gland carcinoma: analysis of prognostic factors. *Ann Otol Rhinol Laryngol* 1998;107:969
2. Cross RR, Shapiro MD, Som PM. MRI of the parapharyngeal space. *Radiol Clin North Am* 1989;27:353
3. McGurk M, Hussain K. Role of fine needle aspiration cytology in the management of the discrete parotid lump. *Ann R Coll Surg Engl* 1997;79:198
4. Wheelis RF, Yarington CT Jr. Tumors of the salivary glands: comparison of frozen section diagnosis with final pathologic diagnosis. *Arch Otolaryngol* 1984;110:76
5. Hillel AD, Fee WE Jr. Evaluation of frozen section in parotid gland surgery. *Arch Otolaryngol* 1983;104:230
6. Witt RL. Facial nerve monitoring in parotid surgery: the standard of care? *Otolaryngol Head Neck Surg* 1998;119:468
7. Tu G, Hu Y, Jiang P, Qin D. The superiority of combined therapy in parotid cancer. *Arch Otolaryngol* 1982;108:710
8. Matsuba HM, Thawley SE, Devineni VR, et al. High grade malignancies of the parotid gland: effective use of planned combined surgery and irradiation. *Laryngoscope* 1985;95:1059
9. Griffin TW, Pajak TF, Laramore GE, et al. Neutron vs. photon irradiation of inoperable salivary gland tumors: results of an RTOG-MRC cooperative randomized study. *Int J Radiat Oncol Biol Phys* 1988;15:1085
10. Phillips PP, Olsen KD. Recurrent pleomorphic adenoma of the parotid gland: report of 126 cases and a review of the literature. *Ann Otol Rhinol Laryngol* 1995;104:100

The Parotid Neoplasm

CHAPTER 66

Ehab Y. Hanna and James Y. Suen

Most parotid masses represent benign neoplasms, most commonly pleomorphic adenoma, originating from the superficial lobe of the gland. Surgical excision is usually all that is required to provide both definitive diagnosis and adequate treatment. Despite this relatively simple algorithm, management of other types of parotid neoplasms is challenging because of their relative infrequency, inconsistent classification, and highly variable biologic behavior. These factors present some difficulty when one attempts to compare data from various institutions describing their experience with parotid tumors. However, some general features can be drawn from the literature regarding the incidence, pathology, and patterns of behavior of benign and malignant tumors of the parotid gland. Despite the large volume of literature describing these salient features, substantial controversy remains regarding several aspects of management of parotid tumors. Some of these controversies concern the role of fine-needle biopsy and high-resolution imaging in the diagnosis of parotid masses. Other controversies exist regarding the extent of resection in benign parotid tumors, management of the facial nerve, the role of elective neck dissection, and the indications of adjuvant radiotherapy. This chapter discusses some of these controversial issues.

Fine-Needle Aspiration Biopsy

The accuracy of fine needle aspiration biopsy (FNAB) in the diagnosis of salivary tumors has been well established. During the past 5 years, several studies from various countries have reported an exceptionally high degree of sensitivity and specificity. Examples of such studies are summarized in Table 66–1. The overall sensitivity ranges from 85.5% to 99%, and the overall specificity ranges from 96.3% to 100%.[1-6] Diagnostic accuracy depends greatly on the experience of the cytopathologist, which in turn depends on the overall volume of patients with salivary neoplasms evaluated in any given institution. The reported sensitivity and specificity were slightly lower in community hospitals than at large academic centers.[7] The most common source of diagnostic error is inadequate sampling. Among 582 FNABs of major and minor salivary glands, lack of cytologic and histologic correlation was noted in 21 cases. Of these, the cause in 10 FNABs was inadequate cytologic sampling of the lesion.[8]

In addition to being accurate, FNAB is safe, simple to perform, and relatively inexpensive. However, one essential question is worth asking. Is FNAB really necessary in the evaluation of parotid masses? Would it change the course of management based on clinical assessment? In an attempt to answer this question, Heller et al.[9] performed a study to determine the impact of FNAB on patient management. In this study, 101 patients underwent FNAB of the major salivary gland masses. The physician's initial clinical impression was compared with the FNAB diagnosis and the final diagnosis in each case. Overall, FNAB prompted a change in the clinical approach to 35% of patients. Examples of such changes in the planned management included avoiding a relatively large resection for lymphomas and sialadenitis. FNAB leads to better informed preoperative counseling of patients, alleviating an already high level of anxiety both to them and to their families.[2] On the

TABLE 66–1
Sensitivity and Specificity of Fine-Needle Aspiration Biopsy

Study/Year	Country	Total Patients	Patients with Malignancy	Sensitivity %	Specificity %
Orell[1] (1995)	Australia	325	—	85.5	99.5
Candel et al.[2] (1993)	USA	163	15	95.7	100
Roland et al.[3] (1993)	UK	92	—	90.9	100
Bhatia[4] (1993)	India	101	34	99	100
Chan et al.[5] (1992)	Hong Kong	112	36	86	99
Abad et al.[6] (1992)	Spain	97	18	90	96.3

basis of these findings, the performance of FNAB may be helpful in treatment planning for patients who present with parotid masses.[9]

Imaging Studies

The routine use of imaging in small well-defined masses of the superficial lobe of the parotid gland is probably not warranted, because imaging in such instances rarely alters the planned management. However, tumors presenting with clinical findings suggestive of malignancy, tumors arising from the deep lobe of the parotid gland, or tumors extending to the parapharyngeal space are better evaluated with high-resolution imaging. Computed tomography (CT) and magnetic resonance imaging (MRI) give a better understanding of the location and extent of the tumor, its relation to major neurovascular structures, perineural spread, and skull base invasion. Conventional radiography and sialography are rarely used because they provide little useful information. Nuclear imaging using technetium-99m pertechnetate is helpful only with oncocytic and Warthin's tumors.[10] Because aspiration needle biopsy can provide better information, nuclear imaging is rarely obtained. High-resolution ultrasound is useful in the hands of experienced radiologists and may detect calculi, abscesses, and cysts; it has been reported to assess up to 90% of benign versus malignant tumors correctly.[11] Imaging modality of choice in evaluating parotid masses remains somewhat controversial among clinicians. Most of this controversy represents either personal or institutional bias, and there is a paucity of published data comparing the merits of different imaging modalities in the evaluation of parotid tumors. Some of these data are outlined herein.

CT AND MRI

Both CT and MRI provide information superior to that provided by other imaging techniques or by physical examination.[12] To obtain the maximum amount of information possible, CT scanning should be performed with intravenous injection of contrast material. The normal parotid gland has a high fat content and is easily visualized on both CT and MRI; therefore, both techniques can demonstrate whether a mass is intra- or extraglandular. Generally, CT/MRI do not provide information regarding the specific histologic diagnosis, except rarely. An example of such a rare scenario is with lipoma of the parotid gland. However, CT/MRI can give useful information that may differentiate benign from malignant tumors. In contrast to benign tumors, which invariably have well-defined margins, malignant tumors usually exhibit irregular margins. Extension of the tumor beyond the confines of the gland can be adequately seen on both CT and MRI. Bony destruction of the mandible or skull base is best visualized on CT, whereas bone marrow involvement is better demonstrated on MRI. Both studies can adequately evaluate the neck for metastatic adenopathy. CT has the advantage of being less expensive and more available than MRI. However, CT images are more susceptible to degradation by dental artifact.[12] MRI is superior to CT in demonstrating the internal architecture of salivary gland tumors in a multiplanar fashion, and in delineating the interface between tumor and normal salivary gland.[13]

Perineural spread of parotid malignancy along the facial nerve have a profound negative impact on survival and can drastically change the therapeutic plan, including the surgical approach and adjuvant therapy.[14] Although perineural spread may present as abnormal nerve function, it often is asymptomatic. High-resolution imaging may be helpful in such cases in detecting perineural involvement. The criteria of nerve involvement on CT rely on bony changes along the course of the facial nerve. These changes include bone erosion, sclerotic margins, and widening of the normal diameter of the fallopian canal or stylomastoid foramen. However, these findings are late indicators of perineural spread. Perineural spread can be detected earlier on MRI, because of the better soft tissue delineation. The capability of MRI to detect the different signal intensity of tumor, fat, and nerve allow for better assessment of perineural spread. The criteria of nerve involvement on MRI include replacement of normal perineural fat with tumor, enhancement with gadolinium (regardless of size), and increased size of the nerve in question (regardless of enhancement). Using these criteria, MRI is more sensitive and specific in evaluating perineural spread than CT.[14]

Although parapharyngeal space masses are well visualized by both techniques, they are better delineated with MRI than CT. This is because of the different signal intensity of tumor, fat, and muscle on MRI. Most salivary tumors have low to intermediate T1 signal intensities and intermediate to high T2 signal intensities. The differential diagnoses of parapharyngeal masses include deep lobe parotid tumors, minor salivary gland tumors, and neurogenic and vascular tumors. Deep lobe parotid tumors and minor salivary gland tumors of the parapharyngeal space lie in the prestyloid compartment, anterior to the carotid artery, and displace the parapharyngeal fat medially. Deep lobe tumors are connected to the parotid gland at least in one imaging section. Minor salivary gland tumors are completely surrounded by fat.[12] By contrast, neurogenic tumors and glomus tumors lie in the poststyloid compartment, posterior to the carotid artery, which is displaced anteriorly. Neurogenic tumors usually enhance intensely with gadolinium, whereas glomus tumors have a characteristic serpiginous flow voids (salt-and-pepper appearance) on MRI.

OTHER IMAGING STUDIES

Ultrasonography

Ultrasonography has the advantage of being inexpensive, noninvasive, and simple to perform; it is also virtually free of complications.

It can be used to differentiate solid from cystic masses in the parotid gland. Its use is limited by its ability to visualize only relatively superficial masses.[12] Its value in evaluating the deep lobe of the parotid and the parapharyngeal space is hampered by the intervening mandibular ramus. Ultrasound guidance may improve the diagnostic accuracy of FNAB in complex masses of the parotid gland.

Color Doppler Sonography

Color duplex scanning is a noninvasive procedure that may be of help in the preoperative assessment of salivary gland tumors.[15] Color doppler sonography has been recently used to evaluate the vascular anatomy of the salivary glands. It can distinguish between the physiologic changes that occur during salivary stimulation in normal subjects, and the flow alterations that occur in diseased glands. Specific patterns of peak systolic vascular shifts were described in various pathologic processes including Sjögren's syndrome, pleomorphic adenoma, and malignant tumors.[16]

Positron Emission Tomography

A recent study evaluated the ability of positron emission tomography (PET) to differentiate benign from malignant lesions of the salivary glands before surgery.[17] Salivary gland masses were evaluated in 26 patients, using PET scans after the administration of fluorine-18-fluorodeoxyglucose (FDG). PET findings helped correctly differentiate benign from malignant masses in 69%, but were false-positive for malignancy in 31% of patients. The investigators concluded that FDG PET is not useful in classifying salivary gland tumors as benign or malignant.[17]

Extent of Resection for Benign Tumors

Pleomorphic adenomas (benign mixed tumors) form the majority of neoplasms arising from the parotid gland. Pleomorphic adenomas should not recur after adequate surgical excision. Most recurrences can be traced to enucleation of the mass with no appreciation of the pseudopodia-like extensions of tumor. Although it appears encapsulated, if a surrounding cuff of normal tissue is not removed along with the tumor, the risk of recurrence is high.[18] Recurrences frequently occur in multiple sites and are significantly more difficult to treat. Consequently, the treatment of choice for a pleomorphic adenoma of the parotid gland is excision of tumor with a surrounding cuff of normal tissue. Because 90% of pleomorphic adenomas arise lateral to the plane of the facial nerve, the treatment usually involves a complete or partial excision of the superficial lobe of the parotid gland. The extent of dissection of the facial nerve and the amount of parotid tissue resection depend on the size, location, and histology of the tumor.[18] Small adenomas located in the tail of the parotid gland may only require dissection of the lower division of the facial nerve with removal of the tumor and the surrounding parotid tissue, avoiding unnecessary dissection of the upper division. Larger tumors of the superficial lobe usually require a complete superficial parotidectomy. Deep lobe tumors usually require a total parotidectomy, with facial nerve preservation. Although there is some controversy regarding the extent of resection of normal tissue surrounding a pleomorphic adenoma, there is universal agreement that capsular penetration should be avoided in order to minimize the risks of recurrence.

Recurrent pleomorphic adenomas may present a more complex problem. The scarring and altered anatomy in such cases place the facial nerve at greater risk of surgical injury during the dissection. Under such circumstances, facial nerve monitoring during revision surgery may be helpful in reducing the risk of damage to the facial nerve. Frequently there are multiple foci of recurrence, and they may continue to manifest over several years. Provided that a recurrence is nonprogressive and asymptomatic, it may be prudent to observe such stable recurrent disease for sometime. During this period of observation, other recurrences may become manifest and, in such cases, multiple surgeries can thus be avoided.[18] Another reason for observing small asymptomatic recurrent pleomorphic adenomas is the increased risk to the facial nerve during revision surgery. Radiotherapy may be considered in the treatment of recurrent pleomorphic adenoma when surgery is no longer a feasible option.

Facial Nerve Management

One of the most crucial decisions in the planning of surgical treatment of parotid gland malignancy is management of the facial nerve. Several decades of controversy in the literature regarding the optimal management of the facial nerve have resulted in a better definition of the indications for preserving, sacrificing, and reconstructing the facial nerve. The current consensus is that the facial nerve should be dissected and preserved, unless it is directly involved by tumor.[18,19] Preoperative weakness or paralysis of the facial nerve usually indicates tumor involvement, and in these instances, the nerve should be sacrificed.[20] The nerve should also be sacrificed if there is intraoperative evidence of gross invasion or microscopic infiltration of the nerve by tumor, even in the presence of normal preoperative facial nerve function. This is more likely to occur with larger and high-grade tumors, and in tumors that extend from the superficial to the deep lobe transgressing the plane of the facial nerve.[18] Surgical margins on both the distal and proximal nerve stumps should be checked because of the possibility of perineural spread for some distance from the area of the primary tumor.[14] In certain cases, achieving negative surgical margins on the proximal stump of the facial nerve may require a mastoidectomy and facial nerve dissection along its course in the temporal bone. If the facial nerve is sacrificed, nerve repair may be done by using either direct neurorrhaphy of the cut edges, or a cable graft, depending on the length of the resected segment. Immediate rehabilitation of the paralyzed face requires diligent eye care to prevent exposure keratitis. This involves liberal use of artificial tears, lubricating ointment, and protection with an appropriate eye dressing and eyewear. A temporary tarsorrhaphy may be needed for patients with lower eyelid ectropion. A gold weight implant may be needed in patients with corneal exposure. If the facial nerve is not repaired or grafted, one or more of the surgical procedures for static or dynamic facial rehabilitation of the paralyzed face may be indicated.[18]

Neck Dissection

There is universal agreement in the literature that a neck dissection is indicated when there is clinical evidence of metastatic disease from the parotid gland to the cervical lymph nodes. This usually involves a comprehensive cervical lymphadenectomy, either a modified radical or radical neck dissection, depending on the extent of disease.[18] However, the surgical management of the clinically negative neck (N0) remains controversial. Both the indications and type of elective neck dissection are not well defined in the literature.

In an effort to define the indications for elective neck treatment, Armstrong et al.[21] studied the incidence of clinical and occult nodal disease in 474 patients with salivary gland cancer. Overall, clinically occult but pathologically positive nodes occurred in 12% of patients. In view of the low frequency of occult metastases in the entire group, routine elective treatment of the neck was not recommended. However, tumor size, and histologic grade significantly influenced the incidence of occult metastatic disease. Tumors of ≥4 cm had a 20% risk of occult metastases compared with a 4% risk for smaller tumors. High-grade tumors (regardless of histologic type) had a 49% risk of occult metastases compared with a 7% risk for intermediate-grade or low-grade tumors. Rodriguez-Cuevas et al.[22] also found an increased risk (50%) of occult node metastases in patients with high grade carcinomas, while no cases were found in low-grade carcinomas. These findings demonstrate that the incidence of occult regional disease in patients with large and/or high-grade tumors is relatively high; therefore, an elective neck dissection should be considered in these patients. A selective (supraomohyoid) neck dissection may be used as a staging procedure in such cases. Suspicious nodes should be sent for frozen-section diagnosis; if positive for metastatic carcinoma, a comprehensive neck dissection is performed. Elective neck dissection is probably not indicated for low-grade malignancy of the parotid gland.[21,22]

Radiotherapy

ADJUVANT RADIOTHERAPY

Several reports suggest that the use of adjuvant radiotherapy in conjunction with surgery is superior to surgery alone in the treatment of high-grade and/or advanced cancers of the parotid gland. Theriault and Fitzpatrick[23] reported the outcome of 271 with parotid carcinomas. Among these were 64 (24%) mucoepidermoid carcinomas, 50 (18%) adenocarcinomas, 40 (15%) malignant mixed tumors, 39 (14%) adenoid cystic carcinomas, 37 (14%) undifferentiated, 21 (8%) acinic, and 20 (7%) squamous cell carcinomas. The prognostic characteristics were similar for the 67 (25%) patients treated by surgery and for the 169 (62%) patients treated with surgery and postoperative radiotherapy. Patients treated with combined therapy had a 10-year relapse-free rate of 62% compared with 22% for those treated by surgery alone. Borthne et al.[24] demonstrated that radiation therapy lowered the recurrence rates after surgery and controlled approximately one-third of the inoperable tumors. Their data suggested that a dose-response relationship exists for salivary gland cancers and that the radiation dose should not be <70 Gy in 7 weeks.

Although the addition of adjuvant radiotherapy should not be considered an adequate substitute for clear surgical margins, in many instances it is not possible to obtain negative margins of resection. In such cases, the use of postoperative radiation may enhance local control. In 1994, Sakata et al.[25] described 17 patients with positive surgical margins after resection of cancer of the major salivary glands. All patients received postoperative radiotherapy. Overall local control at 5 years was 65%. Shingaki et al.[26] compared 22 patients with salivary gland malignancy treated with surgery alone with 22 patients treated with combination surgery and radiotherapy. In the surgery group, local recurrence developed in all 8 patients with evidence of residual disease at the surgical margins, whereas local control was achieved in 7 of 15 patients with positive surgical margins in the combination group, and the control rate was related to the amount of residual disease.

In conclusion, postoperative radiotherapy is generally recommended for patients with poor prognostic indicators, including high-grade tumors, large primary lesions, perineural invasion, bone invasion, cervical lymph node metastasis, and positive margins. Although a clear-cut survival advantage has not been established, the addition of postoperative radiotherapy improves locoregional control for patients with such adverse prognostic parameters.

RADIOTHERAPY FOR INOPERABLE TUMORS

Over the past decade, there has been substantial evidence that fast-neutron radiation therapy provides higher rates of locoregional control of unresectable salivary gland cancer compared to photon or electron radiation therapy[27-31] and perhaps should be considered the initial treatment of choice in such cases.[32] Buchholz et al.[33] reported the outcome of 53 patients with locally advanced salivary gland malignant neoplasms treated with fast neutron radiation therapy. All patients received treatment for gross inoperable, residual unresectable, or recurrent disease. With a median follow-up of 42 months and a minimum follow-up of 1 year, the overall locoregional tumor control rate was 77%. The 5-year actuarial overall locoregional control rate was 65%. Grouping patients according to prior treatment status, actuarial 5-year locoregional control rates were 92% for patients treated definitively (without a prior surgical procedure), 63% for those treated postoperatively for gross residual disease, and 51% for those treated for recurrent disease after a surgical procedure. This study suggested that neutron irradiation alone may be the therapy of choice in the treatment of advanced-stage unresectable salivary gland tumors, and that surgery should be limited to those patients in whom disease-free margins can be obtained. The potential morbidity of a debulking surgical procedure before neutron irradiation is not accompanied by an improvement in locoregional control over that achievable with neutron therapy alone.[33] These impressive results are encouraging; however, the use of fast-neutron radiotherapy is hampered by its lack of widespread availability. Currently, only few facilities are equipped with the technology and expertise of delivering fast-neutron radiotherapy.

Other investigators described their experience with photon-beam radiotherapy for the treatment of unresectable salivary gland cancer, and reported comparable results to those obtained by fast-neutron therapy. Wang and Goodman[34] presented their experience with 24 patients with inoperable and/or unresectable cancer of the parotid (9 patients), or the minor salivary glands (15 patients) treated by photon irradiation. The 5-year actuarial local control of parotid gland lesions after photon irradiation was 100%, and the survival rate was 65%. For the minor salivary gland lesions, the 5-year actuarial local control was 78% and the survival rate with or without disease was 93%. All lesions were irradiated by accelerated hyperfractionated photons (bid) with 1.6 Gy per fraction, intermixed with various boost techniques, including electron beam, intraoral cone, interstitial implant, and/or submental photons for a total of 65 to 70 Gy.

The Radiation Therapy Oncology Group (RTOG) in the United States and the Medical Research Council (MRC) in Great Britain sponsored a study comparing the efficacy of fast neutron radiotherapy versus conventional photon and/or electron radiotherapy for unresectable malignant salivary gland tumors. In 1993, Laramore et al.[35] published the final report on this study, demonstrating that at 10-year follow-up, there was a statistically significant improvement in local/regional control for the neutron group (56% vs 25%, $P = 0.009$), but there was no difference in survival between both arms of the study. Distant metastases accounted for the majority of failures in the neutron arm, and local/regional failures accounted for most failures in the photon arm. Although the incidence of morbidity graded "severe" was greater on the neutron arm, there was no significant difference in life-threatening complications. This well-executed study suggested that fast neutron radiotherapy may be a reasonable treatment option for patients with inoperable primary or recurrent malignant salivary gland tumors. It is hoped that fast-neutron therapy will be more widely available for patients with unresectable salivary gland malignancy.

Conclusion

1. Most parotid masses represent benign neoplasms, most commonly pleomorphic adenoma, originating from the superficial lobe of the gland. In this clinical scenario, surgical excision is usually all that is required to provide both definitive diagnosis and adequate treatment.
2. FNAB is helpful in treatment planning for patients presenting with parotid masses. The accuracy of this technique depends on sample adequacy, tumor cellularity, and the experience of the cytopathologist.
3. The routine use of imaging in small well-defined masses of the superficial lobe of the parotid gland is probably not warranted. However, tumors presenting with clinical findings suggestive of malignancy, tumors arising from the deep lobe of the parotid gland, or tumors extending to the parapharyngeal space are better evaluated with high-resolution imaging.
4. During parotid gland surgery for excision of malignant tumors the facial nerve is usually dissected and preserved, unless there is evidence of gross invasion or microscopic infiltration of the nerve by tumor, or there was evidence of preoperative facial weakness or paralysis.
5. The incidence of occult nodal metastasis in patients with large and/or high-grade malignant tumors is relatively high; therefore, an elective neck dissection should be considered in these patients.
6. Postoperative radiation therapy is generally recommended for patients with poor prognostic indicators including high-grade tumors, large primary lesions, perineural invasion, bone invasion, cervical lymph node metastasis, and positive margins.
7. Fast-neutron radiotherapy is a promising treatment option for patients with inoperable primary or recurrent malignant salivary gland tumors.

REFERENCES

1. Orell SR. Diagnostic difficulties in the interpretation of fine needle aspirates of salivary gland lesions: the problem revisited. *Cytopathology* 1995;6:285–300
2. Candel A, Gattuso P, Reddy V, Matz G, Castelli M. Is fine needle aspiration biopsy of salivary gland masses really necessary? *Ear Nose Throat J* 1993;72:485–489
3. Roland NJ, Caslin AW, Smith PA, et al. Fine needle aspiration cytology of salivary gland lesions reported immediately in a head and neck clinic. *J Laryngol Otol* 1993;107: 1025–1028
4. Bhatia A. Fine needle aspiration cytology in the diagnosis of mass lesions of the salivary gland. *Indian J Cancer* 1993;30:26–30
5. Chan MK, McGuire LJ, King W, et al. Cytodiagnosis of 112 salivary gland lesions. Correlation with histologic and frozen section diagnosis. *Acta Cytol* 1992;36:353–363
6. Abad MM, G-Macias C, Alonso MJ, et al. Statistical evaluation of the predictive power of fine needle aspiration (FNA) of salivary glands. Results and cytohistological correlation. *Path Res Pract* 1992;188:340–343
7. Pitts DB, Hilsinger RL Jr, Karandy E, et al. Fine-needle aspiration in the diagnosis of salivary gland disorders in the community hospital setting. *Arch Otolaryngol Head Neck Surg* 1992;118:479–482
8. MacLeod CB, Frable WJ. Fine-needle aspiration biopsy of the salivary gland: problem cases. *Diagn Cytopathol* 1993;9:216–224; discussion 224–225
9. Heller KS, Dubner S, Chess Q, et al. Value of fine needle aspiration biopsy of salivary gland masses in clinical decision-making. *Am J Surg* 1992;164:667–670
10. Higashi T, Shindo J, Everhart FR, et al. Technetium-99m pertechnetate and gallium-67 imaging in salivary gland disease. *Clin Nucl Med* 1989;14:504–514
11. Gritzman N. Sonography of the salivary glands. *Am J Roentgenol* 1989; 153:161–155
12. Heller KS. Salivary gland cancer-diagnostic evaluation. In: Johnson JT, Didolkar, eds. *Head and Neck Cancer.* Vol III. New York: Elsevier Science; 1993;589–594
13. Kaneda T, Minami M, Ozawa K, et al. Imaging tumors of the minor salivary glands. *Oral Surg Oral Med Oral Path* 1994;78: 385–390
14. Hanna E, Janecka I. Perineural spread in head and neck and skull base cancer. *Crit Rev Neurosurg* 1994;4:109–115
15. Ajayi BA, Pugh ND, Carolan G, et al. Salivary gland tumours: is colour Doppler imaging of added value in their preoperative assessment? *Eur J Surg Oncol* 1992;18:463–468
16. Martinoli C, Derchi LE, Solbiati L, et al. Color Doppler sonography of salivary glands. *Am J Roentgenol* 1994;163:933–941
17. Keyes JW Jr, Harkness BA, Greven KM, et al. Salivary gland tumors: pretherapy evaluation with PET. *Radiology* 1994; 192:99–102
18. Hanna E, Suen JY. Neoplasms of the salivary glands. In: Cummings CW, Fredrickson JM, Harker LA, Kraus CJ, Schuller DE, Richardson MA, eds. *Otolaryngology–Head and Neck Surgery.* Vol II. 3rd Ed. St. Louis, MO: CV Mosby; 1998; 1255–1302
19. Woods JE. The facial nerve in parotid malignancy. *Am J Surg* 1983;146:493–496
20. Woods JE, Chong GC, Beahrs OH. Experience with 1,360 primary parotid tumors. *Am J Surg* 1975;130:460–462
21. Armstrong JG, Harrison LB, Thaler HT, et al. The indications for elective treatment of the neck in cancer of the major salivary glands. *Cancer* 1992;69:615–619
22. Rodriguez-Cuevas S, Labastida S, Baena L, et al. Risk of nodal metastases from malignant salivary gland tumors related to tumor size and grade of malignancy. *Eur Arch Oto Rhinol Laryngol* 1995;252:139–142
23. Theriault C, Fitzpatrick PJ. Malignant parotid tumors: prognostic factors and optimum treatment. *Am J Clin Oncol* 1986; 9:510–516
24. Borthne A, Kjellevold K, Kaalhus O, et al. Salivary gland malignant neoplasms: treatment and prognosis. *Int J Radiat Oncol Biol Phys* 1986;12:747–754
25. Sakata K, Aoki Y, Karasawa K, et al. Radiation therapy for patients of malignant salivary gland tumors with positive surgical margins. *Strahlenther und Onkol* 1994;170: 342–346
26. Shingaki S, Ohtake K, Nomura T, et al. The role of radiotherapy in the management of salivary gland carcinomas. *J Craniomaxillofac Surg* 1992;20:220–224
27. Stelzer KJ, Laramore GE, Griffin TW, et al. Fast neutron radiotherapy. The University of Washington experience. *Acta Oncol* 1994;33:275–280
28. Koh W, Laramore G, Griffin T, et al. Fast neutron radiation for inoperable and recurrent salivary gland cancers. *Am J Clin Oncol* 1989;12:316–319
29. Saroja KR, Mansell J, Hendrickson FR, et al. An update on malignant salivary gland tumors treated with neutrons at Fermilab. *Int J Radiat Oncol Biol Phys* 1987;13:1319–1325
30. Catterall M, Errington RD. The implications of improved treatment of malignant salivary gland tumors by fast neutron radiotherapy. *Int J Radiat Oncol Biol Phys* 1987;13: 1313–1318
31. Henry LW, Blasko JC, Griffin TW, et al. Evolution of fast neutron teletherapy for advanced carcinomas of the major salivary glands. *Cancer* 1979;44:814–818

32. Laramore GE: Fast neutron radiotherapy for inoperable salivary gland tumors: is it the treatment of choice? *Int J Radiat Oncol Biol Phys* 1987;13:1421–1423
33. Buchholz TA, Laramore GE, Griffin BR, et al. The role of fast neutron radiation therapy in the management of advanced salivary gland malignant neoplasms. *Cancer* 1992; 69:2779–2788
34. Wang CC, Goodman M. Photon irradiation of unresectable carcinomas of salivary glands. *Int J Radiat Oncol Biol Phys* 1991;21:569–576
35. Laramore GE, Krall JM, Griffin TW, et al. Neutron versus photon irradiation for unresectable salivary gland tumors: final report of an RTOG–MRC randomized clinical trial. *Int J Radiat Oncol Biol Phys* 1993;27:235–240

SUGGESTED READINGS

Hanna and Suen—CHAPTER 66

Armstrong JG, Harrison LB, Thaler HT, et al. The indications for elective treatment of the neck in cancer of the major salivary glands. *Cancer* 1992;69:615–619

Hanna E, Suen JY. Neoplasms of the salivary glands. In: Cummings CW, Fredrickson JM, Harker LA, Kraus CJ, Schuller DE, Richardson MA, eds. *Otolaryngology–Head and Neck Surgery* Vol II. 3rd Ed. St. Louis, MO: CV Mosby; 1998;1255–1302

Heller KS, Dubner S, Chess Q, et al. Value of fine needle aspiration biopsy of salivary gland masses in clinical decision–making. *Am J Surg* 1992;164:667–670

Laramore GE, Krall JM, Griffin TW, et al. Neutron versus photon irradiation for unresectable salivary gland tumors: final report of an RTOG–MRC randomized clinical trial. *Int J Radiat Oncol Biol Phys* 1993;27:235–240

23

Pediatric Chronic Rhinosinusitis Assessment and Management

"Whereas most clinicians would easily accept that a chronic sinus condition exists when a single process persists for more than several months, there is little evidence to suggest that this occurs in young children at a rate beyond rarely. By contrast, the pediatric sinus is frequently, and sometimes continually, assailed by the multitude of respiratory pathogens typical of the day-care flora."

Michael D. Poole

"There is little doubt that sinuslike symptoms occur in children with large obstructive adenoid pads. If the obstructive adenoid pad is not removed, the nasal cavity cannot become healthy. Several studies indicate that adenoidectomy improves the signs and symptoms of sinusitis. Good prospective studies designed to assess the efficacy of adenoidectomy in well-documented cases of sinusitis are needed".

Rodney P. Lusk

"There are virtually no data indicating the optimum duration of antimicrobial therapy for chronic rhinosinusitis in children, although many clinicians recommend a minimum course of 3 to 6 weeks. In general, antibiotic therapy extended 1 week beyond the time that symptoms resolve provides an opportunity for eradication of all bacteria. If, however, there is no symptomatic response after 5 to 7 days of antimicrobial therapy, the antibiotic should be changed."

Richard N. Hubbell

Pediatric Chronic Rhinosinusitis Assessment and Management

CHAPTER 67

Michael D. Poole

This chapter is intended to guide the sophisticated consumer of otolaryngology literature through many of the challenging clinical problems for which there are no straightforward answers, no definite proofs of efficacy, and no consensus. Pediatric sinusitis, particularly those aspects that pertain to surgical therapy, is an ideal topic for such a work, especially because so few published pertinent works are intellectually sound, scientifically rigorous, and unbiased in their conclusions. Nonetheless, pediatric sinusitis is a common and important entity, and clinicians can better manage patients, families, and other clinicians through improved understanding of the diagnostic and therapeutic dilemmas we face. This review includes a brief historic overview and then considers controversies and problem areas in the definition, diagnosis, and treatment of disease. It is my intent to pull no punches, but rather to expose the reader to the range of critical opinions about current literature and practice.

A Brief History of Pediatric Sinusitis

Before the 1980s, pediatric sinusitis, especially in the young child or infant, was rarely entertained as a distinct clinical entity. Most cases were apparently dismissed as an unimportant "allergy" or a "cold" and were rarely treated with anything beyond decongestants or antihistamines, or both, perhaps not an altogether bad approach. Through a series of well-designed and executed studies, Dr. Ellen Wald and her associates in Pittsburgh established a logical framework for diagnosing and treating children with sinus infections.[1,2] These and other studies, many with pharmaceuticals industry support, demonstrated the efficacy of antimicrobial therapy.[3,4]

During the late 1980s the recognition of the value of coronal computed tomography (CT) and sinus telescopes led to the rise of "osteomeatal fundamentalism" as a predominant sinus doctrine, especially among rhinologic surgeons. Obstruction of the osteomeatal complex (OMC), recognized as being involved in selected cases of persistent or chronic sinusitis, was put forward as a unifying event in acute, recurrent, and chronic sinusitis. Initially focusing on adult disease, support for OMC doctrine proliferated, as did endoscopic sinus surgery courses and surgical cases.

During the early 1990s, several individuals and groups began performing and reporting hundreds of cases of pediatric endoscopic sinus surgery (mostly infants and young children).[5-9] Applied enthusiasm for the procedure made more than a few pediatric otolaryngologists wealthy. The excitement for the procedure, among surgeons, was understandable—suddenly, the most common childhood illness (rhinitis/sinusitis) could be viewed as a surgical disease. The surgical indications were, in general, some type of sinus symptomatology, with rhinorrhea the most common, and CT evidence of mucosal disease, and sometimes simply an abnormal CT. This occurred before the nature of the "sinus disease" was defined or understood, in terms of etiology or pathogenesis. A number of otolaryngologists went on record against this trend, and the topic was the subject of the 1994 Great Debate in Otolaryngology at the Annual Meeting of the American Academy of Otolaryngology[10,11] Over the past 3 years, the number of pediatric and infantile cases has moderated substantially, and several of the busiest surgeons have withdrawn support for the operation, at least for nonmorbid indications.

The 1990s saw an explosion in the number of oral antimicrobial agents that might be used in sinusitis, but also a dramatic rise in resistance to those antimicrobials. This decade has seen an increase in our understanding of the pharmacokinetic and pharmacodynamic properties of antimicrobials that contribute to their clinical effectiveness in respiratory infections. Recent and forthcoming recommendations from consensus panels have reflected that understanding and the outcome from a few comparative trials—making a handful of antimicrobials "winners" and the rest either "also-rans" or losers. The array of antimicrobial choices, resistance issues, and selection considerations has complicated the selection process.[12]

Problems in Definitions

SINUSITIS, RHINOSINUSITIS, OR NASOPHARYNGITIS?

The organisms classically associated with acute bacterial respiratory infections—*Streptococcus pneumoniae, Haemophilus influenzae,* and *Moraxella catarrhalis*—are not usually considered pathogens of abscess cavities. Rather, they are mucosal pathogens that have proclivities for thriving on damaged respiratory epithelium, whether in the cigarette smoke–damaged lungs of the adult with chronic bronchitis or in the virally damaged airway of the child in daycare. Unfortunately, any attempt to use bacterial samples from the nasal specimens, as opposed to maxillary antral aspirates, would prompt critics to decry the results on the grounds that (1) nasal cultures do not correlate with antral cultures, and (2) the organisms recovered are considered "normal" nasal flora, particularly in children and infants.

To the critics, we might respond by asking, Who cares what is in the maxillary sinus? Our job is to characterize the disease present in the symptomatic patient. Although typical sinusitis pathogens may be present in low to modest numbers in the asymptomatic patient, it appears difficult to classify as "normal" a symptomatic nasal airway with significant damage to the epithelial ultrastructure, a heavy concentration of acute inflammatory cells, and the presence of pathogenic bacteria in high concentrations. This condition may be common, and often self-limiting, but it is certainly not normal. A more accurate differentiation of significant from insignificant bacterial infection should probably be based on quantitative bacteriology combined with an assessment of the inflammatory and immunologic responses, and not by the specific sinus involved. Easier said than done, perhaps, but to assume otherwise leads us clinically astray. The above considerations can be turned into a case for the use of nasal cultures of visible purulence when that purulence is persistent, has failed empirical therapy and is thought to be related to the disease process of interest. Purulent secretions probably have some, but not absolute, predictive value for bacterial infection versus viral processes. Some viral infections can present with thick purulent secretions, especially in the morning, after nocturnal stasis of the nasal secretions.[1]

WHY THE MAXILLARY SINUS?

Although the frontal and sphenoid sinuses have long been recognized as occasional sites of clinically important disease, the maxillary sinus has traditionally been the focus for defining bacterial sinusitis. Emphasis on the OMC has only recently shifted new attention to the importance of the ethmoidal cells. In retrospect, it was our ability to "image" the maxillary sinuses satisfactorily with standard radiographic equipment, that led to that site as the gold standard for assessing the microbiology and efficacy issues surrounding sinusitis. The insistence by established sinus investigators and regulatory agencies, such as Food and Drug Administration (FDA), that sinusitis primarily be considered by maxillary investigations is not consistent with our current understanding. In all likelihood, for most cases of symptomatic acute sinusitis, mucosal disease in the ethmoids and nasal cavity accounts for more symptoms than what transpires in the maxillary sinus, especially in children.

WHAT IS "CHRONIC" PEDIATRIC SINUSITIS?

Whereas most clinicians would easily accept that a chronic sinus condition exists when a single process persists for more than several months, there is little evidence to suggest that this occurs in young children at a rate beyond rarely. By contrast, the pediatric sinus is frequently, and sometimes continually, assailed by the multitude of respiratory pathogens typical of the day-care flora. It appears that a number of clinicians have extrapolated certain diagnostic and therapeutic approaches from otitis media to the assessment and management of pediatric sinusitis. At first glance, the rationale appears sound—the same organisms, similar respiratory epithelium, closed-space infections, and the like. The two major inconsistencies relate to the failure to differentiate accurately between the various clinical types of sinusitis and the failure to understand the real pathophysiologic basis of pediatric rhinosinusitis.

Most cases of pediatric endoscopic sinus surgery are performed after a period of chronicity or multiple sinus infections. Some clinicians have advocated protocols in which sinus surgery was recommended after failure of an adenoidectomy to control the disease.[13] But what is the definition of failure, and what is the process responsible for these clinical failures? Is it persistent bacterial infection? Perhaps—but that, we believe, can be completely eliminated as a problem by effective antimicrobial use, even considering today's resistance problems (see Treatment Issues, below). Is it uncontrolled allergic disease? I am not aware of anyone admitting to recommending pediatric sinus surgery for allergic disease (without polyps). Most chronic disease actually represents the reemergence of symptoms related to intercurrent new viral and bacterial respiratory infections. Perhaps just as important as a determinant of which child receives aggressive sinus management is the presence of a family member who is uncommonly focused on, and intolerant of, sinus symptoms. Those symptoms and associated findings are typically identical to those of thousands of other children who are receiving no specific care for their rhinosinusitis.

IS PEDIATRIC RHINOSINUSITIS AN OBSTRUCTIVE PROCESS?

The role of OMC obstruction, and therefore of sinus surgery, has been restated so often that the doctrine has rarely been challenged—at least by otolaryngologists. However, proof of a role for ostial obstruction in the routine case of sinusitis is lacking. An occasional case of pediatric sinus disease has an obvious obstructive component. Most cases, however, do not. It has been our impression that children with widely patent (postsurgical) sinus ostia do not differ significantly in the incidence of acute rhinosinusitis or the radiographic presentation of individual cases from that of children without enlarged ostia. In other words, mucosal disease, with damage to the ultrastructural integrity, is the key pathologic change in acute rhinosinusitis, and will be largely unaffected by ostial surgery.

Problems in Diagnosis

HETEROGENEITY OF SINUSITIS

The onset of acute sinusitis typically involves an antecedent mucosal insult, such as one of a wide variety of viral infections or atopic inflammation, followed by infection caused by one of several different bacterial species. Because a large number of host factors add to the variance related to multiple viral and bacterial causes of sinusitis, clinicians dealing with this entity are actually faced with a wide and very heterogeneous group of processes with significant differences in severity of illness, natural history, and response to a given intervention. In all probability, if we were to try to lump such a huge array of processes together at any other anatomic site and attempt to develop logical and consistent diagnostic or therapeutic algorithms, we would be laughed out of academic medicine. In short, sinusitis is a vague description of inflammatory processes involving the sinuses. It is now clear that viruses can cause "rhinosinusitis," as well as bacteria, as can, in all likelihood, some types of atopic disease.

The clinically indistinct nature of sinusitis has allowed for the "disease" to be twisted to the advantage of special interest groups. The pharmaceuticals industry would like us to believe that all cases of clinically defined sinusitis warrant the use of the latest antimicrobial. The allergists would have us believe that all the patients require an allergic evaluation. The surgeons point to the central role of the osteomeatal complex in the pathogenesis of the disease. All have used their arguments to increase their own business and profit.

WHEN IS SINUSITIS PRESENT?

Many lecturers try to convince their audiences that unless the signs and symptoms of pediatric sinusitis have been present and unabated for 7 to 10 days, the chance of having "sinusitis" is remote. This notion is false. More accurately, the likelihood of having significant bacterial infection in the maxillary sinus is small. However, most patients with a cold or respiratory virus actually do have rhinosinusitis, at least according to histopathologic and radiologic criteria. We have traditionally ignored "viral rhinosinusitis" because we had no effective therapy, and because the disease was usually uncomplicated and spontaneously resolving—although the degree of morbidity and length of symptoms varies widely. Consider now that we are on the threshold of possessing prescription drugs active against influenza or the common "cold" that will shorten the period of symptomatology and viral shedding. Suddenly, we are in the business of diagnosing diseases that have, for several generations, been intentionally ignored. We can only refine our therapeutics when we refine our diagnostic abilities.

WHEN SHOULD RADIOLOGIC EVALUATIONS BE ORDERED?

Because of the very high incidence of abnormal CT scans in young children,[14] a scan cannot rationally be used to determine the need for sinus surgery. Most abnormal CT findings are related to routine (self-limiting) viral and bacterial infections or to postinfectious inflammatory changes that are not related to any particular symptomatology. CT scans, or perhaps other imaging studies, are reasonably ordered with a clinical suspicion of complications (periorbital, intracranial) or in the face of significant symptoms that may be related to sinusitis (e.g., marked worsening of bronchospasm) without findings specific for sinusitis. Children with abnormal nasal symptoms (e.g, rhinorrhea, congestion) will, in the vast majority of cases, have a scan with abnormal findings. Does one type of CT finding make the patient a better surgical candidate than another set of findings? Some surgeons prefer to consider patients with mucosal disease limited to the OMC, whereas others prefer their surgical candidates to have pansinusitis. If one views sinusitis as a mucosal disease, neither preference makes much sense. An unbalanced emphasis on CT finding has caused any number of families to focus on those findings as if the CT findings were a disease themselves, regardless patient's clinical status.

WHAT ABOUT ALLERGY, IMMUNODEFICIENCY, AND REFLUX?

By the time a child arrives in the otolaryngologist's office for evaluation of "chronic" sinusitis, someone in the family will have raised the issue that "this is all due to allergy." In many situations, the nature of the rhinorrhea and congestion does resemble that seen in atopic patients. However, microscopic and immunologic analyses of the secretions are not consistent with what is seen in IgE-mediated rhinitis. Rather, the findings are those of acute infectious inflammation. Whereas some reports report a higher incidence of sinusitis in atopic children, concerns about reporting biases and biases in the allergy practices reporting such findings raise concerns about the validity of the reports. The primary risk factors for such disease are primarily related to exposure to other children, as in day care. The prompt response to effective antimicrobials also weighs against allergy being of primary importance. As a child grows beyond 3–5 years of age, the incidence of IgE-mediated disease rises and becomes more important in the differential diagnosis. Although the rationale for atopic mucosa increasing the likelihood of bacterial infection appears sound, many of our adults with the worst allergic rhinitis are never affected by bacterial sinusitis.

Some allergists maintain that the main culprit is an IgG-mediated allergy or food allergy. Although that may occasionally be the case, the scientific evidence for food allergy contributing to pediatric sinusitis is weak.

The role of testing for immunodeficiencies in patients with problematic pediatric sinusitis is controversial. Mild age-related immunodeficiency is common, but a specific therapy for this is not currently available or practical. The same applies for IgG subclass deficiencies. We do not generally order such tests unless a child is severely affected or shows evidence of chronic infections elsewhere.

Reflux esophagitis is said to be an underlying cause of chronic pediatric sinusitis with a frequency ranging from almost always to rarely.[15,16] Testing or empirical therapy for reflux may be appropriate in children with associated symptoms of reflux or in cases in which other forms of medical therapy have not been successful.

In approaching the child with "chronic sinusitis," we find it useful to try to classify the patients as having one or more of the common sinus "syndromes" (in the approximate order of frequency):

1. Relatively normal rhinosinusitis with an excessively concerned family
2. Frequently recurrent rhinosinusitis (day-care syndrome)
3. Purulent rhinosinusitis unresponsive to empirically selected oral antimicrobials
4. Rhinosinusitis associated with posterior nasal obstruction (adenoid enlargement)
5. Sinusitis with reflux
6. Significant component of IgE-mediated rhinitis/sinusitis

Treatment Issues

ANTIMICROBIAL ISSUES

There have been no recent clinical trials pitting one antibiotic versus another for pediatric sinusitis. The major reason has to do with the perceived need to obtain bacteriologic data by means of maxillary antral taps. Still, the lack of direct comparative evidence does not diminish the compelling evidence from other sources about the relative efficacy of available antimicrobials against the pathogens of interest. Young children with persistent bacterial rhinosinusitis often harbor multiple relatively resistant pathogens, making empirical therapy with a single agent problematic. Even the more potent agents (e.g., amoxicillin-clavulanate, cefuroxime axetil, cefpodoxime proxetil) will fail against some of strains of *S. pneumoniae* and *H. influenzae*. Resistance to sulfa drugs and the macrolides (including azithromycin and clarithromycin) is relatively common among those same organisms. Even pneumococcal resistance to clindamycin is increasing. However, if a given strain is isolated and susceptibility testing is performed, an astute clinician can usually find at least one oral agent that is active against that organism. Ceftriaxone, when given for more than 3 to 5 doses is currently active (in the respiratory tract) against virtually all strains of pneumococci, *Haemophilus*, and *Moraxella*. In an important recent study, 90% of surgical candidates were cured by potent antimicrobial therapy.[17]

If a patient still has suspected bacterial rhinosinusitis, and a culture has not been obtained or is not helpful, empirical therapy with 5 to 10 days of ceftriaxone can be expected be effective in well over 90% of cases (in older children, the addition of anti-staphylococcal and anaerobe coverage should be considered, e.g., clindamycin). Other potent empirical combinations include high-dose amoxicillin-clavulanate (approximately 90 mg/kg/day of the amoxicillin component, maintaining a 14:1 ratio of amoxicillin to clavulanate), clindamycin plus a third-generation cephalosporin (e.g., ceftibuten), or one or more shots of ceftriaxone followed by high-dose amoxicillin. Recently available conjugated pneumococcal vaccines may reduce the likelihood of colonization or infection with drug-resistant strains of pneumococci, making third generation cephalosporins (e.g., cefpodoxime proxetil or cefdinir) relatively more attractive. The interested reader is directed elsewhere or to papers related to antimicrobial therapy for otitis media.

SURGICAL OPTIONS

Adenoidectomy is the most commonly recommended procedure for young children with problematic sinusitis. That procedure may alleviate posterior nasal obstruction or reduce the reservoir of pathogenic bacteria. A number of clinicians still routinely perform therapeutic lavages of the maxillary sinuses of affected children,[18] whereas a number never perform this procedure. We have found it neither useful nor necessary.

Pediatric endoscopic sinus surgery (PESS) has been reported to yield satisfactory results in 80 to 95% of cases.[17, 23] We know from the otitis media literature that almost two-thirds of infants and children identified as prone to otitis on historic grounds no longer continue that pattern, with placebo providing dramatic improvement. Pediatric rhinosinusitis should be no different. In a study of chronic pediatric maxillary opacification, almost all resolved spontaneously.[19]

Most surgeons routinely administer intravenous antibiotics along with performing the surgery, obscuring the efficacy of surgery alone. Furthermore, PESS has not been directly compared with enlightened nonsurgical management. Notably, hundreds to thousands of otolaryngologists feel capable of managing these same cases without PESS.

In cases of sinusitis complicating asthma, PESS has been reported to significantly improve the course of the asthma.[20] A number of clinicians have used that information to lower the threshold for PESS in the presence asthma. The real conclusion should be that effective therapy for sinusitis assists in the management of asthmatics. A number of us achieve the same improvement without surgery.

PROBLEMS AND COMPLICATIONS OF PESS

For most sinus surgeons, the scope of PESS has been reduced sufficiently that it is now a relatively safe and well-tolerated procedure. Some concerns remain. Most importantly, the surgery may not achieve the expected results. For example, we have seen many children who have undergone one or more sinus surgeries with a period of improvement, only to exhibit similar radiographic and clinical findings again, and to become surgical candidates once again. In these cases, what are the goals of surgery in a patient who continues to have episodic pansinusitis whose sinus ostia are already widely patent?

The true incidence of nasal synechiae or other abnormal intranasal scars is unknown but is undoubtedly underreported. Most of the pediatric intranasal synechiae that we have seen have not been reported to the family by the operating surgeon. An occasional case of PESS becomes markedly dysfunctional. This patient, who initially may have had relatively limited OMC mucosal disease during an episodic case of rhinosinusitis develops chronic staphylococcal, pseudomonal, or fungal sinusitis and osteitis after PESS, with years of symptomatology, intravenous antibiotics (usually unsuccessful), and multiple operations. There may be important functional and protective reasons that sinus ostia developed in such anatomically protected locations. Most of us caring for a significant number of sinus surgery cases note the creation of a small number of "sinus cripples." They exist in two varieties. The first type is the patient with the unrelenting opportunistic infection in a sinus that has been operated on, as described above. The second type, seen in patients or their families, reflects a reinforced obsession about the sinonasal symptoms, CT scans, or various treatments. We have to wonder how many of those cases could have been avoided by a more balanced and conservative management.

The impact of PESS on facial growth has received a fair amount of attention since Maier and colleagues reported that intranasal surgery on piglets interfered with growth of the midface.[21] Abnormal growth, particularly midface hypoplasia, has been reported anecdotally in children.[22, 24] The significance of this problem has been downplayed by some surgeons, noting that facial growth in piglets was much greater than in humans over the period of infancy to adulthood, and therefore, the impact on cosmesis was significantly less in humans. Although the alterations in facial growth may not be obvious to the casual observer in most cases, alterations in maxillary growth will probably impact dental occlusion—a problem that has not been investigated.

PEDIATRIC SINUS SURGERY—A STINGING ASSESSMENT

Having fielded comments about sinus surgery from hundreds of otolaryngologists, I am left with several impressions about PESS and otolaryngologists. First, although otolaryngology attracts some of the brightest medical students and clinicians into the specialty, we surgeons are still willing and capable of embracing new surgical procedures and indications enthusiastically, without adequate analysis or discussion. Because of the financial and academic incentives associated with propagating a new procedure, as opposed to a cheaper established approach, the "pro-surgery" voice and interest in generating pertinent (usually poor) literature is usually the loudest.

The advocates of a surgical approach actively excluded their detractors from self-organized consensus panels, papers, and discussions, while the pediatric and sinus leadership turned a blind and ineffectual eye. In the case of PESS, surgeons are advocating a procedure that has no proven efficacy over nonsurgical management and that may have no proven rationale. The procedure is associated with significant costs, possible complications, and a likelihood of at least occasionally adversely affecting facial growth. Sinusitis, as a vague and poorly defined clinical entity, is a "dream come true" for the unscrupulous or less-than-thoughtful clinician.

REFERENCES

1. Wald ER. Purulent nasal discharge. *Pediatr Infect Dis J* 1991;10:329–333
2. Wald ER, Milmoe GJ, Bowen A, et al. Acute maxillary sinusitis in children. *N Engl J Med* 1981;304:749–754
3. Wald ER. Antimicrobial therapy of pediatric patients with sinusitis. *J Allergy Clin Immunol* 1992;90(3 pt 2):469–473
4. Wald ER, Chiponis D, Ledesma-Medina. Comparative effectiveness of amoxicillin and amoxicillin-clavulanate potassium in acute paranasal sinus infections in children: a double-blind, placebo-controlled trial. *J Pediatr* 1986;77:795–800
5. Gross CW, Lazar RH, Gurucharri MJ. Pediatric functional endonasal sinus surgery. *Otolaryngol Clin North Am* 1989;22: 733–738
6. Lazar RH, Younis RT, Gross CW. Pediatric functional endonasal sinus surgery: review of 210 cases. *Head Neck* 1992; 14:92–98
7. Lusk RP, Muntz HR. Endoscopic sinus surgery in children with chronic sinusitis: a pilot study. *Laryngoscope* 1990;100:654–658
8. Manning SC. Surgical management of sinus disease in children. *Ann Otol Rhinol Laryngol* 1992;155(suppl):42–45
9. Parsons DS, Phillips SE. Functional endoscopic surgery in children: a retrospective analysis of results. *Laryngoscope* 1993; 103:899–903
10. Jones NS. Current concepts in the management of paediatric rhinosinusitis. *J Laryngol Otol* 1999;113:1–9
11. Poole MD. Pediatric endoscopic sinus surgery: the conservative view. *Ear Nose Throat J* 1994;73:221–227
12. Poole MD. Antimicrobial therapy for sinusitis. *Otolaryngol Clin North Am* 1997;30:331–339
13. Rosenfeld RM. Pilot study of outcomes in pediatric rhinosinusitis. *Arch Otolaryngol Head Neck Surg* 1995;121:729–736
14. Manning SC, Biavati MJ, Phillips DL. Correlation of clinical sinusitis signs and symptoms to imaging findings in pediatric patients. *Int J Pediatr Otorhinolaryngol* 1996;37:65–74
15. Halstead LA. Role of gastroesophageal reflux in pediatric upper airway disorders. *Otolaryngol Head Neck Surg* 1999; 120:208–214
16. Ulualp SO, Toohill RJ, Hoffmann R, Shaker R. Possible relationship of gastroesophagopharyngeal acid reflux with pathogenesis of chronic sinusitis. *Am J Rhinol* 1999;13:197–202
17. Buchman CA, Yellon RF, Bluestone CD. Alternative to endoscopic sinus surgery in the management of pediatric chronic rhinosinusitis refractory to oral antimicrobial therapy. *Otolaryngol Head Neck Surg* 1999;120:219–224
18. Stankiewicz JA. Pediatric endoscopic sinus surgery: thoughts about therapy for chronic sinusitis. *Vanderbilt Univ Sinus Newsl* 1997
19. Floris WA, van Aarem A, Grote JJ. Long-term follow-up of chronic maxillary sinusitis in children. *Int J Pediatr Otorhinolaryngol* 1991:22:81–84
20. Manning SC, Wasserman RL, Silver R, Phillips DL. Results of endoscopic sinus surgery in pediatric patients with chronic sinusitis and asthma. *Arch Otolaryngol Head Neck Surg* 1994;120:1142–1145
21. Mair EA, Bolger WE, Breisch EA. Sinus and facial growth after pediatric endoscopic sinus surgery. *Arch Otolaryngol Head Neck Surg* 1995;121:547–552
22. Kosko JR, Hall BE, Tunkel DE. Acquired maxillary sinus hypopiasia: a consequence of endoscopic sinus surgery? *Laryngoscope* 1996;106:1210–1213
23. Hebert RL II, Bent JP. Meta-analysis of outcomes of pediatric functional endoscopic sinus surgery. *Laryngoscope* 1998;108: 796–799
24. Wolf G, Anderhuber W, Kuhn F. Development of the paranasal sinuses in children: implications for paranasal sinus surgery. *Ann Otol Rhinol Laryngol* 1993;102:705–711

Pediatric Chronic Rhinosinusitis Assessment and Management

CHAPTER 68

Rodney P. Lusk

There are significant controversies regarding the diagnosis and management of pediatric sinusitis. Space does not allow an in-depth discussion of each potential controversy, but several areas warrant discussion.

Imaging Studies

The diagnosis of acute and chronic sinusitis remains primarily a clinical diagnosis.[1] Although it is now clear that plain films do not adequately image the pediatric sinuses, some clinicians continue to use plain films in the acute setting.[2] In general, plain films are not warranted to make the diagnosis of acute sinusitis.[1] This approach, however, is not accepted in many parts of the developed world.

In Europe, ultrasound continues to be used to make the diagnosis of acute sinusitis and to follow its resolution.[3] Haapaniemi[4] recently reported that a negative ultrasound finding excludes the presence of sinusitis. The study was more useful if the findings were negative; positive results were not of significant use. A major flaw of this study[4] is that ultrasound was compared with plain films of the maxillary sinus, and previous studies have not supported the accuracy of plain films.[2] Unfortunately, ultrasound and plain films image only the maxillary sinus, and we know from previous studies that the ethmoids are involved with equal frequency and that approximately 25% of affected children will have only ethmoid disease.[5,6] In the acute setting, we would expect these studies to be positive, and therefore of little use, because the infection is not limited to the nasal cavity. Gwaltney's and Glasier's work showed a high incidence of opacification of the anterior ethmoid and maxillary sinuses with acute rhinovirus infections.[7,8]

Culture

In general, cultures of the nasal cavity have not been readily used in the pediatric population. The primary reasons are poor patient compliance and the inability to obtain an uncontaminated specimen. Recently cultures of the middle meatus have shown a high correlation with antral punctures.[9] In the cooperative patient, endoscopically directed cultures of the middle meatus may be very useful, particularly in communities with increased resistance. Cultures of the maxillary sinus in patients who have complicated acute sinusitis or in those who fail to respond appropriately are indications that a culture should be obtained by antral puncture.[1]

Pathophysiology

The multifactorial cause of sinusitis continues to fuel the controversy regarding the underlying pathophysiologies of chronic sinusitis. Age is clearly one of the most significant factors in pediatric sinusitis. The younger the child, the higher the incidence of sinusitis and the more likely the maxillary sinus will be diseased.[6,10] Children also have an immature immune system, making them more likely to develop upper respiratory tract viral infections and associated acute sinusitis. There is a strong association between sinusitis and respiratory viral infections.[11] The viral infections cause mucosal edema that obstructs the ostium and increases the risk of bacterial infection in the sinuses. As the infundibulum is one of the narrowest drainage sites, the adjacent anterior ethmoid sinuses and maxillary sinuses would be the most likely to be involved with sinusitis. Van der Veken and Clement and colleagues,[6] and Lusk et al.[5] found that this indeed is the case and that the maxillary sinus takes the longest to clear. Viral infections are also thought to cause significant ciliary dysfunction by decreasing the ciliary beat frequency[12] or destroying the ciliary blanket.[13] Poor ciliary function would increase the chance of bacterial infection through stasis of the secretions and the inability to move these secretions from the sinus.[14] As the sinus clears, there is corresponding improvement in the ciliary function.[13]

The role of allergy and sinusitis remains controversial. Rachelefsky and colleagues[15-17] were the first to point out an association between allergic symptoms and sinusitis in children. The highest incidence of sinusitis and allergic symptoms does not show a high degree of correlation, however. Numerous studies show that approximately 50% of children with sinusitis also have allergies, but the cause and effect have not been demonstrated satisfactorily. Some patients do appear to bear out a well-founded association between allergy and fungal sinusitis.[18-20]

Without a doubt, the increasing resistance of bacteria, especially *Streptococcus pneumoniae*, has made medical treatment of chronic sinusitis more difficult. This problem is unfolding, and the ultimate impact on medical and surgical management is uncertain. With continued use of broad-spectrum antibiotics in the treatment of chronic sinusitis, it seems logical that resistance will increase, rather than decrease. The ramifications of this problem remain unknown, but it will likely mean less effective medical management and perhaps an increase in the number of surgical procedures performed. The incidence of complicated acute sinusitis may also increase significantly.

Gastroesophageal reflux disease (GERD) can be associated with chronic sinusitis.[21] The incidence of GERD in children is unknown, but Barbero[21] is convinced that it is present in most patients. There is a paucity of information on the subject in the literature. Over the past 4 years, only 14 articles in the literature have associated gastroesophageal reflux and sinusitis in their titles or abstracts. Most of these articles have concentrated on airway disease as the primary manifestation of reflux. Clearly, there are cases of patients with sinusitis and GERD, and treatment of the GERD is associated with improvement in their sinus symptoms. In our experience to date, it is not frequent and usually associated with additional symptoms such as cough or airway disease. Because both sinusitis and GERD can be associated with chronic cough, it is very difficult to differentiate between the two. The disease should diagnosed with a 24-hour pH probe study. If present, therapy should consist of a prokinetic agent such as metaclopramide, 0.1 to 0.2 mg/kg/dose three to four times a day; an H_2-blocker such as ranitidine, 1 to 4 mg/kg/dose; and/or a H_2-blocker such as omeprazole 20 mg h.s. The prokinetic agent cisapride was removed from the market July 14, 2000. Like most studies in chronic sinusitis, good prospective data are needed to elucidate the role of GERD in sinusitis when the study is performed.

Anatomic Abnormalities

VARIATIONS

The importance of anatomic abnormalities as a cause of sinusitis remains an area of significant controversy, especially in the pediatric population. It is best to think of these anatomic structures as variants of normal, and not as abnormalities. This issue is of some importance because if anatomic variations are not associated with increased sinusitis, the cause of sinusitis is more likely to be systemic, and possibly more amenable to medical management. If the problem is more systemic, conservative surgical procedures may be adequate. The anatomy is most effectively assessed by computed tomography (CT) scans.

Most anatomic variations are found equally in control and sinusitis patients.[22,23] There is convincing evidence that the incidence of anatomic variations increases with age.[20] In general, anatomic variations are not associated with increased sinusitis[24] and the incidence of anomalies is similar in diseased and control patients.[22] The variations thought to be most likely associated with increased sinusitis are septal deviation, infraorbital cells, choncha bullosa, and a narrowed middle meatus or infundibulum. Jones et al.[24] found no association between sinusitis and these anatomic variations in adults and children. Because the incidence of variations is low, their 100 cases may not be high enough to demonstrate an association.

Septal deviation increases with age. Septal deviation could cause narrowing of the middle meatus on the side of the deviation and be associated with an increased incidence of sinusitis. Elahi et al.[25] found an association between a higher incidence of ostiomeatal complex (OMC) obstruction and sinusitis and increasing nasoseptal deviations. In children, the deviation is rarely significant enough to cause disease or warrant surgical intervention.

Infraorbital cells could easily close the natural maxillary ostium with increasing size. The incidence ranges form 5.2% in pediatric patients[26] to 45.1% in adults.[23] Stackpole and Edelstein[27] graded the size of infraorbital cells and correlated it with radiologic evidence of sinusitis. As the size of the infraorbital cell increased there was a higher incidence of maxillary sinusitis. In children, the bulk of the infraorbital cells are small and our data do not show a correlation.

A choncha bullosa could be associated with significant narrowing of the middle meatus and infundibulum. Once again the evidence is mixed. The incidence varies from 5.5%[20] to 53%[28] and the incidence increases with age.[6] Calhoun et al.,[29] Jorissen et al.,[22] and Scribano et al.[30] found the concha bullosa was associated with an increased risk of sinusitis. Lam et al.,[31] Zinreich et al.,[32] Tonai and Baba,[33] Jones et al.,[24] and Bolger et al.[23] found no evidence of increased sinus disease with concha bullosa. Nadas et al.[28] sized and defined the location of concha bullosa and correlated it with the incidence of sinusitis. These investigators found that the usually accepted hypothesis that the concha bullosa may contribute to the pathogenesis of inflammatory sinus disease seems doubtful.

The uncinate bulla is more common than is generally appreciated at about 12%.[34] In children, it is not readily diagnosed. Studies looking at this variation and sinusitis have not been performed. Narrowing of the middle meatus on CT scan did not show a higher incidence of sinusitis.[24] The exception to this is narrowing secondary to scarring of the middle meatus after surgery. In the pediatric patient the middle meatus is likely more prone to scarring because of the dimensions.

MEDICAL MANAGEMENT

Much is unknown about antibiotic therapy and chronic sinusitis. Prospective studies are lacking in the use of antihistamines and decongestants. Theoretically, decongestants would decrease the amount of edema and open the ostia. This has not been proved, however. Topical steroids have been shown to decrease edema within 2 weeks and may be of modest benefit. If reflux is present, it should be aggressively treated before surgical intervention is attempted.

Increasing resistance of *S. pneumoniae* is of increasing concern. It is the most common organism to cause acute sinusitis, but it has become dramatically more resistant. The current recommendations for treatment of cultured resistant bacteria are high-dose amoxicillin (80 to 90 mg/kg/day), azithromycin, clindamycin, and rifampin.[35] In patients with resistant bacteria, surgery may be necessary to improve drainage.

SURGICAL MANAGEMENT

There is little doubt that sinus-like symptoms occur in children with large obstructive adenoid pads. If the obstructive adenoid pad is not removed, the nasal cavity cannot become healthy. Several studies indicate that adenoidectomy improves the signs and symptoms of sinusitis.[36,37] Good prospective studies designed to assess the efficacy of adenoidectomy in well-documented cases of sinusitis are needed.

The use of maxillary sinus irrigation and nasal antral windows is not a routine approach primarily because these techniques address only the maxillary sinus and do not show good results.[38] Endoscopic sinus surgery is currently the primary method of treatment for chronic sinusitis. The indications for endoscopic sinus surgery remain controversial. The Consensus Panel[1] preferred to divide their indications into absolute and possible indications.

Absolute indications include (1) complete nasal airway obstruction in cystic fibrosis due to massive polyposis or closure of the nose by medialization of the lateral nasal wall; (2) antrochoanal polyp; (3) intracranial complications; (4) mucoceles and mucopyoceles; (5) orbital abscess; (6) traumatic injury to the optic canal; (7) dacryocystorhinitis due to sinusitis and resistant to medical treatment; (8) fungal sinusitis; (9) some meningoencephaloceles; and (10) some neoplasms.

Relative or possible indications include the vast majority of patients, such as chronic rhinosinusitis that persists despite optimal medical management, and after the exclusion of any systemic disease. Optimal management includes 4 to 6 weeks of adequate antibiotics and treatment of any concomitant diseases. The Consensus Panel[1] holds that only a small fraction of all children suffering from chronic sinusitis will require surgery.

Some investigators believe that endoscopic surgery is rarely indicated.[39,40] Increasing experience has prompted many surgeons to modify their surgical approach to one that is less aggressive.[41-43] Many investigators have now found that endoscopic ethmoidectomy can be performed safely in children, with an efficacy of around 80%.[36,42-50] Extensive sphenoethmoidectomy is usually not justified in children unless they have symptomatic polyps secondary to cystic fibrosis or allergic fungal sinusitis.

Many areas of surgical management of sinusitis need further investigation, but none is more important than the impact on facial growth. Piglet models have shown interruption of facial growth on the side of endoscopic surgery, but the animals did not show clinical evidence of abnormal growth.[51,52] Lund et al.[53] have reported evidence that very aggressive surgical management of midface lesions is not associated with interruption of facial growth. We have performed and reported, but not yet published, a retrospective age-matched cohort 10-year outcome study on facial growth.[54] The study group consisted of 46 children who underwent FES surgery, and 21 children who did not undergo FES surgery. Quantitative anthropomorphic analysis was performed using standard measurements and criteria, as well as qualitative facial analysis performed by a facial plastic expert. Quantitative anthropomorphic measurements obtained showed no statistical significance between FES-surgery and no-FES-surgery groups. There is no evidence that facial growth alteration will be clinically significant 10 years after FES surgery.

Research in the area of pediatric sinusitis will continue to be difficult because of the multifactorial nature of the disease. Large clinical studies are needed to further elucidate the pathophysiology and management of sinusitis.

REFERENCES

1. Clement PA, Bluestone CD, Gordts F, et al. Management of rhinosinusitis in children: consensus meeting, Brussels, Belgium, September 13, 1996. *Arch Otolaryngol Head Neck Surg* 1998;124:31–34
2. McAlister WH, Lusk RP, Muntz HR. Comparison of plain radiographs and coronal CT scans in infants and children with recurrent sinusitis [see comments]. *Am J Roentogenol* 1989; 153:1259–1264
3. Landman MD. Ultrasound screening for sinus disease. *Otolaryngol Head Neck Surg* 1986;94:157–164
4. Haapaniemi J. Comparison of ultrasound and X-ray maxillary sinus findings in school-aged children. *Ear Nose Throat J* 1997;76:102–106
5. Lusk RP, McAlister WH, Fouley A. Anatomic variations in pediatric chronic sinusitis. *Otolaryngol Clin North Am* 1996;29:75–76
6. van der Veken PJ, Clement PA, Buisseret T, et al. CT-scan study of the incidence of sinus involvement and nasal anatomic variations in 196 children. *Rhinology* 1990;28:177–184
7. Gwaltney JM Jr, Phillips CD, Miller RD, Riker DK. Computed tomographic study of the common cold. *N Engl J Med* 1994;330:25–30
8. Glasier CM, Ascher DP, Williams KD. Incidental paranasal sinus abnormalities on CT of children: clinical correlation. *Am J Neuroradiol* 1986;7:861–864
9. Gold SM, Tami TA. Role of middle meatus aspiration culture in the diagnosis of chronic sinusitis. *Laryngoscope* 1997;107: 1586–1589
10. Diament MJ, Senac MO Jr, Gilsanz V, Baker S, Gillespie T, Larsson S. Prevalence of incidental paranasal sinuses opacification in pediatric patients: a CT study. *J Comput Assist Tomogr* 1987; 11:426–431
11. Daele JJ. Chronic sinusitis in children. *Acta Otorhinolaryngol Belg* 1997;51:285–304
12. Joki S, Toskala E, Saano V, Nuutinen J. Correlation between ciliary beat frequency and the structure of ciliated epithelia in pathologic human nasal mucosa. *Laryngoscope* 1998;108:426–430
13. Guo Y, Majima Y, Hattori M, et al. Effects of functional endoscopic sinus surgery on maxillary sinus mucosa. *Arch Otolaryngol Head Neck Surg* 1997;123:1097–1100
14. Guo Y, Majima Y, Hattori M, et al. A comparative study of the ciliary area of the maxillary sinus mucosa and computed tomographic images. *Eur Arch Otorhinolaryngol* 1998;255:202–204
15. Rachelefsky GS, Katz RM, Siegel SC. Diseases of paranasal sinuses in children. *Curr Probl Pediatr* 1982;12:1–57
16. Rachelefsky GS. Sinusitis in children—diagnosis and management. *Clin Rev Allergy* 1984;2:397–408
17. Rachelefsky GS, Katz RM, Siegel SC. Chronic sinusitis in the allergic child. *Pediatr Clin North Am* 1988;35:1091–1101

18. Bartynski JM, McCaffrey TV, Frigas E. Allergic fungal sinusitis secondary to dermatiaceous fungi—curvularia lunata and alternaria. *Otolaryngol Head Neck Surg* 1990;103:32–39
19. Manning SC, Mabry RL, Schaefer SD, Close LG. Evidence of IgE-mediated hypersensitivity in allergic fungal sinusitis. *Laryngoscope* 1993;103:717–721
20. Nguyen KL, Corbett ML, Garcia DP, et al. Chronic sinusitis among pediatric patients with chronic respiratory complaints. *J Allergy Clin Immunol* 1993;92:824–830
21. Barbero GJ. Gastroesophageal reflux and upper airway disease. *Otolaryngol Clin North Am* 1996;29:27–38
22. Jorissen M, Hermans R, Bertrand B, Eloy P. Anatomical variations and sinusitis. *Acta Otorhinolaryngol Belg* 1997;51:219–226
23. Bolger WE, Butzin CA, Parsons DS. Paranasal sinus bony anatomic variations and mucosal abnormalities: CT analysis for endoscopic sinus surgery. *Laryngoscope* 1991;101:56–64
24. Jones NS, Strobl A, Holland I. A study of the CT findings in 100 patients with rhinosinusitis and 100 controls. *Clin Otolaryngol Appli Sci* 1997;22:47–51
25. Elahi MM, Frenkiel S, Fageeh N. Paraseptal structural changes and chronic sinus disease in relation to the deviated septum. *J Otolaryngol* 1997;26:236–240
26. Milczuk HA, Dalley HA, Wessbacher RW, Richardson MA. Nasal and paranasal sinus anomalies in children with chronic sinusitis. *Laryngoscope* 1993;103:247–252
27. Stackpole SA, Edelstein DR. The anatomic relevance of the Haller cell in sinusitis. *Am J Rhinol* 1997;11:219–223
28. Nadas S, Duvoisin B, Landry M, Schnyder P. Concha bullosa: frequency and appearances on CT and correlations with sinus disease in 308 patients with chronic sinusitis. *Neuroradiology* 1995;37:234–237
29. Calhoun KH, Waggenspack GA, Simpson CB, et al. CT evaluation of the paranasal sinuses in symptomatic and asymptomatic populations. *Otolaryngol Head Neck Surg* 1991;104:480–483
30. Scribano E, Ascenti G, Loria G, et al. The role of the ostiomeatal unit anatomic variations in inflammatory disease of the maxillary sinuses. *Eur J Radiol* 1997;24:172–174
31. Lam WW, Liang EY, Woo JK, et al. The etiological role of concha bullosa in chronic sinusitis. *Eur Radiol* 1996;6:550–552
32. Zinreich SJ, Mattox DE, Kennedy DW, et al. Concha bullosa: CT evaluation. *J Comput Assist Tomogr* 1988;12:778–784
33. Tonai A, Baba S. Anatomic variations of the bone in sinonasal CT. *Acta Otolaryngol (Stockh)* 1996;525(suppl):9–13
34. Gumusburun E, Aykut M, Muderris S, Adiguzel E. The uncinate bulla. *Okajimas Folia Anat Jpn* 1996;73:101–103
35. Wald ER. Sinusitis. *Pediatr Ann* 1998;27:811–818
36. Rosenfeld RM. Pilot study of outcomes in pediatric rhinosinusitis. *Arch Otolaryngol Head Neck Surg* 1995;121: 729–736
37. Vandenberg SJ, Heatley DG. Efficacy of adenoidectomy in relieving symptoms of chronic sinusitis in children. *Arch Otolaryngol Head Neck Surg* 1997;123:675–678
38. Muntz HR, Lusk RP. Nasal antral windows in children: a retrospective study. *Laryngoscope* 1990;100:643–646
39. Poole MD. Otitis media complications and treatment failures: implications of pneumococcal resistance. *Pediatr Infect Dis J* 1995;14:S23–26
40. Otten FW, van Aarem A, Grote JJ. Long-term follow-up of chronic maxillary sinusitis in children. *Int J Pediatr Otorhinolaryngol* 1991;22:81–84
41. Setliff RC III. Minimally invasive sinus surgery: the rationale and the technique. *Otolaryngol Clin North Am* 1996;29:115–124
42. Lusk RP. Endoscopic approach to sinus disease. *J Allergy Clin Immunol* 1992;90:496–505
43. Parsons DS, Phillips SE. Functional endoscopic surgery in children: a retrospective analysis of results. *Laryngoscope* 1993; 103:899–903
44. Gross CW, Gurucharri MJ, Lazar RH, Long TE. Functional endonasal sinus surgery (FESS) in the pediatric age group. *Laryngoscope* 1989;99:272–275
45. Haltom JR, Cannon CR. Functional endoscopic sinus surgery in children. *J Miss State Med Assoc* 1993;34:1–6
46. Hellmich S. Surgical treatment of sinusitis. *Acta Otorhinolaryngol Belg* 1983;37:624–634
47. Lazar RH, Younis RT, Gross CW. Pediatric functional endonasal sinus surgery: review of 210 cases. *Head Neck* 1992;14:92–98
48. Lazar RH, Younis RT, Long TE. Functional endonasal sinus surgery in adults and children. *Laryngoscope* 1993;103:1–5
49. Lusk RP, Muntz HR. Endoscopic sinus surgery in children with chronic sinusitis—a pilot study. *Laryngoscope* 1990;100:654–658
50. Manning SC, Wasserman RL, Silver R, Phillips DL. Results of endoscopic sinus surgery in pediatric patients with chronic sinusitis and asthma. *Arch Otolaryngol Head Neck Surg* 1994; 120:1142–1145
51. Mair EA, Bolger WE, Breisch EA. Sinus and facial growth after pediatric endoscopic sinus surgery. *Arch Otolaryngol Head Neck Surg* 1995;121:547–552
52. Carpenter KM, Graham SM, Smith RJ. Facial skeletal growth after endoscopic sinus surgery in the piglet model. *Am J Rhinol* 1997;11:211–217
53. Lund VJ, Howard DJ, Wei WI, Cheesman AD. Craniofacial resection for tumors of the nasal cavity and paranasal sinuses—a 17-year experience. *Head Neck* 1999;20:97–105
54. Bothwell M, Piccirillo J, Ridenour B, Lusk R. Long-term outcome of facial growth after functional endoscopic sinus surgery. Paper pesented at: American Academy of Otolaryngology–Head and Neck Surgery research forum; September 25, 2000; Washingtown, DC

Pediatric Chronic Rhinosinusitis Assessment and Management

CHAPTER 69

Richard N. Hubbell and Judith M. Skoner

The diagnosis of pediatric rhinosinusitis often proves challenging due to the overlap of the symptoms of this disease with various other nasoadenoidal problems, including the common cold. The confusion exists because rhinosinusitis is part of a continuum of disease. Most cases of rhinosinusitis in children actually begin as a viral upper respiratory infection (URI) in the nasal mucosa, eventually progressing to a secondary bacterial infection involving the paranasal sinuses.[1,2]

The continuum of disease theory explains why rhinosinusitis cannot be differentiated from viral rhinitis on clinical grounds alone, and why isolated rhinitis probably exists, yet isolated sinusitis is rare.[3] Because of the resulting inconsistencies in the interpretation of a child's symptoms, the management of pediatric rhinosinusitis itself is often inconsistent.

Further confounding the assessment and management of this disease is the fact that the natural history of chronic pediatric rhinosinusitis is not well understood. Thus, as opinions regarding etiology vary, so do opinions regarding appropriate treatments. The therapeutic spectrum ranges from no intervention, to maximal medical management, to aggressive surgical intervention. At the conservative end are those who support minimal to no intervention. This is based on evidence that argues that spontaneous resolution of chronic pediatric rhinosinusitis is the norm.[4,5] At the other end of the spectrum are those favoring earlier surgical intervention. Controversies, however, still revolve around the definition of maximal medical management, clear indications for surgery, the extent and timing of surgery, postoperative care, and potential surgical risks. Although advances are being made in understanding this disease process, data directing management is still limited. There are no prospective studies to date comparing medical with surgical therapy in this population to serve as a decision-making guide.

Embryology and Anatomy

In children, the precise anatomy of the paranasal sinuses is complex and quite variable, however, some consistencies do exist. There are four groups of paranasal sinuses: maxillary, ethmoid, frontal, and sphenoid. All the paranasal sinuses develop as nasal chamber outpouchings, eventually extending into their respective bony vaults to varying degrees. The paired maxillary sinus develops early during the second trimester of fetal life and is fully developed by 3 years of age, up to which time the respective cavities are growing in width and height.[3,6] Ultimately, the floor of the maxillary sinus is determined by the eruption of teeth.

The ethmoid sinus develops during the fourth gestational month, although matures at a slower pace than the maxillary sinus. The ethmoid sinus exists as paired groupings of individual cells or compartments subdivided anatomically on the basis of their locations, usually with 5 to 15 cells per side.[3] Aeration of ethmoid cells is variable, producing a honeycombed radiographic appearance. The thin lateral walls of the ethmoid labyrinth are intimately related to the medial orbit.

Development of the typically paired frontal sinus is quite variable. After 4 years of age, the frontal sinus is in a supraorbital position; however, it is radiologically indistinguishable from the ethmoid sinus until 6 to 8 years of age. Growth then continues for another 8 to 10 years before reaching full adult development.[3] The sphenoid sinus is present at 3 years of age and is generally fully developed by 12 years of age. Its slow growth and relative isolation in the skull base may preserve it from frequent infection, as isolated sphenoid sinusitis is uncommon in children.[3]

Physiology and Pathophysiology

The paranasal sinuses and their pathways are lined by mucosa composed of ciliated pseudostratified columnar epithelium. The cilia beat consistently in a fluid medium, moving sinus secretions out toward the natural ostia, along the drainage pathways, and eventually into the nasopharynx. It is this interplay of ostial patency, mucociliary functioning, and fluid secretions that allows for normal paranasal sinus physiology. When one or more of these elements is impaired, the potential for sinus dysfunction exists.

Patency of the paranasal sinus ostia with maintenance of drainage pathways is a key element in normal sinus physiology. The posterior ethmoid cells drain secretions through the superior meatus, and the sphenoid sinus drains into the sphenoethmoidal recess. The frontal sinuses, anterior ethmoid sinuses (agger nasi cells and both supra- and infraorbital ethmoids), and maxillary sinuses drain into the osteomeatal complex (OMC). This area consists of the hiatus semilunaris, frontal recess, anterior ethmoid cells, ethmoid bulla, anterior wall of the middle turbinate, and the infundibulum. The infundibulum is a troughlike space just anterior to the anterior ethmoid cells, which acts as a common drainage pathway. Because of these anatomic and physiologic relationships, OMC or anterior ethmoid disease can induce mucosal edema and functional obstruction of the infundibulum and drainage of its related sinuses.[7] Mechanical factors, as well as functional factors, may also precipitate obstruction, although viral URI with secondary mucosal swelling is by far the most frequent cause of ostial obstruction.[3]

Once the sinus ostia become obstructed, ventilation is impaired and there is a transient increase in intrasinal pressure, followed by a negative intrasinal pressure.[8] The negative pressure within the sinus relative to the atmospheric pressure may allow nasal flora to flow against the mucosal ciliary beat patterns and enter the typically sterile sinus cavity. Sniffing, sneezing, and nose-blowing, associated with altered intranasal pressure, may also facilitate entry of bacteria into the sinus from a colonized nasal chamber.[3] As nasal congestion increases, nasal breathing decreases; decreased gas exchange produces a decreased partial pressure of oxygen intrasinally, which favors multiplication of certain bacterial species. An acidic pH may also develop, promoting anaerobic conditions. As the immune system responds to the bacterial invasion, tissue congestion worsens secondary to the inflammatory response, further perpetuating the cycle of obstruction.

Normal mucociliary functioning usually protects respiratory epithelium from bacterial invasion, however, certain respiratory viruses appear to exert a direct cytotoxic effect on the cilia.[3] Alteration of the number, morphology, and function of cilia in the respiratory epithelium may facilitate secondary bacterial infection of the paranasal sinuses. Ciliary activity may also be impaired with alterations in mucosal secretions, as cilia can only beat in a fluid medium. Thickened secretions typically seen in systemic disorders such as cystic fibrosis or asthma have the potential to impair ciliary movement. Purulent secretions from an infected sinus may also affect ciliary movement, however, reports on this are conflicting.[9,10]

Ostial obstruction thus initiates a vicious circle, with self-mediated mucosal edema and hyperplasia, obstruction of sinus drainage, retention of secretions, and ciliary dysfunction, cumulatively creating an environment ideal for long-standing infection. In children, OMC obstruction is recognized as a critical factor in chronic rhinosinusitis, however, it is unclear whether this is the primary cause of the disease.

Perhaps critical to our further understanding of this unique pathophysiologic model is the concept that there is rarely a single isolated cause. A number of conditions have been identified as predisposing to chronic rhinosinusitis in children, although an acute viral illness—the common cold—appears to be the most frequently recognized association.[11,12] Data suggest children average 6 to 8 upper respiratory infections (URIs) per year, and acute sinusitis complicates 5 to 10% of cases.[13,14] The precise mechanism whereby viruses predispose to rhinosinusitis is unknown, but it may involve local immune defense destruction and a subsequent increase in bacterial attachment to epithelial cells.[15] An immature immune system and lack of previous exposures presumably make children more susceptible to common viral URIs, especially in settings where close contact with other children facilitates infectious transfers.[16] Also, the smaller size of developing sinuses and a shorter distance between ostial mucosal surfaces may further facilitate OMC obstruction, and encourage the development of rhinosinusitis after a viral URI in children.[16] Potentially modifiable predisposing factors involved in the pathogenesis of this disease have also been identified, and are addressed later in the chapter.

Definitions

According to the most recent consensus meeting in Brussels,[17] chronic rhinosinusitis in children is defined as a sinus infection with low-grade symptoms and signs that persists for longer than 12 weeks. This definition allows for a diagnosis without the previously mandatory computed tomography (CT) scan, based on the consensus panel's belief that imaging all children with suspected chronic rhinosinusitis is not feasible.[17] Patients with acute exacerbations of chronic rhinosinusitis may have multiple acute episodes in addition to persistent low-grade symptoms and signs that do not resolve completely between acute episodes.

Symptoms and Signs

A thorough history is the most critical component in the evaluation of rhinosinusitis. Symptoms most commonly associated with chronic rhinosinusitis in children have been described by Parsons and Phillips as "the seven cardinal symptoms."[18] These include chronic nasal congestion (100% occurrence), purulent nasal discharge (90%), head pain/discomfort (90%), cough (71%), fetid breath (67%), postnasal drainage (63%), and behavioral changes (63%).[18] The cough, most often secondary to postnasal drainage, is typically worse in the evening for younger children, and in the early morning for adolescents. Infrequent symptoms reported in less than 20% of the study population include recurrent odynophagia, intermittent fever, nausea, hoarseness, facial puffiness, epistaxis, dizziness, impaired smell, epiphora, and localized pain in the ear, eye, or maxillary teeth.[18,19]

A complete head and neck examination should be performed in all children with suspected rhinosinusitis. It is especially important to rule out other possible etiologies of a child's symptoms, such as adenoid hypertrophy and obstruction, foreign body, tumor, choanal stenosis or atresia, and deviated nasal septum.[7] On physical examination, the signs of chronic rhinosinusitis are not specific, and there are no direct means of examining the paranasal sinuses. The examination itself is challenging in the pediatric patient, but it may be accomplished in a simple way by tilting the tip of the nose upward. Anterior rhinoscopy with the use of an otoscope provides even better visualization. These methods permit assessment of the inferior (and possibly middle) turbinate and mucosa; the nasal septum; the presence or absence of crusts, secretions, and lesions; and the overall patency of the nasal airway.[20] Findings suggestive of rhinosinusitis include boggy edematous mucosa with significant obstruction, along with various amounts and types of nasal discharge. Other physical findings may include cobbling of the posterior pharyngeal lymphoid follicles, posterior nasal discharge, and slightly tender enlarged cervical lymph nodes.[7,21] Intranasal polyps are principally seen in association with cystic fibrosis or allergy.[3] Investigators also report widening of the nasal bridge in some children with chronic rhinosinusitis, producing a pseudohypertelorism.[3]

Although virtually impossible in the very young child, nasal endoscopy can sometimes be performed in patients 6 years of age or older. It is helpful to prepare the nose first with a topical decongestant (0.25% phenylephrine) and topical anesthetic (3% lidocaine) administered via an atomizer. The 0- and 30-degree rigid pediatric endoscopes provide the most complete view of the nasal mucosa, nasopharynx, and middle meatus and enable the clinician to obtain cultures and tissue samples in select cases.

Flexible nasopharyngoscopy is better tolerated and allows good visualization of the nasal cavity and nasopharynx; this method, however, does not yield sufficient information about the middle meatus, which is the site of the osteomeatal complex, a key concept in the pathophysiology of rhinosinusitis.[22]

Diagnosis

The most commonly used basis of diagnosing chronic pediatric rhinosinusitis is clinical judgment. Transillumination of the sinuses in children is difficult to perform and unreliable, especially in patients younger than 10 years of age because of increased thickness of both the soft tissue and the bony vault.[3,23] The value of ultrasonography is controversial, and has a very limited or no role in evaluating rhinosinusitis in children[20,24-26] Similarly, plain radiographs have limited value in this setting;[27] interpretation in infants and young children is often difficult, there is poor correlation with ethmoid disease, and the significance of sinus clouding is uncertain.[28] Furthermore, plain sinus films do not provide visualization of the osteomeatal complex, a cornerstone in the diagnosis of rhinosinusitis.[12] In a study comparing plain sinus films with coronal CT scans taken within hours of each other in children displaying symptoms compatible with chronic rhinosinusitis, there was a lack of correlation between the two methods in 74% of the patients.[22] The investigators concluded that plain films both over- and underestimate sinus findings.[22] Radiographic examination of the nasopharynx, however, may be adjunctively helpful in determining the size of the adenoids, yet this does not replace nasopharyngoscopy; adenoidal tissue size alone does not necessarily correlate with chronic inflammation.[15]

Imaging is not necessary to diagnose uncomplicated pediatric chronic rhinosinusitis. When indicated, however, fine-cut coronal CT is the imaging modality of choice because of its ability to resolve both bone and soft tissue.[29] The need for caution when considering CT evaluation must be emphasized, as the incidence of bony or mucosal disease of the paranasal sinuses in asymptomatic children may be as high as 50% on imaging.[30,31] In children with symptoms and signs compatible with chronic rhinosinusitis, CT scanning is most frequently performed if surgery is being considered, or if the patient has a complicated course or a systemic disorder. According to the Brussels consensus meeting, the complete list of indications for CT scanning in the assessment of pediatric rhinosinusitis includes:[17]

1. Evaluation of the surgical candidate
2. Presence of suppurative intraorbital or intracranial complications (excluding orbital cellulitis)
3. Symptomatic immunocompromised host
4. Severe illness or toxic condition
5. Acute illness that does not improve with medical therapy in 48 to 72 h

In comparison to CT, magnetic resonance imaging (MRI) provides optimal visualization of soft tissues but has no bone resolution. This imaging modality thus has no use in routine evaluation of the paranasal sinuses, and cannot be used reliably as a preoperative guide. MRI is most often reserved for children with suspected neoplasm, congenital mass, intraorbital/intracranial complications, or intravenous contrast allergy.[32,33]

Microbiologic assessment is not necessary in cases of routine evaluation of uncomplicated chronic rhinosinusitis in children, although it does have a role in recalcitrant and complicated disease. Results of most surface cultures have no predictive value, and thus nose, throat, and nasopharyngeal cultures cannot be recommended as guides to the bacteriology on therapy for chronic rhinosinusitis.[25] Cultures of pus taken directly from the middle meatus do, however, correlate well with maxillary antral and ethmoid cultures,[34,35] although there is no consensus regarding whether middle meatal cultures can substitute for sinus aspirations.[17] Indications for maxillary sinus aspiration or puncture in children parallel indications for CT scanning and include symptomatic sinus disease in an immunocompromised host, suppurative complications, severe illness or a toxic condition, and acute illness unresponsive to therapy within 48 to 72 h.[17] This technique is best performed transnasally to avoid injury to dentition and the natural ostium. After sterilization of the puncture site, a needle on a syringe is directed beneath the inferior turbinate and advanced through the lateral nasal wall.[2] Aspirated secretions are submitted for gram stain and aerobic and anaerobic cultures. Bacterial counts of greater than 10^4 colony-forming units (CFU)/ml reflect a high degree of confirmation of infection, rather than contamination.[3]

Predisposing Factors

Chronic pediatric rhinosinusitis is recognized as a multifactorial disease with various predisposing factors that change over time. Once the diagnosis of rhinosinusitis is suspected in a child, underlying modifiable contributors to sinonasal inflammation must be identified and managed appropriately. Once this is accomplished, the infectious disease aspect which actually may be secondary, can then be more effectively treated.[7] Although their roles are still being defined, conditions that are currently recognized as potential predisposing factors for rhinosinusitis include allergy,[27] immunodeficiency,[35-38] cystic fibrosis,[39,40] primary ciliary dyskinesia,[41,42] environment,[43,44] and gastroesophageal reflux.[45-47]

ALLERGY

Allergy is one of the most common causes of problematic nasal mucosa edema[48] and is implicated as a contributing factor in rhinosinusitis.[49] Some investigators consider allergy in children the most important predisposing element in pediatric chronic rhinosinusitis,[50,51] although its true role in this disease process is still under debate. Controlled studies comparing the incidence of sinusitis in allergic groups with nonallergic groups are very scarce, especially in pediatric populations. One study found no difference in the involvement of the sinuses of atopic children in comparison to nonallergic children with chronic nasal complaints.[52] The same investigators showed the prevalence of rhinosinusitis to decrease after 8 years of age, and the prevalence of atopy to increase with age.[52] Together, these findings suggest that allergy may not be a primary cause of chronic pediatric rhinosinusitis.[44] Interestingly, however, the prevalence of rhinosinusitis in allergic children is higher than in nonallergic patients.[44,53]

Identification of the allergic child is important in patient evaluation, and a complete medical and family history is the most critical aspect of this process. Symptoms suggestive of allergy include nasal congestion, pruritic nasal and ocular mucous membranes, clear rhinorrhea, paroxysmal sneezing (often exacerbated by inhaled dust or animal exposure), and rhinosinusitis during allergy season.[17,27] The history may also include infantile eczema, asthma, food allergy, or a previous good response to antihistamines or intranasal anti-inflammatory agents.[17] Family history is important because children of two allergic parents have a 65 to 75% incidence of significant atopy, and children with one atopic parent have a 35% incidence of allergy.[54] The likelihood of allergies is also increased in children with an atopic sibling.[54]

If any elements of the history or physical examination suggest atopy, allergic assessment should be performed.[17] Some investigators assert that allergy testing should be obtained in every child with chronic rhinosinusitis who responds poorly to initial management, regardless of whether the history is positive for atopy.[48] This is based on the high occurrence rate of allergic disease in rhinosinusitis patients.[48] Acceptable methods of assessment include skin-prick testing, nasal smear, radioallergosorbent testing, or treatment trials.[17] Intradermal skin testing is reported to be the most sensitive study, but some in vitro blood tests have been found to be accurate within 5 to 8% of the intradermal results.[48,55]

IMMUNODEFICIENCY

Young children all have a relative physiologic immunodeficiency because of a slow continual rise in plasma immunoglobulins (IgG, IgM, IgA) until 6 to 10 years of age, when adult levels are finally reached.[29] Thus, children are theoretically more susceptible to infection during this period. Immunologic assessment is typically not warranted in all children with chronic rhinosinusitis; however, the clinician must have a low threshold of suspicion for primary or secondary immune deficiency in patients with recalcitrant disease. Chronic rhinosinusitis is reportedly the most common clinical presentation of common variable immune deficiency (CVID),[56] a disorder characterized by reduced levels of at least two serum immunoglobulin classes, usually IgG and IgA. IgG subclass deficiency also may manifest as chronic rhinosinusitis.[56] Less common childhood immunodeficiencies are X-linked agammaglobulinemia, C_4 deficiency, ataxia-telangiectasia, and hyper-IgM immunodeficiency.[56] Evaluation for immunodeficiency should include serum immnunoglobulin levels, IgG subclasses, and assessment of response to immunization with protein antigens (i.e., diphtheria and tetanus toxoid) and polysaccharide antigens (i.e., pneumococcal vaccine).[44,57] Recommendations for this workup in children with chronic rhinosinutis are the following:[57]

1. History of infections at other sites
2. Inadequate response to appropriate antimicrobial therapy
3. Sinus cultures exhibiting unusual pathogens
4. Persistent rhinosinusitis despite surgical intervention and restoration of sinus ventilation and mucociliary transport

GENETIC DISORDERS

An association between cystic fibrosis, nasal polyposis, and chronic rhinosinusitis is recognized.[58] Studies indicate that nasal polyposis generally occurs after 5 years of age, although mucopyosinusitis of the maxillary sinus can occur as early as 3 months of age.[59] The maxillary sinus seems to be the first sinus affected by cystic fibrosis,[59] although eventual pansinusitis is the norm. A positive family history and nasal polyposis in a child are indications for sweat testing to rule out cystic fibrosis; nasal polyps are otherwise uncommon in the pediatric population. Characteristic CT findings of this disease are pansinusitis with uncinate process demineralization and bilateral medial displacement of the lateral nasal wall.[60] Despite management of the underlying disorder, cystic fibrosis is a progressive disease. Cystic fibrosis may be associated with massive polyposis and complete nasal obstruction, and is frequently an indication for endoscopic sinus surgery; unfortunately, recurrence of disease is to be expected.[44]

Primary ciliary dyskinesia is an autosomal recessive disease characterized by the lack of dynein arms on the peripheral doublets of cilia. The manifestations at birth classically include sinusitis, bronchiectasis and situs inversus, a triad known as Kartagener syndrome. The simultaneous presence of all three findings is variable, however. Situs inversus is not always present, and a neonatal form of this disease does not manifest sinusitis or bronchiectasis until later in infancy.[44] Because of the difficulty in diagnosis based on history and examination this disorder should always be considered in infants with respiratory or otolaryngologic problems of unknown origin. Tracheal or nasal mucosa biopsy submitted for electron microscopy confirms the diagnosis.

ENVIRONMENT

An increase in the prevalence of chronic rhinosinusitis has been shown in children staying in day care centers compared with children staying at home.[61] The cleanliness and size of the day care group are important, as large number facilities have a potentially increased viral URI burden predisposing to rhinosinusitis.[2,48,60] Secondary smoke and inhaled irritant exposure have also been implicated as contributing factors to rhinosinusitis, again perhaps by increasing a child's risk of URI.[60]

GASTROESOPHAGEAL REFLUX

Gastroesophageal reflux (GER) has been suggested as another important factor contributing to rhinosinusitis in some children.[45-47] This concept is based on the theory that there is reflux into the nasopharynx, and that when low pH gastric contents contact upper respiratory mucosa, edema and irritation result, potentially leading first to obstruction of the eustachian tubes or sinus ostia, and eventually to rhinosinusitis. Most children do not exhibit typical GER symptoms such as heartburn or regurgitation, however; in these cases, the history is often not suggestive of the condition.

In a child with chronic rhinosinusitis, the potential for GER as an underlying condition may be addressed by empirically optimizing positional and dietary factors. Reflux precautions are advised to all patients and include head-of-bed elevation, and avoidance of caffeine/spicy foods/pre-bedtime meals. An antacid trial may be initiated as well if the diagnosis of GER is under consideration. If a child does provide a history or symptoms compatible with GER, a histamine blocker to decrease gastric acidity and a prokinetic agent to increase gastric emptying may be initiated if more conservative measures are unsuccessful. The diagnosis may be confirmed by 24-h gastric pH probe monitoring, although less specific, scintiscanning and barium swallow studies may also provide diagnostic insight.[20] In our practice, diagnostic studies for GER are not performed routinely; rather, these are reserved for children with recalcitrant chronic rhinosinusitis failing adequate medical therapy and conservative measures.

Medical Management

ANTIBIOTICS

The goals of therapy in chronic pediatric rhinosinusitis are to eradicate the infection, provide reversal of sinus obstruction, and return effective mucociliary clearance.[62] After all factors predisposing to this disease have been appropriately pursued, and the positive findings addressed, antibiotic therapy remains the cornerstone of treatment in children with rhinosinusitis. The choice of antibiotic is most often empirical, as representative cultures are difficult to routinely obtain in children. Selective cultures, however, are indicated for complicated cases (see Diagnosis).

Ideally, antimicrobial therapy is aimed at eradicating the most commonly found pathogens associated with a particular disease process. However, the microbiology of chronic sinusitis in children has received very limited study, and discrepancies exist in the bacterial results of several investigations.[3] Some studies implicate respiratory anaerobic organisms as the predominant pathogens of chronic rhinosinusitis,[63] whereas other investigators identify *Streptococcus pneumoniae, Haemophilus influenzae, Moraxella catarrhalis*, α-hemolytic streptococci, and occasional staphylococcal species as the predominant organisms in chronic disease.[7,64,65] Unfortunately, several of the bacteriologic studies were conducted after antibiotic therapy, making interpretation difficult. It is possible that the different groups of organisms identified may actually reflect both acute exacerbations and chronic inflammation. Despite the lack of microbiologic data, an important inference may be made from the findings that do exist—that chronic rhinosinusitis is often polymicrobial, with anaerobes and penicillin-resistant organisms potentially contributing to its chronicity; treatment may therefore require several different antibiotics before a satisfactory response is achieved.[60]

In the choice of antibiotics, the list of suitable agents for chronic rhinosinusitis is reportedly the same as that for acute disease[3,17,27] (Table 69–1). However, because many children with chronic rhinosinusitis present to the otolaryngologist with protracted symptoms or after multiple failed antibiotic trials, several investigators suggest that the antibiotic agent chosen should provide activity against β-lactamase-producing bacteria.[3,6,27,48] Examples of appropriate antimicrobials include amoxicillin/ clavulonic acid, clindamycin, or second- and third-generation cephalosporins.[66,67] First-generation cephalosporins lack sufficient activity against *H. influenzae* and are therefore inappropriate for treatment of rhinosinusitis.

There are virtually no data indicating the optimum duration of antimicrobial therapy for chronic rhinosinusitis in children, although many clinicians recommend a minimum course of 3 to 6 weeks.[2,3,27,68] In general, antibiotic therapy extended 1 week beyond the time that symptoms resolve provides an opportunity for eradication of all bacteria.[68,69] If, however, there is no symptomatic response after 5 to 7 days of antimicrobial therapy, the antibiotic should be changed.

Prophylactic antibiotics have not gained uniform acceptance in pediatric rhinosinusitis in the absence of systemic disorders.[27,70] Currently, there are no randomized controlled trials to support the efficacy of prophylaxis for chronic rhinosinusitis.

SUPPLEMENTAL MEDICAL THERAPY

Additional medical therapies are often used in conjunction with antimicrobial agents to decrease sinonasal edema and reestablish a more normal functioning nasal environment. No controlled studies have been performed to document their efficacy in chronic pediatric rhinosinusitis. Investigators report that buffered hypertonic nasal irrigation provides rapid and effective cleansing of nasal debris, decreases mucosal edema, and may improve mucociliary flow patterns by decreasing ciliary transit times.[7,48] Although frequent nasal irrigation with this solution may allow for a healthier sinonasal tract, the improvement lasts only hours.

For longer-lasting nasal decongestion in children with chronic rhinosinusitis, several Consensus Panel members support intranasal steroid sprays,[17] which may be even more effective when used after hypertonic saline irrigation.[48] These agents reduce cholinergic receptor sensitivity, reduce the number of basophils and eosinophils in nasal mucosa, and inhibit the

TABLE 69–1
Antibiotics for Use in Pediatric Rhinosinusitis

Antimicrobial	Dose	Specifications
Amoxicillin	40 mg/kg/day divided tid	*Streptococus, Haemophilus influenzae, Moraxella catarrhalis*; β-lactamase unstable
Amoxicillin-clavulanate	45 mg/kg/day divided bid	*S. pneumoniae, H. influenzae, M. catarrhalis*; anaerobes; staphylococcus; β-lactamase stable
Cefaclor	40mg/kg/day divided tid	*S. pneumoniae* (side effects include serum sicknesslike reaction)
Cefprozil	30 mg/kg/day divided bid	*S. pneumoniae, H. influenzae, M. catarrhalis* (Staphylococcus resistant)
Cefuroxime axetil	20-30 mg/kg/day divided bid	Staphylococcus; β-lactamase stable
Cefixime	8 mg/kg/day qd or divided bid	Gram-negative organisms; β-lactamase stable (not active vs. *Staphylococcus* or *Pneumococcus*)
Cefpodoxime proxetil	10 mg/kg/day divided bid	*Staphylococcus, streptococcus, H. influenzae, M. catarrhalis* (β-lactamase stability not proven)
Clindamycin	15–40 mg/kg/day divided tid	*Staphylococcus*; anaerobes (poor *influenzae* coverage)
Loracarbef	30 mg/kg/day divided bid	*Staphylococcus*; anaerobes; β-lactamase stable
Clarithromycin	15 mg/kg/day divided bid	*H. influenzae M. catarrhalis, S. pneumoniae*; β-lactamase stable
Erythromycin-Sulfisoxazole	(50/150) mg/kg/day divided qid	*Staphylococcus* (side effects include blood dyscrasias and hepatorenal toxicity)
Trimethoprim-sulfamerhoxazole	(8/40) mg/kg/day divided bid	*S. pneumoniae, H. influenzae, M. catarrhalis*; β-lactamase unstable (side effects include blood dyscrasias, anemia, and hepatorenal toxicity)

Modified from Gungor A, Corey J. Pediatric sinusitis: a literature review with emphasis on the role of allergy. *Otolaryngol Head Neck Surg* 1997;116:4–15. qd, once a day; bid, twice a day; tid, three times a day; qid, four times a day.

late-phase reaction after exposure to antigen.[71] Accordingly, steroid nasal sprays are especially useful in children with allergic rhinitis or nasal polyps or both. Nasal sprays containing ipatropium bromide have a different mechanism of action, and no studies have been done to validate the efficacy of this drug in rhinosinusitis.

Humidification may also be a simple means by which to moisturize sinonasal mucosa, thin nasal secretions, and facilitate mucociliary transport. Care must be taken, however, to minimize potential fungal overgrowth in the humidifier, as this may actually worsen or precipitate rhinosinusitis. Mucolytic agents such as guaifenesin serve to thin mucus, potentially reducing stasis and promoting clearing of secretions. Their efficacy in children has not been established in rhinosinusitis. Antihistamines are inappropriate in chronic rhinosinusitis unless allergy is involved.[44]

Topical decongestants, typically an α_2-agonist such as oxymetazoline, provide rapid symptom relief; nevertheless, they should not be used for longer than 1 week because of their potential to decrease local blood flow,[29] exert a ciliotoxic influence,[72] and produce a potential rebound congestion.[22] Oral decongestants in children are less appropriate, and their role is unclear.[50]

To summarize, in our practice, medical management consists of the following: at least one 4- to 7-week course of an empirical broad-spectrum β-lactamase-resistant antibiotic, 5 days only of a topical decongestant at initiation of therapy, daily saline nasal irrigations and nasal steroid sprays, antihistamines in patients with positive allergy profiles, room humidification, and judicious use of mucolytics if they afford symptomatic benefit to the patient. In addition, appropriate medical therapy includes evaluation for the multifactorial predisposing factors to rhinosinusitis, with treatment of positive findings. Without proper management of the primary condition initiating sinonasal edema, rhinosinusitis symptoms in children often cannot be controlled, even with aggressive interventions.

Surgical Management

As our knowledge of the natural history of chronic rhinosinusitis in children is limited, it is often challenging to identify those patients who will experience spontaneous regression of their disease with time, and those who will require more aggressive interventions. A study of 40 children with chronic rhinosinusitis and no history of allergy showed spontaneous resolution of symptoms in 95% by the age of 7 years,[24,73,74] which is presumed to be reflective of the immature immune system in the younger child. These findings thus support that uncomplicated rhinosinusitis in children is usually self-limiting. The potential for self-resolution of disease with maturation must always be kept in mind when considering more invasive therapies or surgical management in chronic pediatric rhinosinusitis. Unfortunately, the existing literature evaluating surgical management in this disease is confusing and lacks studies that would provide a clear decision-making guide.

ADENOIDECTOMY

After the multifactorial causes of rhinosinusitis have been addressed and adequate medical management has continually failed to yield effective responses, the clinician may then consider a more interventional approach to therapy. Adenoidectomy offers promise as a simple, effective, and relatively safe procedure that may affect the sinuses indirectly.[75] Clinical trials have shown adenoidectomy to be effective in alleviating symptoms in some patients,[76,77] although definite conclusions cannot be drawn, owing to the limited size of these studies. Different theories have been described to explain the relationship between adenoids and the symptoms of chronic rhinosinusitis. One theory is that adenoid hypertrophy with chronic nasal obstruction and stasis may merely mimic signs and symptoms of rhinosinusitis; with adenoidectomy, the effective relief of symptoms may be so great that further aggressive intervention is unneccessary.[7,78] Another theory asserts that an adenoidal bed of any size may act as a bacterial reservoir that serves as a nidus for chronic infection.[79] Studies have been conducted in which adenoidectomy produced a positive response in pediatric rhinosinusitis patients, in both the presence and absence of adenoid hypertrophy.[75,79] To establish a causal relationship, more investigations are needed. Although there is no consensus on the timing of adenoidectomy, it appears to be a reasonable first surgical step before performing functional endoscopic sinus surgery (FESS) in children with chronic rhinosinusitis, regardless of adenoid size[75] (see Endoscopic Sinus Surgery, below). Children with overt or submucous cleft palate, however, would not be candidates for adenoidectomy.

Endoscopy may also be performed while the child is anesthetized for adenoidectomy. This allows for assessment of the nasal cavities with particular attention directed to anatomic abnormalities and the patency of the maxillary ostium. Also during thus evaluation, middle meatal cultures may be obtained, although their correlation with sinus bacteriology is still under debate.

NASAL ANTRAL WINDOW

The nasal antral window, or inferior meatal antrostomy, no longer plays a role in the management of uncomplicated pediatric chronic rhinosinusitis.[2,80-82] This technique is unsuccessful in part because the cilia continue to beat toward the obstructed natural ostium, and because it does not address ethmoid disease. The current indication for the inferior antrostomy is in primary ciliary dyskinesia, as normal ciliary patterns do not exist, and the goal is gravitational drainage.

ANTRAL LAVAGE

Antral lavage is another procedure that is not a viable therapy for chronic rhinosinusitis in children.[17,83,84] This technique requires multiple irrigations, each under general anesthesia, and does not address the ethmoid disease common in pediatric rhinosinusitis. It does, however, remain a useful diagnostic tool in severe complicated disease that is based primarily in the maxillary sinus. The indications for antral lavage are identical to those for sinus puncture as described earlier (see Diagnosis).[17]

ENDOSCOPIC SINUS SURGERY

When prolonged maximal medical therapy and adenoidectomy both fail to provide adequate relief in a child with at least 6 months of severe symptoms of chronic rhinosinusitis, the child may be a potential candidate for functional endoscopic sinus surgery (FESS).[78,85] The Caldwell-Luc procedure is essentially contraindicated in young children due to the potential for damage to unerupted teeth.[29,44] Indications for FESS in pediatric rhinosinusitis remain poorly defined and shrouded in controversies. The Consensus Meeting in Brussels defined their indications in the context of "absolute" and "possible" and are as follows.[17]

Absolute indications

- Complete nasal obstruction in cystic fibrosis due to massive polyposis or medialization of the lateral nasal wall
- Antrochoanal polyp
- Intracranial complications
- Mucoceles and mucopyoceles
- Orbital abscess
- Traumatic injury in the optic canal (decompression)
- Dacryocystorhinitis due to sinusitis resistant to appropriate medical management
- Fungal sinusitis
- Some meningoencephaloceles
- Some neoplasms

Possible indications

- Chronic rhinosinusitis that persists despite optimal medical management, and after exclusion of systemic disease (optimal medical management includes 2 to 5 weeks of appropriate antibiotics and treatment of concomitant diseases)

Patients with cystic fibrosis and other systemic disorders are more likely to require surgery; thus, the indications for these children are unique. The details are beyond the scope of this chapter.

To evaluate the potential surgical candidate, coronal CT scans are necessary.[44] The scans should be obtained while the child is still receiving treatment, yet nearing the completion of at least 4 weeks of appropriate antibiotic therapy[48] with concurrent treatment of associated conditions. This approach is necessary to minimize false-positive readings secondary to edema or untreated acute infection. Based on the scans, anatomic abnormalities and mucosal derangements identified in the paranasal sinuses help direct the surgical management plans.

The goals of FESS are to open the osteomeatal complex (OMC), eliminate ethmoid disease, and open the occluded natural sinus ostia when appropriate, in order to reestablish normal mucociliary clearance of the sinuses.[86] Frontal and sphenoid sinuses are rarely entered in children.[2] According to Lusk,[78] dissection into the frontal recess is not performed unless there is extensive disease. Although the appropriate extent of surgery is controversial, a limited procedure is usually all that is necessary in pediatric rhinosinusitis patients. The maxillary and anterior ethmoid sinuses are the primary sites of disease in children; accordingly, the most common FESS procedures in these cases are anterior ethmoidectomy with removal of the entire uncinate process, and possibly maxillary antrostomy with conservative enlargement of the natural ostium.[2] Tissue biopsies and cultures are also obtained at surgery to guide continued medical therapy. Currently, gelatin film stenting of the ethmoid cavity is commonly performed to decrease synechiae and granulation tissue and is removed 2 weeks later under a general anesthesia for a second-look procedure. Few studies have addressed the role for the second-look procedure, although some investigators conclude that this procedure may not offer any advantages.[87,88] Postoperatively, antibiotics and adjunctive medical management are commonly continued for at least 2 to 3 weeks.

Technically, endoscopic sinus surgery in children is potentially more challenging than in adults because of the relatively restricted anatomy. Because the nasosinal structures are still developing, preservation of unaffected structures is very important, and every attempt must be made to preserve normal mucosa. Also, concerns have been raised that surgery on the middle meatus could lead to possible disturbances of midface growth; thus far, no studies confirm these concerns.[89] However, the risk-to-benefit ratio must always be carefully considered when embarking on pediatric FESS.

Various studies have reported good FESS outcomes in children, with success rates in the 80% range.[2,66,78,90,91] A recent meta-analysis of pediatric FESS outcomes reports an 88.4% positive outcome with a 0.6% major complication rate in patients with chronic rhinosinusitis refractory to appropriate medical therapy.[91] There are no standardized criteria for defining success, however, and more long-term prospective studies are needed for an effective assessment of the outcomes of this surgical approach in children.

Summary

Chronic pediatric rhinosinusitis is a multifactorial disease process that continues to be a topic of considerable controversy. Although many predisposing factors have been identified, the complete natural history of this disease is still unknown. It is recognized, however, that there is a spontaneous tendency toward recovery in children after the age of 6 to 8 years.[24,73,74] Thus, with maturation of a child's immune system and developing anatomy, chronic rhinosinusitis may indeed resolve, warranting a conservative approach to treatment. As our understanding of this disease process advances, it is becoming increasingly apparent that chronic pediatric rhinosinusitis is medically treatable in most cases and that surgery is very rarely indicated in infants and children (Table 69-2).

TABLE 69–2

Stepwise Summary of Assessment Management and Management of Uncomplicated Chronic Pediatric Rhinosinusitis

Step 1:	Thorough history and physical examination suggesting chronic rhinosinusitis "Cardinal symptoms":[18] chronic nasal congestion purulent nasal discharge, head, pain, cough, fetid breath, postnasal drainage, behavioral changes Boggy edematous turbinates with obstruction; polyposis; posterior pharyngeal cobbling; postnasal discharge; tender cervical adenopathy Symptom duration of 12 weeks or more
Step 2:	Evaluation for predisposing factors and concomitant diseases, with treatment of positive findings Allergy/atopy Immune deficiency Cystic fibrosis Ciliary dyskinesia Enviromnent (smoking, day care) Gastroesophageal reflux
Step 3:	Medical management of rhinosinusitis Appropriate treatment of concomitant diseases/predisposing factors At least one 4- to 6-week course of appropriate antibiotics Limited (5-day) use of topical decongestant (weight-appropriate dosage) at initiation of therapy Daily nasal saline irrigations and nasal steroid sprays Antihistamines in atopic patients Room humidification Judicious use of mucolytics, if patient is afforded symptomatic relief
Step 4:	Adenoidectomy with concurrent nasal endoscopy and middle meatal culture
Step 5:	With continued symptoms Reevaluate diagnosis and possible predisposing factors Consider repeating STEP 3, using different antibiotic(s) Consider CT scan while medical treatment continues, if symptoms persist for $>$ 6 months and the patient is a potential surgical candidate If positive bony/mucosal derangements on CT with the above criteria met, *carefully* consider the possibility for limited FESS (depending on patient and parental expectations/desires)

CT, computed tomography; FESS, functional endoscopic sinus surgery.

REFERENCES

Hubbell and Skoner—CHAPTER 69

1. Gwaltney J, Philips C, Miller R, et al. Computed tomographic study of the common cold. *N Engl J Med* 1994;330:25–30
2. Lusk R, Stankiewicz, J. Pediatric rhinosinusitis. *Otolaryngol Head Neck Surg* 1997;117:S53–S57
3. Wald E. Rhinitis and acute and chronic sinusitis. In: Bluestone C, Stool S, Kenna M, eds. *Pediatric Otolaryngology.* 3rd Ed. WB Saunders: Philadelphia; 1996:843–858
4. Poole M. Pediatric endoscopic sinus surgery: the conservative view. *Ear Nose Throat J* 1994;73:221–227
5. Otten F, Van Aarem A, Grote J. Long-term follow-up of chronic maxillary sinusitis in children. *Int J Pediatr Otorhinolaryngol* 1991;22:81–84
6. April M, Zinreich S, Baroody F, Naclerio R. Coronal CT scan abnormalities in children with chronic sinusitis. *Laryngoscope* 1993;103:985–990
7. Parsons D, Wald E. Otitis media and sinusitis. *Otolaryngol Clin North Am* 1996;29:11–25
8. Aust R, Drettner B, Falck B. Studies of the effect of peroral phenylpropanolamine on the functional size of the human maxillary ostium. *Acta Otolaryngol (Stockh)* 1979;88:455
9. Ohashi Y, Nakai Y. Functional and morphological pathology of chronic sinusitis mucous membrane. *Acta Otolaryngol (Stockh)* 1983;397:11
10. Reimer A, von Mecklenburg C, Tormalm N. The mucociliary activity of the upper respiratory tract. III. A functional and morphological study of human and animal material with special reference to maxillary sinus disease. *Acta Otolaryngol (Stockh)* 1978;355:3
11. Giebink G. Criteria for evaluation of antimicrobial agents and current therapies for acute sinusitis in children. *Clin Infect Dis* 1992;14(suppl 2):S212–S215
12. Kennedy D, ed. *Sinus Disease. Guide to First-Line Management.* Philadelphia: Health Communications; 1994:1–44
13. Wald E, Gurerra N, Byers C. Upper respiratory tract infection in young children, duration of and frequency of complications. *Pediatrics* 1991;87:129–133
14. Wald E. Sinusitis in children. *N Engl J Med* 1992;326: 319–323
15. Stenfors L, Raisanen S. Abundant attachment of bacteria to nasopharyngeal epithelium in otitis-prone children. *J Infect Dis* 1992;165:1148–1150
16. Benninger M, Anon J, Mabry R. The medical management of rhinosinusitis. *Otolaryngol Head Neck Surg* 1997;117(suppl): S41–S49
17. Clement P, Bluestone C, Gordts F, et al. Management of rhinosinusitis in children. Consensus Meeting, Brussels, Belgium, September 13, 1996. *Arch Otol Head Neck Surg* 1998;124: 31–34
18. Parsons D, Phillips S. Functional endoscopic surgery in children: a retrospective analysis of results. *Laryngoscope* 1993; 103:899–903
19. Parsons D, Pransky S. Functional endoscopic sinus surgery in infants and young children. *Instruct Courses Am Acad Otol Head Neck Surg* 1992;5:159–164
20. Dolitsky J. Management of sinusitis in adolescent children. In: Schaefer S (ed). *Rhinology and Sinus Disease. A Problem-Oriented Approach.* St Louis, MO: CV Mosby; 1998: 135–142
21. Wilner A, Lazar R, Younis R, et al. Sinusitis in children: current management. *Ear Nose Throat J* 1994;73:45–90
22. Lusk R, Lazar R, Muntz H. The diagnosis and treatment of recurrent and chronic sinusitis in children. *Pediatr Clin* 1989;36:1411–1421
23. Otten F, Grote J. The diagnostic value of transillumination for maxillary sinusitis in children. *Int J Pediatr Otorhinolaryngol* 1989;18:9–11
24. Van Buchem F, Peeters M, Knottnerus J. Maxillary sinusitis in children. *Clin Otolaryngol* 1992;17:49–53
25. Wald E, Milmoe G, Bowen A, et al. Acute maxillary sinusitis in children. *N Engl J Med* 1981;304:749–754
26. Shapiro G, Furukawa C, Pierson W, et al. Blinded comparison of maxillary sinus radiography and ultrasound for diagnosis of sinusitis. *J Allergy Clin Immunol* 1986;77:59–64
27. Gungor A, Corey J. Pediatric sinusitis: a literature review with emphasis on the role of allergy. *Otolaryngol Head Neck Surg* 1997;116:4–15
28. McAllister W, Herman T, Wippold F. Imaging of sinusitis in infants and children. In: Lusk R (ed). *Pediatric Sinusitis.* New York: Raven Press; 1992:15–42
29. Manning S. Pediatric sinusitis. *Otolaryngol Clin North Am* 1993;26:623–638
30. Van tier Veken P, Clement P, Buisseret T, et al. CT scan study of the incidence of sinus involvement and nasal anatomic variation in 196 children. *Rhinology* 1990;28:177–184
31. Diament M. Prevalence of incidental paranasal sinus opacification in pediatric patients. A CT study. *J Comput Assist Tomogr* 1987;11:426–431
32. Manning S. Paranasal sinus disease in children. *Curr Opin Otolaryngol Head Neck Surg* 1993;1:171–176
33. Zinreich S, Borders J, Eisele D, et al. The utility of magnetic resonance imaging in the diagnosis of intranasal meningoencephaloceles. *Arch Otolaryngol Head Neck Surg* 1992;118: 1253–1256
34. Duplechain J, Miller R. Pediatric sinusitis: diagnosis and treatment with endoscopic techniques. *South Med J* 1994;143: 7–13
35. Orobello P, Park R, Belcher R, et al. Microbiology of chronic sinusitis in children. *Arch Otolaryngol Head Neck Surg* 1991; 117:980–983
36. Lusk R, Polmar S, Muntz H. Endoscopic ethmoidectomy and maxillary antrostomy in immunodeficient patients. *Arch Otolaryngol Head Neck Surg* 1991;117:60–63

37. Shapiro G, Virant F, Furukawa C, et al. Immunologic defects in patients with refractory sinusitis. *Pediatrics* 1991;87:311–316
38. Kurono Y, Fujiyoshi T, Mogi G. Secretory IgA and bacterial adherence to nasal mucosal cells. *Ann Otol Rhinol Laryngol* 1989;98:273–277
39. Ramsey B, Richardson M. Impact of sinusitis in cystic fibrosis. *J Allergy Clin Immunol* 1992;90:547–552
40. Drake-Lee A, Morgan D. Nasal polyps and sinusitis in children with cystic fibrosis. *J Laryngol Otol* 1989;103:753–755
41. Karja J, Nuutinen J. Immotile cilia syndrome in children. *Int J Pediatr Otorhinolaryngol* 1983;5:275–279
42. Scheeren R, Keehnen R, Meijer C, et al. Defects in cellular immunity in chronic upper airway infections are associated with immunosuppressive retroviral p15E-like proteins. *Arch Otolaryngol Head Neck Surg* 1993;119:439–443
43. Koltai P. Effects of air pollution on the upper respiratory tract of children. *Otolaryngol Head Neck Surg* 1994;111:9–11
44. Clement P. Management of sinusitis in infants and young children. In: Schaefer S, ed. *Rhinoloy and Sinus Disease: A Problem-Oriented Approach.* St. Louis: CV Mosby; 1998:105–134
45. Hamilos D. Gastroesophageal reflux and sinusitis in asthma. *Chin Chest Med* 1995;16:683–697
46. Holinger L, Sanders A. Chronic cough in infants and children: an update. *Laryngoscope* 1991;101:596–605
47. Barbero G. Gastroesophageal reflux and upper airway disease: a commentary. *Otolaryngol Clin North Am* 1996;29:27–38
48. Parsons D. Chronic sinusitis: a medical or surgical disease? *Otolaryngol Clin North Am* 1996;29:1–9
49. Cook P, Nishioka G. Allergic rhinosinusitis in the pediatric population. *Otolaryngol Clin North Am* 1996;29:39–56
50. Furukawa C, Shapiro GG, Rachelefsky G. Children with sinusitis. *Pediatrics* 1983;71:133–134
51. Sharpe M, Furukawa C, Bierman C, et al. Allergic patients have more frequent sinus infections than nonallergic patients (abstract). *J Allergy Clin Immunol* 1992;751:332
52. Van der Veken P, Clement P, Buisseret T, et al. Age-related CT-scan study of the incidence of sinusitis in children. *Am J Rhinol* 1992;6:45–48
53. Iwens P, Clement P. Sinusitis in allergic patients. *Rhinology* 1994;32:65–67
54. Abdulrazzaq Y, Bener A, DeBuse P. Association of allergic symptoms in children with those in their parents. *Allergy* 1994;49:737–743
55. Williams P, Dolen W, Koepke J, et al. Comparison of skin testing and three in vitro assays for specific IgE in the clinical evaluation of immediate hypersensitivity. *Ann Allergy* 1992;68:34–45
56. Polmar S. Sinusitis and immune deficiency. In: Lusk R, ed. *Pediatric Sinusitis.* New York: Raven Press; 1992:53–58
57. Sethi D, Leopold D. Diagnosis and management of chronic recurrent sinusitis and immunoglobulin deficiency. *Curr Opin Otolaryngol Head Neck Surg* 1995;3:21–25
58. Shwachman H, Kulczycki L, Mueller H, et al. Nasal polyposis in patients with cystic fibrosis. *Pediatrics* 1962;30:389–401
59. Brihaye P, Clement P, Dab I, et al. Pathological changes of the lateral nasal wall in patients with cystic fibrosis (mucoviscidosis). *Pediatr Otorhinolaryngol* 1994;28:141–147
60. Rosenfeld R. Sinusitis in children. In: Gates G, ed. *Current therapy in otolaryngology head and neck surgery.* 6th Ed. St. Louis: CV Mosby; 1998:354–358
61. Bjuggren G, Kraepelien S, Lind J, et al. Occult sinusitis in children. *Acta Otolaryngol (Stockh)* 1952;42:287–310
62. Lanza D, Kennedy D. Nose and sinus mucosal inflammation and infection, including medical therapy. *Curr Opin Otolaryngol Head Neck Surg* 1994;2:27–32
63. Brook I. Bacteriologic features of chronic sinusitis in children. *JAMA* 1981;246:967–969
64. Muntz H, Lusk R. Bacteriology of the ethmoid bullae in children with chronic sinusitis. *Arch Otolaryngol Head Neck Surg* 1991;117:179–181
65. Tinkelman D, Silk H. Clinical and bacteriologic features of chronic sinusitis in children. *Am J Dis Child* 1989;143:938–941
66. Lazar R, Youmis R, Gross C. Pediatric functional endonasal sinus surgery: review of 210 cases. *Head Neck* 1992;14:92–98
67. Haltom J, Cannon C. Functional endoscopic sinus surgery in children. *J Miss State Med Soc* 1993;34:1–6
68. Dunham M. New light on sinusitis. *Contemp Pediatr* 1994;11:102–117
69. Wald E. Antimicrobial therapy of pediatric patients with sinusitis. *J Allergy Clin Immunol* 1992;90:469–973
70. Manning S. Surgical management of sinus disease in children. *Ann Otol Rhinol Laryngol* 1992 101(suppl 155):42–45
71. Pipkorn U, Proud D, Lichtenstein L, et al. Inhibition of mediator release in allergic rhinitis by pretreatment with topical glucocorticosteroids. *N Engl J Med* 1987;316:1506–1510
72. Ingels K, Meeuwsen F, Graamans K, et al. Influence of sympathetic and parasympathetic substances in clinical concentrations on human nasal ciliary beat. *Rhinology* 1992;30:149–160
73. Yaniv E, Oppenheim D, Fuchs C. Chronic rhinitis in children. *Int J Pediatr Otorhinolaryngol* 1992;23:51–57
74. Clement P, Van der Veken P, Iwens P, et al. X-ray, T-scan, MR-imaging. In: Mygind N, Nacleirio R, eds. *Allergic and Nonallergic Rhinitis: Clinical Aspects.* Copenhagen Munksgaard; 1993:58–65
75. Vandenberg S, Heatley D. Efficacy of adenoidectomy in relieving symptom of chronic sinusitis in children. *Arch Otolaryngol Head Neck Surg* 1997;123:675–678
76. Takahashi H, Fujita A, Honjo I. Effect of adenoidectomy on otitis media with effusion, tubal function, and sinusitis. *Am J Otolaryngol* 1989;10:208–213
77. Rosenfeld R. Pilot study of outcomes in pediatric rhinosinusitis. *Arch Otolaryngol Head Neck Surg* 1995;121:729–736
78. Lusk R. Chronic sinusitis: surgical management. In: Bluestone C, Stool S, Kenna M, eds. *Pediatric otolaryngololgy.* 3rd Ed. Philadelphia: WB Saunders; 1996:859–865

79. Lee D, Rosenfeld R. Adenoid bacteriology and sinonasal symptoms in children. *Otolaryngol Head Neck Surg* 1997;116: 301–317
80. Muntz H, Lusk R. Nasal antral windows in children: a retrospective study. *Laryngoscope* 1990;100:643–646
81. Lund V. Fundamental considerations of the design and function of intranasal antrostomies. *Rhinology* 1985;23:231–236
82. Lund V. Inferior meatal antrostomy. Fundamental considerations of design and function. *J Laryngol Otol* 1988;15(suppl):1–18
83. Maes J, Clement P. The usefulness of irrigation of the maxillary sinus in children with maxillary sinusitis on the basis of the Water's X-ray. *Rhinology* 1987;25:259–264
84. Lusk R, Lazar R, Muntz H. The diagnosis and treatment of recurrent and chronic sinusitis in children. *Pediatr Clin North Am* 1989;36:1411–1485.
85. Younis R, Lazar R. Criteria for success in pediatric functional endonasal sinus surgery. *Laryngoscope* 1996;106:869–873
86. Manning S, Wasserman R, Silver R, et al. Results of endoscopic sinus surgery in pediatric patients with chronic sinusitis and asthma. *Arch Otolaryngol Head Neck Surg* 1994;120:1142–1145
87. Walner D, Falciglia M, Willging J, et al. The role of second-look nasal endnscopy after pediatric functional endoscopic sinus surgery. *Arch Otolaryngol Head Neck Surg* 1998;124: 425–428.
88. Mitchell B, Pereira K, Younis R. et al. Pediatric functional endoscopic sinus surgery: is a second-look necessary? *Laryngoscope* 1997;107:1267–1269
89. Lund V, Neijens H, Clement P, et al. Symposium. The treatment of chronic sinusitis: a controversial issue. *Int J Pediatr Otolaryngol* 1995; 32(suppl):S21–S35
90. Lusk R, Muntz H. Endoscopic sinus surgery in children with chronic sinusitis: a pilot study. *Laryngoscope* 1990;100: 654–658
91. Hebert R, Bent J. Meta-analysis of outcomes of pediatric functional endoscopic sinus surgery. *Laryngoscope* 1998;108: 796–799

24

Management of the Unilateral Atretic Ear

"No one would argue that surgery for congenital aural atresia has the same potential for hearing restoration as does stapedectomy; few middle ear procedures involving the middle ear ossicles do. But is the success rate so modest that unilateral cases are best observed, at least until the individual is an adult and can make his or her own decision?"

Paul R. Lambert

"We cannot overemphasize the importance of complete audiologic evaluation even in the child with unilateral atresia with or without microtia."

Antonio De la Cruz

"The routine use of the facial nerve monitor supplements the surgeon's knowledge of temporal bone anatomy, the information provided by the preoperative HRCT, and provides another asset in making unilateral aural atresia repair safer for the patient."

Daniel I. Choo

Management of the Unilateral Atretic Ear

CHAPTER 70

Paul R. Lambert

Most otologic surgeons, even experienced ones, would agree that surgery for congenital aural atresia is challenging. Some submit that this procedure is inappropriate for unilateral cases, whereas others express no hesitation in recommending intervention to selected patients. The basis for this controversy has not been clearly articulated in the literature. In many cases, the bias has simply been inherited as part of the philosophy of one's training program. In order to provide more objectivity to this issue, several possible areas of concern need to be explored: (1) impact of unilateral hearing loss, (2) probability of achieving binaural hearing with surgery and stability of hearing results over time, and (3) surgical risks, especially to the facial nerve. The purpose of this chapter is to analyze these issues and draw conclusions regarding surgery for the unilateral atretic ear.

Issue 1: Impact of Unilateral Hearing Loss

In the past, clinicians expressed little concern about unilateral loss of hearing. Recently, research has shown that children with a significant unilateral sensorineural hearing loss—and presumably a significant unilateral conductive hearing loss—do experience a variety of auditory, linguistic, and cognitive difficulties that may impact educational progress.[1] Impaired sound localization[1-3] and speech recognition in background noise do occur with unilateral hearing loss and may underlie these difficulties. Interestingly, the speech recognition problem occurs regardless of whether the speech stimuli are directed toward the normal or hearing-impaired ear.[4,5] These findings have obvious implications for the student in the typical classroom environment.

Both clinical and animal research have shown evidence of auditory brainstem abnormalities in the setting of unilateral conductive hearing loss. For example, Moore et al.[6] have experimentally induced unilateral conductive hearing losses in ferrets during critical periods. Various abnormalities in the development of binaural neural elements in the auditory brainstem pathways were noted. Clinical studies of adults with unilateral conductive hearing loss using auditory brain stem responses (ABR) and the masking-level difference (MLD) have also documented abnormalities in brain stem auditory processing.[7] Specifically, delays in wave V and in I to V and III to V interwave intervals were noted. The MLD, a behavioral test that measures the sensitivity of the auditory system to interaural differences of time and amplitude, was reduced, and they correlated significantly with the ABR abnormalities. These changes were similar to those observed in children with chronic otitis media with effusion.

Issue 2: Probability of Achieving Binaural Hearing and the Stability of Hearing over Time

No one would argue that surgery for congenital aural atresia has the same potential for hearing restoration as does stapedectomy; few middle ear procedures involving the middle ear ossicles do. But is the success rate so modest that unilateral cases are best observed, at least until the individual is an adult and can make his or her own decision?

Within the first postoperative year, a hearing level of ≥30 dB has been achievable in approximately 70% of patients[8-13] (Table 70–1). This degree of success compares favorably with

TABLE 70–1
Aural Atresia: Hearing Status during the First Postoperative Year

Source/Year	No. of Patients	Hearing Parameter	Success (%)
Nager and Levin (1980)[8]	23	Hearing level ≤ 30 dB	70
Bellucci (1981)[9]	45	Hearing level ≤ 30 dB	73
De la Cruz et al. (1985)[10]	56	Conductive deficit ≤ 30 dB	73
Schuknecht (1989)[11]	30	Hearing Level ≤ 30 dB	50
Jahrsdoerfer et al. (1992)[12]	86	Hearing level ≤ 25 dB	71
Lambert (1998)[13]	50	SRT ≤ 25 dB	60
		SRT ≤ 30 dB	70

TABLE 70–2
Aural Atresia: Longer-Term Hearing Status

Source/Year	No. of Patients	Follow-up (yr)	Hearing Parameter	Success (%)
Bellucci (1981)[9]	45	≥2	Hearing level ≤30 dB	53
Chandrasekhar et al. (1995)[14]	42	Mean 2.6	Conductive deficit ≤30 dB	60
Lambert (1998)[13]	46	Mean 2.8 (range 1–7.5)	SRT ≤30 dB	50

many tympanoplasty procedures involving reconstruction of the ossicular chain. Like chronic ear surgery, some decrement in hearing is to be expected over time[9,13,14] (Table 70–2) and revision surgery may be necessary. In my experience, approximately 60% of patients will achieve an excellent initial hearing result of 10 to 25 dB SRT. Approximately 75% of these individuals will maintain this level of hearing longer term (follow-up: mean 2.8 years, range 1 to 7.5 years). Considering all patients, revision surgery will be necessary in approximately one-third of cases. The most frequent complication requiring secondary surgery is stenosis of the external ear canal. Even for the highly successful stapedectomy, approximately 20% of patients will experience a significant recurrent conductive hearing loss after successful air–bone gap closure if follow up extends beyond 5 years.[15]

Issue 3: Surgical Risks

Injury to the facial nerve is, perhaps, the most feared complication in otologic surgery. In chronic ear disease the facial nerve may be partially obscured by granulation tissue and the infectious process may have eroded areas of the fallopian canal. The facial nerve is placed at jeopardy in cases of aural atresia because of the abnormal development of the temporal bone. This vulnerability can be minimized, however, by recognizing the anomalies likely to be encountered. Anterior and lateral displacement of the mastoid segment and dehiscence of the tympanic segment should be anticipated. The former anomaly is of particular concern when enlarging the new canal posteroinferiorly.[16]

Appropriate patient selection, surgical technique predicated on a thorough understanding of abnormal facial nerve development, and judicious use of facial nerve monitoring will permit aural atresia surgery with minimal morbidity. In my personal experience of 50 primary and 17 revision surgeries, one patient developed a temporary facial paresis. A series of 1000 patients was recently reported by Jahrsdoerfer and Lambert[17] and an approximate 1% incidence of facial paresis or paralysis was reported. Postoperative facial nerve dysfunction can therefore, be expected in 1.0 to 1.5% of patients, an incidence which approximates that encountered during mastoid and middle ear surgery for cholesteatoma.

Concern about labyrinthine injury has not usually been discussed with the same emotion as facial nerve injury, nor has it been emphasized as a strong deterrent to aural atresia surgery. Acoustic trauma to the ear and direct violation of the labyrinthine capsule, however, should be acknowledged as definite risks. Although their potential for occurrence is greater than that for facial nerve injury, the actual incidence of sensorineural hearing loss, or vertigo, or both, remains small in published reports.

Acoustic trauma to the inner ear can result from direct manipulation of the ossicular chain or through conduction of the acoustic energy by the dense atretic bone during drilling. A mild hearing loss in the frequencies 4000 to 8000 Hz can be expected to occur in approximately 15% of cases.[16,18] In my experience, a more significant loss in the speech frequencies or decrease in speech discrimination occurs in approximately 2% of cases.[13] This incidence is similar to that anticipated for stapes surgery, where the occurrence of significant sensorineural hearing loss has been reported to be 0.6 to 3.0%.[19,20]

In summary, the risk of facial nerve injury or sensorineural hearing loss, or both, must be considered in surgery for aural atresia. These complications can be minimized with appropriate patient selection (discussed below) and a thorough understanding of the abnormal temporal bone anatomy that will be encountered at surgery. The low incidence of these complications reported by experienced surgeons documents a favorable risk/benefit ratio for operating on congential aural atresia.

Patient Selection

Appropriate patient selection is critical to the arguments supporting unilateral atresia surgery. It is obviously important as well for surgical intervention in bilateral cases, although the criteria are less strict in this latter circumstance.

Most patients undergoing atresia repair will have a residual conductive deficit of ≥10 dB. Sensorineural function should, therefore, be normal in order to maximize the potential for achieving binaural hearing. Normal or near-normal sensorineural function in the contralateral ear is also important to avoid operating on the better-hearing ear.

Although audiometric criteria can be defined quantitatively, the true art of patient selection is centered on computed tomographic (CT) evaluation of the middle ear and mastoid. Hypoplasia of the middle ear space, ranging from mild to severe, occurs in most cases of aural atresia, and ossicular development can be expected to correlate directly with middle ear size. The risk of surgical complications will be minimized and the chances for a successful hearing result increased if the middle ear and mastoid are aerated and at least two-thirds of the normal size, and if all three ossicles (although deformed) can be identified. Rarely, a well-developed middle ear/mastoid containing fluid will be encountered. To rule out a resolving otitis media or temporary eustachian tube dysfunction, a repeat scan 6 to 12 months later is recommended. Persistent middle ear fluid is a contraindication to surgery, although reassessment when the child is a teenager is reasonable.

It is important to demonstrate a patent oval window on CT. An absent oval window is more common in minor malformations[21] (i.e., mild microtia, external auditory canal and tympanic membrane normal or only slightly small, conductive hearing loss) but can occur in aural atresia. Drilling a neo-fenestra, especially when the tympanic segment of the facial nerve is displaced inferiorly, and reconstructing with a prosthesis are associated with increased risks and decreased probability of long-term hearing improvement.

The position of the vertical segment of the facial nerve on the CT scan should be noted. Particular attention is paid to the area of the second genu. Extreme anterior displacement of the vertical segment restricts access to the middle space, increasing the chance of facial nerve injury during drilling of the canal and reducing the chance of a successful hearing result.

Recently, Jahrsdoerfer et al.[12] developed a grading system that quantifies the developmental status of the atretic ear. This 10-point scale has been shown to predict postoperative hearing results. Using these strict selection criteria, only about 60% of patients with unilateral aural atresia are surgical candidates. The one exception to the audiometric and CT criteria reviewed above is the case of cholesteatoma developing in a severely stenotic external auditory canal. In such cases, surgery to address the cholesteatoma is mandatory; restoration of the conduction system depends on the degree of middle ear development and sensorineural function.

Surgical Considerations

It is not the purpose of this chapter to detail the surgical technique for aural atresia. It is important, however, to emphasize several key points that will minimize morbidity and optimize long-term hearing success.

ANTERIOR SURGICAL APPROACH

As opposed to the mastoid approach, the anterior approach avoids a mastoid cavity with its attendant problems of debris accumulation and infection, and it facilitates placement of the split-thickness skin graft (STSG).

IDENTIFY MALLEUS–INCUS HEAD

To minimize potential labyrinthine or facial nerve injury, the initial drilling should be focused superiorly and anteriorly. The middle cranial fossa dura is identified and followed medially into the epitympanic space, where the fused heads of the ossicles are noted. Identifying the middle ear in this manner will help protect the facial nerve, which always lies medial to the ossicular mass in the epitympanum. It will also prevent drilling into the lateral semicircular canal, and avoid mistaking it for part of the atretic bone.

CAREFUL POSTERIOR INFERIOR CANAL ENLARGEMENT

The facial nerve is especially vulnerable to injury, as the external canal is enlarged in the posteroinferior direction. In this area, the nerve may actually lie lateral to the middle ear cavity, in addition to being anteriorly displaced. As drilling through the atretic bone in this area proceeds, one looks for the facial nerve in a manner similar to that used when identifying that structure in the mastoid, during chronic ear surgery.

MAINTAIN OSSICULAR CHAIN INTACT

The stapes may be partially obscured because of the contracted middle ear space, the malformed lateral ossicular mass, and/or the overlying facial nerve. Usually, enough of the stapes can be seen to assess its mobility and the integrity of the incudostapedial joint. The lateral ossicular mass is maintained in position and not removed to obtain a better view of the stapes. In most cases, the ossicular chain, although deformed, is mobile. Hearing results may be better when the chain is left intact, instead of interposing a prosthesis or autograft material.[13] Prostheses are vulnerable to fixation because of the small size of the middle ear space and the reduced clearance between them and the bony walls of the tympanum.

APPROPRIATE TYMPANIC MEMBRANE AND STSG IMMOBILIZATION

Because the malleus handle is shortened or absent, it is difficult to anchor the fascia graft to this ossicle. To prevent laterization, the STSG should overlap the fascia graft by at least several millimeters and a Silastic button should be contoured to the circumference of the canal and placed on top of the new tympanic membrane. The Silastic button will also help maintain an anterior sulcus. The skin graft and fascia are further stabilized by Merocel wicks placed within the canal and hydrated with Cortisporin suspension.

CREATE A LARGE MEATUS

Stenosis of the external canal or meatus, or both, is the most frequent complication requiring revision surgery. In my experience, this occurs in 20% of patients.[13] To minimize this problem, the meatal opening should be approximately twice the normal size. The soft tissue is debulked from the area around the meatus to limit the length of the membranous canal and its propensity to collapse. An anteriorly based, full-thickness skin flap from the conchal area of the reconstructed auricle could also be used to line a portion of the anterior external canal to obviate a circumferential suture line at the meatal opening.

Summary

Most otologic surgeons would explore the middle ear of a child with a unilateral conductive hearing loss secondary to trauma, infection, or presumed ossicular fixation (e.g., malleus or stapes). Why, then, the reluctance, or controversy, regarding aural atresia, which, fortunately, is unilateral in most patients? Certainly, the hearing loss resulting from aural atresia is significant both in terms of severity (i.e., maximal conductive deficit) and, as discussed above, in its potential impact on auditory and linguistic development.

The concerns appear to focus on surgical risks and hearing outcome. These issues have been addressed in this chapter. Specifically, it has been documented in the literature that approximately 70% of patients will achieve a hearing threshold of at least 30 dB after surgery, and about 75% of these patients will maintain this level over a longer term. The surgery can be accomplished with minimal morbidity, and a mastoid cavity with its potential for long-term care is not created.

This level of predictability—in terms of both hearing results and complications—is predicated on experience in patient selection and surgical technique. Just as all otolaryngologists, or even otologists, are not equally trained in the various facets of major skull base surgery, the same must be acknowledged for atresia surgery. Optimal treatment for patients with unilateral aural atresia will be realized as more surgeons become trained in managing these patients and as referrals to centers experienced with this condition become a priority.

REFERENCES

Lambert—CHAPTER 70

1. Bess FH. The unilaterally hearing-impaired child: a final comment. *Ear Hearing* 1986;7:52–54
2. Humes LE, Allen SK, Bess FH. Horizontal sound localization skills of unilaterally hearing-impaired children. *Audiology* 1980;19:508–518
3. Viehweg R, Campbell RA. Localization difficulty in monaurally impaired listeners. *Trans Otol Soc* 1960;48:339–350
4. Tharpe AM, Bess FH. Identification and management of children with minimal hearing loss. *Int J Pediatr Otorhinol* 1991;21:41–50
5. Bess FH, Tharpe AM, Gibler AM. Auditory performance of children with unilateral sensorineural hearing loss. *Ear Hearing* 1986;7:20–26
6. Moore DR, Hutchings ME, King AJ, et al. Auditory brainstem of the ferret: some effects of hearing with unilateral ear plug on the cochlea, cochlear nucleus, and projections to the inferior colliculus. *J Neurosci* 1989;9:1213–1222
7. Ferguson MO, Cook RD, Hall JW III, et al. Chronic conductive hearing loss in adults: effects on the auditory brainstem response and masking-level difference. *Arch Otolaryngol Head Neck Surg* 1998;124:678–685
8. Nager GT, Levin LS. Congenital aural atresia: embryology, pathology, classification, genetics, and surgical management. In: Paparella MM, Shumrick D, eds. *Otolaryngology*. Philadelphia: WB Saunders; 1980:1303
9. Bellucci RJ. Congenital aural malformations: diagnosis and treatment. *Otolaryngol Clin North Am* 1981;14:95–124
10. De la Cruz A, Linthicum FH Jr, Luxford WM. Congenital atresia of the external auditory canal. *Laryngoscope* 1985;95:421–427
11. Schuknecht HG. Congential aural atresia. *Laryngoscope* 1989;99:908–917
12. Jahrsdoerfer RA, Yeakley JW, Aguilar EA, et al. Grading system for the selection of patients with congenital aural atresia. *Am J Otolaryngol* 1992;13:6–12
13. Lambert PR. Congenital aural atresia: stability of surgical results. *Laryngoscope* 1998;108:1801–1805
14. Chandrasekhar SS, De la Cruz A, Garrido E. Surgery of congenital aural atresia. *Am J Otol* 1995;16:713–717
15. Glasscock ME, Storper IS, Haynes DS, Bohrer PS. Twenty-five years of experience with stapedectomy. *Laryngoscope* 1995;105:899–904
16. Lambert PR. Complications of surgery for congenital atresia. In: Eisele DW, ed. *Complications in Head and Neck Surgery*. St Louis, MO: CV Mosby; 1993:660–665
17. Jahrsdoerfer RA, Lambert PR. Facial nerve injury in congenital aural atresia surgery. *Am J Otol* 1998;19:283–287
18. Jahrsdoerfer RA. External auditory canal atresia. In: Lalwani AK, Grundfast KM, eds. *Pediatric Otology and Neurotology*. Philadelphia: Lippincott-Raven; 1998:533–540
19. Sheehy JL, House HP. Causes of failure in stapes surgery. *Laryngoscope* 1962;72:10–31
20. Hough JVD. Recent advances in otosclerosis. *Arch Otolaryngol* 1966;83:379–390
21. Lambert PR. Congenital absence of the oval window. *Laryngoscope* 1990;100:37–40

Management of the Unilateral Atretic Ear

CHAPTER 71

Antonio De la Cruz and Bradley W. Kesser

Congenital aural atresia results from a failure of canalization of a solid core of epithelial cells that extends from the developing auricle to the tympanic ring and middle ear cleft. The incidence of congenital aural atresia is 1 per 10,000 to 20,000 live births.[1] Approximately one-third of cases are bilateral.[2] The child with unilateral congenital aural atresia and a normally-functioning contralateral ear will develop language normally and have no significant cognitive, developmental, or social deficits, even without the use of a hearing aid in the affected ear.[1,11,12] As such, the decision to operate on the child with unilateral atresia is controversial.

Most cases of atresia of the external auditory canal are accompanied by some form of microtia, although isolated middle ear ossicular anomalies do occur and may not be diagnosed until the child is several years old. Aural atresia can be associated with other craniofacial anomalies (e.g., Treacher Collins, hemifacial microsomia) or can occur as an isolated congenital anomaly. Jafek reported a 14% positive family history;[2] atresia is seen in families, although no genetic inheritance pattern has been demonstrated.

Surgery for aural atresia involves a number of steps, with the ultimate goal of creating a healed, dry ear canal with liberation of the ossicles to restore the middle ear conductive mechanism. The following steps give a general overview of the procedure:

1. A postauricular incision followed by standard T-shaped periosteal incision is made to identify the atretic bone.
2. Using surface landmarks, including the glenoid fossa, linea temporalis, and cribriform areas, the new ear canal is drilled.
3. The middle ear ossicles are identified and freed from the surrounding bone.
4. A tympanic membrane graft is fashioned from temporalis fascia and lain over the mobile ossicles.
5. A split thickness skin graft is used to line the new bony ear canal.
6. A meatoplasty is created and the skin graft pulled through and sutured to the skin of the native or reconstructed auricle.

Children with bilateral aural atresia have maximal conductive hearing deficits (50 to 60 dB hearing loss [HL]), and if the anatomy is favorable, surgery at age 6 is performed in an attempt to gain hearing. Cholesteatoma will be found in 8 to 14% of children with atretic ear canals.[3,4] Stenosis of the external auditory canal is associated with a higher incidence of cholesteatoma than is complete atresia. One series of 50 patients (54 ears) with an average canal diameter of $\leq$ 4 mm found a 50% incidence of cholesteatoma.[5] No cholesteatoma was found in patients less than 3 years old. The more stenotic (especially $<$ 2 mm) canals had the greater incidence of cholesteatoma. Regardless of middle and inner ear anatomy, patients with cholesteatoma require an operation to clean the ear and eradicate the disease.

Controversy exists, however, in the management of the unilateral atretic ear without cholesteatoma, as the surgery itself is challenging and has potential complications. In addition, the predictability of the final hearing result has been questioned. Improvement in the hearing threshold to $\geq$ 20 dB eliminates the handicap of unilateral hearing loss;[6] achieving that result cannot be guaranteed. The heart of the issue lies in the ability to predict preoperatively which patients have the potential to achieve closure of the air–bone gap to within 20 to 30 dB.

Although the incidence of major complications (total sensorineural hearing loss, facial nerve paralysis, restenosis) has decreased significantly over the years, other complications (high-tone sensorineural hearing loss [SHL], tympanic membrane lateralization) have essentially remained the same. The postoperative ear must be cleaned and debrided regularly (every 6 to 12 months). The postoperative draining ear requires extra attention and cleanings along with restrictions on swimming, exercise, and moisture/water in the ear. An argument can easily be made against operating on the unilateral atretic ear, so long as the contralateral ear is in good health and functioning well.

Nevertheless, thoughtful evaluation and preparation before surgery and advances in surgical techniques have made atresia surgery results more predictable. Patients are carefully chosen for surgery on the basis of motivation, cooperation, and anatomy, as demonstrated on high-resolution computed tomography (CT) scanning. The well-healed postoperative ear is treated normally; we even allow patients to swim. Older patients who have developed presbycusis or patients who suffer hearing loss in the unaffected ear are potentially excellent candidates and may reap the rewards of surgery. Given the improved predictability of results of atresia surgery, we feel that the benefits of binaural hearing, sound localization, and improved hearing in noise outweigh the risks of surgery. In the hands of an experienced atresia surgeon, we favor atresiaplasty in the unilateral atretic ear, if the patient is motivated, cooperative, and a good candidate (minor malformations) anatomically.

Embryology

The human external auditory canal is derived from the first branchial groove. A primitive meatus is initially formed in the fifth week of gestation from an invagination of ectoderm medially toward the endoderm of the first pharyngeal pouch. This primitive meatus becomes the cartilaginous ear canal. The surface ectoderm also gives rise to a core of epithelial cells called the meatal plate which extends medially toward the tympanic cavity (pharyngeal pouch). The most medial ectodermal cells of the meatal plate form the superficial layer of the tympanic membrane. A layer of mesenchymal growth between the meatal plate and pharyngeal endoderm forms the middle fibrous layer of the tympanic membrane. Pharyngeal endoderm contributes to the medial mucosal layer.

In the third month of gestation, the medial canal is formed by ossification of the tympanic bone around the core of epithelial cells. Malformation of this bone medially results in atretic bone at the tympanic membrane and atresia of the bony ear canal. Similarly, if the core of epithelial cells does not grow toward the pharyngeal groove, tympanic bone is allowed to ossify producing atretic bone. The epithelial core canalizes late in development—the seventh month. Failure of these cells to absorb can result in a normal tympanic membrane and bony canal, with an atretic or stenotic cartilaginous ear canal. In 313 patients with major congenital ear malformations, Jahrsdoerfer,[1] found atresia far more common than stenosis, in a ratio of 7 : 1. Pneumatization of the mastoid bone is also a late embryologic event and continues into postnatal life. As discussed later, size of the mastoid air cell system and tympanic cleft are crucial in evaluating candidacy for atresia surgery.

The pharyngeal pouch persists medially as the tubotympanum and widens laterally to form the tympanic cavity. Interestingly, the eustachian tube generally develops normally, and patients with aural atresia have no increased incidence of eustachian tube dysfunction.[6] The ossicles develop from the first and second branchial arches. The head of the malleus and body of incus are formed from Meckel's cartilage of the first branchial arch, while the manubrium of the malleus, long process of incus, and stapes superstructure are derived from Reichert's cartilage of the second branchial arch. The stapes footplate is a product of Reichert's cartilage and otic capsule bone; it develops normally, and is rarely fixed in aural atresia. Ballachandra[7] gives an excellent review of developmental anatomy of the outer and middle ears.

The derivation of inner ear structures including the membranous labyrinth is from the ectodermal otocyst and is completely separate from the embryology of the middle and outer ears. As a result, vestibular function and sensorineural hearing in these patients is usually normal. Inner ear abnormalities, both anatomic and functional, can exist in patients with aural atresia, however, and may be a relative contraindication to atresiaplasty.

Patient Evaluation

The diagnosis of aural atresia is most often made secondary to a deformed auricle (microtia). Microtia does not always accompany atresia, however, and unilateral cases without microtia may not be diagnosed until the child fails a school hearing test. The history should search for problems in the prenatal, including exposures (tobacco and alcohol included), infections, and overall maternal health; birth; and postnatal periods.

Speech and motor development and family history not just of ear problems, but other associated craniofacial disorders should be assessed as well. Physical examination should include otoscopy with attention to grading the caliber of the ear canal and searching for debris/canal cholesteatoma. Facial musculature and nerve function of all branches is critical to test and document. Tuning fork testing should be performed if the child is able to cooperate. An overall otolaryngologic examination should be performed to look for associated craniofacial or branchial arch anomalies, including cleft lip/palate, hemifacial microsomia, and mandibular hypoplasia.

We cannot overemphasize the importance of complete audiologic evaluation even in the child with unilateral atresia with or without microtia. The infant with bilateral or unilateral atresia/microtia should undergo brain stem auditory response testing of both ears early in infancy to evaluate sensorineural function. Bone conducting hearing aids should be placed on the child with bilateral atresia as early as possible. In addition to inner ear anomalies that are occasionally seen with atresia cases, there is a reported incidence of conductive hearing loss in the apparently normal contralateral ear of up to 27%, with a sensorineural loss in as many as 18%.[4]

Radiologic Evaluation

High-resolution computed tomography (HRCT) in the coronal and axial projections at age 6 is the radiologic study of choice. HRCT provides excellent images for the assessment of inner ear structures, mastoid pneumatization, middle ear ossicular status, patency of the oval window, course of the facial nerve, and presence of cholesteatoma. If a cholesteatoma is suspected, earlier imaging with operative intervention is warranted. HRCT is mandatory in the preoperative evaluation of the atresia patient.

Good hearing results in atresia surgery are dependent on the anatomy of the ear as documented in the HRCT. We have traditionally used three very important anatomic criteria to evaluate a patient's candidacy for surgery: (1) mastoid/middle ear pneumatization, (2) normal appearance of inner ear structures, and (3) relationship of the facial nerve to a patent oval window and stapes footplate. With adequate pneumatization of the temporal bone, a normal inner ear, and a facial nerve in its normal course over (or perhaps slightly anterior, but always superior and posterior to) an open oval window/footplate, we have achieved excellent hearing results. Seventy-three percent of patients have achieved closure of the air–bone gap to within 30 dB.[3]

Jahrsdoerfer et al.[8] reported an anatomic grading system to evaluate a patient's candidacy for surgery. In his system, one point is given each for patency of the oval window, middle ear space, facial nerve, malleus/incus complex, mastoid pneumatization, incus-stapes connection, round window, and appearance of the external ear. Two points are given for the appearance of the stapes. Preoperative grade was predictive of postoperative hearing result, as 80% of patients with a score of ≥ 8/10 achieved closure of the air–bone gap to within 25 dB; 72% of patients with a grade 7 achieved closure to within 25 dB, 41% of patients with grade 6, and no patient (only 3 operated on) with a grade 5 achieved closure of the air–bone gap to within 25 dB. In cases of bilateral atresia, it is not unreasonable to operate on a grade 5 patient so that some serviceable hearing may be recovered; however, in cases of unilateral atresia, we do not recommend atresiaplasty for these anatomically marginal patients, as the hearing result may not provide useful hearing.

Timing of Surgery

Children with bilateral aural atresia generally undergo atresiaplasty at the age of 6. Bone conducting hearing aids are essential until such time. If auricular reconstruction is to be performed, consultation with the reconstructive surgeon is necessary to coordinate timing. Microtia repair is performed before atresia repair, as the costal cartilage graft is dependent on a field free of scar tissue and an intact vascular supply. We recommend completion of the auricular reconstruction, and 2 months later, the atresiaplasty. This timing ensures precise placement of the meatus and a well-vascularized cartilage graft.[9]

Older patients in whom mild presbycusis in the contralateral ear has begun to develop, or patients who suffer hearing loss in the normal ear, often seek surgical evaluation for correction. They realize how important binaural hearing is to them once the hearing becomes compromised in the normal ear. These patients, with favorable anatomy, are certainly candidates for atresiaplasty. Our oldest atresia patient was 61 years of age.

Surgical Technique

The general surgical technique for atresiaplasty has been described elsewhere.[3,10] A few selected highlights are discussed below.

Facial nerve monitoring is used for every case. We always use the anterior approach—the most direct approach to the epitympanum and ossicular mass. Before drilling the external auditory canal, we explore the posterior bony wall of the temporomandibular joint to guide the proper angle of drilling, to locate the anterior extent of drilling, and to ensure that the facial nerve does not exit the temporal bone through the joint. Drilling is started at the cribriform area. The mastoid tegmen/middle fossa plate is identified and followed medially. We recommend a cylinder with a diameter of 12 mm for size. Care is taken to open as few mastoid air cells posteriorly as possible. The facial nerve can take an aberrant course and be encountered posteriorly or inferiorly while drilling. Preoperative planning and identification of the entire course of the facial nerve on the HRCT will eliminate any surprises. If the facial nerve is too far anterior in the tympanic segment/second genu (i.e., coursing over the footplate), the patient may not be a candidate for atresia surgery. We do not recommend facial nerve rerouting in these cases.

The epitympanum is next opened and the malleus/incus complex is identified. At this point, drill trauma to the ossicular mass must be minimized or a high tone sensorineural deficit may result (approx. 5% incidence[4]). The laser has been very useful in freeing the ossicles from bony adhesions and ligamentous attachments in the middle ear space. The ossicular chain must be mobile; we prefer to graft over the malleus/incus complex whenever possible, rather than remove it and place an ossicular replacement prosthesis. Freeing the ossicular mass from all attachments, as well as drilling bone away from the mass, is crucial in preventing refixation.

The reconstructive technique of Jahrsdoerfer has withstood the test of time.[1,20] A 0.009-inch split-thickness skin graft is harvested from the hypogastrium and is prepared by cutting 4 to 5 triangles in one edge. The tips of the triangles are marked for placement medially on the temporalis fascia. The fascia is cut to a 20 × 15-mm oval, and small tabs are cut anteriorly and superiorly for placement under the protympanic periosteum to prevent lateralization. The fascia is lain over the ossicular mass, and the bony canal is completely lined by the skin graft with the triangles and marks placed over the fascia. The entire bony canal must be covered with skin. A thin disk of Gelfilm is used to hold the skin and fascia in place and to create an anterior tympanomeatal angle. The canal is lined with two small strips of Silastic sheeting and packed with a Cortisporin-soaked Ambrus wick.

The meatoplasty is made 10 mm in diameter by removing cartilage, and the skin graft is brought through and sutured to the native skin. Interrupted tacking sutures of 5-0 Ticron are used at the four quadrants, followed by a running suture of 6-0 fast absorbing gut placed between the Ticrons. A second Ambrus wick is used to secure the meatus. Improvements in tympanoplasty grafting, the addition of the laser to minimize drill trauma and ossicular manipulation, and facial nerve monitoring have significantly improved surgical results over the last 10 years.

Postoperative Care

Postoperative care is critical in maintaining a clean, dry ear canal. Annual and sometimes semiannual cleanings are necessary, and the patient must be cooperative. We see the patient the morning after surgery for mastoid dressing removal and inspection of the ear. The next appointment is 1 week later for aspiration of the meatal Ambrus wick and Silastic sheeting. At this point, we want aeration of the canal. Two weeks later, the packing and medial Ambrus wick are removed; and at this time, the ear is generally well healed. We then repack the lateral ear with Cortisporin-soaked Gelfoam and have the patient use Cortisporin Otic drops bid for the next 2 months. Dry ear precautions are necessary up to this point. After the ear has healed, it can be treated as a "normal" ear. We even allow patients to swim and get the ear wet; we recommend a couple drops of alcohol in the ear after swimming to dry the canal.

Discussion

Surgery for atresia of the external auditory canal has undergone vast evolution since the first documented attempt at correction by Kiesselbach in 1883.[1] Improvements in imaging and thus patient selection, facial nerve monitoring, grafting techniques, and drill technology have enabled many children to attain functional hearing without the use of amplification. Closure of the air–bone gap to within 30 dB has been achieved in upward of 80% of selected patients.[3,8] Nevertheless, not all children are candidates for atresiaplasty. Contraindications to atresiaplasty include poor sensorineural function as documented on brainstem evoked response audiometry, a closed oval window, a facial nerve that courses on the oval window, no aeration of the middle ear space,[18] and a poorly pneumatized mastoid (best seen on HRCT in the coronal projection).

Controversy remains over whether children with unilateral atresia should undergo surgery. In the past, Schuknecht,[11] Crabtree,[12] and Bellucci[13] have recommended against operating on children with unilateral atresia, arguing that the benefit to be gained is minimal and unappreciated in the presence of a contralateral normal hearing ear. Hearing results at that time were unpredictable and often did not approach the 20-dB air–bone gap needed for useful hearing in the atretic ear.[11] Risks of surgery, including facial nerve injury, also precluded operating on the unilateral atretic ear. In a recent review of more than 1000 operations for aural atresia with and without cholesteatoma, 10 patients (1%) suffered facial nerve injury.[17] In nine patients, recovery had occurred by 7 months; the last patient had a facial nerve transection during the skin incision. These investigators identified five situations in which the facial nerve was most vulnerable: (1) skin incision, (2) dissecting in the glenoid fossa, (3) during the canalplasty, (4) transposing the facial nerve, and (5) dissecting soft tissue of the preauricular area.[17]

Other investigators have advocated atresiaplasty when the patient is old enough to give his own consent.[14,19] They have cited moderate rates of restenosis and otorrhea (especially with the mastoidectomy approach) that argue against opening the ear; this approach often results in a draining radical cavity.

Complications of atresia surgery include high frequency sensorineural hearing loss (5%), total sensorineural hearing loss (2%), facial nerve palsy (1%), tympanic membrane graft lateralization (5 to 15%), and restenosis (5 to 15%).[3,4] The incidence of major complications (total SNHL and facial nerve injury) has decreased over the years, but the other complication rate has essentially remained unchanged. The decision to operate on the unilateral atretic ear must weigh these potential complication rates along with the possibility of a draining ear. Nevertheless, with excellent preoperative imaging, improved surgical techniques, and advances in technology (i.e., laser), we believe that the results of atresia surgery are now more predictable. Closure of the air–bone gap to within 30 dB in the properly selected patient can be consistently achieved. A recent review examining the long-term stability of hearing results in patients operated on for aural atresia shows some dropoff in hearing thresholds (SRT) over time, however.[16] Additional long–term follow-up studies are necessary to document and confirm these hearing results.

Wound complication rates, including otorrhea and restenosis, have stabilized or dropped over time. These potential complications can often be averted with office care. We stress the importance of a cooperative patient in the postoperative setting. Cleaning and manipulation of the ear are necessary; a beautiful result lost in the postoperative period from poor patient follow-up or cooperation serves no one. Most children do very well with cleaning, but an assessment should be made before surgery as to the child's willingness to sit in the chair and have the ears examined.

Using similar grading systems, De la Cruz, (Chandrasekhar et al.[4]) and Jahrsdoerfer[8] have argued for atresia surgery in selected children with unilateral atresia. A recent literature review also supports this position.[15] Again, anatomic candidacy is predicated on temporal bone pneumatization, facial nerve course, inner ear morphology, stapes/oval window appearance on HRCT, as well as documentation of the functional integrity of the inner ear. In the hands of an experienced otologic atresia surgeon with an anatomically favorable patient who (with the parents) understands the risks of potential complications and need for postoperative care, atresiaplasty in the patient with unilateral atresia is a rewarding operation for both surgeon and patient. The healed ear can be treated as a "normal" ear without restrictions on perspiration or water. Surgical correction of unilateral aural atresia offers the benefits of a clean, dry ear with binaural hearing, including sound localization and improved hearing in noise.

REFERENCES

De la Cruz and Kesser—CHAPTER 71

1. Jahrsdoerfer RA. Congenital atresia of the ear. *Laryngoscope* 1978;88:1
2. Jafek BW, Nager GT, Strife J, et al. Congenital aural atresia: an analysis of 311 cases. *Trans Am Acad Ophthalmol Otolaryngol* 1975;80:588
3. De la Cruz A, Linthicum FH Jr, Luxford WM. Congenital atresia of the external auditory canal. *Laryngoscope* 1985;95:421
4. Chandrasekhar SS, De la Cruz A, Garrido E. Surgery of congenital aural atresia. *Am J Otol* 1995;16:713
5. Cole RR, Jahrsdoerfer RA. The risk of cholesteatoma in congenital aural stenosis. *Laryngoscope* 1990;100:576
6. Lambert PR. Congenital aural atresia. In: Byron J. Bailey, eds. *Head and Neck Surgery—Otolaryngology*. Philadelphia: JB Lippincott; 1993:1579
7. Ballachandra BB. Developmental anatomy of the outer ear. In: BB Ballachanda, ed. *The Human Ear Canal*. San Diego: Singular Publishing; 1995:8
8. Jahrsdoerfer RA, Yeakley JW, Aguilar EA, et al. Grading system for the selection of patients with congenital aural atresia. *Am J Otol* 1992;13:6
9. Jahrsdoerfer RA, Kesser BW. Issues on aural atresia for the facial plastic surgeon. *Facial Plast Surg* 1995;11:274
10. Malony TB, De la Cruz A. Surgical approaches to congenital atresia of the external auditory canal. *Otolaryngol Head Neck Surg* 1990;103:991
11. Schuknecht HG. Congenital aural atresia. *Laryngoscope* 1989; 99:908
12. Crabtree JA. Congenital atresia: case selection, complications, and prevention. *Otolaryngol Clin North Am* 1982; 15:755
13. Bellucci RJ. Congenital aural malformations: diagnosis and treatment. *Otolaryngol Clin North Am* 1981;14:95
14. Mattox DE, Fisch U. Surgical correction of congenital atresia of the ear. *Otolaryngol Head Neck Surg* 1986;94:574
15. Trigg DJ, Applebaum EL. Indications for the surgical repair of unilateral aural atresia in children. *Am J Otol* 1998; 19:679
16. Lambert PR. Long-term hearing results in congenital aural atresia surgery. *Laryngoscope* 1998;108:1801
17. Jahrsdoerfer RA, Lambert PR. Facial nerve injury in congenital aural atresia surgery. *Am J Otol* 1998;19:283
18. Lambert PR. Major congenital ear malformations: surgical management and results. *Ann Otol Rhinol Laryngol* 1988; 97:641
19. Glasscock ME III, Scwaber MK, Nissen AJ, Jackson CG. Management of congenital ear malformations. *Ann Otol Rhinol Laryngol* 1983;92:504
20. Jahrsdoerfer RA. Congenital malformations of the ear: analysis of 94 operations. *Ann Otol Rhinol Laryngol* 1980; 89:348

Management of the Unilateral Atretic Ear

CHAPTER 72

Christopher J. Hartnick and Daniel I. Choo

Unilateral congenital aural atresia represents one of the most complex and challenging problems that an otolaryngologist may have to face. The surgical procedure itself is fraught with potential pitfalls such as facial nerve paralysis and sensorineural hearing loss. There are differing schools of thought concerning the repair of congenital unilateral aural atresia; one school of thought is represented by Crabtree,[1] who states that "one does not usually operate in cases of unilateral atresia until the patient is an adult and expresses the desire for surgery." The other school of thought is represented by Jahrsdoerfer et al.[2] who writes that "whether the ear malformation is unilateral or bilateral plays no part in our selection process. Because we believe that hearing results are predictable, we operate on unilateral atresia patients routinely." The underpinnings of and the differences between these two surgical beliefs are in part philosophical, but another part rests in technological advances that have allowed for greater facility in predicting the results of surgery. This chapter, discusses the controversy over managing patients with unilateral congenital aural atresia by describing the preoperative evaluation that goes into formulating a treatment algorithm and our rationale for offering unilateral atresia repair to pediatric patients and their families.

Embryology and Epidemiology

The incidence of congenital aural atresia is 1:10,000 to 20,000.[3] Unilateral atresia is five to six times more common.[1] The embryologic basis of aural atresia is the failure of the external auditory canal to recanalize during the sixth and seventh months of gestation. The external auditory canal is derived from the first branchial groove. In the developing embryo, an epithelial core of cells arises and fills the external auditory canal. It is the failure of these cells to canalize that gives rise to aural atresia. Aural atresia occurs either together with, or in isolation from, external or middle ear malformations. It is important to note that middle ear malformations are much more common in the atretic ear where there is also microtia present; they are also more common in the normal ear where the other ear canal is atretic than if there are two normal ears.[1]

Surgical Considerations

As it is not the purpose of this chapter to present a technical manual of aural atresia surgery, the extensive details of the surgical procedure are not discussed in this chapter. However, an alternative approach to the anterior atresiaplasty that is now commonly advocated is presented. As described by several surgeons,[3-5] the anterior approach involves skeletonizing the posterior temporomandibular joint in order to define the anterior extent of the future canal. Drilling superiorly and following the tegmen medially allows the surgeon to expose the ossicular mass directly and minimize the risk to the facial nerve that will run deep to the ossicles. Initiating the dissection anteriorly and superiorly allows the surgeon to begin creation of the new ear canal (directly) lateral to the middle ear cleft without necessarily creating a large mastoid bowl while still allowing purposeful identification of the facial nerve (as required in all otologic procedures). Alternatively, the repair of an aural atresia can be performed in a more posteriorly based approach. In the severely atretic ear with a thick bony plate; for example, the only identifiable landmarks available to the surgeon may be the middle fossa dura and the sinodural angle. In these cases, identifying these landmarks may allow the surgeon to determine the level of the lateral semicircular canal and subsequently the position of the fallopian canal. Once these landmarks have been identified, completion of the atresia repair can be performed on the basis of the anatomic limitations of the given ear. Again, careful preoperative evaluation of the high-resolution computed tomography (HRCT) can provide the surgeon with invaluable anatomic information that can be translated directly to reduced surgical risk to the facial nerve. The routine use of the facial nerve monitor supplements the surgeon's knowledge of temporal bone anatomy, the information provided by the preoperative HRCT, and provides another asset in making unilateral aural atresia repair safer for the patient. We stress the routine use of facial nerve monitoring in all otologic cases, as familiarity with the monitoring devices and experience in interpretation of monitor data is essential to obtaining the maximum information from these tools. The remainder of the surgical technique (ossicular mobilization, tympanic membrane construction, and skin grafting) have been well described elsewhere.[3,4]

Decision Making

In the case of bilateral aural atresia, the primary concern is that of the development of normal speech and language. These children should be fitted early on with bone anchored hearing aids, and surgery should be strongly considered. In the case of unilateral aural atresia, a complete audiologic evaluation should be performed. Surgery is only a consideration if there is normal or near-normal sensorineural hearing loss in the atretic ear. Historically it has been felt that if the patient has normal hearing in one ear, then the effect on language and speech will not be greatly affected by the loss of hearing in the other ear. This premise has recently been called into question and there is debate currently over whether unilateral hearing loss can in fact create linguistic and cognitive deficits.[6]

As for the timing of repair of the unilateral atretic ear, there is a range of years during which it is considered acceptable to offer surgery, depending on the co-mitigating factors. In the face of atresia coupled with grade III microtia, we feel that the atresia repair should be delayed until after the auricular reconstruction so that the costal cartilage has a well-vascularized bed in which to be placed. As microtia repairs generally do not occur before the age of 6 years, the subsequent atresia repairs are then delayed until the patient is 7 or 8 years of age. If the atresia is in isolation, some authors (e.g., Crabtree[1]) assert that the repair should take place when the patient is old enough to understand the risks involved. Others believe that it is only necessary for the patient to be able to cooperate so that adequate postoperative care can be delivered.

The fear in operating on patients with unilateral aural atresia has historically rested in the inability to predict surgical success and the danger of injuring the facial nerve. The advent of HRCT imaging and facial nerve monitoring have dramatically reduced these unknowns in atresia surgery and make it possible to offer surgical management based upon objective preoperative data and reasonable expectations of surgical outcome. HRCT has allowed for specific answers to crucial questions that affect the preoperative evaluation, such as the following: Is there a stapes? Is the oval window visible? Is the facial nerve identifiable in a predictable course? Jahrsdoerfer used HRCT to develop a 10-point system to predict the success rate for surgical repair.[2] In his system, 2 points are given for an identifiable stapes, 1 point for the following findings: an open oval window, an identifiable middle ear space, a normal facial nerve, an identifiable malleus-incus complex, a well-pneumatized mastoid, an incus–stapes connection, a normal-appearing round window, and a normal-appearing external ear. A score of 8 signaled an 80% chance of success defined as a postoperative speech reception threshold of 10 to 25 dB. This point grading scheme has proved more clinically useful than Altmann's purely descriptive classification scheme.[7] De la Cruz et al.[4] have also proposed a classification scheme with an eye toward guiding surgical management.

If Jahrsdoerfer's grading system allowed for some measure of predictability in terms of surgical success, the advent of modern facial nerve monitoring has allowed for greater degrees of comfort with respect to avoiding potentially disastrous pitfalls. Although Jahrsdoerfer[8] states that facial nerve monitoring is of little use in atresia surgery, many practicing otologists and otolaryngologists believe that facial nerve monitoring remains an invaluable tool. The incidence of facial nerve injury after atresia surgery approximates 1%.[5] This low incidence is due in part to the use of HRCT and preoperative knowledge of particular facial nerve anatomy. We attribute it to the use of intraoperative facial nerve monitoring, as well. Whether one advocates facial nerve monitoring, it is essential for the surgeon embarking on repair of aural atresia to have a sound knowledge of facial nerve anatomy and its potential aberrations.

Summary

We use a rigorous preoperative evaluation to determine which of our pediatric patients are appropriate candidates for surgery and offer unilateral atresiaplasty to good candidates based upon this evaluation (regardless of the status of the contralateral ear). As in all realms of surgery, the success of aural atresia surgery rests upon the experience of the surgeon in choosing the appropriate patient and knowing how to avoid the potential complications that can occur. The advent of HRCT has allowed for the development of strict criteria for choosing potential surgical candidates. By following these criteria, a reasonable estimation of the probability of surgical success in terms of restoration of hearing can be surmised. The facial nerve monitor is helpful and should be used in all cases, but is no substitute for a detailed knowledge of facial nerve anatomy. Certain conditions, such as occult cholesteatoma, will dictate management and produce a need for early surgical intervention. In other cases, management must be individualized, tailored to the patients and their families' needs and desires, and then carefully planned and orchestrated. Experience has suggested that patients with isolated atresia are more likely to be suitable candidates than are patients with concomitant microtia or other auricular anomalies.[2] For patients who are not suitable candidates, other options such as bone anchored hearing aids should be considered.

REFERENCES

Hartnick and Choo—CHAPTER 72

1. Crabtree JA. Congenital atresia: case selection, complications, and prevention. *Otolaryngolog Clin North Am.* 1982;15:755–762
2. Jahrsdoerfer RA, Yearkley JW, Aguilar EA, et al. Grading system for the selection of patients with congenital aural atresia. *Am J Otol.* 1982;13:6–12
3. Jahrsdoerfer RA. Congenital atresia of the ear. *Laryngoscope* 1978;88:1
4. De la Cruz A, Linthicum FH, Jr, Luxford WM. Congenital atresia of the external auditory canal. *Laryngoscope* 1985; 95:421–427
5. Jahrsdoerfer RA, Lambert PR. Facial nerve surgery in congenital aural atresia surgery. *Am J Otol* 1998;19:283–287
6. Bess FH. The unilaterally hearing-impaired child: a final comment. *Ear Hearing* 1986;7:52–54
7. Altmann F. Congenital atresia of the ear in man and animals. *Ann Otol Rhinol Laryngol* 1955;64:824–858
8. Jahrsdoerfer RA. Surgical Correction of Congenital Malformations of the Sound Conducting Mechanism. In: Glasscock ME, Shanbaugh GE Jr, eds. *Surgery of the Ear.* 4th Ed. Philadelphia: WB Saunders; 1990:321–334

25

Airway Management of the Retrognathic Patient

"Although positioning may be successful in some patients, alternative measures have been necessary in other children in order to enable retrognathic children to grow and develop normally. The literature is polarized over this issue, and clinical decisions seem to be based as much on emotion as on scientific data."

Charles M. Myer III

"Patients may be discharged home early, provided that their parents are taught NP intubation, suctioning, tracheotomy care, appropriate feeding techniques, cardiopulmonary resuscitation, and the use of apnea monitor and pulse oximetry."

George H. Zalzal

"The first step in managing the airway of the retrognathic patient with known airway compromise is to assess the severity and urgency of the obstruction. Historically, retrognathia in association with emergent airway compromise has been necessarily addressed in neonates and infants born with syndromes associated with posterior positioning of the mandible and/or micrognathia."

Eve Bluestein

Airway Management of the Retrognathic Patient

Charles M. Myer III

CHAPTER 73

In general, most children with retrognathia have some degree of airway obstruction as part of their anomaly. In managing these children, physicians should attempt to minimize any airway obstruction present while promoting normal neurologic development and ensuring appropriate weight gain. Although positioning may be successful in some patients, alternative measures have been necessary in other children in order to enable retrognathic children to grow and develop normally. The literature is polarized over this issue, and clinical decisions seem to be based as much on emotion as on scientific data. This chapter is intended to help the clinician decide which retrognathic patients warrant operative intervention and those who should be managed conservatively.

Several potential etiologic factors in airway obstruction with retrognathia have been described, including (1) posterior displacement of a normal-size tongue; (2) loss of support of the genioglossus muscle; and (3) development of negative pressure within the upper aerodigestive tract during deglutition and inspiration resulting in glossoptosis. These events cause airway obstruction by means of four different mechanisms: (1) antero/posterior collapse secondary to posterior movement of the tongue against the posterior pharyngeal wall; (2) posterior/superior displacement of the tongue, prompting contact between the tongue, velum, and pharyngeal wall in the superior oropharynx; (3) pharyngeal obstruction secondary to prolapse of the medial walls of the pharynx; and (4) constriction of the pharynx in a circular manner with movement of the tongue as well as both lateral pharyngeal walls. In some children with retrognathia, brain stem immaturity may lead to apnea and hypoxia from vagal overactivity and esophageal motor abnormalities.[1-3]

The need for intervention in retrognathic children is driven by the potential consequences of unrecognized and inappropriately managed obstruction (i.e., hypoxia, cor pulmonale), failure to thrive, and embarrassment of central nervous system (CNS) activities. It is essential to remember that children with retrognathia may have significant hypoxia without apparent obstructive episodes.[4] These may occur more frequently with advancing age as the child's metabolic demands increase associated with increasing physical activity. Similarly, the degree of obstruction and resultant hypoxia may worsen with superimposed upper respiratory infections. Thus, vigilant observation is mandatory in order to prevent the potentially devastating growth and neurologic sequelae of prolonged hypoxia.

Once a patient is recognized as being at risk of airway obstruction with retrognathia, an appropriate evaluation should be undertaken in order to optimize management. In addition to performing continuous pulse oximetry and serial polysomnography (as necessary),[4] a full endoscopic evaluation of the upper aerodigestive system should be considered, to rule out other possible treatable causes of obstruction.[1] An evaluation for gastroesophageal reflux disease (GERD) may be appropriate, as GERD may worsen known airway compromise. Children with retrognathia are at risk of GERD because of the increased negative intrathoracic pressure often found in this population of children. Both a pH probe and a gastric emptying scan should be obtained to quantify any potential problems.[4]

Although airway obstruction often improves with time as infants develop voluntary tongue control and progressive mandibular growth occurs, this may take months. It is clearly impractical to keep children hospitalized until these events occur, assuming they take place. Thus, as a result of economic issues and the desire to establish family integrity, it is necessary for physicians to develop a rational plan for airway management at home.[5] Should a child be premature or have associated medical problems that mandate hospitalization, definitive intervention may be delayed until discharge planning begins.

In making a determination about whether a patient needs intervention, one should consider whether the patient has isolated retrognathia or retrognathia associated with a syndrome. A classic example is provided by examining children with Pierre Robin sequence (PRS), who have either isolated Robin sequence (IRS) or Robin sequence with a syndrome (RSS). Associated malformations have been reported in up to 82% of children with PRS. Categorization is important prognostically as one group found that there was a 22.8% mortality in RSS but only a 5.9% mortality in those with IRS.[6] Another method of categorization places patients into groups with mild obstruction (airway obstruction resolves with posture alone; supine nursing possible), moderate obstruction (utilization of nasopharyngeal airway and prone positioning for feeding after removal of nasopharyngeal airway), and severe obstruction (long-term management with nasopharyngeal airway or tracheotomy).[7] There are probably more children with mild obstruction than are recognized generally since most studies only involve hospitalized children. PRS patients in the general population may be managed conservatively at home in most circumstances and therefore would not be included in most studies. As a result, the percentage of children with PRS who require surgical intervention is overestimated in the literature. In one study of 125 hospitalized patients with PRS, 45% had mild obstruction, 32% had moderate obstruction, and 23% had major respiratory difficulties.[6]

Several different methods have been described for airway management in children with retrognathia and symptomatic airway obstruction. These include lateral and prone positioning, use of intraoral devices, use of a nasopharyngeal airway, intubation, glossopexy (including tongue–lip adhesion [TLA]), mandibular expansion by traction, and tracheotomy.[8] Advantages and disadvantages are present in each of these techniques, and their relative merits will be compared and contrasted.

In the retrognathic patient with acute obstruction, prone positioning may be effective if the airway obstruction is secondary to glossoptosis. This allows the effects of gravity to prevent the tongue from falling into the hypopharynx. In addition, this will minimize the effects of negative intrathoracic pressure during swallowing and inspiration, which cause the tongue to prolapse posteriorly due to its lack of voluntary muscular control.[9] Although positioning may be effective on a short-term basis, it is not physiologic on a long-term basis. This will also prevent the normal parental–child physical contact needed for bonding to take place. In fact, at the Center for Craniofacial Disorders (CCFD) in the Bronx, New York, all patients who needed positioning or a nasopharyngeal airway greater than 30 days required surgical intervention. If feeding can be accomplished readily with the patient who requires prone positioning, this may be an appropriate solution for a relatively short time. However, if the feeding process becomes laborious, the joys of parenting may decrease significantly and make this an exhausting process. In that situation, an alternative method of airway control is necessary.[3,10,11]

The use of a nasopharyngeal airway is appropriate in some children with retrognathia who require airway support for a short period of time. However, at the CCFD any child who required support for more than 30 days needed a surgical procedure. It is interesting that in a review of several articles from the CCFD there are contradictory reports regarding timing of abandonment of management with a nasopharyngeal airway. Specifically, different physicians from the same center have indicated that the decision to abandon use of a nasopharyngeal airway should be made at 7 to 10 days or at 8 weeks, even with the supporting data that any child requiring a nasopharyngeal airway for longer than 4 weeks required surgical intervention.

Use of a nasopharyngeal airway may be problematic because of placement of the tube at an inappropriate level. Accidental dislodgment of the tip of the tube from the correct position in the pharynx may precipitate gagging and vomiting if it slips inferiorly into the pharynx, while airway obstruction may be noted if it dislodges superiorly. Although some patients are discharged with a nasopharyngeal airway as a primary form of long-term therapy, some feel this is unstable for long-term management and is extremely risky.[3,10,12]

Similar to the CCFD experience, clinicians from San Diego have discharged patients successfully using a nasopharyngeal airway with a Tunstal connector to provide stability and minimize motion. This device is attached to the patient's forehead and connects to the nasal tube. These physicians use flexible laryngoscopy and bronchoscopy to rule out other causes of airway obstruction and define the level of obstruction before placing the tube under direct vision, ensuring that the top of the tube is distal to the site of obstruction. In general, polyvinyl chloride (PVC) tubes are used, as opposed to rubber tubes, because of their increased rigidity. The patients are discharged with pulse oximetry, a suction machine, oral airways, and extra nasopharyngeal tubes. The parents have been taught cardiopulmonary resuscitation skills, suctioning, oxygen saturation monitoring, and the method for placing oral and nasopharyngeal airways. The parents will be familiar with gavage feeding if that is appropriate, and antimicrobial prophylaxis is often recommended to minimize inflammatory processes in the ears or sinuses. This group cautions that discharge of these patients may not be appropriate without cooperative, enthusiastic, and intelligent families.[1]

Another possible alternative for airway management is glossopexy, the type most frequently employed being a TLA. Although relatively simple in concept, the procedure has been known to fail in the hands of many experienced surgeons, often due to the button/suture cutting through the tongue. In addition, an anterior tongue mass can be created, which may block the airway itself. If the tongue is pulled too far anteriorly, it may tether the epiglottis and lead to possible aspiration. Other possible complications include wound infections, wound dehiscence, injuries to Wharton's ducts, and scar deformation of the lip, chin, and floor of mouth. Though feeding problems are not common with TLA, the procedure is not physiologic and it may lead to difficulties with oral intake.[13] If not taken down before eruption of the teeth, significant dental abnormalities can occur, including retrodisplacement of the central and lateral mandibular incisors.

An adjunct to the TLA is the use of mandibular traction. This technique uses a conformer from the trunk with support bars to maintain an elevated midline bar (outrigger bar). An elastic band connection between the mandible and the outrigger bar allows the newborn to move the head laterally, but it discourages hyperextension because this motion will increase tension and pain. Easter et al.[13] believe that this device is necessary for up to 2 months during the healing phase of TLA. Frohberg and Lange[8] describe the use of circumferential mandibular wiring as a means of mandibular expansion in their study. The wires are attached to weights for three weeks and their index case demonstrated improvement in oxygen saturation with a diminution in the apnea index. However, careful review of their case demonstrates that the child still had a significantly elevated apnea index (22/hour) when they removed the mandibular traction. Although this method of therapy does address specifically the causative anomaly, we would disagree with the authors who consider this method physiologic. In addition, Frohberg and Lange[8] advocate waiting until 18 months of age to repair a cleft palate associated with retrognathia, allowing for more airway growth. Although there may not be subsequent airway problems when waiting this length of time to close the palate, there are other issues that must be considered in regard to facial growth. Another alternative for airway management in this population is hyomandibulopexy. However, once this is accomplished, the larynx is more anterior and more difficult to intubate should that be necessary following surgical repair. In addition, there may be interference with mandibular growth[6] and even problems with difficulty closing the mouth.

Another method that has been described for airway management is the use of an adapted bed that employs a forehead rest and occipital splint. The patient is placed in the prone position with a headrest maintaining the head. Patients have been sent home with this arrangement understanding that failure may necessitate surgical intervention. Continuous positive airway pressure (CPAP) may be necessary in some of these patients. Caouette-Laberg et al.[6] use a subperiosteal release of the floor of mouth musculature on the mandible when the adapted bed previously described does not work. Although they are unable to offer an explanation regarding the success of the procedure, the operation involves removal of the genioglossus insertion from its mandibular attachment. This results in decreased glossoptosis with improved laryngeal position and, subsequently, less airway obstruction.

Shprintzen and Singer[2] and Sher[3] offer alternatives for airway management depending on the site of obstruction. At the CCFD, the investigators feel that a procedure to keep the tongue forward, such as a TLA, is likely to be successful only if the obstruction is secondary to the tongue blocking the airway. At this center, when the tongue presses against the palate, long-term use of a nasopharyngeal airway may be appropriate while awaiting vertical growth of the craniofacial structures. If growth occurs during the first several months of life, this may allow the tube to be removed or a glossopexy then may be successful. When there is collapse of the pharyngeal walls, long-term use of a nasopharyngeal airway may be appropriate while awaiting maturation, characterized by improved muscle tone, weight gain, and improved neurologic function. When no improvement occurs, a tracheotomy is deemed appropriate. These same guidelines are utilized when there is sphincter closure of the airway. As mentioned previously, the decision to intervene surgically at the CCFD is made at 1 to 8 weeks of age.

The results of a survey of pediatric otolaryngology fellowship training programs in regard to their management of the airway in PRS patients mirrors the controversy seen in the literature.[14] This study, conducted by the Department of Otolaryngology at Children's Hospital Medical Center, Cincinnati, Ohio, found no unanimity among respondents in the decision-making process when positioning and observation are no longer sufficient to prevent apneic episodes and oxygen desaturation in the neonate or infant with PRS. However, a clear trend was seen toward the use of a tracheotomy for long-term airway management. In the collection of the data for this report, it became obvious that the responses often were based on emotions as much as on scientific data. In point of fact, no studies have been done in which the different forms of airway management in PRS have been subjected to comparative analysis, thus leading to the multitude of anecdotal reports and pronouncements. Unfortunately, the lack of a large number of cases at any one center prohibits individual comparative trials and makes multi-institutional investigations mandatory. With a topic that is marked by such prejudice, implementation of a cooperative study is virtually impossible.

The following algorithm summarizes the thought process that should be employed by the clinician in the management of a child with PRS. One should note that this algorithm is for the child with isolated retrognathia. If there is an associated syndrome, I am more inclined to do a tracheotomy because of the higher mortality rate (Fig. 73–1). In addition, one might consider use of a nasogastic feeding tube to break the seal created by the glossoptosis. In some cases, this may eliminate the need for further airway intervention. Similarly, feeding difficulties may be addressed with either a nasogastric tube or a gastrostomy tube.

Conclusion

Management of the child with retrognathia is a clinical challenge. If there is no associated syndrome, the decision for intervention can be based on the results of polysomnography in addition to objective assessment of growth parameters. If there is compromise in either area, intervention is necessary. Positioning and observation may be appropriate on a short-term basis. However, if this fails, placement of a nasopharyngeal airway may be successful. If the child has continued symptoms after 3 weeks, placement of a tracheotomy is indicated. Although I will send patients home with positioning and observation, I am reluctant to send children home with nasopharyngeal airways. In the retrognathic child with a syndrome, I go through a similar thought process, but I am much quicker to place a tracheotomy because of the high morbidity and mortality associated with these conditions. In most circumstances, obstruction improves between 6 and 9 months of age, and one can begin the process of withdrawing airway support.[1,2,7,15]

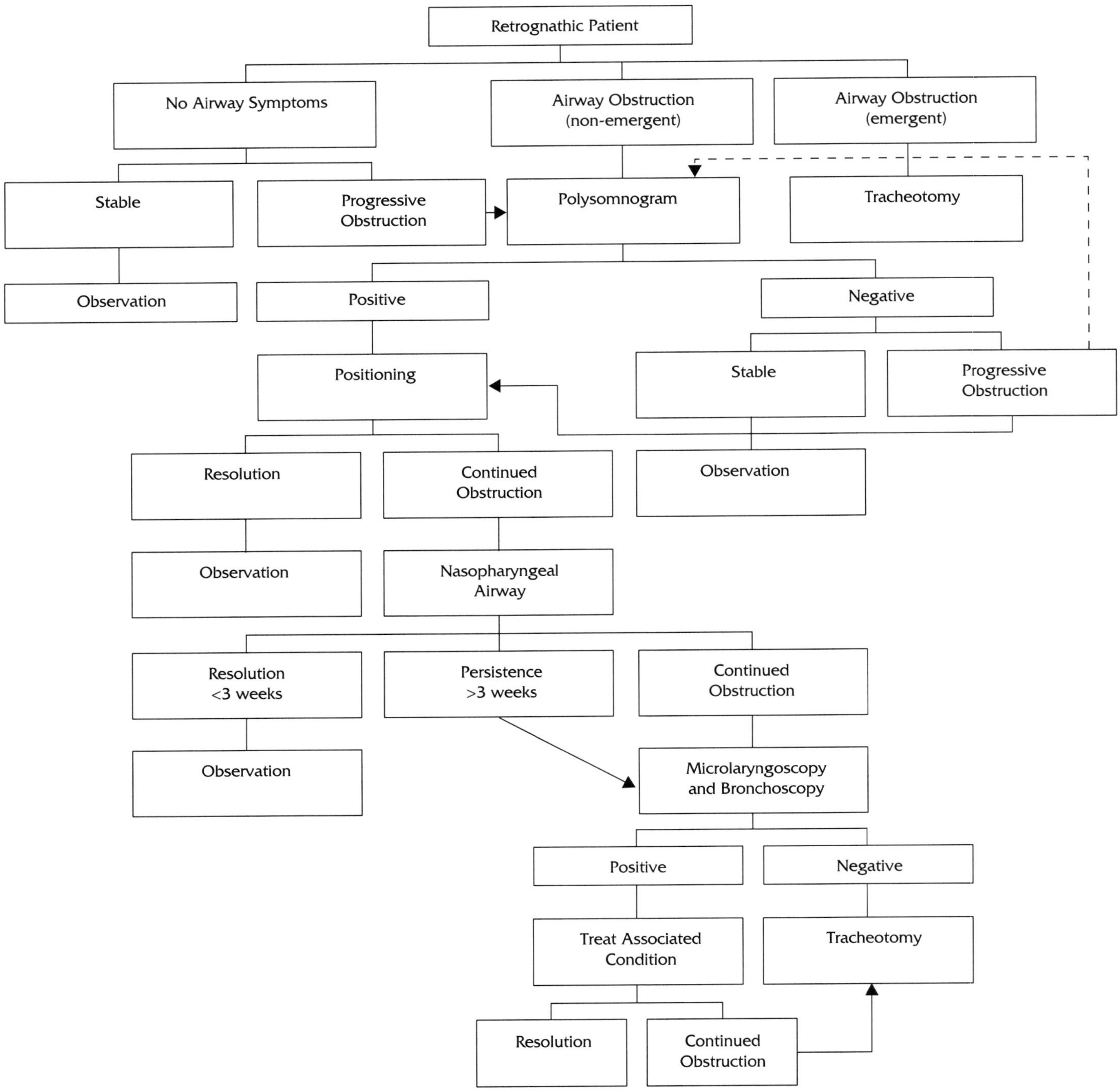

Figure 73–1 Algorithm for the management of the retrognathic patient.

REFERENCES

Myer III—CHAPTER 73

1. Olson TS, Kearns DB, Pransky SM, Seid AB. Early home management of patients with Pierre Robin sequence. *Int J Pediatr Otorhinolaryngol* 1990;20:45–49
2. Shprintzen RJ, Singer L. Upper airway obstruction and the Robin sequence. *Anesthesiology Clin* 1992;30:109–114
3. Sher AE. Mechanisms of airway obstruction in Robin sequence: implications for treatment. *Cleft Palate Craniofac J* 1992;29:224–231
4. Bull MJ, Givan DC, Sadove AM, et al. Improved outcome in Pierre Robin Sequence: effect of multidisciplinary evaluation and management. *Pediatrics* 1990;86:294–301
5. Gilhooly JT, Smith JD, Howell LL, et al. Bedside polysomnography as an adjunct in the management of infants with Robin sequence. *Plast Reconstr Surg* 1993;92:23–27
6. Caouette-Laberge L, Bayet B, Larocque Y. The Pierre Robin sequence: review of 125 cases and evolution of treatment modalities. *Plast Reconstr Surg* 1994;93:934–942
7. Benjamin B, Walker P. Management of airway obstruction in the Pierre Robin sequence. *Int J Pediatr Otorhinolaryngol* 1991;22:29–37
8. Frohberg U, Lange R. Surgical treatment of Robin sequence and sleep apnea syndrome: case report and review of the literature. *J Oral Maxillofac Surg* 1993;51:1274–1277
9. Augarten A, Sagy M, Yahav J, Barzilay Z. Management of upper airway obstruction in the Pierre Robin syndrome. *Br J Oral Maxillofac Surg* 1990;28:105–108
10. Shprintzen RJ. The implications of the diagnosis of Robin sequence. *Cleft Palate Craniofac J* 1992;29:205–209
11. Argamaso RV. Glossopexy for upper airway obstruction in Robin sequence. *Cleft Palate Craniofac J* 1992;29:232–238
12. Singer L, Sidoti EJ. Pediatric management of Robin sequence. *Cleft Palate Craniofac J* 1992;29:220–223
13. Easter B, Wood C, Eppley BL, Sadove AM. Mandibular traction system for adjunctive management of airway insufficiency in infants with Pierre Robin malformation sequence. *Am J Occup Ther* 1991;45:941–943
14. Myer III CM, Reed JM, Cotton RT, et al. Airway management in Piere Robin sequence. *Otolaryngol Head Neck Surg* 1998;118:630–635
15. Tomaski SM, Zalzal GH, Saal HM. Airway obstruction in the Pierre Robin sequence. *Larygoscope* 1995;105:111–114

Airway Management of the Retrognathic Patient

CHAPTER 74

George H. Zalzal and LenhAnh P. Tran

As otolaryngologists, we are often requested to evaluate newborns, infants, and children with upper airway obstruction. Nasal pyriform aperture stenosis, posterior choanal stenosis or atresia, Pierre Robin sequence (PRS), craniofacial anomalies, and laryngotracheal disorders are among the etiologies of upper airway obstruction. PRS is classically known as a triad of micrognathia, glossoptosis, and cleft palate. In PRS, the mandible may be of normal size, but it is displaced posteriorly. Retrognathia, lack of support of the genioglossus muscle, and negative pharyngeal pressure during inspiration lead to of the compromise upper airway.

Positioning, oropharyngeal airway, nasopharyngeal (NP) airway, tongue–lip adhesion (TLA), glossopexy, prosthesis placement, endotracheal intubation, and tracheotomy are many nonsurgical and surgical airway interventions. Choosing the most effective, reliable, and safe airway intervention for retrognathic patients is as challenging as it is controversial.

Background

Pierre Robin, a French stomatologist, was acknowledged for his recognition of the triad with the associated respiratory and nutritional problems.[1] PRS affects 1 in every 2000[2] to 30,000[3] live births. Randall et al.[1] observed true micrognathia in only two-thirds of their PRS patients and suggested that mandibular retrognathia is a more important cause of upper airway obstruction than micrognathia. The cleft palate, when present, is usually a U-shaped palatal defect. During embryogenesis, the malpositioned mandible prevents the tongue from descending below the palatal plane and interferes with the palatal fusion in the midline. Although the tongue is of normal size, it is prolapsed into the nasopharynx and posterior oropharynx. Whether this process occurs as a result of hereditary influence, chromosomal disorder, intrauterine position, trauma, or infections remains to be determined.

PRS may occur as an isolated condition or in association with other syndromes, such as Stickler, velocardiofacial (VCF), fetal alcohol, or Treacher Collins, and other unique patterns of malformation. The incidence of associated syndromes may be observed in up to 83%[4] of PRS patients. In addition to retrognathia and glossoptosis, many other factors may complicate the respiratory obstruction, including skull base abnormalities (Stickler, Treacher Collins), nasopharyngeal hypotonia (VCF), nasal stenosis (VCF, Treacher Collins), or neurologic compromise (VCF, fetal alcohol syndrome).

Most retrognathic infants and children manifest the obstructive respiratory symptoms at birth or days to weeks after birth. The severity of obstruction, ranges from minimal upper airway sounds to severe respiratory distress, failure to thrive, and cor pulmonale. Thus, airway management of PRS patients should be a systematic approach based on the site(s), severity of upper airway obstruction, and associated diseases involving other organs.

Discussion

Attempts have been made to classify PRS patients based on the severity or type of upper airway obstruction. Benjamin and Walker[5] divided their patients into three groups based on their responses to the treatment protocol, which included neonatal intensive care unit (NICU) monitoring, pulse oximetry, and sequential use of all airway interventions (i.e., posturing, NP tube, endotracheal intubation, tracheotomy). Benjamin and Walker[5] reported patients with mild and moderate obstruction were managed successfully with posturing and NP airway, respectively. Patients with severe obstructive symptoms requiring endotracheal intubation or tracheotomy tended to have associated congenital anomalies and severe micrognathia. Freed et al.[6] and Bull et al.[7] used polysomnography (PSG) as an objective measurement of upper airway obstruction, in deciding the type of airway intervention, and in evaluation of treatment efficacy. Although they did not use the same criteria, both groups believed that oxygen desaturation, carbon dioxide retention, and obstruction during sleep were critical indicators of severe airway obstruction. Bull et al.[7] observed PRS infants with multiple congenital anomalies were affected with greater degrees of obstruction and oxygen desaturation, feeding complications, gastroesophageal reflux disease, and developmental impairment, hence the necessity for surgical intervention.

Sher[8] described four types of upper airway obstruction on endoscopy. Type I obstruction was due to the posterior tongue protrusion and contact with the posterior pharyngeal wall. Type II obstruction was the impaction of the posterior tongue and velum to the posterior pharyngeal wall. Lateral pharyngeal wall prolapse resulted in type III obstruction. Type IV obstruction is a circular and sphincteric pattern of movement. The authors commented that glossopexy was effective in treating type I obstruction. Whereas type II obstruction was partially improved by glossopexy, types III and IV obstructions would not. Type I obstruction was often observed in patients with Stickler syndrome, whereas the other types of obstruction were frequently seen in patients with Treacher Collins, fetal alcohol, and VCF syndromes and in those with a unique pattern of malformation.

The difference in number and type of PRS patients (i.e., isolated PRS vs PRS with associated syndromes), inconsistent objective measurements of upper airway obstruction, frequent subjective surgical indications, and variable airway interventions make interpretation of the data difficult. Myer et al.[9] demonstrated such inconsistencies and controversies in their survey of 23 pediatric otolaryngology fellowship programs in the United States and Canada. Most programs evaluated 6 to 10 patients per year. Seventeen of 23 programs supported at least a selective use of PSG, either as single or serial studies. One program used PSG routinely on all children before discharge. The indications for PSG were to screen or to detect the severity of obstruction, to decide on airway treatment options, and to determine the timing of decannulation. The preferred long-term airway interventions (tracheotomy, positioning, NP airway, TLA, oral airway, continuous positive airway pressure [CPAP]) differed vastly among the programs.

We begin our evaluation of PRS patients with close monitoring in the NICU and a complete head and neck examination. Signs and symptoms of airway obstruction including respiratory sounds, substernal or intercostal retraction, pectus excavatum, oxygen desaturation, and feeding problems are documented. Quiet respiration should not be mistaken as normal respiration. Complete airway obstruction may be present despite persistent thoracoabdominal muscular movements. Flexible nasopharyngolaryngoscopy to identify the obstructive site(s), chest radiographs, high-kilovolt lateral and anteroposterior neck radiographs, and electrocardiogram (ECG) should be performed. If the high-kilovolt airway radiographs are abnormal, rigid laryngobronchoscopy is recommended to detect any subglottic or tracheobroncheal lesions. Airway management continues with continuous pulse oximetry, apnea monitoring, and selective PSG to objectively evaluate the severity of airway obstruction. A multidisciplinary team approach that consists of cardiology, pulmonary, genetics, and ophthalmologic and plastic surgical consultations is critical to evaluate for disorders involving other organs.

In 1995, the largest retrospective chart review on airway management pediatric PRS patients (n = 90) was carried out at our institution.[10] Isolated PRS patients (group I) made up 30% of all patients, whereas patients with Stickler syndrome (group II), unique pattern of malformation (group III), and named syndromes (group IV) were 35%, 18%, and 17%, respectively. Eighty-eight percent of all PRS patients were managed with conservative measures: 71% with positioning (77.8% of group I, 75% of group II, 62% of group III, 60% of group IV), and 17% with NP airway (18.5% of group I, 21.9% of group II, 20% of group IV). TLA and other glossopexy procedures were not performed. Tracheotomy was performed on 11 patients (12% of all PRS patients): 1 in group I, 1 in group II, 6 in group III, and 3 in group IV patients. All tracheotomized patients failed conservative treatment and had associated airway abnormalities (laryngomalacia, subglottic stenosis, facial dysostosis) or neurologic abnormalities. Duration from tracheotomy to decannulation ranged from 14 months to 5 years (average of 3.1 years). Most PRS patients who responded to conservative airway treatment also tolerated cleft palate nipple feeding (77% of group I, 81.3% of group II, 12.5% of group III, 33.5% of group IV). Others required either gavage feeding, nasogastric tube, or gastrostomy tube placement. The mortality in this series was 2.2%, a lower rate than previously reported by Dykes et al.[11] (19%) and Benjamin and Walker[5] (19.2%). In summary, when grouped PRS patients are considered, group I and II patients faired better in both airway obstruction and feeding difficulties than did group III and IV patients.

Other studies by Sher,[8] Benjamin and Walker,[5] and Perkins et al.[12] shared similar positive results with conservative management. These studies included patients with isolated PRS, Stickler syndrome, named syndromes, and unique pattern of malformation in different proportions, thus it would be difficult to compare their successes with various airway interventions. Sher[8] and Benjamin and Walker[5] reported 38% and 58% of their patients who had favorable responses to positioning and NP airway. Perkins et al.[12] reported that 14 of 50 PRS patients (28%) did not require any airway intervention, whereas 46% of all patients improved with positioning and NP airway. The remaining 13 patients (26%) underwent a variety of surgical procedures (adenotonsillectomy, endotracheal intubation, glossopexy, tracheotomy). Surgically treated patients were those who failed NP airway,[5] required prolonged NP airway,[5,8] or had associated congenital anomalies.[5,8,12] Provided that the airway is secured, the upper airway obstruction should improve with time as a result of mandibular growth.[13] Nevertheless, the unpredictable mandibular growth[5] may cause PRS patients, especially those with associated congenital anomalies, to require prolonged tracheotomies.[12]

When considering surgery, attention must be given to anesthetic management. Rasch et al.[14] recommended preoperative laryngoscopy to determine the severity of upper airway obstruction. Inhalation induction may be safely performed if glottic opening is easily visualized. On the other hand, if glottic visualization is difficult, other anesthetic techniques such as awake oral or nasal intubation, fiberoptic intubation, or elective tracheotomy should be considered. A surgeon experienced in pediatric tracheotomy should be available for possible tracheotomy.

Patients may be discharged home early, provided that their parents are taught NP intubation, suctioning, tracheotomy care, appropriate feeding techniques, cardiopulmonary resuscitation, and the use of apnea monitor and pulse oximetry. Close follow-up management and reevaluation with the otolaryngologist, geneticist, plastic surgeon, ophthalmologist, and other specialists in the craniofacial team are important.

Summary

Retrognathia patients may have isolated PRS or PRS with Stickler syndrome, unique pattern of malformation, or other named syndromes (i.e., Nager, Treacher Collins, VCF, and fetal alcohol syndromes). PRS patients with associated syndromes or malformations tend to have other factors that complicate the upper airway obstruction: skull base anomalies, nasal stenosis, neuromuscular hypotonia, and cardiac and CNS defects. While patients are closely monitored in the NICU, a systematic airway management should include thorough history and physical examination, evaluation of the airway to determine the site(s) of obstruction (i.e., airway radiographs, endoscopy), objective measurement of the severity of obstruction (i.e., PSG), and other associated congenital disorders. In general, isolated PRS and Stickler patients should benefit from conservative airway intervention (positioning, NP airway). Those patients with named syndromes or unique pattern of malformation are at higher risk of more severe obstruction and tracheotomy because of associated airway anomalies or neurologic deficits, or both. Decannulation is expected as the mandibular growth occurs.

REFERENCES

Zalzal and Tran—CHAPTER 74

1. Randall P, Krogman WM, Jahina S. Pierre Robin and the syndrome that bears his name. *Cleft Palate* 1965;2:237–246
2. Olson TS, Kearns DB, Pransky SM, et al. Early home management of patients with Pierre Robin sequence. *Int J Pediatr Otorhinolaryngol* 1990;20:45–49
3. Salmon MA. *Developmental Clefts and Syndromes.* Aylesbury, England: HM Publishers; 1978:42
4. Shprintzen RJ. The implications of the diagnosis of Robin Sequence. *Cleft Palate Craniofac J* 1992;29:205–209
5. Benjamin B, Walker P. Management of airway obstruction in the Pierre Robin sequence. *Int J Pediatr Otorhinolaryngol* 1991;22:29–37
6. Freed G, Pearlman MA, Brown AS, Barot LR. Polysomnographic indications for surgical intervention in Pierre Robin sequence: acute airway management and follow-up studies after repair and take-down of tongue-lip adhesion. *Cleft Palate J* 1988;25:151–155
7. Bull MJ, Givan DC, Sadove AM, et al. Improved outcome in Pierre Robin sequence: effect of multidisciplinary evaluation and management. *Pediatrics* 1990;86:294–301
8. Sher AE. Mechanisms of airway obstruction in Robin sequence: implications for treatment. *Cleft Palate Craniofac J* 1992;29:224–231
9. Myer CM, Reed JM, Cotton RT. Airway management in Pierre Robin sequence. *Otolaryngol Head Neck Surg* 1998; 118:630–635
10. Tomaski SM, Zalzal GH, Saal HM. Airway obstruction in the Pierre Robin sequence. *Laryngoscope* 1995;105:111–114.
11. Dykes EH, Raine PA, Arthur DS, et al. Pierre Robin syndrome and pulmonary hypertension. *J Pediatr Surg* 1985;20: 49–52
12. Perkins JA, Sie KC, Milczuk H. Airway management in children with craniofacial anomalies. *Cleft Palate Craniofac J* 1997;34:135–140
13. Pruzansky S, Richmond JB. Growth of mandible in infants with micrognathia clinical implications. *Am J Dis Child* 1954; 88:29–42
14. Rasch DK, Browder F, Barr M, et al. Anaesthesia for Treacher Collins and Pierre Robin syndromes: a report of three cases. *Can Anaesth Soc J* 1986;33:364–370

Airway Management of the Retrognathic Patient

Eve Bluestein

CHAPTER 75

Retrognathia, or posterior positioning of the mandible relative to the cranial base, is a complex condition that may have various etiologies and effects on patients of all age groups. The range of those affected spans from neonates born with congenital conditions or syndromes to adults who suffer from growth abnormalities, systemic disease, or posttraumatic deformities. The consequences of retrognathia are many and vary in severity from mild aesthetic abnormalities to emergent airway obstruction. Within this range of consequences exist an entire spectrum of effects on the upper airway.

The airway compromise, regardless of the degree, may result in part, entirely, or not at all from the retrognathia itself. Discerning the precise role played by posterior mandibular positioning in a particular case of airway obstruction is both challenging and controversial. Accurate determination of the contribution of the retrognathia to the airway compromise is paramount to appropriate treatment planning. Once the diagnostic challenge is surmounted, even greater controversies and challenges present in determining the optimum short-term and long-term strategies for managing the patient's airway. This paper presents a general approach to airway management in the retrognathic patient (Fig. 75–1).

Background

Understanding the factors that determine mandibular positioning enhances one's ability to identify the retrognathic mandible and its effects on the upper airway. The mandible articulates with the petrous portions of the temporal bones via bilateral temporomandibular joints. The size, location, and orientation of the petrous portions of the temporal bones affect the position of the mandible in both anteroposterior and superoinferior planes of space.[1] The base of the skull, therefore, is the first variable affecting mandibular positioning. From this articulation forward, the size and morphology of the mandibular condyles, rami, bodies, and symphysis determine the size and position of the mandible relative to the cranial base. This size and position have been shown to have important effects on the upper airway[2] via various mechanisms. One such mechanism is that of tongue position. Tongue position is affected by virtue of the space available for the tongue to rest as dictated by mandibular size, and by the genioglossus muscle[3] pull, which is affected by the anteroposterior location of the genial tubercles located on the lingual cortex of the anterior mandible. Other means by which mandibular position affects the upper airway are by various muscle attachments from the mandible to other structures that affect the airway. Most important are the attachments of the genioglossus muscle, the geniohyoid muscle, and the anterior bellies of the digastric muscles.[4]

Discussion

Because mandibular position frequently plays an important role in airway patency,[2,4,5] one should always question the status of the airway in any patient with retrognathia (Fig. 75–1-a). If airway obstruction is not known to be present, the patient should be questioned and examined for signs and symptoms of obstructive sleep apnea (Fig. 75–1-b). If there is a high index of suspicion for some degree of obstruction, further evaluation, such as polysomnography, cardiovascular and pulmonary examinations, and in some cases, laboratory tests and additional studies, is warranted (Fig. 75–1-c).

The first step in managing the airway of the retrognathic patient with known airway compromise is to assess the severity and urgency of the obstruction (Fig. 75–1-d). Historically, retrognathia in association with emergent airway compromise has been necessarily addressed in neonates and infants born with syndromes associated with posterior positioning of the mandible and/or micrognathia.[6,7] Such congenital conditions include, but are not limited to, Pierre Robin sequence, Treacher Collins syndrome, Goldenhar syndrome, and isolated first and second branchial arch syndromes.[8,9] It is in this subset of congenitally affected patients that emergent airway obstruction secondary to retrognathia, either isolated or in combination with cranial base and/or soft tissue abnormalities, is most likely to be seen.

In the case of emergent airway obstruction, endotracheal intubation should be attempted (Fig. 75–1-e). The next step in management would be either elective (if intubated) or emergent surgical establishment of the airway via either a tracheostomy or cricothyroidotomy (Fig. 75–1-f), the specific method being dependent upon the age of the patient, the operator's skills, and the anticipated length of time the surgical airway will be needed.

Cases of known nonemergent airway obstruction in the retrognathic patient may be encountered in the aforementioned patient population, as well as in patients with obstructive sleep apnea, systemic diseases such as rheumatoid arthritis, temporomandibular joint pathology, and traumatic injuries. Among these patients, those who most frequently suffer from airway compromise associated with retrognathia are infants and patients with obstructive sleep apnea.

Multiple methods of stabilizing the airway have been advocated in the presence of nonemergent airway compromise. A spectrum of such interventions has included prone or lateral positioning, placement of nasopharyngeal airways, continuous positive airway pressure (CPAP), intubation, and tracheostomy[4,10] (Fig 75–1-g).

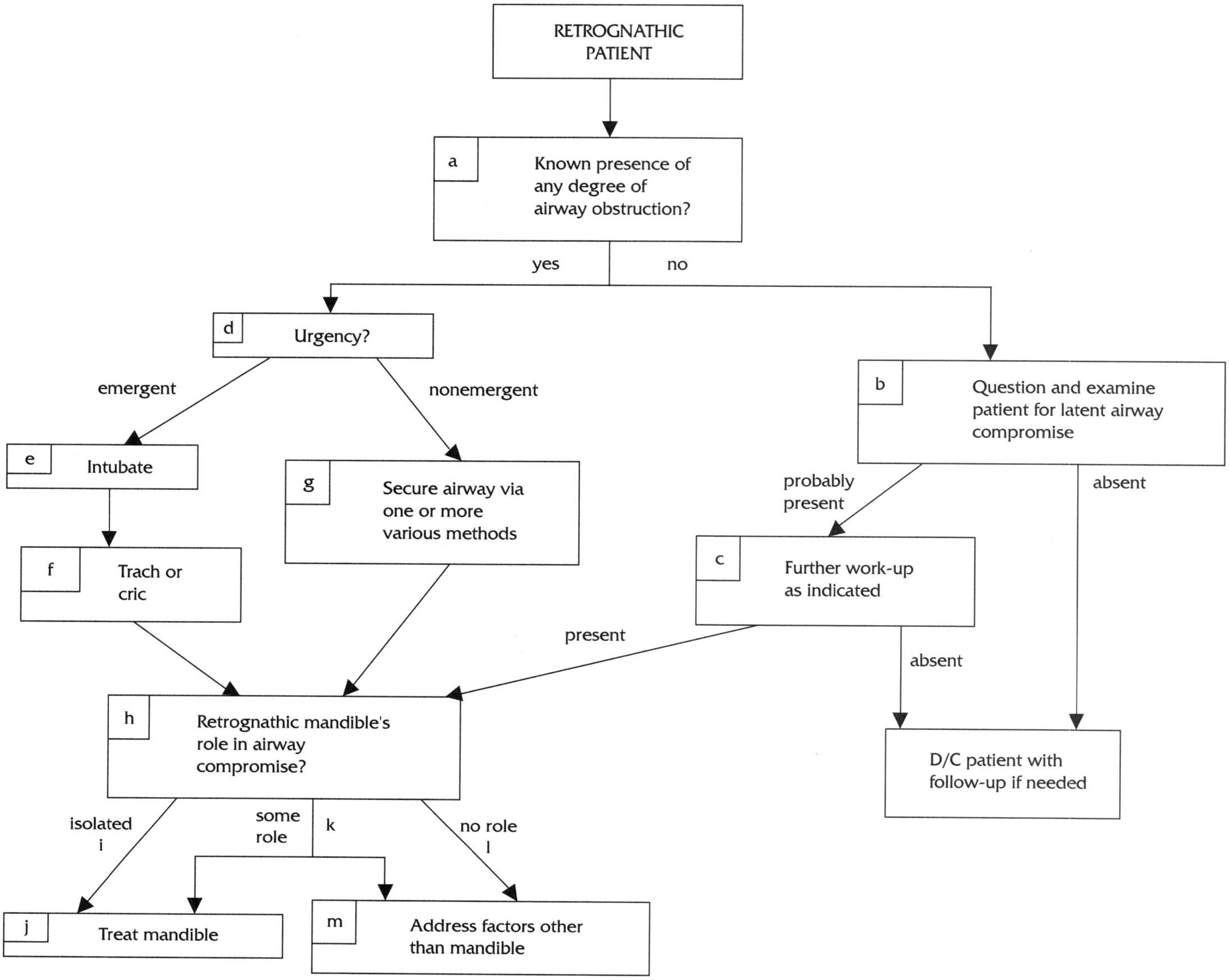

Figure 75–1 General approach to airway management in the retrognathic patient.

Once the airway is secure, the practitioner must assess the precise role that the mandibular retrognathia plays in the airway obstruction (Fig. 75–1-h). Airway patency is affected by many variables in addition to mandibular position, including skull base positioning, soft tissue location and quantity, submucosal tissue composition, and neurologic tone.[3,5] As with any medical condition, it is important to accurately identify the etiology of the problem so that appropriately directed therapy may be instituted.

Sher[3] utilized flexible fiberoptic nasopharyngoscopy in patients with craniofacial anomalies and obstructive sleep apnea, and identified four different mechanisms of airway obstruction. These four types of airway obstruction provide a framework that may be used to aid in the identification of the mandible's role in airway compromise, and thus, subsequent treatment planning.

Sher's type I airway obstruction consists of posterior movement of the tongue such that anteroposterior obstruction occurs by the dorsal aspect of the tongue contacting the posterior pharyngeal wall. It is in this type of obstruction that retrognathia may play the largest isolated role (Fig. 75–1-i). Directing treatment toward the mandible in these patients may yield excellent results.

Many options exist for managing the mandible, the specific details of which are beyond the scope of this chapter. Some options, however, include the use of mandibular positioning devices,[11] orthodontic/orthopedic forces, glossopexy, genial tubercle advancement, genioplasty, bilateral sagittal split osteotomy, distraction osteogenesis, and maxillomandibular advancement.[10-13] (Fig. 75–1-j). The decision as to which specific treatment modality to employ is dependent on many factors, including the severity of the airway obstruction; the remaining mandibular growth potential; the presence or absence of teeth; and the occlusion, if applicable; facial aesthetics; and the presence or absence and degree of facial asymmetry.

Retrognathia and the resulting posterior tongue positioning may also play an influential role in type II airway obstruction. In this type of obstruction, the tongue moves posteriorly, but instead of contacting the posterior pharyngeal wall itself, as in type I obstruction, it pushes the soft palate against the posterior pharyngeal wall.[3] Thus, retrognathia may contribute to the obstruction in these patients, but the position of the velum must be addressed as well (Fig. 75–1-k). Maxillomandibular surgery may be an excellent treatment modality for these patients if an abnormal angle of the cranial base exists.[5]

In type III obstruction, the lateral pharyngeal walls move medially causing them to appose one another. Finally, in type IV obstruction, pharyngeal constriction occurs in a circular or sphincteric manner. The tongue does not contact the posterior pharyngeal wall in either of these types of obstruction. While retrognathia may play a small role in airway obstruction in patients with type III and IV obstruction, it is not a major contributing factor in the obstruction, unlike in types I and II[3] (Fig. 75–1-l). Therefore, airway management in the patient with retrognathia and types III or IV airway obstruction should not focus on treating the retrognathia (Fig. 75–1-m).

Summary

Retrognathia is seen in many different patient populations. The mandible's position has a range of effects on the upper airway in terms of its role in airway compromise as well as in the resulting severity of obstruction. As such, one should have a high degree of suspicion for apparent or subtle airway obstruction when evaluating a patient with retrognathia. Varying degrees of airway compromise may result from retrognathia itself, or from the effects of the posteriorly positioned mandible in combination with other factors. In the presence of any degree of airway compromise and concomitant retrognathia, the etiology of the airway compromise must be determined, and the precise role of the mandible defined. In some patients, the retrognathia may be found to be incidental; in this patient population, addressing the mandible as the source of the airway obstruction will prove futile. However, retrognathia will represent a significant component of upper airway compromise for many other patients. These patients may benefit greatly by various interventions directed at treating the retrognathic mandible.

REFERENCES

Bluestein—CHAPTER 75

1. Peterson LJ, Indresano AT, Marciani RD, Roser SM. *Principles of Oral and Maxillofacial Surgery.* Philadelphia: JB Lippincott; 1992:1228
2. Bacon WH, Turlot JC, Krieger J, et al. Cephalometric evaluation of pharyngeal obstructive factors in patients with sleep apnea syndrome. *Angle Orthod* 1989;60:115–121
3. Sher AE. Mechanisms of airway obstruction in Robin Sequence: implications for treatment. *Cleft Palate Craniofac J* 1992;29: 224–231
4. Guyette RF, Waite PD. *Oral and Maxillofacial Surgery Clinics.* Vol 7. Philadelphia: WB Saunders; 1995:301–310
5. Waite PD, Shettar SM. *Oral and Maxillofacial Surgery Clinics.* Vol 7. Philadelphia: WB Saunders; 1995:327–336
6. Augarten A, Sagy M, Yahav J, Barzilay Z. Management of upper airway obstruction in the Pierre Robin syndrome. *Br J Oral Maxillofac Surg* 1990;28:105–108
7. Tomaski SM, Zalzal GH, Saal HM. Airway obstruction in the Pierre Robin sequence. *Laryngoscope* 1995;105:111–114
8. Neville BW, Damm DD, Allen CM, Bouquot JE. Developmental defects of the oral and maxillofacial region. In: Neville BW et al. *Oral Maxillofacial Pathology.* Philadelphia: WB Saunders; 1995:34–40
9. Gorlin RJ, Cohen MM, Levin LS. Syndromes of the head and neck. 3rd Ed. New York: Oxford University Press; 1990
10. Myer CM III, Reed JM, Cotton RT, et al. Airway management in Pierre Robin sequence. *Otolaryngol Head Neck Surg* 1998;118:630–635
11. Frohberg U, Lange R. Surgical treatment of Robin sequence and sleep apnea syndrome: case report and review of the literature. *J Oral Maxillofac Surg* 1993;51:1274–1277
12. Peterson LJ, Indresano AT, Marciani RD, Roser SM. *Principles of Oral and Maxillofacial Surgery.* Philadelphia: JB Lippincott; 1992:1539–1546
13. Easter B, Wood C, Eppley BL, Sadove AM. Mandibular traction system for adjunctive management of airway insufficiency in infants with Pierre Robin malformation sequence. *Am J Occup Ther* 1991;45:941–943

26

Otitis Media: To Treat or Not to Treat

"The first objective in the effective management of otitis media is not whether or when to treat, but to accept that this is a disorder that is still badly diagnosed and that adequate diagnosis is the keystone to adequate management."

Robin T. Cotton

"Otitis media is a multifactorial disease process involving immunology, infectious disease, anatomic considerations, social and socioeconomic issues, and genetics, among other factors. Before physicians can attain a clear understanding of otitis media, a clear universally accepted classification system will need to be developed."

Brian J. Wiatrak

"Even though most patients will improve spontaneously without the benefit of an antimicrobial agent, the clinician cannot determine at the onset of the infection who will and will not be at risk of developing these complications. Thus, all patients require treatment."

Charles D. Bluestone

Otitis Media: To Treat or Not to Treat

CHAPTER 76

Michael J. Rutter and Robin T. Cotton

There have been few true advances in the treatment of otitis media since Armstrong's reintroduction of the tympanostomy tube in 1954.[1] Management decisions have revolved around three primary options: not to treat, to use antibiotics, or to recommend tympanostomy tubes. Other modalities have been suggested, some shown to be of little benefit (decongestants, antihistamines),[2] and others to have a limited degree of efficacy (Xylitol gum, Otovent balloons, steroids).[3-7] However, with the millenium, there is the promise of new treatment options (laser myringotomy, vaccination), coexistent with the rapid proliferation of drug resistant *Streptococcus pneumoniae.*

Otitis media management has always been dogged by controversy. Any disorder in the United States alone that is estimated to cost $5 billion year,[8] yet for which the benefits of intervention are often not evidence-based, is bound to generate controversy. It remains the commonest cause for visits to the doctor in the pediatric population (24.5 million visits/year in the United States), generating the largest number of antibiotic prescriptions (23.6 million).[9]

Otitis media research also has the potential to confuse and confound as much as it contributes to our knowledge. There are three main reasons for this. First, clinical research has to deal with so many coexistent factors (e.g., season, age, child care, upper respiratory tract infections [UTI]) that significance tends to be diluted, unless very large numbers are involved. Second, much research deals with surrogate outcomes (effusion resolution for example), while long-term true outcomes (e.g., IQ, employment status) are much harder to come by. Meta-analysis is particularly amiss when it comes to grouping subtly disparate studies. Finally, we are overwhelmed by definitions, and what seems very obvious is not always so. For example, Hayden[10] illustrated this nicely when he surveyed 165 pediatricians, who had 147 different definitions for acute otitis media.

Background

References to the treatment of otitis media date back to Hippocrates. Myringotomy as a treatment was in vogue in the eighteenth and nineteenth centuries before its resurgence in the present day.[11] The primary concern during the preantibiotic era was the potential for intracranial complications of acute otitis media.[12] Historically, this was a significant cause of mortality; 70 years later, mortality from ear disease is so rare as to be occasionally—and regrettably—forgotten in the multitude of treatment paradigms available.

The current emphasis is more on otitis media with effusion (of the persistent or chronic variety) and on its long-term consequences. There is a general common sense consensus that long-term untreated otitis media with effusion is an undesirable state, but it has been remarkably hard for this to be proved conclusively. There is indirect evidence to back this view,[13-16] as well as the usual contrary opinion.[17] This is not an area suited to randomized double-blind controlled study, as nontreatment or placebo control cannot be justified in the management of long standing OME.

Acute Otitis Media

Acute otitis media (AOM) is a disorder that lacks a well-accepted universal definition. This problem significantly compromises the comparability of many studies. However, a purulent middle ear effusion with systemic signs of illness (e.g., pain, fever) is a useful yardstick. Systemic signs of illness, such as fever, with the presence of a middle ear effusion (which may be incidental), is not sufficient to necessarily warrant the diagnosis of AOM. Similarly, a not-infrequent incidental finding is of a cloudy or purulent effusion in an otherwise symptomless child—also not enough to warrant a label of AOM. AOM is not always an easy diagnosis to make (or refute!) which may partly explain why it is one of the most overdiagnosed conditions in pediatric practice.

AOM may be further subdivided into simple AOM, AOM with complications, resistant or prolonged AOM, recurrent AOM, or recurrent AOM with a background of otitis media with effusion (OME). It is prudent not to lump these many categories together when arguing the pros and cons of treating, or not treating, AOM. In this context, treatment implies antibiotics, though in a symptomatic child acetaminophen may be an equally and certainly more rapidly effective intervention.

Although rare, AOM does have serious complications, and otolaryngologists are more likely to have exposure to a few a year, as opposed to a few in a practicing lifetime. Untreated or partially treated AOM may result in facial nerve palsy, meningitis, mastoiditis, petrositis, labyrinthitis, sigmoid sinus thrombosis, and extradural, subdural, or cerebral abscesses. No one will argue the need to treat aggressively under these circumstances. The dilemma is that the incidence of these complications has plummeted, coincident—but surely not coincidental—with the onset of the antibiotics era. Currently, a body of opinion holds that we are over-using antibiotics and that we should not necessarily treat AOM. If so, are we on the threshold of returning to the era of the midnight cortical mastoid? Probably not. There is a body of mainly European literature on the nonantibiotic treatment of AOM.[18-20] For the most part, complication risks are low and may often be intercepted. Similarly, the incidence of antibiotic use in AOM varies widely, from 98% in Australasia and the United States, to 31% in the Netherlands, with no discernable difference in the incidence of complications.[21]

There are two goals in treatment: the prevention of complications, and alleviation of symptoms. Symptomatically at 24 hours 60% of children are pain free whether on antibiotic or placebo, although antibiotics have a small symptomatic advantage at 1 week, and help prevent contralateral AOM.[22] The high natural resolution rate of AOM is the primary argument for the nonantibiotic treatment of AOM. But as the complications may have profound consequences, who and when should we treat? There is no black-and-white answer to this but, in general, consensus opinion has it that a child who is symptomatic warrants antibiotic treatment. So when not to treat? It is reasonably common to observe a child who has been symptomatic but who arrives in your office totally asymptomatic despite a purulent effusion. It is implicit that the child should be closely monitored and timely intervention initiated if there is any deterioration.

The social setting of the child must also play a role in decision-making. An increasing number of families are now reliant on two working parents, often without an extended family for child care support. Day care for even the very young is now commonplace and is a significant risk factor for the onset of AOM,[23] with a much higher incidence of resistant organisms than in the rest of the community. Most child care facilities will not tolerate a sick child, necessitating that a parent take time off from work. This problem increases the pressure to treat. Even a small advantage with antibiotics may be of significance to a working parent.

How long to treat? Recent articles suggest that 5 days of antibiotics is sufficient in the treatment of simple AOM in a child over 2 years, and that 10 days is prudent in a child under age 2.[24] The minimum effective course is the aim both in terms of this environment of increasing antibiotic resistance, and because antibiotics treatment is not necessarily benign.[9,22]

Recurrent AOM may be treated on an episode-to-episode basis, with the expectation that, as the eustachian tube matures, the tendency to AOM will steadily reduce. However, many cases warrant further intervention, whether by prophylactic antibiotics or by tympanostomy tubes. Both are designed to buy time while the eustachian tube matures. The use of prophylactic antibiotics, whether for AOM or any other condition, is a very contentious area especially when viewed in the light of increasing antibiotic resistance.[25-27] A meta-analysis of nine papers by Williams et al.[28] suggests a small benefit compared with placebo, particularly in children with multiple episodes of AOM. However, nine children needed treatment to benefit one. There is also evidence that if breakthrough AOM occurs while on prophylaxis, there is a much higher incidence of resistant organism recovery. Meanwhile, tympanostomy tubes usually require a general anesthetic and may be associated with discharging ears, or infrequently with a persistent perforation of the tympanic membrane. They are particularly appropriate in the very young, as recurrent AOM in children younger than 1 year of age significantly predisposes to ongoing AOM and OME problems for the next 6 or 7 years.[29]

The role of tympanocentesis remains an area of controversy. It is not a common procedure in the United States, unlike parts of Europe. The advantages of tympanocentesis are the confirmation of the diagnosis of otitis media and provision of a middle ear specimen to culture.[30] It does not significantly aerate the middle ear, and in most circumstances, even with a myringotomy, the puncture site closes within hours to days. Opponents of the widespread use of tympanocentesis are concerned that there may be damage to other structures in the middle ear space (i.e., the ossicular chain, oval window, dehiscent jugular bulb, aberrant carotid artery). The reported incidence of such complications is very low, although there is potential for a reporting bias. It would seem reasonable that anyone who is suitably trained and who appreciates the anatomy could perform this procedure (which in some respects is comparable to a lumbar puncture). If the anatomy is unclear, the physician should know when to refer. When is tympanocentesis appropriate? In the research setting, in neonates, in the immunocompromised, when there is strong need for a microbiologic diagnosis and sensitivities, and in severe, persistent, or prolonged AOM.

Otitis Media with Effusion

Although, strictly speaking, AOM is a subset of OME, by implication OME describes a nonacutely infected middle ear effusion. Chronic OME is defined as an effusion persisting for more than 3 months' duration, and is a rather limiting term—perhaps a better description is persistent OME. Synonyms include serous otitis, secretory otitis, glue ear, and middle ear catarrh. Unlike AOM, OME is probably underdiagnosed and may present a diagnostic challenge, especially if otoscopy alone is used. Pneumatic otoscopy, especially if complimented by tympanometry, is sensitive in experienced hands. The natural history of this disorder is for spontaneous resolution in the majority of cases—more than 80% resolution by 2 months.[31] It is the small number of children who continue to have effusions after 2 or 3 months that are of concern. An even smaller percentage will have an underlying predisposing pathology, such as Down syndrome, cleft palate, immunoglobulin deficiency, or ciliary dyskinesia.

Although balance and behavioral changes are not uncommon with OME, it is the compromise to hearing that is of greatest concern. In a small percentage of children, chronic middle ear effusions may have a role in the development of retraction pockets, ossicular erosion, and cholesteatoma formation. However, these are more likely consequences of chronic eustachian tube dysfunction (which predisposed to the effusion) than the effusion per se. A dense effusion typically may confer up to a 30-db hearing loss, which represents a significant barrier to learning. It is unknown for what duration an effusion must be present, and at what ages, to be of long-term consequence. It may well be that an effusion acts as a cofactor with other influences such as young age, low socioeconomic status, or poor teacher-to-child ratios, and that these factors act synergistically. The literature is highly suggestive that prolonged effusions are of long-term significance.[13-16]

Until recently, it was believed that for OME to be of concern, it had to be bilateral, and that there had to be at least a

15-dB hearing loss (pure-tone average) to possibly affect education.[32] In fact, the Agency for Health Care Policy and Research (AHCPR) guidelines in 1994 recommended that a 20-db threshold or worse be present in the better hearing ear before the placement of tympanostomy tubes.[33] There is now evidence that binaural hearing is advantageous and that children with normal pure-tone thresholds despite bilateral effusions may, in fact, still be hearing impaired. In a small but elegant study, Rosenfeld et al.[34] looked at children with bilateral effusions and normal pure tone averages, who were then tested with sound field audiology with and without background noise. These investigators found that word recognition was slightly compromised at normal (50-db) conversational levels and markedly compromised at soft (35-db) conversational levels, and that with background noise, there was a marked further deterioration (as poor as 38% word recognition at 35 db with background noise). More impressively, after tympanostomy tube insertion, there was a marked improvement in word recognition. Sadly, sound-field audiology is usually practical only after the age of 4, whereas the population presumed most at risk are those even younger.

Two recent meta-analyses have come to a similar conclusion, namely that antibiotics have a small but distinct advantage over placebo in the treatment of persistent OME.[28,35] It is notable that with the same premise, these two articles did not examine exactly the same set of studies, and their conclusions were not identical. Interestingly they appeared shortly after another attempted meta-analysis on the same topic was abandoned as being an area inappropriate for meta-analysis.[36] There is, however, no conclusive evidence in these or any other article that one antibiotic has a distinct therapeutic advantage over any other. This is in part due to the "Pollyanna" effect, namely that in a spontaneously resolving condition in which antibiotics have only a comparatively small influence on outcome, extremely large numbers are required to show an advantage of one product over another, with the corollary being that a new product can easily be shown to be as good (or statistically no worse) as any other, particularly if the power is low.[37] Similarly, there is little good evidence in the literature that any one duration of treatment offers an advantage over another, though there is a trend toward a longer duration of antibiotic treatment being more efficacious.[28] The advantage of antibiotics relates only to the short-term resolution of OME, with the effects progressively diluted out by remission and spontaneous resolution the longer a study population is followed.

In children presenting with OME of presumed short duration, and who have otherwise normal otoscopic findings, antibiotic therapy is not required. Just when antibiotic therapy is required is debated, but Bluestone's 2-month recommendation is reasonable.[38] The exceptions are adults, who do not tolerate effusions at all well, and are usually insistent on intervention at a much earlier interval. This does not mean that children necessarily have fewer symptoms, but rather that they cannot express or represent themselves as effectively. The ideal duration of an antibiotic course remains unclear, but most recommendations are between 10 days and 4 weeks.

The antibiotic to use in first-line treatment of OME or AOM is hotly debated currently. There is little direct evidence to show that one has a distinct advantage over another, so it is logical to choose an agent that is tried and true, achieves good middle ear concentrations, has reasonable activity against a significant percentage of potential middle ear pathogens, is well tolerated, tastes good, has a convenient dosing schedule, is reasonably stable, and is not too ludicrously priced. Currently, Amoxil and trimethoprim/sulfamethoxazole best fit these criteria, with a variety of second-line agents. Amoxil has had an additional resurgence with the increasing percentage of *Streptococcus pneumoniae* that are multiply drug resistant, as many are intermediately sensitive to high-dose Amoxil. Current guidelines suggest that initial treatment (especially in AOM) with Amoxil at up to 90 mg/kg/day in two divided doses is efficacious against most resistant *S. pneumoniae*.[39,40]

If antibiotic therapy is not effective, the usual options are to observe, to continue the current course, to change antibiotics, or to consider tympanostomy tubes. The first three options are all probably of similar efficacy, although definitive data are lacking. There is, however, a vast experience with tubes accrued over the last 45 years, with nearly one million sets of tubes placed each year in the United States alone. This is the commonest operation in the world, one of the safest, and one of the most effective. The complications are well known, with ear discharge and residual perforation being the most significant. There are a plethora of different tubes from which to select, with virtually all balancing length of duration against residual perforation rate.

The other common intervention is adenoidectomy with or without tube insertion. There is little doubt that adenoidectomy is an effective therapy,[41-44] probably as a result of ridding the nasopharynx of a chronic focus of infection (rather than the size of the adenoid obstructing the eustachian tube). In a proportion of children however, the size of the adenoid is also of significance.[45] However, adenoidectomy is a much more invasive operation than tube insertion, with significant risks in children younger than 3 years of age that usually outweigh its benefit. Less than 20% of children receiving a first set of tubes will ever have recurrent problems of a magnitude to justify a second set. Bluestone et al.[46] again provide sage advice when recommending that adenoidectomy be a consideration in the child older than 3 years of age at the time of insertion of a second set of tubes. Adenoidectomy in this population probably reduces by one-half the requirement of ultimately placing a third set of tubes.

Several other treatment options are available, most aimed at restoring the function of the eustachian tube by reducing edema at the tube orifice. Systemic antihistamines and decongestants have not proved beneficial,[2] and topical decongestants and topical steroids, although having considerable theoretical appeal, so far have little evidence of efficacy. Systemic steroids, in combination with antibiotics, do appear to be effective, but the studies performed to date have been small enough that even meta-analysis still leaves wide confidence intervals that include 0.[7] There are also some theoretical risks (lessening with the arrival of the varicella vaccine), such that systemic steroids should not be considered a routine therapy, but rather be reserved for selected patients on a case-by-case basis.

The most intriguing new player is the Otolam (laser assisted myringotomy), a recently introduced flashscan laser that delivers a very precise spiral of laser energy in around one-fifth of 1 second. The depth and circumference of the burn can be preselected. In fact laser myringotomy is not at all new,[47] although the technology and, more importantly, the anesthetic and marketing techniques are. The use of 16% tetracaine topically is most impressive although it may take up to 45 min to have its full effect. The attraction of the laser is that the resultant myringotomy heals in around 3 weeks, as opposed to months for a tube, or hours to days for a standard myringotomy. The tetracaine and the speed and precision of the burn allow this to be performed in the office even in infants. The most obvious candidates for such technology are patients in whom a temporary myringotomy will suffice, with OME (for which 3 weeks will allow the Eustachian tube to recover, i.e., break the disease cycle) being the most obvious example. Other applications include persistent or severe AOM, hyperbaric oxygen candidates, as a bloodless method of tympanocentesis, or as a bloodless port for telescopic examination of the middle ear cleft. Tubes can obviously be inserted at the same time if desired. The initial results with the laser have been a 70% cure rate, with cure constituting a healed tympanic membrane with no effusion.[48] However, this is a most expensive tool, and the economics to justify its existence have not yet been investigated. In fact, the science to justify its use, although in progress, also remains to be seen.

The next goal on the horizon is the development of an effective otitis media vaccine, aimed mainly at *S. pneumoniae*, a project into which considerable effort is being poured, although there are still very significant hurdles to overcome.[49]

Summary

The first objective in the effective management of otitis media is not whether or when to treat, but to accept that this is a disorder that is still badly diagnosed and that adequate diagnosis is the keystone to adequate management. Even as simple a step as the routine use of the pneumatic otoscopy would be a major advance. The significant recent change in management results from the increasing prevalence of drug resistant *S. pneumoniae*, and the realization that we have brought this upon ourselves from inappropriate overuse of antibiotics.[40,50,51] However, we still have the opportunity to reverse the trend, should we have the fortitude.[52] It is important to remember that more than 50% of antibiotics used in the pediatric population in the United States is for the treatment of otitis media.[53] If we do not take on board that restrictions in antibiotic utilization are required, the trend will not be reversed.

What is encouraging in this endeavor is that limiting antibiotics usage will not alter the clinical outcome for most of our patients. Accurate diagnosis of AOM, and a higher threshold for the use of prophylactic antibiotics with recurrent AOM, are achievable aims. Limiting initial antibiotic exposure in OME is also essential. To quote Rosenfeld, "Children with OME fall into two groups—those who get better in a few months no matter what treatment they receive, and those who don't."[54]

REFERENCES

Rutter and Cotton—CHAPTER 76

1. Armstrong BW. A new treatment for chronic secretory otitis media. *Arch Otolaryngol* 1954;59:653–654
2. Mandel EM, Rockette HE, Bluestone CD, et al. Efficacy of amoxicillin with and without decongestant-antihistamine for otitis media with effusion in children. Results of a double-blind, randomized trial. *N Engl J Med* 1987;316:432–437
3. Uhari M, Kontiokari T, Koskela M, Niemela M. Xylitol chewing gum in prevention of acute otitis media: double blind randomised trial. *BMJ* 1996;313:1180–1184
4. Uhari M, Kontiokari T, Niemela M. A novel use of xylitol sugar in preventing acute otitis media. *Pediatrics* 1998;102 (4 Pt 1):879–884
5. Blanshard JD, Maw AR, Bawden R. Conservative treatment of otitis media with effusion by autoinflation of the middle ear. *Clin Otolaryngol Allied Sci* 1993;18:188–192
6. Stangerup SE, Sederberg-Olsen J, Balle VH. Treatment with the Otovent device in tubal dysfunction and secretory otitis media in children. [In Danish.] *Ugeskrift Laeger* 1991;153:3008–3009
7. Rosenfeld RM. New concepts for steroid use in otitis media with effusion. *Clin Pediatr* 1992;31:615–621
8. Gates GA. Cost-effectiveness considerations in otitis media treatment. *Otolaryngol Head Neck Surg* 1996;114:525–530
9. Ruben RJ. Sequelae of antibiotic therapy for acute otitis media and otitis media with effusion. In: Lim DJ, et al., ed. *Sixth International Symposium on Recent Advances in Otitis Media.* Fort Lauderdale, FL: BC Decker; 1995:369–373
10. Hayden GF. Acute suppurative otitis media in children: diversity of clinical diagnostic criteria. *Clin Pediatr* 1981;20:99–104
11. Weir N. *Otolaryngology: An Illustrated History.* 1st Ed. London: Butterworths; 1990
12. Rudberg R. Sulfonamide and penecillin in acute otitis media. *Acta Otolaryngol (Stockh)* 1954;44(suppl):45–65
13. Ruben RJ, Wallace IF, Gravel J. Long-term communication deficiencies in children with otitis media during their first year of life. *Acta Otolaryngol (Stockh)* 1997;117:206–207
14. Stewart IA, Silva PA, Williams S. Relationships of otitis media with effusion in early childhood to educational and behavioural disadvantage during the teenage years. In: Lim DJ, et al., ed. *Sixth International Symposium on Recent Advances in Otitis Media.* Fort Lauderdale, FL: BC Decker; 1995:337–339
15. Teele DW, Klein JO, Chase C, et al. Otitis media in infancy and intellectual ability, school achievement, speech, and language at age 7 years. Greater Boston Otitis Media Study Group. *J Infect Dis* 1990;162:685–694

16. Teele DW. Long-term sequelae of otitis media: fact or fantasy? *Pediatr Infect Dis J* 1994;13:1069–1073
17. Roberts JE, Burchinal MR, Clarke-Klein SM. Otitis media in early childhood and cognitive, academic, and behavior outcomes at 12 years of age. *J Pediatr Psychol* 1995;20:645–660
18. van Buchem FL, Peeters MF, van't Hof MA. Acute otitis media: a new treatment strategy. *BMJ* 1985;290:1033–1037
19. Van Buchem FL. Antibiotics for otitis media [letter]. *J R Coll Gen Pract* 1987;37:367
20. Claessen JQ, Appelman CL, Touw-Otten FW, et al. A review of clinical trials regarding treatment of acute otitis media. *Clin Otolaryngol Allied Sci* 1992;17:251–257
21. Froom J, Culpepper L, Grob P, et al. Diagnosis and antibiotic treatment of acute otitis media: report from International Primary Care Network. *BMJ* 1990;300:582–586
22. Del Mar C, Glasziou P, Hayem M. Are antibiotics indicated as initial treatment for children with acute otitis media? A meta-analysis. *BMJ* 1997;314:1526–1529
23. Froom J, Culpepper L. Otitis media in day-care children. A report from the International Primary Care Network. *J Fam Pract* 1991;32:289–294
24. Kozyrskyj AL, Hildes-Ripstein GE, Longstaffe SE, et al. Treatment of acute otitis media with a shortened course of antibiotics: a meta-analysis. *JAMA* 1998;279:1736–1742
25. Klein JO. Preventing recurrent otitis: what role for antibiotics? *Contemp Pediatr* 1994;11:44–60
26. Paradise JL. Managing otitis media: a time for change. *Pediatrics* 1995;96(4 Pt 1):712–715
27. Roark R, Berman S. Continuous twice daily or once daily amoxicillin prophylaxis compared with placebo for children with recurrent acute otitis media. *Pediatr Infect Dis J* 1997;16:376–381
28. Williams RC, Stange KC, Chalmers FT, Bowlin SJ. Use of antibiotics in preventing recurrent acute otitis media and in treating otitis media with effusion. A meta-analytic attempt to resolve the brouhaha. *JAMA* 1993;270:1344–1351
29. Ryding MK, Kalm O, Prellner K. Sequelae of recurrent acute otitis media. Ten-year follow-up of a prospectively studied cohort of children. *Acta Paediatr* 1997;86:1208–1213
30. Hoberman AP, Wald ER. Tympanocentesis technique revisited. *Pediatr Infect Dis J* 1997;16:S25–26
31. Teele DW, Klein JO, Rosner BA. Epidemiology of otitis media in children. *Ann Otol Rhinol Laryngol* 1980;89(3 Pt 2)(suppl):5–6
32. Bachmann KRA. Early identification and intervention for children who are hearing impaired. *Pediatr Rev* 1998;19:155–165
33. Managing otitis media with effusion in young children. Agency for Health Care Policy and Research. *Clin Pract Guidel Quick Ref Guide Clin* 1994;12:1–13
34. Rosenfeld RM, Madell JR, McMahon A. Auditory function in normal-hearing children with middle ear effusion. In: Lim DJ, et al., ed. *Sixth International Symposium on Recent Advances in Otitis Media.* Fort Lauderdale, FL: BC Decker; 1995:354–356
35. Rosenfeld RM, Post JC. Meta-analysis of antibiotics for the treatment of otitis media with effusion. *Otolaryngol Head Neck Surg* 1992;106:378–386
36. Bodner EE, Browning GG, Chalmers FT, Chalmers TC. Can meta-analysis help uncertainty in surgery for otitis media in children. *J Laryngol Otol* 1991;105:812–819
37. Marchant CD, Carlin SA, Johnson CE, Shurin PA. Measuring the comparative efficacy of antibacterial agents for acute otitis media: the "Pollyanna phenomenon." *J Pediatr* 1992;120:72–77
38. Bluestone CD. Modern management of otitis media. *Pediatr Clin North Am* 1989;36:1371–1387
39. Otitis Media Guideline Committee. Evidence based clinical practice guideline for otitis media in children under 6 years of age. In: Health Policy and Clinical Effectiveness Clinical Practice Guidelines, Children's Hospital Medical Center, Cincinnati, March 1999
40. Dowell SF, Giebink GS, et al. Acute otitis media: management and surveillance in an era of pneumoccocal resistance—a report from the drug-resistant *Streptoccocus pneumoniae.* Therapeutic Working Group. *Pediatr Infect Dis J* 1999;18:1–9
41. Gates GA, Muntz HR, Gaylis B. Adenoidectomy and otitis media. *Ann Otol Rhinol Laryngol* 1992;155(suppl):24–32
42. Gates GA. Adenoidectomy for otitis media with effusion. *Ann Otol Rhinol Laryngol* 1994;163(suppl):54–58
43. Maw AR, Bawden R. Does adenoidectomy have an adjuvant effect on ventilation tube insertion and thus reduce the need for re-treatment? *Clin Otolaryngol Allied Sci* 1994;19:340–343
44. Paradise JL, Bluestone CD, Rogers KD, et al. Efficacy of adenoidectomy for recurrent otitis media in children previously treated with tympanostomy-tube placement. Results of parallel randomized and nonrandomized trials. *JAMA* 1990;263:2066–2073
45. Sade J, Luntz M. Adenoidectomy in otitis media. A review. *Ann Otol Rhinol Laryngol* 1991;100:226–231
46. Bluestone CD, Gates GA, Paradise JL, Stool SE. Controversy over tubes and adenoidectomy. *Pediatr Infect Dis J* 1988;7(11 suppl):S146–S149
47. Goode RL. CO_2 laser myringotomy. *Laryngoscope* 1982;92:420–423
48. Siegel G, Brodsky L, Waner M, Shaha S. Office-based laser assisted tympanic membrane fenestration in adults and children: pilot data to support an alternative to traditional approaches to otitis media. *Int J Otorhinolaryngol* 2000;53(2):111–120
49. Giebink GS. Vaccination against middle-ear bacterial and viral pathogens. *Ann NY Acad Sci* 1997;830:330–352
50. Arason VA, Kristinsson KG, Sigurdsson JA, et al. Do antimicrobials increase the carriage rate of penicillin resistant pneumococci in children? Cross sectional prevalence study. *BMJ* 1996;313:387–391
51. Dowell SF, Schwartz B. Resistant pneumococci: protecting patients through judicious use of antibiotics. *Am Fam Physician* 1997;55:1647–1654, 1657–1658
52. Boken DJ, Chartrand SA, Goering RV, et al. Colonization with penicillin-resistant *Streptococcus pneumoniae* in a child-care center. *Pediatr Infect Dis J* 1995;14:879–884
53. McCaig LF, Hughes JM. Trends in antimicrobial drug prescribing among office-based physicians in the United States. [published erratum appears in *JAMA* 1998;279:434]. *JAMA* 1995;273:214–219
54. Rosenfeld RM. Amusing parents while nature cures otitis media with effusion. *Int J Pediatr Otorhinolaryngol* 1998;43:189–192

Otitis Media: To Treat or Not to Treat

CHAPTER 77

Brian J. Wiatrak

Otitis media is one of the most common ailments of childhood and is the most common complaint that brings a child to the health care provider.[1] Approximately 70% of children below the age of 3 will develop an episode of otitis media[2] and by the age of 7 years, 65 to 95% of children will experience one or more episodes of acute otitis media. Approximately $3.5 billion per year is spent on the management of otitis media in the United States.[3] A large portion of this is spent on antimicrobial therapy. With such a significant impact on our health care system, it is not surprising that numerous controversies exist regarding the medical and surgical management of otitis media.

It is apparent from review of the literature regarding otitis media that a clear, descriptive classification system does not exist. Otitis media is a multifactorial disease process involving immunology, infectious disease, anatomic considerations, social and socioeconomic issues, and genetics, among other factors. Before physicians can attain a clear understanding of otitis media, a clear universally accepted classification system will need to be developed.

Although it is clear that serious bacterial infections should be treated with antibiotics, it is not clear that all otitis media is an infectious process necessitating treatment with antimicrobial therapy. In addition, evidence is emerging that the traditional 10-day treatment course for treatment for acute otitis media may not be necessary and that shorter treatment courses may be satisfactory. The role of antibiotic prophylaxis for recurrent acute otitis media has also come under criticism due to the emergence of resistant strains of *Streptococcus pneumoniae,* which may be related to the overutilization of antimicrobial therapy for children with upper respiratory tract infections.[4]

In addition to the controversy surrounding antimicrobial therapy for otitis media, numerous other medical therapeutic options have been described in the literature that also tend to complicate a clear understanding of the management of this disease process. Some of these treatment options include antihistamine/decongestants, inhalation or systemic corticosteroids, desensitization for inhalation or food allergies, and alternative medicine treatment modalities. The role of vaccinations is gaining significant exposure in both the medical literature and lay press.

Surgical treatment options for otitis media are also not without controversy. The standard surgical treatment modality of myringotomy with placement of tympanostomy tubes has recently[5] been called into question and the role of alternative surgical options (i.e., the role of adenoidectomy as well as laser myringotomy) has also been examined in recent years. An attempt will be made to address some of these controversial issues and to make recommendations regarding the appropriate treatment for otitis media.

Classification of Otitis Media

The terminology in the literature associated with otitis media is complex and quite variable. Most classification systems for otitis media attempt to describe the disease process on the basis of the duration of the process, the type of inflammatory fluid involved, the presence of tympanic membrane perforation, the presence of suppurative or nonsuppurative disease and other criteria.[6] The confusion in the literature regarding classification impedes our ability to describe the disease process and thus complicates clinical research and our ability to communicate effectively about otitis media.[7]

For the purposes of this chapter, the following terminology is used:

1. *Acute otitis media:* Suppurative or purulent middle ear process associated with purulent middle ear effusion with one or more of the following signs: otalgia, otorrhea, fever, and acute onset of irritability. Otoscopic findings demonstrate purulent middle ear effusion and a bulging tympanic membrane with loss of tympanic landmarks; possibly with the presence of an acute draining perforation.
2. *Recurrent acute otitis media:* Repetitive bouts of acute otitis media, separated by asymptomatic periods and clearing of middle ear effusion.
3. *Chronic otitis media with effusion:* The presence of middle ear effusion, regardless of symptomatology, that has been present for 90 days or longer. The fluid may be categorized into serous, purulent, or mucoid middle ear effusion.

Microbiology of Otitis Media

The microbiology of otitis media has been carefully elucidated by numerous studies.[8-12] However, with the increased use of antimicrobial agents, the emergence of resistant bacteria has become a significant problem related to otitis media. Data from studies performed by Bluestone and Klein[9] demonstrate that *Streptococcus pneumoniae* remains the primary bacterial cause of otitis media, followed by *Haemophilus* (38%), *Haemophilus influenzae* (27%), and *Moraxella caterrhalis* (10%). In this same study, 28% demonstrated no bacteria or nonpathogenic bacteria. Approximately 30 to 40% of patients with acute otitis media demonstrate respiratory viruses that may be present in combination with bacterial pathogens.[13] Respiratory syncytial virus has recently been implicated as a major viral pathogen in otitis media.[14] In recent years, the incidence of resistant bacteria has increased in cases of otitis media. First noted was the advent of β-lactamase-producing *Haemophilus influenzae* and *Moraxella caterrhalis.* More recently, the incidence of penicillin-resistant pneumococci has increased.[15] The resistance mechanism for each of these resistance types is quite different. Studies performed throughout the 1990s have demonstrated increased incidence of resistance by both β-lactamase-producing bacteria and *Streptococcus pneumonia.*[15-20] The increased prevalence of bacterial resistance may alter the way we treat otitis media in children, with respect to both antimicrobial therapy and surgical intervention.

Treatment Options for Otitis Media

To understand fully when it is appropriate to treat otitis media in children, the pathophysiology of the various subtypes of otitis media should be understood and the appropriate diagnosis must be made. In addition, various treatment modalities for otitis media—both medical and surgical—may benefit a particular patient. The importance of individualization of treatment for every patient with otitis media must be emphasized. Otitis media is a multifactorial process. Different treatment modalities may be warranted in patients based on their particular social situation, immunologic status, age, associated medical problems, or other factors. Various treatment modalities for otitis media will be briefly discussed to help the practitioner decide which patient should be treated, and by what particular treatment strategy.

Medical Management Options for Otitis Media

ANTIBIOTICS

Antimicrobial therapy has continued to be a mainstay of therapy for patients with otitis media. Recently, there has been evidence that over usage of antimicrobial therapy has led to an increased incidence of bacterial resistance in common pathogens related to otitis media. Most notably, *St. pneumoniae, H. influenzae,* and *M. caterrhalis.*[15] Children frequently presenting to primary physicians with viral upper respiratory tract infections may be treated with antimicrobials, whether or not the patient has simultaneously developed otitis media.[4] We know from prior microbiologic studies[13,14] that a significant number of middle ear effusion cultures contain predominantly viruses that would not benefit from antimicrobial therapy. It is apparent from these prior studies that many children with otitis media may not benefit from antimicrobial agents, as the cause of otitis media in many cases is nonbacterial, or some cases of bacterial otitis media may resolve without pharmacologic therapy. Approximately 60% of cases of acute otitis media may resolve spontaneously; however, spontaneous resolution is less common in cases of *S. pneumoniae*, approximately 20%.[21,22] Although there are advocates of withholding antimicrobial therapy in cases of otitis media,[17] this management strategy is not recommended because of the 20 to 40% incidence of persistent otitis, often caused by *S. pneumoniae* in nontreated cases. In addition, in cases of untreated otitis media, there is a risk of development of intratemporal or intracranial complications.

Currently, approximately 16 approved antimicrobials may be used for the treatment of otitis media.[23] The recommended first line antibiotic for treatment of otitis media continues to be amoxicillin.[24,25] In situations of treatment failures or drug allergy to amoxicillin, other antimicrobials should be considered. In cases where agents which have high activity against β-lactamase-producing *H. influenzae* and *M. caterrhalis*-effective antimicrobials include amoxicillin and clavulanate potassium, cefixime, cefpodoxime proxetil, and cefuroxime axetil. In cases in which resistant *Pneumococcus* is suspected or has been diagnosed, high-dose amoxicillin may be beneficial with doses ranging from 60 to 90 mg/kg/day. This regimen may also be used in combination with amoxicillin/shill clavulanate. Obviously, without tympanocentesis, it is difficult to obtain a true diagnosis of the bacteriologic agents in any specific case of otitis media. Unfortunately, tympanocentesis continues as a rather invasive and often uncomfortable procedure that may be difficult to perform in the office setting. A child's parents may also be quite resistant to the possibility of performing this procedure, especially if they are aware of the alternative of empirical antimicrobial treatment. In the future, it may be that as more resistant bacteria emerge from the continued overusage of antimicrobials in our society, there may be an increased role for tympanocentesis for more bacterial-specific treatment for cases of otitis media. Currently, we reserve the role of tympanocentesis for children who have extreme symptomatology and need decompression for immediate relief, for treatment failures, or for children with underlying immunologic disorders who require specific bacteriologic assessment before treatment.

A patient with physical diagnostic findings of acute purulent otitis media with significant symptomatology and fever should be treated with antimicrobial therapy. By contrast, a patient, with a viral upper respiratory tract illness, with evidence of middle ear effusion that is nonpurulent with insignificant otologic symptomatology may initially be treated symptomatically without antimicrobial therapy. If progression of symptoms occurs, antimicrobials could be initiated subsequently.

The duration of treatment with antimicrobials for otitis media has traditionally been 7 to 10 days. However, with the advent of newer antibiotics, such as azithromycin, 5-day treatment courses have been advocated.[26] Therapy of shorter duration with other antibiotics has also been recommended by some investigators.[1,27,28] Single-dose therapy with ceftriaxone has also demonstrated efficacy.[29,30]

A controversial area in the treatment of otitis media involves chemoprophylaxis with antimicrobial agents in otitis-prone children. Otitis-prone children who tend to completely clear middle ear effusion after appropriate medical therapy for acute otitis media and have no suspected significant hearing loss are candidates for chemoprophylaxis, typically using low-dose amoxicillin and sulfasoxazole. Numerous studies have looked at this issue with no definite conclusions having been determined.[31] Williams et al.[31] performed a meta-analysis of prior chemoprophylaxis studies, specifically looking at the efficacy of chemoprophylaxis in otitis media. The study did demonstrate a small short-term benefit for the management of recurrent otitis media. However, there did not appear to be any long-term benefit to this treatment strategy. Paradise[16,32] stated that physicians should reexamine the role of chemoprophylaxis and the treatment of recurrent otitis media due to the increased incidence of bacterial resistance. He advocates refraining from administration of chemoprophylaxis altogether, or possibly limiting the role of chemoprophylaxis in otitis-prone children just during upper respiratory tract infections.

Children who have significant problems with recurrent acute otitis media requiring multiple courses of antimicrobials may be candidates for chemoprophylaxis. This is a treatment modality that should be individualized to the patient and should be pursued after consultation with the patient's primary care physician. Because of increasing antimicrobial resistance, early placement of tympanostomy tubes may be preferable to long-term chemoprophylaxis.

Alternative Medical Treatment Options

Other medical modalities recommended for the treatment of otitis include corticosteroids, administered orally or intra nasally;[33-36] antihistamines; and/or decongestants. Although there is evidence that orally administered corticosteroids may help clear chronic middle ear effusion, there is no evidence that this provides a long-term benefit in patients with chronic otitis media with effusion.[35] In addition, there is the risk of potential side effects from utilization of cortocosteroids. Intranasal steroids may play a role in patients with chronic middle ear effusion.[36] However, there is no evidence of efficacy in the treatment of acute otitis media. Antihistamine/decongestant preparations have been used in the past for treatment of otitis media with effusion. However, there is no evidence that this accelerates clearance of middle ear effusion and there appears to be no role for these medications in the treatment of acute otitis media.[37] In children who have significant symptoms of nasal congestion and rhinorrhea related to upper respiratory tract infection or allergic rhinitis, there may be a role for these preparations. In older patients with a history of recurrent otitis media of chronic otitis media with effusion when there is symptomatology or family history suggestive of inhalant allergies, an allergy evaluation should be recommended. In addition, there is evidence that second-hand smoke exposure may be an etiologic factor in chronic otitis media in children,[38,39] and this should be addressed by parental education, to decrease the patient's exposure.

Surgical Management Options

The primary surgical therapy for chronic otitis media remains placement of tympanostomy tubes for pressure equalization and drainage of the middle ear space. Numerous publications have demonstrated the efficacy of tympanostomy tubes for the treatment of chronic otitis media with effusion and recurrent otitis media.[38,40-43] The Academy of Otolaryngology, in its 1995 Clinical Indicators Compendium,[44] listed the following indications for placement of tympanostomy tubes: (1) middle ear effusion present for 3 months or more; (2) otitis media with effusion associated with hearing loss of > 30 db; (3) chronic severe tympanic membrane retraction; (4) impending intracranial complications associated with otitis media; and (5) recurrent otitis media with more than three episodes within a 6-month period, or more than four episodes within a 12-month period. It should be emphasized that these indications are guidelines and a decision to place tympanostomy tubes should be individualized for each patient, based on their particular situation. Because of the increasing prevalence of resistant bacteria in communities around the United States, there may be a role for earlier placement of myringotomy tubes in situations of recurrent acute otitis media and chronic otitis media with effusion to avoid long-term antimicrobial therapy.

Other surgical options may be considered in children with chronic otitis media. Adenoidectomy has clearly been demonstrated as a useful adjunctive surgical procedure that may decrease the incidence of otitis media. This procedure may performed with myringotomy alone, or with myringotomy and placement of tympanostomy tubes.[45-49] Adenoidectomy should be considered for children with chronic otitis media who are candidates for tympanostomy tube placement and who have symptoms of chronic adenoid hypertrophy, such as hyponasal speech and chronic mouth-breathing. Adenoidectomy should also be considered in children requiring multiple sets of tympanostomy tubes, regardless of symptomatology, as it has been demonstrated that adenoidectomy may accelerate the resolution of chronic otitis media regardless of the size of the adenoid pad.[50,51]

Finally, the recently publicized Otolam laser-assisted myringotomy has been advocated as a treatment option for the management of chronic otitis media with effusion. This may provide immediate symptomatic relief and potentially avoid placement of tympanostomy tubes. This may be performed under local anesthesia in the office setting. No long-term studies have been performed to investigate this particular treatment modality. However, clinical trials are currently in progress.

Conclusion

The question of whether to treat otitis media is complex because of the multifactorial etiology of otitis media the complex microbiology involved, and changing antibiotic-prescribing patterns within the United States. It is important to remember that individualization should take place whenever treating a child with otitis media. Antimicrobial therapy is warranted in cases of acute otitis media with significant symptomatology. However, cases associated with upper respiratory tract infections and minimal otologic symptoms may not require antimicrobial therapy. Chemoprophylaxis should be discouraged due to the increased incidence of bacterial resistance in the United States. However, selective use of chemoprophylaxis for upper respiratory tract infections, during the winter months, may be beneficial in some cases. Tympanostomy tubes continue to be the mainstay of surgical treatment for otitis media and for refractory cases of chronic otitis media with effusion and recurrent otitis media. Earlier tube placement to avoid possible bacterial resistance may be warranted to avoid long-term antimicrobial therapy for patients with chronic otitis media.

REFERENCES

Wiatrak—CHAPTER 77

1. Kozyrskyj AL, Hildes–Ripstein GE, Longstaffe SE, et al. Treatment of acute otitis media with a shortened course of antibiotics: a meta-analysis. *JAMA* 1998;279:1736–1742
2. Teele DW, Klein JO, Rosner B. Epidemiology of otitis media during the first seven years of life in children in greater Boston: a prospective, cohort study. *J Infect Dis* 1989;160:83–94
3. Stool SE, Field MJ. The impact of otitis media. *Pediatr Infect Dis J* 1989;8:S11–S14
4. Nyquist AC, Gonzales R, Steiner JF, Sande MA. Antibiotic prescribing for children with colds, upper respiratory tract infections, and bronchitis [published erratum appears in JAMA 1998 3;279:1702]. *JAMA* 1998;279:875–877
5. Kleinman LC, Kosecoff J, Dubois RW, Brook RH. The medical appropriateness of tympanostomy tubes proposed for children younger than 16 years in the United States. *JAMA* 1994; 271:1250–1255
6. Bluestone CD. Pathogenesis of otitis media: role of eustachian tube. *Pediatr Infect Dis J* 1996;15:281–291
7. Harkness P, Topham J. Classification of otitis media (abstract). *Laryngoscope* 1998;108:1539–1543
8. Bluestone CD, Stephenson JS, Martin LM. Ten-year review of otitis media pathogens. *Pediat Infect Dis J* 1992;11:S7–S11
9. Bluestone CD, Klein JO, eds. *Otitis Media in Infants and Children*. Philadelphia: WB Saunders; 1995:56
10. Klein JO. Otitis media. *Clin Infect Dis* 1994;19:823–833
11. Wald ER. Changing trends in the microbiology of otitis media with effusion. *Pediatr Infect Dis* 1984;3:380–383
12. Del Beccaro MA, Mendelman PM, et al. Bacteriology of acute otitis media: a new perspective. *J Pediatr* 1992;120:81–84
13. Heikkinen T, Ruuskanen O. New prospects in the prevention of otitis media. *Ann Med* 1996;28:23–30
14. Heikkinen T, Thint M, Chonmaitree MD. Prevalence of various respiratory viruses in the middle ear during acute otitis media (abstract). *N Engl J Med* 1999;340:260–264
15. McCracken GH Jr. Emergence of resistant *Streptococcus pnuemoniae*: a problem in pediatrics (abstract). *Pediatr Infect Dis J* 1995;14:424–428
16. Paradise JL. Managing otitis media: a time for change. *Pediatrics* 1995;96:712–715
17. Culpepper L, Froom J. Routine antimicrobial treatment of otitis media: is it necessary? (abstract). *JAMA* 1997;278:1643–1645
18. Baquero F. Trends in antibiotic resistance of respiratory pathogens: an analysis and commentary on a collaborative surveillance study (abstract). *J Antimicrob Chemother* 1996;38(suppl A):117–132
19. Rudberg RD. Acute otitis media: comparative therapeutic results of sulphonamide and penicillin administered in various forms (abstract). *Acta Otolarynogol (Stockh)* 1954;113(suppl):9–79
20. Lahikainen EA. Clinico–bacteriologic studies on acute otitis media: aspiration of the tympanum as a diagnostic and therapeutic method (abstract). *Acta Otolaryngol (Stockh)* 1954; 107(supp):1–82
21. Marchant CD, Carlin SA, Johnson CE, Shurin PA. Measuring the comparative efficacy of antibacterial agents for acute otitis media: the “Pollyanna phenomenon.” *J Pediatr* 1992;120:72–77
22. Klein JO. Microbiologic efficacy of antibacterial drugs for acute otitis media [published erratum appears in *Pediatr Infect Dis J* 1994;13:1125]. *Pediatr Infect Dis J* 1993;12:973–975
23. Klein JO. Current recommendations on the therapy of otitis media. *Pediatr Infect Dis J* 1998;17:1058–1059
24. McCracken GH Jr. Considerations in selecting an antibiotic for treatment of acute otitis media (abstract). *Pediatr Infect Dis J* 1994;13:1054–1057
25. Block SL. Causitive pathogens, antibiotic resistance and therapeutic considerations in acute otitis media (abstract). *Pediatr Infect Dis J* 1997;16:449–456
26. Pichichero ME, Cohen R. Shortened course of antibiotic therapy for acute otitis media, sinusitis and tonsillopharyngitis (abstract). *Pediatr Infect Dis J* 1997;16:680–695
27. Chaput de Saintonage DM, Levine DF. Trial of three-day and ten-day courses of amoxicillin in otitis media (abstract). *BMJ* 1982;284:1078–1081
28. Hendrickse WA, Kusmiesz H, Shelton S, Nelson JD. Five vs. ten days of therapy for acute otitis media (abstract). *Pediatr Infect Dis J* 1988;7:14–23
29. Varsano I, Frydman M, Amir J, et al. Single intramuscular dose of ceftriaxone as compared to 7-day amoxicillin therapy for acute otitis media in children. (abstract) *Chemotherapy.* 1988;34(suppl 1):39–46
30. Green SM, Rothrock SG. Single-dose intramuscular ceftriaxone for acute otitis media in children (abstract). *Pediatrics* 1993;91:23–30

31. Williams R, Chalmers T, Stange K, et al. Use of antibiotics in preventing acute otitis media and in treating otitis media with effusion. A meta–analytic attempt to resolve the brouhaha (abstract). *JAMA* 1999;270:1344–1351
32. Paradise JL. Treatment guidelines for otitis media: the need for breadth and flexibility. *Pediatr Infect Dis J* 1995;14: 429–435
33. Podoshin L, Fradis M, Ben-David Y, Faraggi D. The efficacy of oral steroids in the treatment of persistent otitis media with effusion. *Arch of Otolaryngol Head Neck Surg* 1990;116:1404–1406
34. Persico M, Podoshin L, Fradis M. Otitis media with effusion: a steroid and antibiotic therapeutic trial before surgery. *Ann of Otol Rhinol Laryngol* 1978;87:191–196
35. Rosenfeld RM, Mandel EM, Bluestone CD. Systemic steroids for otitis media with effusion in children. *Arch Otolaryngol Head Neck Surg* 1991;117:984–989
36. Tracy JM, Demain JG, Hoffman KM, Goetz DW. Intranasal beclomethasone as an adjunct to treatment of chronic middle ear effusion. *Ann Allergy Asthma Immunol* 1998;80:198–206
37. Cantekin EI, Mandel EM, Bluestone CD, et al. Lack of efficacy of a decongestant–antihistamine combination for otitis media with effusion ("secretory" otitis media) in children. Results of a double-blind, randomized trial. *N Engl J of Med* 1983;308:297–301
38. Etzel RA, Pattishall EN, Haley NJ, et al. Passive smoking and middle ear effusion among children in daycare (abstract). *Pediatrics* 1992;90:228–232
39. Strachan DP, Jarvis MJ, Feyerabend C. Passive smoking, salivary cotinine concentrations, and middle ear effusion in 7-year-old children (abstract). *BMJ* 1989;298:1549–1552
40. Mandel EM, Rockette HE, Bluestone CD, et al. Efficacy of myringotomy with and without tympanostomy tubes for chronic otitis media with effusion. *Pediatr Infect Dis J* 1992; 11:270–277
41. Bluestone CD. Surgical management of otitis media: current indications and role related to increasing bacterial resistance. *Pediatr Infect Dis J* 1994;13:1058–1063
42. Mandel EM, Rockette HE, Bluestone CD, et al. Myringotomy with and without tympanostomy tubes for chronic otitis media with effusion. *Arch of Otolaryngol Head Neck Surg* 1989;115:1217–1224
43. Casselbrant ML, Kaleida PH, Rockette HE, et al. Efficacy of antimicrobial prophylaxis and of tympanostomy tube insertion for prevention of recurrent acute otitis media: results of a randomized clinical trial. *Pediatr Infect Dis J* 1992;11:278–286
44. Anonymous. Abstract. *Clinical Indicators Compendium.* Academy of Otolaryngology:1995
45. Paradise JL, Bluestone CD, Rogers KD, et al. Efficacy of adenoidectomy for recurrent otitis media in children previously treated with tympanostomy-tube placement. Results of parallel randomized and nonrandomized trials. *JAMA* 1990;263: 2066–2073
46. Gates GA, Muntz HR, Gaylis B. Adenoidectomy and otitis media. *Ann of Otol Rhinol Laryngol 1*992;155(suppl):24–32
47. Margolis RH, Hunter LL, Rykken JR, Giebink GS. Effects of otitis media on extended high-frequency hearing in children. *Ann of Otol, Rhinol Laryngol* 1993;102:1–5
48. Rosenfeld RM. Nonsurgical management of surgical otitis media with effusion. *Laryngol Otol* 1995;109:811–816
49. Gates GA, Avery CA, Prihoda TJ, Cooper JC, Jr. Effectiveness of adenoidectomy and tympanostomy tubes in the treatment of chronic otitis media with effusion. *N Engl J M* 1987; 317:1444–1451
50. Antonelli PJ, Juhn SK, Goycoolea MV, Giebink GS. Pseudomonas otitis media after eustachian tube obstruction. *Otolaryngol Head Neck Surgery* 1992;107:511–515
51. Rosenfeld RM. What to expect from medical treatment of otitis media. *Pediatr Infect Dis J* 1995;14:731–737; quiz 738

Otitis Media: To Treat or Not to Treat*

Charles D. Bluestone

CHAPTER 78

Otitis media is now the most common disease diagnosed by clinicians in the United States. Even though these infections primarily affect infants and young children and to a lesser extent, older children and teenagers, the disease is also common in adults. Over the past two decades, there has been a significant increase in the incidence of otitis media in children, especially in the infant age group, which has been attributed to the dramatic rise in attendance in child day care centers.[1]

Currently, there are at least four major controversies related to the management of this highly prevalent disease: (1) to treat or not to treat acute otitis media with antibiotics; (2) to treat or not to treat middle ear effusion that persists after an episode of acute otitis media with antibiotics; (3) to treat or not to treat otitis media with effusion with antibiotics; and (4) which management options are most safe and effective for prevention of recurrent acute otitis media. These controversial issues are primarily due to the ever-increasing rates of antibiotic-resistant bacterial pathogens that cause otitis media, which has been attributed to overuse of antimicrobial agents.

Diagnosis of Otitis Media Related to Treatment

Important in the decision to treat or not treat otitis media, the clinician must appreciate the diagnostic differences between acute otitis media and otitis media with effusion, as the latter condition is usually not treated unless it becomes chronic (Table 78–1).

Acute otitis media is characterized by the rapid, brief onset of signs and symptoms of infection in the middle ear. One or more of the following are present: otalgia (or pulling of the ear in the infant), fever, or irritability of recent onset. The tympanic membrane is full or bulging, opaque, and has limited or no mobility to pneumatic otoscopy. After an episode of acute otitis media, the middle ear may have fluid that remains for weeks to months, which has been termed persistent middle ear effusion.

Otitis media with effusion is a relatively asymptomatic middle ear effusion. Pneumatic otoscopy frequently shows either a retracted or concave tympanic membrane, the mobility of which is limited or absent. However, fullness, or even bulging, may be visualized. In addition, an air-fluid level or bubbles, or both, may be observed through a translucent tympanic membrane.

Microbiologic Etiology Related to Treatment

Related to an accurate diagnosis, there is a difference in the prevalence of bacterial pathogens that are isolated from ears of patients with acute otitis media compared to aspirates of otitis media with effusion. This, in turn, has an impact on the decision to recommend or not recommend antimicrobial therapy.

Pathogenic bacteria are present in approximately 70% of the middle ears of patients who have acute otitis media, and are similar in type in both children and adults.[2,3] *Streptococcus pneumoniae* (40%), *Haemophilus influenzae* (25%), and *Moraxella catarrhalis* (12%) are the most common pathogens isolated. Group A β-hemolytic streptococcus and *Staphylococcus aureus* also cause this infection in both children and adults, but not as frequently as pneumococcus and *H. influenzae.* Respiratory viruses have been cultured from as many as 20% of acute effusions.

The percentage of *H. influenzae* that is β-lactamase-producing varies according to the community in the United States, but the rate is now about 25%. Currently, most, if not all strains of *M. catarrhalis* produce β-lactamase. The rate of isolation of multidrug-resistant *S. pneumoniae* is increasing in this country. At the Children's Hospital of Pittsburgh—a tertiary referral center—the rate

* Maria B. Bluestone provided editorial assistance in the preparation of this manuscript.

TABLE 78–1
Diagnostic Similarities and Differences between Acute Otitis Media and Otitis Media with Effusion

	Otalgia, Fever, Irritability	Middle Ear Effusion	Opaque Drum	Bulging Drum	Impaired Drum Mobility	Hearing Loss
Acute otitis media	Present	Present	Present	Present	Present	Present
Otitis media with effusion	Absent	Present	May be absent (air–fluid level)	Usually absent	Present	Usually present

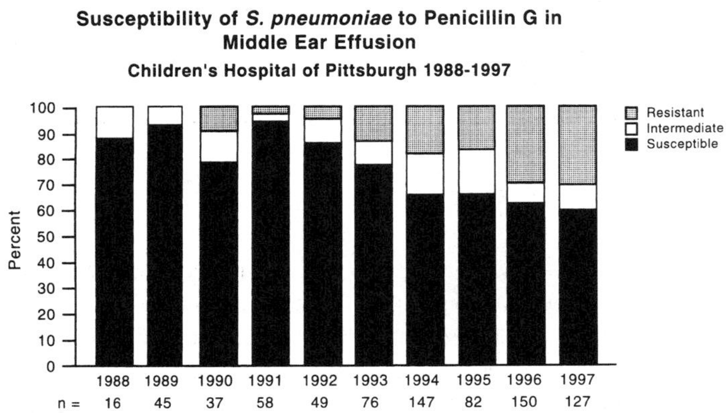

Figure 78–1 Prevalence of penicillin-resistant *Pneumococcus* isolated from the middle ears of infants and children at the Children's Hospital of Pittsburgh from 1988 to 1997.

increased from approximately 10% in 1988 to more than 40% in 1997, and more than one-half of these strains were highly resistant; most likely the rate is lower in community practices (Fig. 78–1).

In contrast to acute otitis media, bacteria considered to be potentially pathogenic can be isolated from only one-third of middle-ear aspirates from patients who have otitis media with effusion. Similar to isolates from acute otitis media, the most common are *S. pneumoniae, H. influenzae,* and *M. catarrhalis*, but the latter two organisms are more commonly isolated than pneumococcus.[4] Resistance rates of these organisms are similar to rates found when these bacteria cause acute otitis media. Recently, these three bacteria have been detected by polymerase chain reaction (PCR) in approximately 70% of chronic middle ear effusions at the time of myringotomy and tympanostomy tube insertion; only about one-third of the organisms were identified using traditional culture methods.[5,6]

Management

ACUTE OTITIS MEDIA

Antibiotic therapy has been the standard treatment for acute otitis media for over half a century, but this widespread practice has now been questioned.

To Treat or Not to Treat Acute Otitis Media with Antibiotics?

With the possibility of increasing the problem of resistant bacterial pathogens, some clinicians, especially in some European countries, question the need for antimicrobial therapy in all patients for treatment of acute otitis media. But most experts in the United States today agree that acute otitis media should be actively treated with an antimicrobial agent. Table 78–2 summarizes four outcomes that provide convincing evidence to support this recommendation and are described in detail below.

TABLE 78–2
Evidence That Antimicrobial Agents Are Indicated for Treatment of Acute Otitis Media

Compared with placebo (or no drug), antimicrobials:

1. Sterilize the middle ear effusion[7]
2. Result in earlier resolution of symptoms of acute infection[8]
3. Shorten time with middle ear effusion (hearing loss)[9]
4. Dramatically decrease suppurative complications[10,11]

Microbiologic Outcome Howie et al.[7] evaluated the microbiologic efficacy with various therapeutic regimens, including a placebo. Although these studies suggest that many cases of infection of the middle ear resolve spontaneously or with the assistance of spontaneous drainage, the data indicate that the most important bacterial pathogens responsible for otitis media will not resolve clinically or microbiologically without medical intervention. A proportion of middle ear effusions that have a positive culture clear the organism without drug intervention (spontaneous clearance). However, in about 20% of infections due to *S. pneumoniae*, and in 50% of infections due to *H. influenzae*, administration of an antimicrobial agent to which these organisms are susceptible results in sterilization of the effusion in almost all the ears.

Symptomatic Outcome Rosenfeld et al.[8] conducted a meta-analysis of 5400 children from 33 randomized trials that addressed the question of efficacy of antimicrobial therapy. These investigators found the spontaneous (without antibiotics or tympanocentesis) rate of primary control to be 81%. However, the rate was 95% when antimicrobial agents were administered. They concluded that "antibiotics have a modest but significant impact on the primary control of acute otitis media."

Middle Ear Effusion Outcome Kaleida and colleagues[9] evaluated amoxicillin or placebo for management of nonsevere acute otitis media. (The distinction between severe and nonsevere disease was based on an otalgia scoring system and the child's temperature; subjects in the severe category were not randomized to receive only placebo.) At the completion of the 2-week amoxicillin treatment, there were statistically fewer children with middle ear effusion (47%) when compared to those who received placebo (63%). Since presence of middle ear effusion is associated with a conductive hearing loss, the administration of an antimicrobial agent reduces the time with hearing loss, which may have implications for child development.

Suppurative Complications Outcome Two important, large clinical trials conducted in Scandinavia during the 1950s, in which patients either were treated with an antibiotic or the agents were withheld, demonstrated that the suppurative complications of otitis media, such as mastoiditis and meningitis, almost exclusively occurred in those children who did not receive antimicrobial agents.[10,11] The rate of suppurative complications of acute otitis media has dramatically fallen with the advent of the widespread use of antimicrobial agents for this infection. Withholding antimicrobial therapy today will most likely result in an increase in complications.

Indeed, the Centers for Disease Control and Prevention and the American Academy of Pediatrics have recently reaffirmed the recommendation to treat all documented cases of acute otitis media with an antimicrobial agent, but stressed the need to make a distinction between acute otitis media and otitis media with effusion, as the latter disease does necessarily require medical treatment.[12]

Selection of an Antimicrobial Agent

Of the 15 antimicrobial agents currently approved for treatment of acute otitis media, amoxicillin is still recommended for initial empiric therapy, as it is relatively safe, effective for most strains of *S. pneumoniae* and *H. influenzae,* and available in a variety of formulations (Table 78–3). The traditional dose of amoxicillin is 40 mg/kg in three divided doses per day, but in communities in which there is a high prevalence of resistant pneumococcus, 80 mg/kg in two doses is now advocated. If the patient is allergic to the penicillins, a combination of erythromycin and sulfisoxazole, or one of the new macrolides, azithromycin or clarithromycin, is advocated; as an alternative, one of the newer cephalosporins (e.g., cefuroxime-axetil, cefpodoxime, loracarbef, ceftriaxone) could be used, if the patient does not have hypersensitivity to these agents, and does not have an immediate hypersensitivity reaction to the penicillins. Trimethoprim-sulfamethoxazole is not a desirable alternative, as it has had an unacceptable safety record. A single parenteral dose of ceftriaxone is the most recent antimicrobial agent approved for treatment. The quinolones, such as ciprofloxacin, are not indicated in children below 18 years of age, and efficacy of these antimicrobial agents has not been reported in adults with acute otitis media.

TABLE 78–3
Antimicrobial Agents Available for Treatment of Otitis Media*

Penicillins	
	Amoxicillin
	Amoxicillin-clavulanate (Augmentin)
Cephalosporins	
	Cefaclor (Ceclor)
	Cefuroxime-axetil (Ceftin)
	Cefpodoxime (Vantin)
	Cefixime (Suprax)
	Ceftibuten (Cedax)
	Cefdinir (Omnicef)
	Ceftriaxone (Rocephin)[a]
Carbapenem	
	Loracarbef (Lorabid)
Macrolides	
	Erythromycin
	Clarithromycin (Biaxin)
	Azithromycin (Zithromax)
Sulfa combinations	
	Erythromycin-sulfisoxazole (Pediazole)
	Trimethoprim-sulfamethoxazole (Bactrim, Septra)

* Includes the oral agents and one parenteral drug available for treatment on an ambulatory basis, whereas there are other parenteral antimicrobial agents effective for treatment of otitis media, usually on an inpatient basis.

[a] Available only in parenteral form.

The traditional 10- to 14-day course of therapy is usually recommended, but there has been a recent proposal to shorten the course to 5 to 7 days in an effort to reduce antibiotic usage.[13] However, there is some evidence that infants should not be treated for a period of fewer than 10 days.[14]

Follow-up Visits

Most cases of acute otitis media improve significantly within 48 to 72 h when appropriate antimicrobial therapy is administered. If signs and symptoms of infection progress despite this treatment, i.e., treatment failure, the patient should be reevaluated within 24 h, since a suppurative complication (e.g., acute mastoiditis) or a concurrent serious infection, such as meningitis, may have developed. Persistent or recurrent pain or fever, or both, during treatment would signal the need for tympanocentesis (for Gram stain, culture, and susceptibility testing), selection of another antimicrobial agent, or both. Selection of an antibiotic at this stage would depend upon the results of the culture and susceptibility testing. If amoxicillin was initially administered, one of the alternative antimicrobial agents to amoxicillin would be reasonable as empiric therapy until the results of the culture are available, or if culture is not obtained. In this era of multidrug-resistant otitic pathogenic bacteria, tympanocentesis should be used as often as possible when a patient is considered to be an antibiotic treatment failure, since it is important to document the causative organism. The procedure can be successfully performed in almost all patients without the need for a general anesthetic. Table 78–4 lists the indications for tympanocentesis (needle aspiration for diagnosis) and myringotomy (drainage of the middle ear).

Patients should be reexamined at the end of the course of antibiotic therapy if they still have any signs or symptoms of acute infection, as further evaluation and therapy may be indicated. If the patient is asymptomatic at the end of therapy, the follow-up visit can be delayed until 4 to 6 weeks after the onset of the attack because further treatment is usually not indicated, even if effusion persists in the middle ear.

To Treat or Not to Treat Persistent Middle Ear Effusion with Antibiotics

After antibiotic therapy for an episode of acute otitis media, middle ear effusion persists in approximately 50% of ears. But the presence of asymptomatic effusion does *not* require further treatment with an antimicrobial agent, since about 90% of these

TABLE 78–4
Recommended Indications for Tympanocentesis (Myringotomy)

1. Otitis media in patients who have severe otalgia, are seriously ill, or appear toxic
2. Unsatisfactory response to antimicrobial therapy
3. Onset of otitis media in a patient who is receiving antimicrobial therapy
4. Otitis media associated with a confirmed or potential suppurative complication
5. Otitis media in a newborn, sick neonate, or immunologically deficient patient, any of whom might harbor an unusual organism

effusions resolve spontaneously during the 3 months after onset. There is a well-founded perception by authorities in the field that too many patients are receiving unnecessary amounts of antibiotics for this condition, which may be related to the growing resistance problem.[12]

Patients who still have a middle ear effusion present at the 4- to 6-week visit should be reevaluated 3 to 4 months after the onset of the infection; those without effusion at 4 to 6 weeks can be discharged. Management of persistent middle ear effusion is similar to that described below for patients who have otitis media with effusion.

OTITIS MEDIA WITH EFFUSION

Appropriate management of relatively asymptomatic otitis media with effusion is controversial.

To Treat or Not to Treat with Antibiotics

Many question the need to treat otitis media with effusion, because the effusion will resolve in most children without active treatment in 2 or 3 months. Nevertheless, treatment may be indicated in some children, because there are possible complications and sequelae associated with this condition. Since hearing loss of some degree usually accompanies a middle ear effusion, treatment may be warranted when longstanding impairment in hearing is present. Although the significance of this hearing loss is still uncertain, such a loss may impair cognitive and language function and result in disturbances in psychosocial adjustment. Important factors that should be considered when deciding to treat or not to treat are listed in Table 78–5.

TABLE 78–5
Factors to Be Considered, on an Individual Basis, Favoring Treatment of Otitis Media with Effusion

1. Significant associated conductive hearing loss
2. Occurrence in young infants, as they are unable to communicate about their symptoms and may have suppurative disease
3. An associated acute suppurative upper respiratory tract infection
4. Concurrent permanent conductive/sensorineural hearing loss
5. Presence of speech/language delay associated with effusion and hearing loss
6. Tinnitus, vertigo, or disequilibrium
7. Alterations of tympanic membrane, such as a retraction pocket
8. Middle-ear changes, such as adhesive otitis media or ossicular involvement
9. Previous surgery for otitis media (e.g., tympanostomy tube placement or adenoidectomy)
10. When episodes recur frequently
11. Effusion that persists for 3 months or longer (i.e., chronic otitis media with effusion, before consideration for tympanostomy tube placement)

Which Treatments Are Effective and Which Are Not?

If active treatment is elected, options are limited. Even though a combination of an oral decongestant and antihistamine was considered effective—and widely used—in the past, studies failed to demonstrate their efficacy in eliminating middle ear effusion.[15] Despite the apparent efficacy of systemic corticosteroid therapy in clinical trials, a recent official government guideline found the risks of this option in children to outweigh its possible benefits.[16] Clinical trials have not been reported that have tested the efficacy of topical nasal corticosteroid treatment, immunotherapy, and control of allergy in children who have nasal allergy and middle ear disease. Nevertheless, this method of management seems reasonable in children who have frequently recurrent or chronic otitis media with effusion and evidence of upper respiratory allergy.

Of all the medical treatments that have been advocated, a trial of an antimicrobial agent would appear to be most appropriate in those children who have not received an antibiotic recently. A meta-analysis of the effect of antimicrobial agents in the treatment of otitis media with effusion was reported by Rosenfeld and Post, which confirmed their efficacy.[17] Two other meta-analyses also verified their short-term effect, but as expected, there was no long-term efficacy.[16,18] Other strategies, such as antimicrobial prophylaxis or surgery, is required for long-term control, since the disease is frequently recurrent due to repeated exposure to upper respiratory tract infections. A 10- to 14-day course of amoxicillin is recommended.[15] Repeated courses of a variety of antibiotics are not appropriate, as this common practice is also probably contributing to the rising resistant bacteria problem.

When the effusion is chronic, surgical intervention should be considered, especially when antimicrobial therapy fails. Two Pittsburgh clinical trials demonstrated that myringotomy and tympanostomy tube insertion was more effective than myringotomy without tube insertion or no surgery for chronic effusions.[19,20] Adenoidectomy, in conjunction with myringotomy with and without tympanostomy tube placement, has been shown to be effective for chronic effusions in two large, well-controlled clinical trials in children.[21,22] Tonsillectomy in conjunction with adenoidectomy for chronic effusions has been shown in a clinical trial in Great Britain to provide no significant benefit over adenoidectomy alone, and is not recommended unless there are other compelling indications, such as frequently recurrent throat infections or severe airway obstruction secondary to grossly enlarged tonsils.[23,24]

RECURRENT ACUTE OTITIS MEDIA

When attacks of acute otitis media are frequent and close together (e.g., three or more episodes in 6 months, or four or more attacks in 12 months, with one being recent), prevention is desirable. The parents/caretakers should be advised to avoid placing the child in a day-care center, or if this is not feasible, a facility should be chosen that has the fewest number of children possible. Also, they should be counseled about the increased risk of recurrent acute otitis media associated with smoking in the household. Although not effective in infants, the administration of the currently available pneumococcal vaccine is also recommended for children above the age of 2 years; the influenza vaccine is also advocated and can be administered to infants.

There is no general agreement today on the other nonsurgical and surgical methods of prevention. Amoxicillin, 20 mg/kg in one dose (given at bedtime), has proved effective.[25] If the child is allergic to the penicillins, a daily dose of sulfisoxazole 50 mg/kg may be substituted. This prophylactic regimen can be continued during the respiratory season. But today, with the growing evidence that long-term, low-dose antimicrobial prophylaxis is associated with the emergence of resistant *Pneumococcus* in infants and young children, a more desirable option would be myringotomy and tympanostomy tube placement, as this operation has been shown to be effective for prevention of otitis media.[25,26] Table 78–6 lists the indications for tympanostomy tube placement. Adenoidectomy may also be an option for those who have had one or more tympanostomy tube insertions in the past.[21]

TABLE 78–6
Recommended Indications for Tympanostomy Tube Insertion

1. Chronic otitis media with effusion, unresponsive to medical management, that has persisted for at least 3 months when bilateral, or 6 months when unilateral
2. Recurrent acute otitis media, especially when antimicrobial prophylaxis fails; minimum frequency for tube insertion would be three or more episodes during previous 6 months, or four or more attacks during previous year, with one being recent
3. Recurrent episodes of otitis media with effusion in which duration of each episode does not meet criteria for chronic disease, but cumulative duration is considered excessive, such as 6 of previous 12 months
4. Suppurative complication is suspected or present; insertion of a tympanostomy tube at time of tympanocentesis/myringotomy can provide more prolonged drainage and aeration of middle ear and mastoid
5. Eustachian tube dysfunction (even in absence of middle ear effusion) when patient has persistent/recurrent signs and symptoms not relieved by medical treatment options, or at the time of reconstructive middle ear surgery; signs and symptoms include hearing loss (usually fluctuating), disequilibrium/vertigo, tinnitus, autophony, severe retraction pocket
6. Barotrauma, especially for prevention of recurrent episodes (e.g., after airplane flying or hypobaric chamber treatment)

Summary

There is a legitimate growing concern today that acute otitis media is being overdiagnosed and that antimicrobial agents are being overused for all stages of otitis media, which is contributing to the ever-increasing rate of antibiotic-resistant otitic bacteria. But there is ample evidence that patients with proven acute otitis media should still be treated with an antibiotic, primarily to prevent suppurative complications. Even though most patients will improve spontaneously without the benefit of an antimicrobial agent, the clinician cannot determine at the onset of the infection who will and will not be at risk of developing these complications. Thus, all patients require treatment. Tympanocentesis (myringotomy) should be performed when patients fail to improve on antimicrobial therapy in an effort to identify the causative organism, which may be resistant to the standard antibiotics.

Patients who have persistent middle ear effusion after an attack of acute otitis media, and most patients who develop otitis media with effusion, do not require treatment with an antibiotic, unless the effusion progresses to the chronic stage. When antibiotic treatment is needed, a 2- to 4-week course should be adequate; the practice of administering multiple courses of a variety of antimicrobial agents in an effort to clear the effusion is to be condemned. Likewise, long-term prophylaxis with low-dose antibiotics for prevention of recurrent otitis media is currently not as desirable as other methods of prevention, including placement of tympanostomy tubes or adenoidectomy, or both. These operations have also been demonstrated to be effective for the treatment and prevention of chronic otitis media with effusion.

Judicious use of antimicrobial agents for treatment and prevention of otitis media should help curtail the growing resistant bacteria problem. The role of surgery in the management of these patients should also be considered, as there is now convincing evidence of the efficacy of these procedures.

REFERENCES

Bluestone—CHAPTER 78

1. Shappert SM. Office visits for otitis media: United States, 1975–90. Vital and Health Statistics of the Centers for Disease Control/National Center for Health Statistics 1992;214:1–18
2. Celin SE, Bluestone CD, Stephenson J, et al. Bacteriology of acute otitis media in adults. *JAMA* 1991;266:2249–2252
3. Bluestone CD, Stephenson JS, Martin LM. Ten-year review of otitis media pathogens. *Pediatr Infect Dis J* 1992;11:S7–S11
4. Riding KH, Bluestone CD, Michaels RH, et al. Microbiology of recurrent and chronic otitis media with effusion. *J Pediatr* 1978;93:739–743
5. Post JC, Preston RA, Aul JJ, et al. Molecular analysis of bacterial pathogens in otitis media with effusion. *JAMA* 1995;273:1598–1604
6. Rayner MG, Zhang Y, Gorry MC, et al. Evidence of bacterial metabolic activity in culture-negative otitis media with effusion. *JAMA* 1998;279:296–299
7. Howie VM, Ploussard JH. Efficacy of fixed combination antibiotics versus separate components in otitis media. *Clin Pediatr* 1972;11:205–214
8. Rosenfeld RM, Vertrees JE, Carr J, et al. Clinical efficacy of antimicrobial drugs for acute otitis media: meta-analysis of 5400 children from thirty-three randomized trials. *J Pediatr* 1994;124:355–367
9. Kaleida PH, Casselbrant ML, Rockette HE, et al. Amoxicillin or myringotomy or both for acute otitis media: results of a randomized clinical trial. *Pediatrics* 1991;87:466–474
10. Lahkainen EA. Clinico-bacteriologic studies on acute otitis media: aspiration of tympanum as diagnostic and therapeutic method. *Acta Otolaryngol (Stockh)* 1953;107(suppl):1–82
11. Rudberg RD. Acute otitis media: comparative therapeutic results of sulfonamide and penicillin administered in various forms. *Acta Otolaryngol (Stockh)* 1954;113:1–79
12. Dowell SF, Marcy SM, Phillips WR, et al. Otitis media-principles of judicious use of antimicrobial agents. In: Dowell SF, ed. Principles of judicious use of antimicrobial agents for pediatric upper respiratory tract infections. *Pediatrics* 1998;101:165–171
13. Kozyrskyj AL, Hildes–Ripstein GE, Longstaffe SE, et al. Treatment of acute otitis media with a shortened course of antibiotics: a meta-analysis. *JAMA* 1998;279:1736–1742
14. Paradise JL. Short-course antimicrobial treatment for acute otitis media: not best for infants and young children. *JAMA* 1997;278:1640–1642
15. Mandel EM, Rockette HE, Bluestone CD, et al. Efficacy of amoxicillin with and without decongestant-antihistamine for otitis media with effusion in children. *N Engl J Med* 1987;316: 432–437
16. Stool SE, Berg AO, Carney CJ, et al. *Otitis Media with Effusion in Young Children.* Clinical Practice Guideline No. 12. AHCPR Publ No. 94-0622. Rockville, MD: Agency for Health Care Policy and Research, Public Health Service, US Department of Health and Human Services; 1994
17. Rosenfeld RM, Post JC. Meta-analysis of antibiotics for the treatment of otitis media with effusion. *Otol Head Neck Surg* 1992;106:378–386
18. Williams RL, Chalmers TC, Stange KC, et al. Use of antibiotics in preventing recurrent acute otitis media and in treating otitis media with effusion. *JAMA* 1993;270:1344–1351
19. Mandel EM, Rockette HE, Bluestone CD, et al. Myringotomy with and without tympanostomy tubes for chronic otitis media with effusion. *Arch Otolaryngol Head Neck Surg* 1989; 115:1217–1224
20. Mandel EM, Rockette HE, Bluestone CD, et al. Efficacy of myringotomy with and without tympanostomy tubes for chronic otitis media with effusion. *Pediatr Infect Dis J* 1992; 11:270–277
21. Paradise JL, Bluestone CD, Rogers KD, et al. Efficacy of adenoidectomy for recurrent otitis media in children previously treated with tympanostomy-tube placement: results of parallel randomized and nonrandomized trials. *JAMA* 1990;263: 2066–2073
22. Gates GA, Avery CA, Prihoda TJ, et al. Effectiveness of adenoidectomy and tympanostomy tubes in the treatment of chronic otitis media with effusion. *N Engl J Med* 1987;317: 1444–1451
23. Maw AR. Chronic otitis media with effusion (glue ear) and adenotonsillectomy: prospective randomised controlled study. *BMJ* 1983;287:1586–1588
24. Paradise JL, Bluestone CD, Bachman RZ, et al. Efficacy of tonsillectomy for recurrent throat infection in severly affected children. Results of parallel randomized and nonrandomized clinical trials. *N Engl J Med* 1984;310:674–683
25. Casselbrant ML, Kaleida PH, Rockette HE, et al. Efficacy of antimicrobial prophylaxis and of tympanostomy tube insertion for prevention of recurrent acute otitis media: results of a randomized clinical trial. *Pediatr Infect Dis J* 1992;11:278–286
26. Bluestone CD. Surgical management of otitis media: current indications and role related to increasing bacterial resistance. *Pediatr Infect Dis J* 1994;11:1058–1063

27

Cochlear Implants in Congenitally Deaf Children

"Some members of the deaf community believe that hearing parents are not capable of making appropriate decisions for their deaf children since they are not members of the same community and culture."

Thomas J. Balkany

"Some children can communicate extremely well using the auditory/oral modality and acquire age-appropriate language skills, whereas other children display only minimal spoken word recognition skills or demonstrate severe language delay, or both. Accounting for this enormous variability in the effectiveness of CIs on a wide range of outcome measures presents the most serious challenge facing cochlear implant clinicians and researchers today."

Richard T. Miyamoto

"Although the early cortical plasticity research could be taken to argue for implantation during the first year of life, it seems to explain why some congenitally deaf children who are implanted early do not make progress. If the auditory cortex and complex brain underpinnings for spoken language cannot be awakened to sensory stimulation in this way, the value of an implant would be expected to be restricted."

Laura W. Kretschmer

Cochlear Implants in Congenitally Deaf Children

Annelle V. Hodges, Thomas J. Balkany, Stacy L. Butts, and Shelly Ash

CHAPTER 79

The use of cochlear implants in children in the United States was first evaluated during the mid-1980s after Food and Drug Administration (FDA) approval of the House/3M single-channel device in adults. A substantial number of children received single-channel cochlear implants during an FDA-controlled multicenter study, beginning in 1983. Also in 1983, the first child received a multichannel device in Melbourne, Australia. Initiation of a pediatric clinical trial of the Nucleus multichannel cochlear implant occurred in 1986 after FDA approval for use of the device in adults in 1985. The clinical trials in children continued over a period of approximately 4 years, with 142 children receiving the device before FDA approval was granted in 1990.[1] Several upgrades of the Nucleus device, as well as several generations of the Advanced Bionics Clarion device, have undergone successful FDA trials; pediatric trials are currently ongoing with the Austrian-made Med-El. Results of these closely controlled studies indicate that cochlear implant manufacturers have made safety and efficacy claims for children that were supported by the trial data.

In addition to FDA trials, the National Institutes of Health (NIH) convened two consensus conferences on cochlear implants, one in 1988, and the second in 1995. In May 1995, nearly 200 professionals and interested parties gathered to assess the status of cochlear implants after 10 years of clinical use. As reflected by the consensus statement, the use of cochlear implants in children has been shown to "result in successful speech perception in children." In addition, it was noted that "a younger age of implantation may limit the negative consequences of auditory deprivation and may allow more efficient acquisition of speech and language."[2]

In spite of repeated FDA approval and NIH support for use of cochlear implants in children, a strong body of opposition to pediatric use of the device has remained. Few if any other proven treatment options for treatment of major pediatric health disorders have received the type and intensity of negative response which has accompanied use of the cochlear implant in children. As suggested by the title of this chapter, opposition has centered on resisting implantation of the congenitally deafened child. That adults and postlinguistically deafened children can benefit from implants has been acknowledged by most of those who continue to oppose its use in the congenitally deaf child. Primary opposition has come from members of the deaf world, a subset of the deaf community who hold more extreme views on the nature of deafness. They hold that deafness is not a disability, but is rather a natural human variation and therefore does not need to be treated medically.[3] Support for their position has also been strong among some educators of the deaf and even among some medical and communication disorders professionals.

Initially, arguments against the cochlear implant were based on claims that congenitally deaf children do not derive benefit from cochlear implants. However, an increasing body of data supports that, given the appropriate circumstances, congenitally deaf children can indeed derive significant benefit from cochlear implants.[4-7] This has led to a revision of the argument to confirm that even though cochlear implants do work for congenitally deaf children, for other moral and ethical reasons, they should not be used in this population. Both concepts will be discussed in this chapter.

Congenitally Deaf Children Cannot Benefit from Implants

Initially, arguments against use of the implant in congenitally deaf children centered on the idea that individuals without prior exposure to speech and language could not make use of the information provided by the implant. Early in its development, the cochlear implant was seen primarily as an aid to speechreading, and there was little expectation that open-set speech recognition without visual cues was a realistic goal. Postlinguistically deafened adults with well-developed oral language were able to use a combination of speechreading and contextual information together with the auditory cues provided by the implant to improve communication abilities. Early results with prelinguistically deafened adults were not as promising, leading some researches to suggest that loss of hearing before speech and language acquisition was a significant deterrent to successful cochlear implant use, possibly due to lasting effects of auditory deprivation.[1]

Studies such as those conducted by Shepherd et al.,[8] Matsushima et al.,[9] Lousteau,[10] and Hartshorn et al.[11] have provided evidence that suggests otherwise. Animal studies have shown that even in the presence of the auditory deprivation caused by congenital deafness, some cochleotopic organization remains and that electrical stimulation may both prevent degenerative changes in the neural pathways and may in fact produce morphologic and physiologic changes that improve function. Obviously, the longer the period of deprivation, the greater the negative impact; the positive benefit of the implant decreases. This has implications when considering implantation of older congenitally deaf children and adolescents who have not been consistent users of amplification.

What at first appeared to be decreased ability to benefit from an implant has generally come to be recognized as a developmental issue. Instead of comparing the information provided by a cochlear implant to an existing store of auditory language as in the case of a postlinguistically deafened user, the congenitally deaf implant recipient must use the information to develop language, as would any infant. The normally hearing infant spends the first year of life listening and receiving language before beginning to use it expressively. Therefore, the time course of 1 to 2 years required to see substantial results with congenitally deaf implant users[12] is developmentally appropriate.

Ethical Opposition to Cochlear Implants in Congenitally Deaf Children

Cochlear implants are one example in which technological advances have come into direct conflict with cultural values. Others include organ transplantation, gene manipulation, and artificial life-support systems. Cochlear implants, viewed as a medical achievement with the potential to alleviate the loss of a major sensory system by the medical community, represent confirmation to members of the deaf community that they are viewed as inferior and should be eliminated from the population. What appears as a solution to a problem by some is viewed as a "final solution" to a people and a way of life by others. Members and supporters of the deaf world consider those who communicate exclusively through American sign language (ASL) to represent an oppressed linguistic minority. They view attempts to provide hearing to deaf children as racist and genocidal.[13] Opposition to cochlear implants from members of the deaf world does not arise out of concern that they do not work, but rather that they work well enough to allow the child to reject deaf culture in favor of mainstream society. We have written extensively on this conflict[14-17] and summarize those works in this discussion.

In order to understand why cochlear implant technology is perceived as a significant threat by the deaf community, it is important to note that 90% of deaf children are born to hearing parents and 97% have at least one hearing parent.[3] If the deaf world is to continue, the children of hearing parents must continue to embrace the language and culture of deafness. Traditionally, this culture and language have been absorbed by deaf children at residential schools where teachers, house parents, and peers are generally themselves members of the deaf community. If parents are given a safe and effective means of enabling their children to remain at home and enter the educational mainstream, many children could be lost to the deaf community. Ultimately, this could have a serious impact on the perpetuation of deaf culture and language. The desire of parents to keep their children at home received national support in the passage by Congress of Public Laws 94-142 and 99-457. These laws ensure that all handicapped children will be educated in the "least restrictive" or most normal environment.

By contrast, deaf world proponents hold the position that children born deaf are ipso facto members of the deaf community and that hearing parents are obliged to allow the child to assume his or her place in that community. This is best accomplished through residential school placement where language, culture, and values are taught by culturally deaf adults, rather than by the parents. This process of "horizontal acculturation" is threatened when children remain in the home and develop the oral language that enables them to be "vertically" acculturated by parents, grandparents, and other family members, as is the norm in our society.

Some members of the deaf community believe that hearing parents are not capable of making appropriate decisions for their deaf children since they are not members of the same community and culture. According to Roz Rosen, past president of the National Association for the Deaf, "hearing parents are not qualified to make decisions about implants."[18] Harlan Lane, a hearing supporter of deaf culture states that hearing parents are "in a conflict of interest with their own child." Furthermore, he has suggested that a culturally Deaf adult should serve as the child's advocate rather than the parent.[13]

This conflict leads to two ethical questions: who should decide for the child? and according to what standards should the decision be made? Regardless of the decision to be made, three well-established standards for surrogate decision making should guide the process. First is the advance directive through which the affected individual has made his or her own wishes known as in the use of a living will. Second is substituted judgment, in which someone close to the individual makes a decision based on what he or she knows to reflect the wishes of the affected individual. Members of the deaf world argue that once the child grows up to be a deaf person with deaf culture values, he or she would not want a cochlear implant. By contrast, no one can in reality foresee what the child may ultimately desire as an adult. Neither of these two standards can realistically be applied to young children. The third standard is that of best interest. In this case the surrogate decision maker is expected to choose a course of action that will ultimately be most beneficial to the affected individual. This standard of surrogate decision making is most appropriate in decisions made for young children.

That the family is in the best position to decide what is in the child's best interest is generally a given in medical ethics. It is assumed that because parents bear the responsibility for all aspects of the child's life and will bear the-long term financial and emotional consequences of any decision made, it is the family who will strive to make the decisions that are in fact in the child's best interest overall. According to Buchanan and Brock,[19] "there must be a clear locus of authority or decision making will lack coherence, continuity, and accountability." Only someone who has responsibility for all aspects of the child's life can provide that continuity and accountability. Decision making by a culturally deaf adult who bears no real responsibility for the child would violate the principle of a clear locus of authority. Only the parents, family, or a legally appointed guardian can fulfill such a role. There is recent evidence that deaf leaders have begun to reconsider and are now willing to concede that the parent is the appropriate surrogate decision maker.[20]

Given that the cochlear implant works and that parents have the right to choose implantation for their child, the conflict that then arises is between the parties who are trying to influence the parental decision. It is vital that parents, in order to make a decision that is in their child's best interest, do it from a well-informed position. The ethical value of truthfulness must be respected by both proponents and opponents of cochlear implants if parents are to be enabled to make a fully informed decision. Cochlear implant surgeons are ethically responsible to obtain an informed consent from parents in which the risks of the surgery are outlined. It is also incumbent on the parents to ensure that parents have a full understanding of not only the benefits but also the limitations of the technology. Parents must be made fully aware of the intensive rehabilitation necessary if the child is to derive maximum benefit. They must also be aware of the many trips that will be required to the implant center over the years, as well as prepared for the inevitable equipment breakdowns, and probably worst of all, they must be informed that the internal device may fail requiring another surgery in the future. No cochlear implant team, which adheres to standards of medical ethics, would lead parents to believe that the implant is an easy fix. Members of cochlear implant teams should inform parents that there is an alternative lifestyle available to their child that they should explore prior to making a decision.

Proponents of that lifestyle (i.e., members of the deaf world) should as well be truthful with parents about both the pros and the cons that face the child entering their community. Members of the deaf community are bonded by their use of ASL, which is a language separate from English, and not merely English in a manual code. They have their own social and political organizations, participate in Deaf Olympics and Miss Deaf pageants. They marry and raise children and attend churches and theater all within their own ASL-based community. To them it is a rich and rewarding life within, but apart from, mainstream culture.

However, just as with cochlear implants, there are negative aspects associated with acculturation into the deaf world of which parents should be made aware. As has been mentioned earlier, the primary avenue of acculturation into the deaf world is through attendance at residential schools for the deaf. When parents of deaf children visit such schools, they need to be informed that the average reading level of a graduate is approximately third grade, and that three out of four graduates cannot read a newspaper.[21] They should also be informed that deafness is associated with the lowest educational level, the lowest family income, the lowest percentage working, and the poorest assessment of well being among all disabilities.[22] Parents considering the benefits of the deaf community for their child should be aware of the gap that inevitably develops between the child and his or her extended, if not immediate, family due to an inability to communicate effectively. Other members of the deaf community in effect become the child's family. Although an individual can indeed live a full life as a member of the deaf community, the child's ability to participate in mainstream society is severely limited by the need for an interpreter in all interactions with hearing persons.

Finally, just as it is important for cochlear implant proponents to acknowledge that there are positive aspects of the deaf community, members of the deaf community have an ethical responsibility to stem the flow of misinformation about cochlear implants, which pervades their intracommunity communication sources. Because there is no written form of ASL, many in the deaf community are dependent on informal sources for information about implants (as well as other newsworthy items). Numerous examples of misleading and pejorative statements have fueled opposition to implants among members of the deaf community:

> There is absolutely no question that our government has a hidden agenda for deaf children much akin to Nazi experiments on Holocaust victims[23]
>
> [the surgeon was] eager to use his skills on 17 Deaf individuals... Three died due to complications and one became mentally ill. The rest were failures.[24]
>
> I feel that cochlear implants are wrong because it makes the recipient a robot with wires sticking out of their head.[25]
>
> Using deaf children as lab rats and medical guinea pigs is profoundly disturbing.[26]

None of these statements has any basis in fact, but each has been used as an effective tool in influencing how deaf people view cochlear implants. The ethical value of truthfulness has clearly been violated by these statements.

Summary

Even as one source of the controversy is resolved, others emerge. There remains little concern about the effectiveness of cochlear implants as a sensory aid for both adults and children. Given appropriate candidate selection and follow-up, cochlear implants provide adequate auditory input to enable a young child to develop functional oral language and speech. Yet the conflict remains. By doing just that, it has been suggested that the use of cochlear implants violates United Nations conventions against limiting the growth of linguistic minorities. The question that must then be answered is: which is more important—the best interest of the individual child, or the best interest of deaf culture? It is a question any parent can easily answer, but it cannot be agreed upon by ethicists.

Another controversy with which cochlear implant teams struggle on a routine basis is that of candidacy criteria. Evidence continues to mount that children in aurally based oral rehabilitation programs derive greater measurable benefit from cochlear implants than do children receiving visually based rehabilitation. Yet, if it is indeed a parental decision as has been argued by implant proponents, can implant teams refuse to implant children based on the rehabilitation mode? Is the implant team's responsibility fulfilled by informing the parents that the child will be unlikely to derive maximum benefit from the device in the current rehabilitation setting, or does the implant team have the right to deny the child an implant based on their own beliefs? An issue that remains controversial today is the age at which children should be considered for implant surgery. For many years, the age of 2 was accepted as the lower limit for implantation. As both implants and means of identifying infant hearing loss have improved, that limit has been challenged. In fact, the FDA recently recommended that the age limit be reduced to 18 months. There seems to be indication that younger is better, but no one is sure if there is a lower age beyond which the benefit decreases. Theories of early critical periods of language learning would seem to support earlier implantation, whereas the difficulty in quantifying and establishing the quality of residual hearing in infants together with surgical concerns continues to remain deterrents to implantation below 18 months.

Controversy has been a fact of pediatric cochlear implantation from the beginning. Efficacy, safety, ethics, and candidacy issues have all been sources of controversy at one time or another. As one source of conflict is resolved, another arises. The future may see controversy arise over such issues as best device choice, use of bilateral implants, and whether to save a better ear for future developments, such as hair cell regeneration.

REFERENCES

1. Clark GM. Historical perspectives. In: Clark GM, Cowan RS, Dowell RC, eds. *Cochlear Implantation for Infants and Children*. London: Singular Publishing Group; Inc. 1997, 9–28
2. National Institutes of Health. *Consensus Statement on Cochlear Implants*. Rockville MD: NIH; 1995
3. Paul PV, Quigley SP. *Education and Deafness*. New York: Longman; 1990
4. Miyamoto RT, Osberger MJ, Robbins AM, et al. Longitudinal evaluation of communication skills of children with single or multichannel cochlear implants. *Am J Otol* 1992:13:215
5. Waltzman SB, Cohen NL, Gomolin R, et al. Long-term results of early cochlear implantation in congenitally and prelingually deafened children. *Am J Otol* 1994;14:9–13
6. Waltzman SB, Cohen NL, Gomolin RH, et al. Open set speech perception in congenitally deaf children using cochlear implants. *Am J Otol* 1997;18:342–349
7. Hodges AV, Dolan-Ash MM, Butts SL, Balkany TJ. Speech perception results in children with cochlear implants: contributing factors. *Otolaryngol Head Neck Surg* 1999;121:31–34
8. Shepherd RK, Hartman R, Heid S, et al. The central auditory system and auditory deprivation: experience with cochlear implants in the congenitally deaf. *Acta Otolaryngol* 1997;532(suppl):28–33
9. Matsushima JI, Shepherd RK, Seldon HL, et al. Electrical stimulation of the auditory nerve in deaf kittens: effects on cochlear nucleus morphology. *Hear Res* 1991;56:133–142
10. Lousteau RJ. Increased spiral ganglion cell survival in electrically stimulated deafened guinea pig cochleae. *Laryngoscope* 1987;97:836–842
11. Hartshorn DO, Miller JM, Altschuler RA. Protective effect of electrical stimulation in the deafened guinea pig cochlea. *Otolaryngol Head Neck Surg* 1991;104:311–319
12. Fryauf-Bertschy H, Tyler RS, Kelsay DM, et al. Performance over time of congenitally deaf and postlingually deafened children using a multichannel cochlear implant. *J Speech Hear Res* 1992;35:913–920
13. Lane H. *The mask of benevolence*. New York: Vintage; 1993
14. Balkany TJ. A brief perspective on cochlear implants. *N Engl J* 1993;328:281–282
15. Balkany TJ. The rescuers and cochlear implantation: habilitation or genocide? *Adv Otorhinolaryngol* 1995;50:4–8
16. Balkany TJ, Hodges AV. Misleading the deaf community about cochlear implantation in children. *Ann Otolaryngol* 1995;104:148–149
17. Balkany TJ, Hodges AV, Goodman KW. Ethics of cochlear implantation in young children. *Arch Otolaryngol Head Neck Surg* 1996;114:748–755
18. Coffey R. Caitlin's story on "60 Minutes." *The bicultural center news* 1992;53:3
19. Buchanan AE, Brock DW. *Deciding for Other: The Ethics of Surrogate Decision Making*. Cambridge: Cambridge University Press; 1989
20. Lane H, Hoffmeister R, Bahan B. *A Journey into the Deaf World*. San Diego: Dawn Sign Press; 1996
21. Conrad R. *The Deaf School Child: Language and Cognitive Functioning*. New York: Harper and Row; 1979
22. Harris JP, Anderson JP, Novak R. An outcome study of cochlear implants in deaf patients. *Arch Otolaryngol Head Neck Surg* 1995;121:398–404
23. Silver A. Cochlear implant: surefire prescription for long-term disaster. *TBC News* 1992;53:4–5
24. Andersson Y. Do we want cochlear implants? *World Fed Deaf News* 1994;1:3–4
25. Gallaudet Student letter to the William House Cochlear Implant Study Group. Committee of the American Academy of Otolaryngology Head and Neck Surgery, 1993
26. Roots J. Deaf Canadian fighting back. *World Fed Deaf News*, 1994;2:2–3

Cochlear Implants in Congenitally Deaf Children*

CHAPTER 80

Richard T. Miyamoto, Karen Iler Kirk, and Laurie S. Eisenberg

In 1990, the Food and Drug Administration (FDA) first gave approval for cochlear implantation in children aged 2 to 18 years. Initially, children who received a cochlear implant (CI) had total profound deafness, and most were older than 5 years of age. Early speech perception results demonstrated that congenitally or prelingually deafened children with a CI displayed substantial closed-set abilities (e.g., wherein children identify a word by selecting from a limited set of response alternatives), but only minimal open-set spoken word recognition abilities (i.e., in which no response alternatives are provided).[1,2] Since then, as cochlear implantation has been extended clinically to younger children, and with continued improvements in electrode design and signal processing,[3-6] pediatric CI recipients have achieved much higher levels of open-set word recognition.[7-13] For example, Eisenberg and colleagues[14] reported mean Phonetically Balanced Kindergarten word lists (PB-K) scores of approximately 50% words correct for oral pediatric CI users. Open-set word recognition is an important diagnostic yardstick for determining cochlear implant success because it indicates that these children have established neural representations of words in their long-term lexical memory, a process that is fundamental to the development of spoken language.[15] Although these average results are very encouraging and clearly establish the efficacy of CIs, individual patients vary greatly in outcome.[1-3,13,16-21] Some children can communicate extremely well using the auditory/oral modality and acquire age-appropriate language skills, whereas other children display only minimal spoken word recognition skills or demonstrate severe language delays, or both.[22-27] Accounting for this enormous variability in the effectiveness of CIs on a wide range of outcome measures presents the most serious challenge facing cochlear implant clinicians and researchers today. Gaining an understanding of the nature of the individual differences and sources of variability in cochlear implant outcomes is crucial for predicting individual benefits before implantation and for selecting appropriate intervention strategies after implantation.

Despite the variability in individual outcomes, cochlear implantation is no longer questioned as a therapeutic option for children with prelingual deafness. However, in part because the outcomes are not guaranteed, controversy exists regarding the appropriate expansion of evolving technology into new patient populations. The current trend toward earlier implantation and the implantation of children with more residual hearing mandates careful documentation of performance limits with cochlear implants as well as with nonsurgical alternatives (e.g., hearing aids). Only through rigorous longitudinal studies will these issues be clarified. This chapter reviews current implant technology, patient selection criteria, and performance results for pediatric cochlear implant recipients and considers the challenges inherent in the broadening of cochlear implant candidacy.

*This work was supported in part by research grants 2 RO1 DC 00064, RO1 DC00423, and K08 DC00126 from the National Institute on Deafness and Other Communication Disorders, National Institutes of Health, and by Psi Iota Xi.

Background

PEDIATRIC COCHLEAR IMPLANT SELECTION CRITERIA

Current selection criteria for pediatric cochlear implantation include the following:

- ≥ 12 months of age
- Severe to profound bilateral sensorineural hearing loss (SNHL)
- Minimal benefit from hearing aids
- No medical contraindications
- High motivation and appropriate expectations
- Enrollment in a program that emphasizes development of auditory skills

COCHLEAR IMPLANT SYSTEMS

The cochlear implant devices available for implantation, as well as the speech processing strategies used, continue to undergo technologic improvements. Currently, three types of multichannel, multielectrode cochlear implant devices are commercially available for children in the United States. These devices have several characteristics in common. All have an electrode array that is surgically implanted into the cochlea and an external unit, consisting of a microphone that picks up sound energy and converts it to an electric signal, and a signal processor that modifies the signal, depending on the processing scheme in use. The processed signal is amplified and compressed to match the narrow electrical dynamic range of the ear. (The typical response range of the ear to electrical stimulation is on the order of only 10 to 20 dB, and even less in the high frequencies.) Transmission of the electrical signal across the skin from the external unit to the implanted electrode array is most commonly accomplished by the use of electromagnetic induction or radiofrequency transmission. The neural elements stimulated appear to be the spiral ganglion cells or axons. These devices use place coding to transfer frequency information in addition to providing temporal and amplitude information.

The Nucleus (Cochlear Corporation, Englewood, CA) family of cochlear implant systems (the 22-channel and 24-channel devices) are currently the most commonly used multichannel system. The Nucleus implantable electrode array consists of platinum-iridium band electrodes placed in a silastic carrier.[28] Several generations of speech processors have been employed with the Nucleus multichannel cochlear implant. The initial Nucleus speech processors used a feature-extraction scheme in which selected key features of speech were presented through the implanted electrode array. An early speech processing strategy, the F0F1F2 strategy, primarily conveyed vowel information, including the first and second formant frequencies and their amplitudes, as well as voice pitch. A later coding scheme, the MULTIPEAK strategy, presented these acoustic features along with additional information from three high-frequency spectral bands to aid in consonant perception. One current Nucleus speech processing strategy is the Spectral Peak (SPEAK) strategy. This strategy uses a vocoder in which a filterbank consisting of 20 filters covering the center frequencies from 200 to 10,000 Hz is employed. Each filter is allocated to an active electrode in the array. The filter outputs are scanned and the electrodes that are stimulated represent filters that contain speech components with the highest amplitude. Depending on the acoustic input, the number of spectral maxima detected, and thus the number of electrodes stimulated, on each scan cycle can vary from one to ten, with an average of six per cycle. The rate at which the electrodes are stimulated varies adaptively at 180 to 300 pulses per second.

The Clarion multichannel cochlear implant (Advanced Bionics, Sylmar, CA) has an eight-channel electrode array that uses a radial bipolar configuration through electrode pairs positioned adjacent to the osseous spiral lamina in a 90-degree orientation.[29] The Clarion multichannel cochlear implant offers two types of speech-processing strategies: simultaneous analog stimulation (SAS) and continuous interleaved sampling (CIS). Both strategies represent the waveform or envelope of the speech signal.[30] The Clarion SAS strategy first compresses the analog signal into the restricted range for electrically evoked hearing and then filters the signal into a maximum of eight channels for presentation to the corresponding electrodes. Speech information is conveyed via the relative amplitudes and the temporal details contained in each channel. The CIS strategy filters the incoming speech into eight bands, obtains the speech envelope, and compresses the signal for each channel. Stimulation consists of interleaved digital pulses that sweep rapidly through the channels at a rate of 833 pulses per second when using all eight channels for a maximum pulse rate of 6664 pulses per second ($8 \times 833 = 6{,}664$). With the CIS strategy, rapid changes in the speech signal are tracked by rapid variations in pulse amplitude. The pulses are delivered to consecutive channels in sequence to avoid channel interaction.

The MED-EL COMBI 40-Cochlear Implant system (Medical Electronics, Innsbruck, Austria) uses the CIS (continuous interleaved sampling) strategy, which provides both spectral and temporal resolution. Up to eight active electrodes can be used. The electrode array used has the capability of deep insertion into the apical regions of the cochlea.[31] The MED-EL has the capacity to provide the most rapid stimulation rate of any of the currently available implants (maximum of 12,000 biphasic pulses per second).[32]

SURGICAL IMPLANTATION

Cochlear implantation in children requires meticulous attention to the delicate tissues and small dimensions. Skin incisions are designed to provide access to the mastoid process and coverage of the external portion of the implant package while preserving the blood supply of the postauricular skin. The incision employed at the Indiana University Medical Center has eliminated the need to develop a large postauricular flap. The inferior extent of the incision is made well posterior to the mastoid tip to preserve the branches of the postauricular artery. From here the incision is directed posterosuperiorly and is then directed superiorly without an superior anterior limb. In children, the incision incorporates the temporalis muscle to give added thickness. A subperiosteal pocket is created for positioning the implant induction coil. A bone well tailored to the device being implanted is created, and the induction coil is fixed to the cortex with a fixation suture or periosteal flaps.

After the development of the skin incision, a mastoidectomy is performed. The horizontal semicircular canal is identified in the depths of the mastoid antrum, and the short process of the incus is identified in the fossa incudis. The facial recess is opened using the fossa incudis as an initial landmark. The facial recess is a triangular area bounded by (1) the fossa incudis superiorly, (2) the chorda tympani nerve laterally and anteriorly, and (3) the facial nerve medially and posteriorly. The facial nerve can usually be visualized through the bone without exposing it. The round window niche is visualized through the facial recess approximately 2 mm inferior to the stapes. Occasionally, the round window niche is posteriorly positioned and is not well visualized through the facial recess or is obscured by ossification. Particularly in these situations, it is important not to be misdirected by hypotympanic air cells. Entry into the scala tympani is best accomplished through a cochleostomy created anterior and inferior to the annulus of the round window membrane. A small fenestra slightly larger than the electrode to be implanted (usually 0.5 mm) is developed. A small diamond burr is used to "blue line" the endosteum of the scala tympani, and the endosteal membrane is removed with small picks. This approach bypasses the hook area of the scala tympani allowing direct insertion of the active electrode array. After insertion of the active electrode array, the round window area is sealed with small pieces of fascia.

SPECIAL SURGICAL CONSIDERATIONS

In cases of cochlear dysplasia, a cerebrospinal fluid (CSF) gusher may be encountered. The senior author prefers to enter the cochlea through a small fenestra and tightly pack the electrode at the cochleostomy with fascia. The flow of CSF has been successfully controlled in this way. In patients with severe malformations of the labyrinth, the facial nerve may follow an aberrant course. In these cases, the most direct access to a common cavity deformity may be by a transmastoid labyrinthotomy approach. The otic capsule is opened posterosuperior to the second genu of the facial nerve, and the common cavity is entered directly. Four patients have been treated in this way with no vestibular side effects.[33]

In cases of cochlear ossification, our preference is to drill open the basal turn and create a tunnel approximately 6 mm in length and partially insert a Nucleus electrode. This approach permits implantation of 10 to 12 active electrodes, yielding very satisfactory results. Gantz et al.[34] described an extensive drill-out procedure to gain access to the upper basal turn. The benefits of this extended procedure are under investigation. Steenerson et al.[35] described the insertion of the active electrode into the scala vestibuli in cases of cochlear ossification. This procedure has merit. However, the scala vestibuli is frequently ossified when the scala tympani is completely obliterated.

RESULTS OF COCHLEAR IMPLANTATION IN CHILDREN

Nucleus Cochlear Implant Systems

Pediatric clinical trials with the Nucleus 22-channel cochlear implant began in 1986, and in 1990 the FDA approved this device for use in children. The children originally implanted with the Nucleus 22-channel system used the F0F1F2 feature extraction speech-processing strategy. Children implanted after 1989 were provided with the Multipeak (MPEAK) strategy, and the Spectral Peak (SPEAK) strategy was approved in 1994. Pediatric clinical trials for the Nucleus 24-channel device with the SPEAK strategy were initiated in April 1997, and FDA approval was granted in June 1998.

One of the first large-scale reports of pediatric performance with the Nucleus cochlear implant was presented by Staller et al.[2] These investigators presented speech perception data from 80 children with the Nucleus 22-channel cochlear implant system who were tested as part of the FDA clinical trials. The mean age at onset of deafness was 2 years, 8 months, and the mean age at implantation was 9 years, 10 months for this group of children. The children's performance was classified by the highest category of speech perception achieved. Comparisons were made between their speech perception performance preimplant and again at 12 months postimplant. After 12 months of cochlear implant use, 63% of children showed significant improvements in the closed-set speech perception tasks and 46% of children demonstrated significant improvements on at least one open-set speech perception task. However, open-set speech abilities were still relatively modest. Similar word-recognition results were reported by Osberger et al.[1] for 28 children. Their results demonstrated that the children's speech perception abilities improved significantly after implantation with the largest gains noted when stimuli were presented in the auditory-plus-visual modality (i.e., with visual and lipreading cues). Thus, most children tested with the early Nucleus cochlear implant processing strategies demonstrated at least some open-set word recognition and performance was generally good when both auditory and visual cues were available.

The introduction of newer-generation Nucleus processing strategies yielded greater speech perception benefits in children, just as in adults. Osberger et al.[36] compared the performance of six children who used the F0F1F2 processing strategy with that of six children who used the MPEAK strategy. The children in each group were matched by age at onset of deafness and age at implantation. After 1 year of implant use, the children with the MPEAK device were significantly better at discriminating vowel height and consonant place of articulation cues on the Minimal Pairs Test. However, the two groups did not differ after 3 years of cochlear implant use. The authors concluded that children show an accelerated rate of learning with improved speech processing strategies. Similar improvements have been noted for children who switch from the MPEAK to the SPEAK processing strategies.[8,12,37] Sehgal et al.[12] compared word-recognition scores for children who switched from an earlier processing strategy with the SPEAK processing strategy. These investigators reported mean monosyllabic word recognition scores increased from 28% words correct with the earlier strategy to 58% words correct with the SPEAK strategy.

Clarion Cochlear Implant System

Pediatric clinical trials of the Clarion multichannel cochlear implant system began in 1995, and the device received FDA approval for use in children in 1997. Zimmerman-Phillips et al.[38] summarized the initial results of the children's preoperative performance with hearing aids compared with their postoperative performance with the Clarion device. The mean age of the group of children implanted by 1996 was approximately 5 years (n = 124). Data were reported for children tested at 3 months postimplant (n = 60) and 6 months postimplant (n = 23). After only 3 months of device use, mean scores were higher than the preimplant performance, and many of the children demonstrated some open-set speech recognition. By 6 months postimplant, mean word-recognition scores were 23% for the PB-K and 38% for a test of word recognition in a sentence context, the Glendonald Auditory Screening Procedure (GASP).[39] In a second study, Osberger et al.[11] examined the performance of children implanted with the Clarion device after the age of 5 years who had at least 6 months of device experience (n = 30). The children were divided into two groups based on communication method. After 6 months of device use, children in the oral group correctly identified an average of 27% of the words on the PB-K. The average PB-K word score for children in the total communication group was 8% correct.

Med-El Cochlear Implant System

Pediatric FDA clinical trials for the Med-El device were initiated in 1998. To date, too few children in the United States have used their devices long enough to draw conclusions regarding the benefits to be received by these children.

Summary of Pediatric Results

Children with multichannel cochlear implants demonstrate significant improvements in closed-set speech discrimination and enhanced lipreading ability, and most obtain some open-set speech understanding with their devices. The rate of auditory skills development seems to be increasing as cochlear implant technology improves and cochlear implant candidacy is broadened to include younger children and children with more residual hearing. For example, early studies reported significant increases in the discrimination of nonsegmental speech cues after only 6 months of implant use. However, significant increases in the discrimination of vowel and consonant features were not evident until 1.5 years of cochlear implant experience and auditory-only open-set skills continued to improve long after this time period. More recent studies have shown that many children achieve open-set speech recognition within the first year of device use,[10,11] but these skills still continue to develop over time.[16,17,36,41,42] In fact, Miyamoto et al.[41] noted continued improvements in spoken word recognition even after 5 years of multichannel cochlear implant use. These findings highlight the need to conduct longitudinal studies in order to determine the ultimate benefits of implant use in children.

DEMOGRAPHIC INFLUENCES ON CI PERFORMANCE IN CHILDREN WITH PRELINGUAL DEAFNESS

Age at implantation, length of cochlear implant use, communication mode, and amount of residual hearing before implantation are all demographic factors that have been shown to influence performance results in children with congenital or prelingual deafness. However, age at onset of deafness does not influence performance for this group of children. The speech perception performance of pediatric CI recipients with congenital deafness is similar to that of their peers with adventitious deafness acquired before age 3 years.[43] These results suggest that both groups of children can benefit from similar intervention strategies.

Age at Implantation

Previous studies have shown that earlier implantation yields superior cochlear implant performance. For example, Fryauf-Bertschy et al.[17] demonstrated that children implanted before age 5 displayed significantly better open-set word recognition than did those implanted at a later age. Similar results were reported by Miyamoto et al.[44] Next, Waltzman and colleagues conducted several studies to examine the speech perception abilities of children who were all implanted before the age of 5 years (2 to 5 years).[45-47] Waltzman et al.[46] reported the performance results of 14 children who were implanted before age 3 years and had used their device for at least 3 years. After 1 year of implant use, seven of the children demonstrated consistent open-set speech perception abilities. After 2 years, this number increased to 13 children. The mean word recognition score at 3-years postimplant was 47% correct. Similar performance results also were reported for a group of 11 children implanted before 2 years of age.[45]

Residual Hearing

The presence of preimplant residual hearing has also been shown to have a positive effect on postimplant speech perception performance. Zwolan and colleagues[48] compared the postoperative performance of 12 children who demonstrated some aided open-set speech recognition preimplant (the borderline candidacy group) with that of 12 matched controls who had no preimplant speech recognition (the traditional candidacy group). Candidacy for the study participation was based on preimplant binaural aided speech testing, and the children were subsequently implanted in their poorer hearing ear. Thus, mean preoperative audiograms did not differ for the implanted ears in the two groups. By 1 year postimplant, children in the borderline group had significantly higher scores than children in the traditional group on all six speech perception measures employed. Zwolan and colleagues suggested that increased auditory experience before implantation facilitated the development of speech perception skills postimplant.

More recently, Gantz et al.[49] demonstrated that children with greater residual hearing before implantation might achieve the highest levels of spoken word recognition with a cochlear implant. Gantz and colleagues suggested that children with limited preimplant residual hearing are better able to use the auditory information provided via a cochlear implant because they have more intact auditory systems, including inner hair cells, dendrites, ganglion cells, and central pathways, than their peers who have no preimplant residual hearing or word recognition.

Discussion

With the goal of universal detection of hearing loss in infants by 3 months of age, and appropriate intervention (e.g., amplification) by 6 months of age,[50,51] it is likely that ever-increasing numbers of very young children will be identified as potential implant candidates. We know that early identification (i.e., by 6 months of age) and early intervention with hearing aids (HAs) have a significant effect on language development in children with hearing loss,[52] but the spoken word recognition and receptive language benefits of early implantation in children with profound deafness have not been quantified, and critical age limits for cochlear implantation have not been identified.

Cochlear implantation earlier than the current FDA accepted age of 12 months is feasible as the target organ, the cochlea, is adult size at birth. The small dimensions of the temporal bone must be accounted for, but the facial recess and mastoid antrum that provide access to the middle ear for electrode placement are adequately developed before the age of 1 year. In fact, several centers have chosen to implant children under 12 months of age. Furthermore, implanting children under the age of 12 months may have substantial advantages when the etiology of deafness is meningitis. Progressive intracochlear fibrosis and ossification may occur, which can preclude standard electrode insertion. A relatively short window exists during which this advancing process can be circumvented.

Nonetheless, implantation of the very young child remains controversial because the audiological assessment and management of this population is extremely challenging. Profound deafness must be substantiated and the inability to benefit from conventional hearing aids demonstrated. However, a compelling argument supporting implantation at the earliest possible time can be made because the development of speech perception, speech production, and language competence normally begins early in infancy. In addition, electrical stimulation has been shown to prevent at least some of the degenerative changes in the central auditory pathways caused by auditory deprivation.[53]

The extension of cochlear implantation to children with ever higher levels of preimplant residual hearing should be approached cautiously. Surgical implantation of the electrode array results in the loss of residual hearing in that ear. Thus, cochlear implantation should not be considered unless it seems likely that a given child will receive more benefit from this device than from conventional amplification. Recently, mounting evidence has been found to suggest that some children with severe hearing loss may derive as much or even more benefit from a cochlear implant than as from a well-fitted HA. In amplifying sound for an individual with hearing loss, an assumption is made that the acoustic–phonetic patterns of speech must be detected before they can be discriminated and recognized. To accomplish this goal, audibility across a broad frequency range is typically prescribed as a means of maximizing speech intelligibility.[54] This, in fact, has been the goal of most standard HA prescriptions. For severe to profound losses, however, supplying adequate gain across a broad frequency range can present a special challenge to the clinician. Moreover, achieving this amount of amplification may cause acoustic feedback, necessitating a reduction in gain and audibility.[55] Another issue concerns the risk of delivering high levels of sound to the impaired ear. According to Macrae,[56,57] the sound pressure level required to achieve audibility for individuals with severe to profound hearing loss has the potential to destroy remaining hair cells due to excessive noise exposure. Thus, a trade-off may exist between providing audible speech and risking increased damage to inner ear structures. Lastly, there is some question as to the extent of benefit that may actually be realized by amplifying high frequencies to audible levels for this magnitude of loss. Recent research has suggested that provision of adequate audibility for losses of > 60 dB HL at ≥ 3000 Hz does not improve speech recognition and may even degrade performance.[58-60] Preliminary research has suggested that some children with cochlear implants obtain spoken word recognition abilities that surpass those of other children with severe hearing loss (i.e., pure tone averages (PTAs) of 70 to 90 dB HL) who use well-fit HAs.[14,61,62] Given the limitations imposed in providing high levels of amplified speech to children with severe to profound hearing loss, the evidence suggests that a cochlear implant could provide added benefit for a select population of children with this magnitude of hearing loss.

The encouraging results obtained with younger children and those who have some useful hearing prior to implantation have led investigators to push the boundaries of cochlear implantation criteria further than ever before. With the continued evolution and expansion of cochlear implant candidacy it is crucial that we develop techniques to quantify hearing loss, to fit both hearing aids and cochlear implants, and to document the effects of implantation in these very young children.

REFERENCES

1. Osberger MJ, Miyamoto RT, Zimmerman-Phillips S, et al. Independent evaluation of the speech perception abilities of children with the Nucleus 22-channel cochlear implant system. *Ear Hear* 1991;12(suppl):66S–80S
2. Staller S, Beiter AL, Brimacombe JA, et al. Pediatric performance with the Nucleus 22-channel cochlear implant system. *Am J Otol* 1991;12:126–136
3. Staller SJ. Clinical trials of the Nucleus 24 in adults and children. Presented at the tenth annual convention of the American Academy of Audiology, Los Angeles, CA; 1998
4. Wilson BS. Signal processing. In: Tyler RS, editor. *Cochlear Implants: Audiological Foundations.* San Diego: Singular; 1993:35–85
5. Wilson BS, Lawson DT, Finley CC, Wolford RD. Coding strategies for multichannel cochlear prostheses. *Am J Otol* 1991;12(suppl 1):56–61
6. Wilson BS, Lawson DT, Finley CC, Wolford RD. Importance of patient and processor variables in determining outcomes with cochlear implants. *J Speech Hear Res* 1993;36:373–379
7. Cowan RSC, DelDot J, Barker EJ, et al. Speech perception results for children with implants with different levels of preoperative residual hearing. *Am J Otol* 1997;18:125–126
8. Cowan RSC, Galvin KL, Klieve S, et al. Contributing factors to improved speech perception in children using the Nucleus 22-channel cochlear prosthesis. In: Honjo I, Takahashi H, editors. *Cochlear Implant and Related Sciences Update.* Advances in Otorhinolaryngology, vol 52. Basel: Karger; 1997:193–197
9. Kirk KI, Pisoni DB, Osberger MJ. Lexical effects on spoken word recognition by pediatric cochlear implant users. *Ear Hear* 1995;16:470–481
10. Miyamoto RT, Kirk KI, Svirsky MA, Sehgal ST. Communication skills in pediatric cochlear implant recipients. *Acta Otolaryngol* (Stockh) 1999;119:219–224
11. Osberger MJ, Fisher L, Zimmerman-Phillips S, et al. Speech recognition performance of older children with cochlear implants. *Am J Otol* 1998;19:152–157
12. Sehgal ST, Kirk KI, Svirsky MA, Miyamoto RT. The effects of processor strategy on the speech perception performance of

pediatric Nucleus multichannel cochlear implant users. *Ear Hear* 1998;19:149–161

13. Zimmerman-Phillips S, Osberger MJ, Robbins AM. *Infant Toddler Meaningful Auditory Integration Scale (IT-MAIS).* Sylmar, CA: Advanced Bionics; 1997
14. Eisenberg LS, Martinez AS, Sennaroglu G, Osberger MJ. Establishing new criteria in selecting children for a cochlear implant: performance of "platinum" hearing aid users. *Ann Otol Rhinol Laryngol.* In press
15. Woodward AL, Markman EM. Early word learning. In: Damon W, Kuhn D, Siegler R, editors. *Handbook of Child Psychology.* Vol 2: *Cognition, Perception and Language.* New York: John Wiley & Sons; 1997:371–420
16. Fryauf-Bertschy H, Tyler RS, Kelsay DM, Gantz BJ. Performance over time of congenitally deaf and postlingually deafened children using a multichannel cochlear implant. *J Speech Hear Res* 1992;35:913–920
17. Fryauf-Bertschy H, Tyler RS, Kelsay DMR, et al. Cochlear implant use by prelingually deafened children: the influences of age at implant and length of device use. *J Speech Hear Res* 1997;40:183–199
18. Miyamoto RT, Osberger MJ, Robbins AM, et al. Comparison of sensory aids in deaf children. *Ann Otol Rhinol Laryngol* 1989;98:2–7
19. Tyler RS, Fryauf-Bertschy H, Gantz BJ, et al. Speech perception in prelingually implanted children after four years. In: Honjo I, Takahashi H, eds. *Cochlear Implant and Related Science Update.* Advances in Otolaryngology, vol 52. Basel: Karger; 1997:187–192
20. Tyler RS, Fryauf-Bertschy H, Kelsay DMR, et al. Speech perception by prelingually deaf children using cochlear implants. *Otolaryngol Head Neck Surg* 1997;117:180–187
21. Tyler RS, Parkinson AJ, Fryauf-Bertschy H, et al. Speech perception by prelingually deaf children and postlingually deaf adults with cochlear implant. *Scand J Audiol* 1997; 26(suppl 46):65–71
22. Bollard PM, Chute PM, Popp A, Parisier SC. Specific language growth in young children using the Clarion cochlear implant. *Ann Otol Rhinol Laryngol* 1999;108(suppl 117):119–123
23. Pisoni DB, Kirk KI, Svirsky MA, Miyamoto RT. Looking at the "stars": a first report on the intercorrelations among measures of speech perception, intelligibility and language in pediatric cochlear implant users. *J Speech Lang Hear Res.* In press
24. Robbins AM, Bollard PM, Green J. Language development in children implanted with the Clarion cochlear implant. *Ann Otol Rhinol Laryngol* 1999;108(suppl 117):113–118
25. Robbins AM, Svirsky MA, Kirk KI. Children with implants can speak, but can they communicate? *Otolaryngol Head Neck Surg* 1997;117:155–160
26. Svirsky MA, Sloan RB, Caldwell M, Miyamoto RT. Speech intelligibility of prelingually deaf children with multichannel cochlear implants. Presented at the seventh symposium on cochlear implants in children, Iowa City, IA; 1998
27. Tyler RS, Tomblin JB, Spencer LJ, et al. How speech perception through a cochlear implant affects language and education. *Otolaryngol Head Neck Surg.* In press
28. Clark G. The University of Melbourne Nucleus multi-electrode cochlear implant. *Adv Otol Rhinol Laryngol* 1987;38:189
29. Schindler RA, Kessler DK, Rebscher SJ, et al. The UCSF/Storz multichannel cochlear implant: patient results. *Laryngoscope* 1986;96:597
30. Wilson BS, Finley CC, Lawson DT, Wolford RD, Eddington DK, Rabinowitz WM. Better speech recognition with cochlear implants. *Nature* 1991;352:236–237
31. Gstöttner WK, Baumgartner WD, Franz P, Hamzavi J. Cochlear implant deep-insertion surgery. *Laryngoscope* 1997;107:544–546
32. Hochmair ES. Clinically relevant aspects of the high-rate cis-speech coding strategy for cochlear implants. Abstracts of the first Asia Pacific symposium on cochlear implant and related sciences. Abst 19. 1996;47
33. McElveen JT, Carrasco VN, Miyamoto RT, et al. Surgical approaches for cochlear implantation in patients with cochlear malformations. In press
34. Gantz BJ, McCabe BF, Tyler RS. Use of multichannel cochlear implants in obstructed and obliterated cochleas. *Otolaryngol Head Neck Surg* 1988;98:72–81
35. Steenerson RL, Gary LB, Wynens MS. Scala vestibuli cochlear implantations for labyrinthine ossification. *Am J Otol* 1990;11:360–363
36. Osberger MJ, Robbins AM, Todd SL, et al. Cochlear implants and tactile aids for children with profound hearing impairment. In: Bess F, Gravel J, Tharpe AM, editors. *Amplification for Children with Auditory Deficits.* Nashville, TN: Bill Wilkerson Center Press, 1996:283–308
37. Cowan RSC, Brown C, Whitford LA, et al. Speech perception in children using the advanced SPEAK speech-processing strategy. *Ann Otol Rhinol Laryngol* 1995;104(suppl 166): 318–321
38. Zimmerman-Phillips S, Osberger MJ, Geier L, Barker M. Speech recognition performance of pediatric Clarion patients. *Am J Otol* 1997;18:5153–5154
39. Erber NP. *Auditory Training.* Washington, DC: Alexander Graham Bell Association for the Deaf; 1982
40. Gantz BJ, Tyler RS, Woodworth G, et al. Results of multichannel cochlear implant in congenital and acquired prelingual deafness in children: five-year follow-up. *Am J Otol* 1994;15(suppl 2):1–8
41. Miyamoto RT, Osberger MJ, Todd SL, et al. Variables affecting implant performance in children. *Laryngoscope* 1994;9: 1120–1124
42. Miyamoto RT, Kirk KI, Robbins AM, et al. Speech perception and speech production skills of children with multichannel cochlear implants. *Acta Otolaryngol* 1996;116:240–243
43. Osberger MJ, Todd SL, Berry SW, et al. Effect of age at onset of deafness on children's speech perception abilities with a cochlear implant. *Ann Otol Rhinol Laryngol* 1991;100:883–888
44. Miyamoto RT, Kirk KI, Robbins AM, et al. Speech perception and speech intelligibility in children with multichannel cochlear implants. In: Honjo I, Takahashi H, eds. *Cochlear Implant and Related Sciences Update.* Advances in Otorhinolaryngology, vol 52. Basel: Karger; 1997:198–203

45. Waltzman S, Cohen NL. Cochlear implantation in children younger than 2 years old. *Am J Otol* 1998;19:158–162
46. Waltzman S, Cohen NL, Shapiro W. Effects of cochlear implantation on the young deaf child. In: Uziel AS, Mondain M, eds. *Cochlear Implants in Children*. Advances in Otorhinolaryngology, vol 50. Basel: Karger; 1995:125–128
47. Waltzman S, Cohen NL, Gomolin R, et al. Perception and production results in children implanted between two and five years of age. In: Honjo I, Takahashi H, eds. *Cochlear Implant and Related Sciences Update*. Advances in Otorhinolaryngology, vol 52. Basel: Karger; 1997:177–180
48. Zwolan TA, Zimmerman-Phillips S, Asbaugh CJ, et al. Cochlear implantation of children with minimal open-set speech recognition skills. *Ear Hear* 1997;18:240–251
49. Gantz B, Rubinstein J, Tyler R, et al. Long-term results of cochlear implants in children with residual hearing. *Ann Otol Rhinol Laryngol*. In press
50. American Academy of Pediatrics. Joint Committee on Infant Hearing Screening. 1994 position statement. *Pediatrics* 1994;95:152–156
51. American Academy of Pediatrics. Task force on newborn and infant hearing. Newborn and infant hearing loss: detection and intervention. *Pediatrics* 1999;103:527–530
52. Yoshinaga-Itano C, Sedey AL, Coulter DK, Mehl AL. Language of early- and later-identified children with hearing loss. *Pediatrics* 1998;102:1161–1171
53. Matsushima JI, Shepard RK, Seldon HL, et al. Electrical stimulation of the auditory nerve in deaf kittens: effects on cochlear nucleus morphology. *Hear Res* 1991;56:133–142
54. Skinner MW, Miller JD. Amplification bandwidth and intelligibility of speech in quiet and noise for listeners with sensorineural hearing loss. *Audiology* 1983;22:253–279
55. Skinner MW, Holden LK, Binzer SM. Aural rehabilitation for individuals with severe and profound hearing impairment: hearing aids, cochlear implants, counseling, and training. In: Valente M, ed. *Strategies of Selecting and Verifying Hearing Aid Fittings*. New York: Thieme Medical; 1996
56. Macrae JH. Permanent threshold shift association with overamplification by hearing aids. *J Speech Hear Res* 1991;34: 403–414
57. Macrae JH. Prediction of deterioration in hearing due to hearing aid use. *J Speech Hear Res* 1991;34:661–660
58. Ching TYC, Dillon H, Byrne D. Speech recognition of hearing-impaired listeners: predictions from audibility and the limited role of high-frequency amplification. *J Acoust Soc Am* 1998;103:1128–1140
59. Hogan CA, Turner CW. High-frequency audibility: benefits for hearing-impaired listeners. *J Acoust Soc Am* 1998;104: 432–441
60. Turner CW. The limits of high-frequency amplification. *Hear J* 1999;52:10–14
61. Boothroyd A. Auditory capacity of hearing-impaired children using hearing aids and cochlear implants: issues of efficacy and assessment. *Scand Audiol* 1997;26(suppl 46):17–25
62. Levi A, Eisenberg LS, Martinez AS, Schneider K. Performance comparisons between cochlear implant and "platinum" hearing aid user: case Study. Presented at the Seventh Symposium on Cochlear Implants in Children, Iowa City, IA; 1998

Cochlear Implants in Congenitally Deaf Children

Laura W. Kretschmer

CHAPTER 81

The history of cochlear implants is a somewhat recent one. The first experimental single-channel implant was provided to a child in 1980, and the first multichannel implant in a child was completed in Australia in 1985, with multisite trials begun with children in the United States the next year. Since the initial experimental work, it is estimated that about 12,000 to 15,000 persons worldwide have received implants, with approximately one-third of those being children. Most children with implants in the United States, in Australia, and in western Europe are deaf as a result of meningitis (45 to 64%). Those children with implants who are identified as having congenital onset of deafness is still a small subset. The push for early identification of hearing loss, and for early fitting of hearing aids, suggests that our attention will invariably be drawn to that subset of children with profound bilateral hearing loss who do not receive substantial benefit from conventional hearing aids, most of whom will have a congenital onset of deafness. It is readily accepted that any child who acquires deafness after the onset of spoken language and who receives limited benefit from amplification is a potential candidate for a cochlear implant. The analogous situation of an older child, adolescent, or adult who is deafened and is considered for an implant also causes little controversy. The question of an implant for the infant, toddler, or young child who has never had auditory experience should raise many cautions for the physician and implant teams, however.

The cochlear implant is not the end of habilitation in children with congenital deafness. Rather, it is just the beginning, constituting only one factor in the effort to promote the child's linguistic, educational, psychosocial, and intellectual development. Deafness may be considered a variation in the human condition by some, or a disability by others, but the most critical aspect of the deaf child's habilitation is the establishment of communication, whether or not an implant is involved. The heavy lifting of language acquisition is accomplished in normal hearing children by the fourth or fifth year of life. In view of the importance of these early years for language acquisition in general, it is an important goal to ensure that the first 4 or 5 years of life are primary language learning years for every child with congenital deafness as well.

The list of controversies surrounding the process of implantation in children with congenital deafness is substantial. The set of controversies discussed in this chapter, although not exhaustive, represents the most publicized and the most vexing issues: (1) advisability of lowering the minimum age for implantation; (2) deciding when benefit from conventional amplification is not sufficient to sustain communication development in a young child; (3) determining whether family and educational resources are sufficient to warrant and support implantation as part of the child's habilitation, including the question of which modes of communication (spoken versus sign language) seem to be most important to implant success; (4) the issue of deaf culture and how it should enter into parents' and professionals thinking about implantation; (5) whether or how the perspectives of the child might be taken into account; (6) the advisability of implantation in children with multiple neurologic and cognitive disabilities, including auditory neuropathy; (7) whether published data reflect the full range of outcomes for children who are implanted, to include those children who do not derive benefit or who voluntarily discard the implant; and (8) the implications of animal research on neural plasticity and cortical reorganization in regard to the use of implants in young children with congenital deafness. The best speech-processing schemes remain controversial among manufacturers and auditory researchers. (See comprehensive reports such as the 1997 Acta Otolaryngology supplement or the 1997 *American Journal of Otology* supplement for detailed information on cochlear implants in children, as well as Parkins[1] for further information about processing schemes.)

Minimum and Maximum Age for Implantation and Hearing Aid Benefit

The minimum age for implantation is currently set at 2 years in the United States, with compassionate exemptions granted for children younger than age 2 who are deafened by meningitis, with the threat of cochlear ossification possibly preventing adequate electrode insertion. Data regarding a small sample of early implanted infants (before 2 years of age) show a lack of surgical complications,[2] whereas others report improved communication outcomes on children with early implantation.[3] The controversy arises when considered with the second issue of how to show hearing aid benefit.

There are both national initiatives and regional efforts to establish universal hearing screening in the United States.[4,5] The stated goal of these initiatives is to identify all infants with early onset of hearing loss by 3 months of age and to accomplish hearing aid fitting by 6 months of age for those infants identified with significant hearing loss. The point of these initiatives is to take advantage of the child's natural facility for the acquisition of speech and language during the first year(s) of life, a facility that does not depend on exposure to spoken language but that applies across any mode of language expression. If spoken language is the goal, we know that the sooner sensory evidence from the aided auditory channel is incorporated into learning for the child with congenital deafness, the better the outcomes will be. According to this argument, implantation during the first year of life, but certainly before 2 years of age, seems logical. If this approach is taken, however, there is the real risk that insufficient time for hearing aid use, inadequate hearing aid fitting, and inadequate definition of the infant's residual hearing will mask the child's aided auditory potential. Infants and toddlers with severe hearing loss who are identified early, and who have the benefits of properly fit hearing aids, as well as family and professional support show clear advantage in the area of communication development.[6]

Children with severe hearing loss (90 to 100 dB bilaterally) who have the advantage of early intervention outperform children who are congenitally deaf and receive implants, particularly in terms of interpersonal communication development.[7] In addition, although accurate and reliable evaluation of hearing sensitivity can be accomplished in infants and toddlers through electrophysiologic and behavioral tests administered by experienced pediatric audiologists, the same cannot be said about the quality of hearing evaluations and habilitation processes everywhere in the United States. Despite the criterion of a minimum of 6 months of hearing aid use before an implant is chosen, children more typically need 1 to 2 years of quality input through a well-fit hearing aid before aided hearing benefits are realized. Implant signal processing is improving, as is hearing aid technology. Because implanted cochleas will be unable to take advantage of present or future hearing aid advances, careful definition of residual hearing, informed fitting of hearing aids, and early intervention that includes appropriate use of amplification must precede any consideration of implantation.

With regard to maximum age for implantation, the data suggest that most children with congenital deafness implanted after age 5, and particularly during or after puberty, will be part-time or nonuser 1 to 2 years postimplant.[8,9]

Some data are available regarding adolescents and adults who are congenitally deaf who, after further progression of hearing loss, elect to switch from hearing aid use to a cochlear implant. The individuals in this subset who were long-term dedicated hearing aid users and possessed spoken language before implantation, seem to derive substantial benefit. These persons would likely resemble typical learners in that audition has played a role in their communication development in the first place.[10] As suggested, evidence regarding implant outcomes in adolescents and adults who were not hearing aid users and/or who were primarily sign language users suggests far less satisfaction. Implantation in persons in this latter category should be approached very carefully, if it is performed at all.

Family and Educational Support

It is well understood that establishing clear expectations for the family about the benefits of a cochlear implant and its place as only one of the elements in their child's habilitation is critical. It is also well accepted that educational programs and families in which spoken language and listening experiences are emphasized are critical to the child's successful use of an implant to aid in developing spoken communication and reading and writing. Establishing communication with, and developing language in, a child with congenital deafness is one of the most challenging problems to confront a family. The vast majority of parents (90%) who have a deaf child do not know anything about the habilitation process and do not know how to use sign language or how to otherwise communicate with their child. Furthermore, outside of populated areas, strong educational programs or intervention teams, or both, are often not available to children and their families. If these support systems cannot be identified, implantation is not advisable. Use of sign language, per se, should not recommend against implantation. Measurable gains in language performance, including acquisition of intelligible speech, have been noted for children with implants who are in programs or homes in which sign language is used in addition to speaking and listening. Sadly, however, most families do not develop into competent communicators with their child in any mode, but particularly when sign language is introduced into the habilitation process. In such families, whether they talk or try to sign, or try both, the cochlear implant is likely to be of questionable benefit.

Luetje and Jackson[11] suggest that socioeconomic factors, poor compliance by families, and family impatience with habilitative training should be considered complications as serious as medical/surgical issues or device failures when implanting children.

Deaf Culture and Cochlear Implants

Since the mid-1980s, there has been a dramatic growth in the so-called deaf power or deaf culture movement in the United States, in which some people who are deaf have worked to legitimize deaf culture and to promote its adherents into positions of responsibility in educational institutions and agencies for the deaf. Among deaf culture adherents in America, American Sign Language (ASL) has been argued to be their natural language. Thus, speaking and English-based sign languages are often rejected as the trappings of "oppression" by people who hear. These trappings also include hearing aids in general and cochlear implants and oral education in particular. The motivations of implant surgeons, audiologists, speech/language pathologists, educators of the deaf, and even parents who support cochlear implants, have been questioned both in the media and in the press.[12] Cohen[13] and Balkany et al.,[14] offer strong counterpoints to those who question the motivations of surgeons and other professionals engaged in the cochlear implant process in young children.

One point in this controversy that must be recognized by any family or professional involved in the implant process, however, is that many people who do not talk (and only use signs) are well educated, literate, and gainfully employed, have a productive family life, raise well-adjusted children whatever their hearing status, and otherwise contribute to society. They would argue that deafness does not have to be considered a condition to be fixed. It should also be recognized that the deaf community is not monolithic. Some parents who are themselves congenitally deaf, who use sign language and function socially in deaf culture, have chosen to have their own congenitally deaf child receive an implant. The expressed reason for this decision is generally the wish that their son or daughter will have options with regard to how and with whom they will communicate as adults. That is, they wish their children to have the benefit of being able to both talk and sign. The social and economic realities of society support the wisdom of this decision.

Perceptions of the Child

As societal perspectives about people with disabilities have been modified, whether through federal legislation or through changes in society itself, we have begun to separate the disability from the person. Reading about the accomplishments of a woman who is both deaf and blind, or having an adult with Down's syndrome on a popular television show, or seeing a Miss America who happens to be deaf successfully handle the complexities of modern press coverage, point out how alike we are and how extraordinary some of us can be despite intellectual or sensory disabilities. It should also highlight the importance of being comfortable with oneself, with one's strengths and limitations. We are beginning to understand more clearly how our earliest experiences affect our adjustment and self-perception as adolescents or adults. How well do we understand the implications of implant surgery on the child's perception of themselves, as someone who needs to be "fixed," rather than accepted as a child who happens to be deaf? The importance of children with congenital deafness viewing themselves as competent people who have a variety of strengths, whatever their hearing status, must be recognized. The role of the implant in this process is not clearly understood. If the child has sufficient communication and cognitive maturity to be interviewed, scales or forms can be employed to examine their attitudes and perceptions about implantation. Clearly, this is not a choice if a child is implanted during the preschool years. Because deafness is not a life-threatening disorder, only a life-altering one, we must be careful not to suppose that we can guarantee adult adjustment by means of a cochlear implant in a very young child.

Implants in Children with Multiple Disabilities and/or Auditory Neuropathy

Our ability to implant children with a cochlear device has no more serious potential for damage and financial waste than in instances in which the child is deaf but has additional disabilities. It must be admitted, if not generally acknowledged, that children with multiple disabilities, including mental retardation or severe language-learning difficulties, have been implanted already. In some children who are deaf and blind but otherwise intact, the decision to implant may be a good one. However, the parents of children with multiple disabilities, including deafness, are among the most vulnerable as they seek help for the child whose future may seem bleak. Everyone must understand the implant's role as only one factor in the habilitation and long-term development of any child with deafness. Unless this is clear to all parents, some well-meaning surgeons will continue to be persuaded that an implant is critical for a particular child. Professional implant teams that include audiologists, speech/language pathologists, educators, psychologists, and social workers can be of help in protecting the surgeon from undue family pressure in this regard. Unfortunately, because the implant is no longer an experimental device for children, parents who are refused by one team will usually be able to find another team that will provide the implant.

Interest in, and ability to, identify infants and children with auditory neuropathy has added to the complexity of the decision about implantation. I am referring to a condition in which both conventional and electophysiologic measures of auditory function show abnormal auditory nerve function with relatively intact cochlear function; that is, the infant, toddler, or child with auditory neuropathy will likely show robust pre-neural evidence of cochlear hair cell function (intact evoked otoacoustic emissions) and absent or grossly abnormal 8th cranial nerve auditory transmissions (measured through evoked electrophysiologic measures, such as auditory brainstem response testing). Conventional behavioral audiometry in these cases generally suggests profound bilateral hearing impairment. The precise site of lesion in many cases of auditory neuropathy can only be inferred, particularly in the absense of a syndrome. Implantation in a cochlea with evidence of normal hair cell function means sacrifice of a normal organ, which presents a serious ethical dilemma. Several of these children have been implanted, with mixed results.[15] If a decision is made to implant a child with auditory neuropathy, the quality of family and educational support must be strong and the expectations of family, educators, and the child carefully tempered.

Outcome Data Controversy

For the past dozen years or so, outcome data for children with cochlear implants have moved from case studies showing considerable promise to both summative and evaluative data for dozens of children with profound hearing loss, including those with congenital deafness. The population of students with implants has grown steadily in schools that emphasize auditory/oral education and may constitute as many as one-half of the children currently enrolled in those programs. Part of the impetus for this trend may be the outcome research showing that many children with multichannel cochlear implants outperform children with profound hearing losses who are considered to be very good hearing aid users on a variety of speech perception and speech and language production tasks.[7,16,17] This research is generally in a quantitative style and provides answers about changes in discrete test performance both pre- and postimplant. Efforts to examine the question of improvement in quality of life, as well as in social communication, have been developed through rating scales such as the Meaningful Auditory Integration Scale (MAIS), reported by Robbins et al.[18]

These data are generally positive but, because the subjects are drawn from families who are satisfied with their children's postimplant progress and are motivated to cooperate with researchers, interpretation of these results as applied to all children with congenital deafness must be cautious. It is more difficult to identify and report on children who do not make progress or who are not using the implant for a variety of reasons.[9] Parents should be made aware that there are always two sides to the outcome question, particularly if the child is congenitally deaf.

Neural and Cortical Plasticity/Reorganization

Animal research in the area of cortical plasticity and reorganization as regards the auditory system is intriguing and bears directly on the last controversy considered in this chapter. The phenomenon of failure to develop perceptual ability, due to early sensory deprivation, has been well recognized for many years, beginning with studies of kittens that were kept in darkness, and including newborn mice that were denied auditory input.[19] The outcomes in those experiments showed lack of development of visual cortex and visual perceptual abilities in the first case and noticeable changes in structure of various nuclei in the auditory pathways of the brainstem and midbrain in the latter instance. More recently, reports on declines in speech perception abilities in the unaided ear of adults who are long-term monaural hearing aid users bring this question to the forefront again. Finally, research on apparent cortical reorganization in newborn cats whose auditory cortex is examined several months after they received lesions in the high-frequency region of their cochleas offers some interesting evidence. Observations in these studies have included the fact that the cortical area that commonly codes a range of frequencies was reorganized to be responsive only to the low-frequency information it was receiving. That is, typical high-frequency coding regions were eroded or recruited to code only low-frequency information. This reorganization was noted after only a few months of deprivation. The question of whether this cortex could be awakened to participate in more typical coding patterns has not been answered, of course. Nonetheless, the question of whether peripheral implants can be processed by auditory cortex that has never been stimulated, as in children with congenital deafness, remains. Data concerning adults who begin to wear a hearing aid on a long unaided ear suggest some answers, as many seem to recover speech perception abilities after a period of accommodation, but these are persons who lose hearing as adults and thus have well-developed auditory and language abilities (and brain organization) to assist with accommodation. Positron-emission tomography (PET) scan studies in cochlear implant users[20] and other research of central auditory effects with electrical stimulation[21] seem to offer the possibility that peripheral stimulation does have the effect of (re)activating central auditory pathways.

Although the early cortical plasticity research could be taken to argue for implantation during the first year of life, it seems to explain why some congenitally deaf children who are implanted early do not make progress. If the auditory cortex and complex brain underpinnings for spoken language cannot be awakened to sensory stimulation in this way, the value of an implant would be expected to be restricted.[22]

Summary

A variety of controversies should be considered by an implant team before recommending cochlear implants in children, adolescents, or even adults who are congenitally deaf. These factors include, but are not limited to, minimum and maximum age for implantation, extent and quality of hearing aid, listening and speaking experience, family financial and emotional support, communication mode in the family and in the educational programs available, role of deaf culture in the family and child's life, the child's own perceptions and ability to participate in the implant decision, advisability of implantation in children with multiple disabilities, extent of outcome data studies, and implications of neural plasticity and cortical reorganization studies.

All these controversies serve to remind the members of the implant team how carefully each family and child must be evaluated and how sensitive the counseling and explanation process must be before the decision to implant is made.

REFERENCES

Kretschmer—CHAPTER 81

1. Parkins CW. Compensating for hair cell loss with cochlear implants. In: Berlin CI, editor. *Neurotransmission and Hearing Loss: Basic Science, Diagnosis, and Management*. San Diego: Singular; 1997:107–135
2. Waltzman SB, Cohen NL. Cochlear implants in children younger than two years. *Am J Otol* 1998;19:158–162
3. Brackett D, Zara CV. Communication outcomes related to early implantation. *Am J Otol* 1998;19:453–460
4. National Institutes of Health. *NIH Consensus Statement: Early Identification of Hearing Impairment in Infants and Young Children*. Washington, DC: US Public Health Service; 1993
5. Joint Committee on Infant Hearing. 1994 position statement. *Pediatrics* 1995;95:152–156
6. Yoshinaga-Itano C. Efficacy of early identification and early intervention. *Semin Hear* 1995;16:115–123

7. Geers A. Comparing implants with hearing aids in profoundly deaf children. *Otolaryngol Head Neck Surg* 1997; 117:180–187
8. Snik AF, Makhdoum MJ, Vermeulen AM, et al. The relationship of age at the time of cochlear implantation and long-term speech perception abilities in congenitally deaf subjects. *Int J Pediatr Otorhinolaryngol* 1997;41:121–131
9. Rose DM, Vernon M, Pool AF. Cochlear implant in prelingually deaf children. *Am Ann Deaf* 1996;141:258–262
10. Boothroyd-Turner D, Boothroyd A. The characteristics and attainment of 8 children who are congenitally deaf and who use cochlear implants. Presented at the Alexander Graham Bell Association Conference, Little Rock, AR; 1998
11. Luetje CM, Jackson K. Cochlear implants in children: what constitutes a complication? *Otolaryngol Head Neck Surg* 1997;117:243–247
12. Lane H. *The mask of benevolence.* New York: Alfred Knopf; 1992
13. Cohen NL. The ethics of cochlear implants in young children. *Am J Otol* 1994;15:1–2
14. Balkany T, Hodges AV, Goodman KW. Ethics of cochlear implantation in young children. *Otolaryngol Head Neck Surg* 1996;114:748–755
15. Fabry LB. Identification and management of auditory neuropathy. Presented at Phonak International Conference. A Sound Foundation through Early Amplification, Chicago, IL; 1998
16. Osberger MJ, Fisher L, Zimmerman-Phillips S, et al. Speech recognition performance of older children with cochlear implants. *Am J Otol* 1998;19:152–157
17. Tyler RS, Fryauf-Bertschy H, Kelsay DM, et al. Speech perception by prelingually deaf children using cochlear implants. *Otolaryngol Head Neck Surg* 1997;117:180–187
18. Robbins A, Renshaw JJ, Berry SW. Evaluating meaningful auditory integration in profoundly hearing impaired children. *Am J Otol* 1991;12(suppl):144–150
19. Webster DB. Effects of neonatal sound deprivation in animal research. *Semin Speech Lang Hear* 1982;3:336–343
20. Naito Y, Hirano S, Honjo I, et al. Sound induced activation of auditory cortices in cochlear implant users with post- and prelingual deafness demonstrated by positron emission tomography. *Acta Otolaryngol* 1997;117:490–496
21. Shepherd RK, Hartmann R, Heid S, et al. The central auditory system and auditory deprivation: experiences with cochlear implants in congenitally deaf children. *Acta Otolaryngol* 532(suppl):28–33
22. Willott JF. Physiological plasticity in the auditory system and its possible relevance to hearing aid use, deprivation effects, and acclimitization. *Ear Hear* 1996;17:665–775

28

Jugular Foramen Tumors

"The advent of stereotactic radiosurgery in recent decades provides a more precise technique for administering high-dose focal radiation, and preliminary reports indicate that this modality may have a role in the treatment of jugular foramen tumors."

Harry R. van Loveren

"Jugular foramen tumors are uncommon lesions, dominated by benign tumors (paragangliomas, schwannomas, neurofibromas, and meningiomas). In spite of their benign histopathology, these lesions are characterized by locally destructive behaviour. Presentation is often insidious and the diagnosis delayed. Radiotherapy is inappropriate for the treatment of these radioresistant lesions in generally otherwise healthy patients. Surgical excision by the lateral otologic approaches in established skull base surgical units permits complete resection of these lesions with minimal morbidity and maximum tumor control."

Ugo Fisch

"This idea of 'expectant waiting' was first proposed to me by a skilled head and neck surgeon whose task it has been to fix defects in pharyngolaryngeal function resulting from surgically induced neuropathies. Although some of us may call this option heretical, I think it makes a lot of sense."

Peter G. Smith

Jugular Foramen Tumors

Harry R. van Loveren, Khaled M. Abdel Aziz, Abhay Sanan, Michael R. Chicoine, and John M. Tew, Jr.

CHAPTER 82

The jugular foramen is the most complex foramen of the skull base. It both contains, and is surrounded by, important neurovascular structures. It is in a deep location, and surgical access poses difficulty for both otolaryngologists and neurosurgeons alike. Despite these anatomic challenges, impressive progress has been made in the surgical management of tumors of the jugular foramen. Advances in neuroradiology, the creation of formal skull base teams, and the utilization of microsurgical techniques have all contributed to a lowered surgical morbidity.

This chapter provides an overview of the relevant skull base anatomy needed to understand approaches to the jugular foramen. Because glomus jugulare tumors are, by far, the most common tumor of the jugular foramen, the bulk of the text is devoted to glomus tumors and their management. Although an overview of the surgical classification and treatment algorithm for jugular foramen tumors is provided, we have specifically described our surgical approach to these tumors.

Anatomy

The term *jugular foramen* is derived from the Latin terms for neck and aperture, respectively.[1] Loosely speaking, this translates into "opening to the neck." The jugular foramen truly is an opening to the neck, an avenue for passage of critical structures to and from the intracranial space of the posterior fossa to the neck.

OSSEOUS ANATOMY

The bony limits of this passageway are the petrous portion of the temporal bone and the condylar portion of the occipital bone.[2] A fibrous bridge divides the jugular foramen in 75 to 92% of cadaveric specimens evaluated, and a bony septum in the remaining 8 to 25%.[2] After the evaluation of human dry cadaveric skulls, it has been determined that the size of the jugular foramen is larger on the right than on the left in approximately 70% of specimens, larger on the left in 20%, and of the same size on both sides in 10%.[2-5] The anterior margin of the jugular foramen is formed by the carotid ridge, which separates the jugular bulb from the C2 segment of the internal carotid artery (ICA)[6] in the carotid canal.

CONTENTS OF JUGULAR FORAMEN

The critical structures traversing the jugular foramen are the sigmoid sinus and jugular bulb, the inferior petrosal sinus (IPS), meningeal branches of the ascending pharyngeal and occipital arteries, and cranial nerves (CN) IX, X, and XI (Fig. 82–1).

In addition, within the foramen are CN ganglia (superior and inferior ganglia of CN IX and X) and CN branches, including the tympanic branch of CN IX (Jacobson's nerve) and the auricular branch of CN X (Arnold's nerve). In close proximity to the jugular foramen are the ICA anteriorly and CN XII posteromedially.

COMPARTMENTS OF THE JUGULAR FORAMEN

Classically, the jugular foramen has been divided into two compartments, as described by Hovelacque in 1934.[7] Later investigators called these two compartments the pars venosum (posterolaterally) and the pars nervosa (anteromedially).[4,8,9] These names are misleading, as the pars venosum contains the jugular bulb, the posterior meningeal artery, as well as CN X and XI, and the pars nervosum contains CN IX and the inferior petrosal sinus. In 1997, Katsuta et al.[2] divided the jugular foramen into three compartments: (1) the posterolateral sigmoid part (sigmoid sinus), (2) the interjugular or neural part (CN IX anteriorly, and CN X, XI posteriorly), and (3) the anteromedial petrosal part (inferior petrosal sinus). Their three-compartment (two venous and one neural or interjugular) classification system was based on observations made in 32 dry skulls and 33 cadaveric jugular foramina.[2] The importance of compartmentalization of the jugular foramen is not to memorize a particular classification scheme, but rather to use these systems as a tool for understanding the anatomy of this region and how it affects the surgical approaches to pathological lesions.

VENOUS COMPONENT OF THE JUGULAR FORAMEN

The venous component of the jugular foramen consists of a large posterolateral venous channel (sigmoid part), which receives flow from the sigmoid sinus, and a smaller anteromedial venous channel (petrosal part), which receives drainage from the IPS. The sigmoid sinus courses anteroinferiorly toward the jugular foramen, continuing as the jugular bulb, and then as the internal jugular vein. The dome of the jugular bulb is located approximately 2 mm inferior to the internal auditory canal. The dome of the jugular bulb may extend superiorly to the posterior wall of the internal auditory canal, in which case it is referred to as a "high jugular bulb"[10,11] (Fig. 82–2).

The IPS courses on the intracranial surface of the petroclival fissure and enters the anteromedial (petrosal) part of the

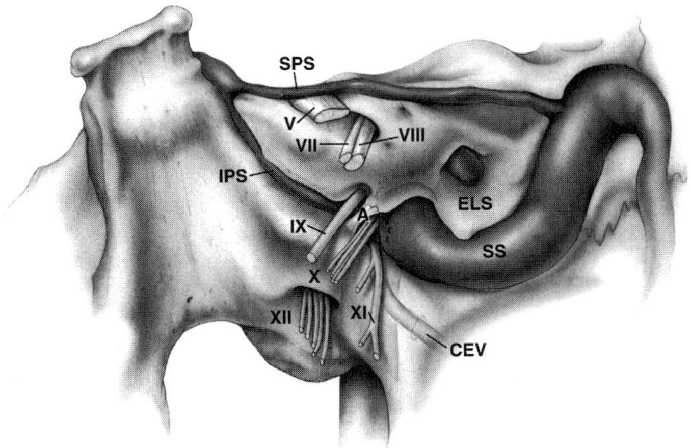

A

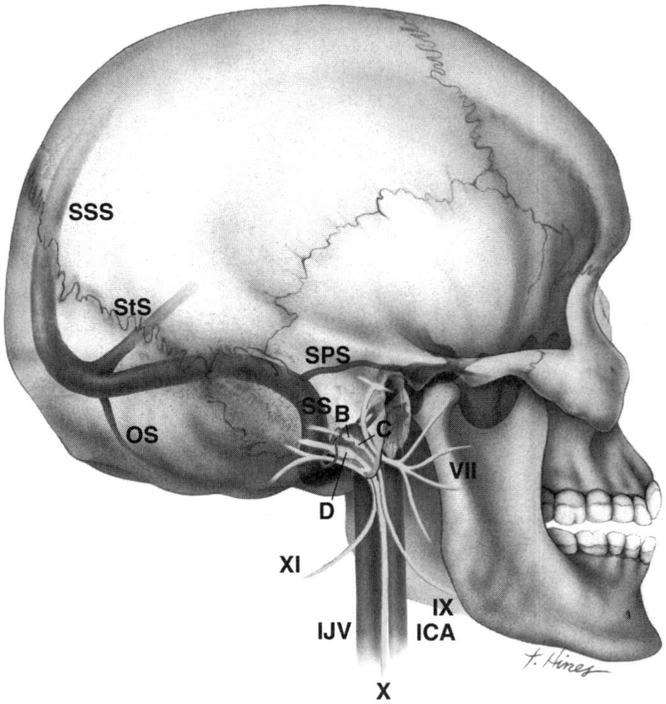

B

Figure 82–1 Endocranial and exocranial views of the jugular foramen. **(A)** Endocranial view shows cranial nerve (CN) IX is separated from CNs X and XI by a dural septum. The inferior petrosal sinus courses inferior to CN IX as the nerve enters the jugular foramen and courses between CN IX and X to drain into the anterior aspect of the jugular bulb. **(B)** Exocranial view of CNs and regional vascular relationships. CN XI courses posterolateral to the internal jugular vein. CN IX is lateral to CNs X and XI and is anchored to the internal carotid artery by a dense fibrous band. ICA, internal carotid artery; IPS, inferior petrosal sinus; SPS, superior petrosal sinus; SS, sigmoid sinus; StS, straight sinus; SSS, superior sagittal sinus; OS, occipital sinus; ELS, endolymphatic sac; CEV, condylar emissary vein; IJV, internal jugular vein; A, dural septum; B, superior ganglion of CN IX; C, inferior ganglion of CN IX; D, superior ganglion of CN X. (Reprinted with permission from the Mayfield Clinic.)

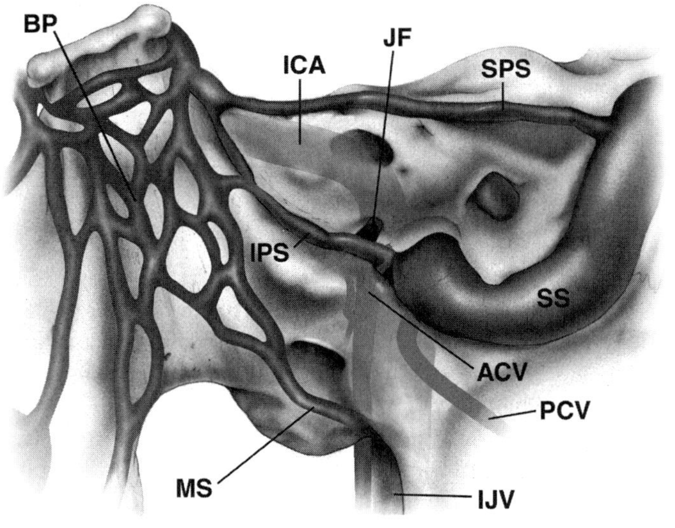

Figure 82–2 Inferior petrosal sinus/anterior condylar vein complex. BP, basilar plexus; ICA, internal carotid artery; IPS, inferior petrosal sinus; JF, jugular foramen; SPS, superior petrosal sinus; SS, sigmoid sinus; ACV, anterior condylar vein; PCV, posterior condylar vein; MS, marginal sinus; IJV, internal jugular vein. (Reprinted with permission from the Mayfield Clinic.)

jugular foramen between CN IX and CN X. The IPS receives tributaries from the inferior petroclival vein (venous plexus in the carotid canal), venous plexus of the hypoglossal canal (anterior condylar vein), posterior condylar vein (emissary vein), and from the vertebral venous plexus. This confluence fills the anteromedial compartment of the jugular foramen, consisting of one or sometimes two main channels that receive drainage from smaller channels.

Shiu et al.[12] described a classification system for the inferior petrosal sinus/anterior condylar vein complex that was further refined by Miller et al.[13] In type I (45% of cases), the IPS drains directly into the jugular bulb and connects with the suboccipital and vertebral venous plexus via a small anterior condylar vein. In type II (24%), the IPS joins an anterior condylar vein of similar size before draining into the jugular bulb. Type III (24%) occurs when the IPS is formed of small venous channels connected to the jugular bulb. In type IV (7%), the IPS is not connected to the jugular bulb, but anastomoses directly with the vertebral and suboccipital venous plexi and may send a small tributary to the internal jugular vein. In summary, the IPS/anterior condylar vein complex forms an anastomosis with the jugular bulb in more than 90% of patients.

INTERJUGULAR COMPARTMENT AND CRANIAL NERVES

The junction of the anteromedial and posterolateral parts of the jugular foramen is a site of two bony prominences, the interjugular processes, on the opposing surfaces of the temporal and occipital bones. These processes are joined by a fibrous septum or, less commonly, an osseous bridge, which forms the interjugular septum between the anteromedial and posterolateral compartments. The dura over this septum has two characteristic perforations: the glossopharyngeal meatus (for CN IX) and the vagal meatus (for CN X and XI). The IPS empties into the jugular bulb between these two openings in approximately 65%, less commonly inferomedial to both openings, and rarely superolateral to them.[13] The dura in the superolateral margins of the interjugular septum is characteristically thick, forming a lip, the plica occipitalis obliqua or jugular dural fold, which becomes less distinct inferomedially over the glossopharyngeal and vagal meatus.[2]

GLOSSOPHARYNGEAL NERVE

Cranial nerve IX arises from the medulla as three or four tiny filaments that quickly collect into one or, rarely, two rootlets passing forward and laterally, ventral to the choroid plexus, to penetrate the glossopharyngeal meatus.[2,14] Cranial nerve IX then turns abruptly anteroinferiorly and, as it traverses the jugular foramen, gives rise to the tympanic branch (Jacobson's nerve) to the tympanic cavity. Along its course in the temporal bone, the tympanic branch of CN IX has many swellings formed by ganglion cells, a potential site of origin for glomus tumors. Cranial nerve IX exits the jugular foramen between the ICA and internal jugular vein and descends lateral to CN X and XI. More distally, CN IX passes anteriorly to cross the lateral surface of ICA deep to the styloid process, where it divides into several branches.

VAGUS NERVE

Cranial nerve X is composed of multiple combinations of small and large rootlets, which are intimately associated with the rootlets of CN IX and XI. These rootlets enter the vagal meatus separated from the glossopharyngeal meatus by a dural septum. During its course in the jugular foramen, CN X gives the auricular branch (Arnold's nerve), which ascends toward the mastoid segment of the facial nerve. Along its course, the auricular branch of CN X has many swellings formed by ganglion cells, which can give rise to glomus tumors. Cranial nerve X exits the jugular foramen vertically with intimate relation to CN XI. Cranial nerves X and XI exit the jugular foramen posterior to CN IX on the posteromedial wall of the internal jugular vein. The main trunk of CN X descends posterior to the ICA within the carotid sheath.[2]

SPINAL ACCESSORY NERVE

Cranial nerve XI has a cranial portion (4 to 16 rootlets) and a spinal portion (6 to 7 rootlets) from C1 to C6 dorsal to the dentate ligament. The cranial and spinal portions of CN XI enter the vagal meatus together; however, they may infrequently be separated by a dural septum. Cranial nerve XI may be indistinguishable from CN X in the jugular foramen. After exiting the foramen, CN XI descends obliquely and laterally between the ICA and internal jugular vein, and then posteriorly across the lateral surface of the vein to reach the sternocleidomastoid and trapezius muscles. In 30% of specimens, CN XI descends alternatively on the medial surface of the internal jugular vein.[2]

HYPOGLOSSAL NERVE

Cranial nerve XII does not traverse the jugular foramen, but joins CN IX, X, and XI as they exit the foramen into the carotid sheath. After passing through the hypoglossal canal, CN XII courses adjacent to CN X and then separates from it and descends laterally in the interval between the ICA and internal jugular vein. At the level of the transverse process of the atlas, the main fibers of CN XII turn abruptly anteriorly along the lateral surface of the ICA en route to the tongue, whereas the remaining fibers, the ansa cervicalis, descend with the major vessels in the neck.

FACIAL NERVE

The vertical portion of the mastoid segment of the facial nerve in the fallopian canal, a critical structure in surgical approaches to the jugular bulb, is separated from the lateral wall of the jugular bulb by the retrofacial and infralabyrinthine air cells. The relationship between the mastoid segment of the facial nerve and the jugular bulb is variable.[15] In approximately 60% of specimens at least one-half of the jugular bulb lies anterior to the facial nerve, and in the remaining 40% only one-third of the jugular bulb lies anterior to the facial nerve.[15] The facial nerve exits the stylomastoid foramen about 5 mm lateral to the lateral margin of the jugular foramen or approximately midway between the styloid process and the anterior part of the digastric groove.

Tumor Classification

Glomus jugulare tumors are the most common tumors of the jugular foramen. Jugular schwannomas and meningiomas, although uncommon, are the other most common tumors affecting the jugular foramen, some series reporting the former and other series reporting the latter as the second most common.[2,14,16] Chordoma,[17,18] chondrosarcoma,[16,19] chondroblastoma,[16] cholesterol granuloma,[20] epidermoid cyst,[20] parotid neoplasm,[16] adenocarcinoma,[16] osteoblastoma,[16] metastasis,[21] plasmacytoma,[22] sarcoidosis,[23] fibrous dysplasia,[24] chondromyxoid fibroma,[25] non-Hodgkin's lymphoma,[26] and amyloidoma[27] are among the other types of lesions reported in the jugular foramen.

Tumors of the jugular foramen may be either intrinsic, arising from within the foramen, or extrinsic, secondarily extending into the jugular foramen.[14] Glomus jugulare is the classic intrinsic jugular foramen tumor, constituting 56 to 77% of jugular foramen tumors in reported series.[14] Schwannomas and meningiomas rarely arise as primarily intrinsic jugular foramen tumors.[14] Extrinsic tumors can penetrate the jugular foramen from four different directions: (1) superiorly, as a downward extension of intracranial schwannomas and meningiomas; (2) inferiorly, as an upward extension of cervical tumors such as glomus vagale tumors, adenocarcinomas, and schwannomas arising in the parapharyngeal space; (3) medially, such as chordomas and chondrosarcomas of the petroclival region; and (4) laterally, from invasive temporal bone tumors such as squamous cell carcinoma and adenomatous tumors.[14]

Glomus Jugulare Tumors

HISTORY

In 1840 Valentin[28] first described paraganglionic tissue near the origin of the tympanic nerve; this was followed in 1878 by Krause,[29] who described the same tissue arising from the temporal bone. However, these early reports received little attention. Subsequently, in the *Anatomic Records* of 1941, Guild[30,31] was the first to use the term *glomus body*, but the significance of this tissue was unknown at that time. Shortly thereafter, in 1946, Rosenwasser[32] described a "carotid body-like" tumor of the middle ear, followed 2 years later by Winship et al.[33] coining the name *glomus jugulare tumor*. Through the 1940s and 1950s, several reports appeared in the literature, but the exact anatomic origin and behavior of this tissue was unknown.[34] The terms *chemodectoma* and *receptoma* were used to refer to these glomus jugulare tumors because of their similarity to carotid body tumors, but unlike carotid body tumors, glomus jugulare tumors have no chemoreceptors.[35] *Paraganglionoma* accurately reflects the origin of these tumors from the paraganglion cells. *Nonchromaffin* was added to the term *paraganglionoma* to convey the lack of positive silver staining by these tumors, but this was inaccurately interpreted to mean that these tumors were nonsecretory.[36]

In the history of the neurosurgical management of cranial neoplastic disease, glomus tumors of the jugular foramen and temporal bone are relatively new. In 1962, Alford and Gilford,[36] in reviewing their own experience (11 cases) and the entirety of cases reported in the literature to date, found only 316 cases of glomus jugulare tumors. In this report, written in the era before modern imaging studies, they defined the natural history of this disease and described a detailed five-tiered classification system based on clinical signs and symptoms.

TABLE 82–1
Fisch Classification of Glomus Tumors*

Class	Description
A	Tympanic (4/23)
B	Tympanomastoid (7/23)
C	Infralabyrinthine (12/23)
D	Intracranial (1/12, recurrence of pt. with type C)
D_1	< 2 cm
D_2	> 2 cm

*From Oldring and Fisch[37] and Jenkins and Fisch.[38]
Series data: 23 patients, 5 M:18 F, mean age 48 years, range 20–69.

CLASSIFICATION SYSTEMS OF GLOMUS TUMORS

Two contemporary anatomically based classification systems of glomus tumors are commonly cited. The first is the four-tiered grouping of Oldring and colleagues[37] of Zurich, first reported in 1979 and subsequently revised in later reports (Table 82–1). The second is the classification initially described in 1982 by Glasscock and Jackson[39] of the Otology Group in Nashville. The latter classification divides glomus tumors into two main groups, glomus jugulare tumors and glomus tympanicum tumors. Each of these two main groups is further subdivided into four subgroups (Table 82–2). These classification systems serve as the standard language by which

TABLE 82–2
Glasscock–Jackson Classification of Glomus Tumors*

Type		Description
A.		**Glomus tympanicum**
	I	Small promontory mass
	II	Fills middle ear
	III	Fills middle ear and extends into mastoid
	IV	Extends into external auditory canal, with or without extension to ICA
B.		**Glomus jugulare**
	I	Small, jugular bulb, middle ear, mastoid
	II	Extends under IAC, with or without intracranial extension
	III	Extends to petrous apex, with or without intracranial extension
	IV	Beyond petrous apex to clivus or infratemporal fossa, with or without intracranial extension

*From Glasscock et al.[39]

these lesions can be described. In addition, preoperative grading of glomus tumors that use these classification schemes and preoperative imaging studies has been shown to be a useful guide for choosing the appropriate surgical approach. Finally, the preoperative grade of the tumor according to these classification systems correlates with the likelihood of attaining a complete surgical resection and as a predictor of postoperative CN morbidity.[14]

BIOLOGY OF GLOMUS TUMORS

Pathology

Macroscopically, glomus jugular tumors are typically tan-gray to purple, encapsulated, vascular, and lobulated masses. Native glomus tissue and glomus tumors are derived from the embryological neural crest cells. Like the normal glomus tissue, glomus tumors are histologically indistinguishable from carotid body tumors and often display the histologic pattern referred to as *Zellballen*, with clusters of chief and sustentacular cells.[5] Nuclear pleomorphism, hyperchromatism, and mitoses may not imply aggressive behavior. Rather, malignancy is defined as the presence of metastasis to an organ without paraganglia (versus multifocal) and occurs in fewer than 10% of cases.[40] The distinction between multifocality and metastasis is illustrated by the example of a patient with a second glomus tumor in the lungs. The pulmonary lesion may not represent metastasis, as native glomus tissue is purported to occur in many locations, including the peribronchial tissue. Because of their slow growth, glomus tumors are somewhat insensitive to radiotherapy, but radiation does afford some degree of tumor control.

Anatomic Origin and Distribution of Glomus Tumors

Rockley and Hawke[41] carefully studied the anatomic distribution of glomus bodies, and concluded that the division of glomus tumors into tympanicum or jugulare types is an arbitrary clinical classification, not reflecting the true anatomic distribution of glomus bodies. These workers proposed that "glomus bodies" are localized along the adventitia of the jugular dome, the tympanic branch of the glossopharyngeal nerve (Jacobson's nerve), and the auricular branch of the vagus nerve (Arnold's nerve).[42] Tumors arising along Jacobson's nerve or the promontory of the middle ear are of the glomus tympanicum type, whereas those arising proximal to Jacobson's nerve in the inferior tympanic canaliculus (adjacent to the jugular bulb) are of the glomus jugulare variety. Glomus bodies located along the course of Arnold's nerve adjacent to the facial nerve account for the occasional tumor in the descending facial canal.[43] Rarely, tumor can arise from glomus tissue in the vagus nerve (i.e., glomus vagale).[44] The ascending pharyngeal artery, through its inferior tympanic branch, is the primary blood supply to glomus tumors.[30,31] Additional blood supply is derived from the postauricular, occipital, internal maxillary, vertebral, and internal carotid arteries.[45]

Glomus jugulare tumors usually arise in the region of the dome of the jugular bulb, gradually filling this region and then expanding into the lateral compartment of the jugular foramen. The fibro-osseus partition in the jugular foramen is generally intact in patients with small and medium-size lesions, thereby leaving the nerves well protected medial to the tumor. This represents a surgically less demanding location, as it is possible to dissect the tumor from this partition without exposing the lower cranial nerves.[14] Large glomus jugulare tumors invade the anterolateral compartment of the jugular foramen and either render the lower cranial nerves dysfunctional or place them in jeopardy during tumor removal. Tumor can transgress the epineurium or even invade the actual nerve substance.[14,46]

Glomus jugulare tumors are locally invasive. After invasion of the temporal bone and middle ear, tumor can extend via the following routes: (1) down through the eustachian tube into the nasopharynx and skull base foramina; (2) along the ICA into the middle cranial fossa; (3) through the tegmen tympani to the middle fossa floor; (4) along the internal jugular vein or the hypoglossal canal into the posterior fossa; and (5) through the round window of the labyrinth with extension via the internal auditory canal into the cerebellopontine angle.[45,47]

Glomus Tumor Hormonal Activity

Glomus tumors may be endocrinologically active. Serum testing shows that approximately 4% of patients with these tumors have elevated catecholamine concentrations.[48] Because of this endocrinologic activity, glomus tumors have been included in the amine and amine-precursor uptake decarboxylase series (APUD) or, by newer terminology, the diffuse neuroendocrine system (DNES).[42,49,50] Immunohistochemistry stains may demonstrate positive numerous markers including neuron-specific enolase (NSE), serotonin, chromogranin, leu-enkephalin, gastrin, substance P, vasoactive intestinal peptide (VIP), somatostatin, bombesin, melanocyte-stimulating hormone (MSH), and calcitonin.[50]

Jugular Schwannoma

Jugular schwannomas, although the second or third most common tumor of the jugular foramen, are relatively rare tumors.[14] Jugular foramen schwannomas originate from CN IX, X, or XI and represent approximately 3 to 4% of intracranial neurinomas.[51,52] In fact, in his 1995 review of his own cases, Samii et al.[51] stated that fewer than 120 cases of schwannomas of CNs IX, X, and XI were previously reported. The term *schwannoma* relates to the cell of origin, the schwann cell, named after Theodor Schwann (1810–1882), the German anatomist credited with its discovery.[53] Schwannomas, in general, are the most common tumor of the petrous temporal bone. In Samii's series, the ratio of acoustic schwannomas to jugular foramen schwannomas was 24 : 1.

Most patients with jugular schwannomas present with vocal cord paralysis; therefore, the vagus nerve is most often described in the literature as the site of origin of these tumors.[14] Theoretically, schwannomas originating from CN X or XI displace

TABLE 82–3
Jugular Schwannoma Classification

Type	Description
A	Primarily limited to cerebellopontine angle, with minimal jugular foramen enlargement
B	Primarily in the jugular foramen, with minimal intracranial extension
C	Primarily extracranial with extension into the jugular foramen
D	Dumbbell-shaped with intra- and extracranial components

From Samii et al.[51]

CN IX laterally toward the surgeon's view (an unfavorable position); conversely, schwannomas originating from CN IX displace CN X and XI medially away from the surgeon's view (a favorable position).[14] In actuality, it is quite difficult to determine intraoperatively the nerve of origin of jugular schwannomas.[54,55]

Samii et al.[51] proposed a four-tiered anatomically based classification system (Table 82–3) of jugular foramen schwannomas similar to classifications systems of other schwannomas such as trigeminal neuromas.[56] Fisch and colleagues[57] proposed a four-tiered anatomically based classification system similar to the one he developed for glomus tumors (Table 82–4).

TABLE 82–4
Jugular Schwannoma Classification

Class	Description
A	Tumor confined to soft tissues of neck
B	Primary involvement of the neck with extension up to jugular foramen
C	Tumor fills jugular foramen, with resultant bone expansion
C1	No involvement of ICA above carotid foramen
C2	Involvement of the vertical segment of ICA
C3	Involvement of the horizontal segment of the ICA
C4	Tumor extending into foramen lacerum
D	Intracranial extension of tumor
D_e	Extradural
D_i	Intradural extension
	≤2-cm extension
	>2-cm extension

From Franklin et al.[57]

Meningiomas

Meningiomas of the jugular foramen are relatively rare, yet they are the second or third most common tumor of this region.[14] Most meningiomas of the jugular foramen invade from adjacent regions: medially, from the lower clivus; laterally, from the sigmoid sinus; superiorly, from the petrous bone or cerebellopontine angle; and inferiorly, from the foramen magnum.[58] Rarely, a meningioma may arise from cells of the arachnoid villi of the jugular bulb.[58] The anatomic relationship of the tumor to the cranial nerves depends on its site of origin. In general, meningiomas of the jugular foramen are thought to be more invasive into surrounding bone and cranial nerves than are glomus tumors; they tend to recur more frequently after surgery as well.[58]

Clinical Presentation of Patients with Jugular Foramen Tumors

GLOMUS TUMORS

Glomus tumors, the most common lesion of the jugular foramen, are most frequently diagnosed in women (female-to-male ratio 2–6 : 1) aged 40 to 60 years.[16,36,40,59] The most common signs and symptoms are tinnitus, hearing loss, and aural mass, but may also include otorrhea, pain, bleeding, vertigo, facial paresis, dysphagia, Horner syndrome, brain stem syndromes, or other abnormalities of lower cranial nerve function.[16,40,48,60] Palpitation, blood pressure lability, flushing, and cephalgia may be indicators of excessive catecholamine release. Classically, there has been a delay in diagnosis of 3 to 6 years from the onset of symptoms,[61] but with the improvement in imaging studies during the past decade one may expect more rapid diagnosis. These tumors are generally slow growing, but because of their critical location, they can cause considerable morbidity.

Glomus tumors may be divided into hereditary and nonhereditary types.[40] The hereditary type is notable for a reversal of the female to male predominance occurring with the nonhereditary type, a higher incidence of multiplicity (25 to 35%), an autosomal dominant pattern of inheritance[62] and younger age at the time of diagnosis.[63] Nonhereditary glomus tumors are associated with bilateral lesions in fewer than 5% of cases, but in up to 11% of cases second glomus tumors at other locations have been reported (e.g., carotid body tumor).[62] Glomus tumors also may be associated with pheochromocytoma,[64] thyroid cancer, and neurofibromatosis types I and II (NF1 and NF2, respectively).[65]

SCHWANNOMAS

Of 21 patients in Samii's series with jugular foramen schwannomas, 5 had NF2. Of the 16 without NF2, there was an 11 : 5 male-to-female ratio, and the mean age of the patients was

43 years. Preoperative cranial nerve deficits were as follows: V (13%), VI (6%), VII (25%), VIII (75%), IX (50%), X (75%), XI (38%), and XII (31%). Forty-four percent of these patients had cerebellar dysfunction at the time of presentation.[51]

Preoperative Imaging and Testing of Jugular Foramen Tumors

Clinical suspicion of a jugular foramen tumor requires radiologic confirmation. Magnetic resonance imaging (MRI) most clearly defines the nature and extent of the lesion,[66] and computed tomography (CT) may be warranted to further define the relevant osseous anatomy. Glomus tumors are generally described as heterogeneously enhancing lesions on gadolinium-enhanced MRI studies. Glomus tumors and meningiomas are typically described as causing irregular enlargement and erosion of the jugular foramen, whereas schwannomas expand the foramen with a smooth margin of bone erosion.

Bilateral carotid angiography is essential in the preoperative evaluation of glomus jugulare tumors to assess tumor vascularity and collateral cerebral blood flow and for consideration of possible preoperative intravascular embolization.[67] Angiography of patients with glomus tumors demonstrates a marked vascular tumor blush with the primary blood supply derived from ascending pharyngeal and occipital artery branches of the external carotid artery. ICA cross-compression and intraluminal balloon occlusion combined with xenon perfusion scanning are useful in the evaluation of collateral blood supply if ICA sacrifice is anticipated. Evaluation of the venous phase of the angiographic study is recommended to determine the dominance of the transverse and sigmoid sinuses and to assess the degree of patency of the jugular bulb and internal jugular vein.

EMBOLIZATION

Preoperative intra-arterial embolization represents a major advancement in the management of glomus jugulare tumors as an adjunct to intraoperative hemostasis, reduced operative time, and facilitation of complete tumor excision.[44,47,68] One retrospective study of 35 patients who underwent surgery for glomus jugulare tumors (18 with preoperative embolization, 17 without) demonstrated that embolization reduced blood loss (by $> 50\%$) and reduced operative time, but did not affect hospitalization time or cranial nerve morbidity.[69] Some surgeons do not advocate preoperative intra-arterial embolization on the grounds that the intraoperative blood loss is primarily venous (from IPS and sigmoid sinus),[61,70] but they probably represent the minority opinion. These surgeons do not feel that the benefits of embolization warrant the risks of stroke or other complications from the use of this technique.

Preoperative catecholamine screening is performed routinely for detection of secretory types of glomus jugulare tumors that require particular perioperative and anesthetic precautions. Elevation of catecholamine concentrations three or more times above normal requires screening for pheochromocytoma. As renal vein sampling may be required for this purpose, catecholamine screening should be performed before bilateral carotid angiography.

Management of Jugular Foramen Tumors

In recent decades, the management of lesions of the jugular foramen has evolved. During the 1940s and 1950s, surgical exposures were often limited to mastoidectomies; therefore, high recurrence rates and postoperative facial nerve deficits were common. Thus, radiotherapy was the treatment of choice. With the development of tomograms and, later, CT, and with refinements in surgical techniques, the 1960s and 1970s saw concentrated efforts toward gross total resections of lesions of the jugular foramen. The addition of intra-arterial embolization and MRI in the 1980s further advanced the capabilities of the surgical management of these lesions. For patients with acceptable surgical risk, complete surgical resection is generally desired for tumors of the jugular foramen. We generally reserve radiotherapy for patients with advanced age, significant comorbidities, or postoperative residual tumor or recurrence.

Surgery for Jugular Foramen Lesions

Seiffert is credited with the first surgical exploration of the jugular foramen for a patient with jugular foramen syndrome secondary to an intraluminal mass of the jugular bulb. Subsequently, numerous variations of the surgical approach to the jugular foramen region have been described.[2,38,51,71-74] Early surgical approaches to large highly vascularized glomus tumors used tumor resection under temporary circulatory arrest,[75] but the addition of preoperative embolization and improved surgical techniques obviates the need for circulatory arrest. The surgical approaches described in the literature combine dissection above and below the jugular foramen to isolate neurovascular structures both proximal and distal to the tumor. Jackson described an algorithm for selection of the appropriate surgical approach for glomus tumors that depend on the Glasscock–Jackson classification of the tumor, which is based on preoperative imaging studies[16,48,61,70,76] (Table 82–5). Fisch[77] described in detail an infratemporal fossa approach to the lateral skull base for tumors of the jugular foramen, and divided this into three variations, types A to C, according to the anatomic limits of the tumor. Samii et al.[51] termed their method for surgical management of jugular schwannomas the "combined cervical-mastoidectomy" approach. Otolaryngologists primarily manage glomus tympanicum tumors. Because this chapter details the neurosurgical perspective on jugular foramen tumors, management of glomus tympanicum tumors is not reviewed. Rather, emphasis is given to the management of glomus jugulare tumors and other lesions of the jugular foramen.

TABLE 82–5
Approach Algorithm for Glomus Tumors

Class	Description
Glomus tympanicum	
I	Transcanal
II	Postauricular
III	Postauricular
IV	Postauricular
Glomus jugulare	
I	Traditional skull base
II	Traditional skull base
III	Modified infratemporal
IV	Modified and/or extended infratemporal

From Jackson et al.[48] and Jackson.[70]

TABLE 82–6
Craniocervical Approach to Jugular Foramen

A. Cervical dissection	
	Internal carotid artery
	Internal jugular vein
	Hypoglossal nerve
	Vagus nerve
	Spinal accessory nerve
	Glossopharyngeal nerve
	Parotid segment of facial nerve
B. Cranial dissection[a]	
	Mastoid decortication
	Antrum
	Digastric ridge
	Lateral semicircular canal
	Posterior semicircular canal
	Fallopian canal
	Sigmoid sinus
	Superior semicircular canal
	Trautmann's triangle
	Suboccipital craniotomy
C. Jugular foramen dissection	
	Ligate jugular vein
	Ligate sigmoid sinus
	Remove jugular vein/sigmoid sinus (preserve medial wall)
	Occlude inferior petrosal sinus
	Identify proximal CN VII to XII

[a] Adapted from Miller et al.[10]

Craniocervical Approach to the Jugular Foramen

We describe the craniocervical approach to the jugular foramen used at the University of Cincinnati. The surgical technique is divided into three parts: (A) cervical dissection, (B) cranial dissection, and (C) jugular foramen dissection. Each part is subdivided into its essential steps (Table 82–6), which are performed by the ENT surgeons and the neurosurgeons. As with all surgery of the skull base, we view these approaches as a series of building blocks, each of which is included or excluded according to the particular lesion upon which we are operating. In the true sense of skull base surgery, our approach to jugular foramen lesions is a collaborative effort between head and neck surgery, neurotology, neurosurgery, neuroradiology, and radiation oncology. Philosophically, our strategy is to control and isolate neurovascular structures proximally and distally. This strategy allows us to follow these structures from areas of intact normal anatomy to areas distorted by tumor, facilitating their dissection and preservation when possible.

POSITION AND SKIN INCISION

The patient is positioned supine with the head fixed in the three-point Mayfield headholder (Ohio Medical Instruments, Cincinnati, OH) and rotated to the side contralateral to the tumor (Fig. 82–3). A crescent-shaped incision is marked extending from above the ear curving posteriorly and inferiorly behind the ear and extending into the neck across the rostral aspect of the sternocleidomastoid muscle. For tumors with significant anterior extension, the external auditory canal may be transected and oversewn into a blind sac during the opening to gain maximal anterior reflection of the musculocutaneous flap.

EXPOSURE IN THE NECK—HEAD AND NECK SURGEON

The head and neck surgeons of our skull base team begin the operation by performing the neck dissection. The internal carotid artery, internal jugular vein, and the cervical portions of CNs VII (parotid segment), IX, X, XI, and XII are exposed and marked with loosely applied vessel loops (Fig. 82–4A).

POSTERIOR PETROSECTOMY—NEUROTOLOGIST

After completion of the cervical exposure, our neurotologist performs the posterior petrosectomy. This is performed under the operating microscope with continuous irrigation and a variety of cutting and diamond bits on a high-speed drill.

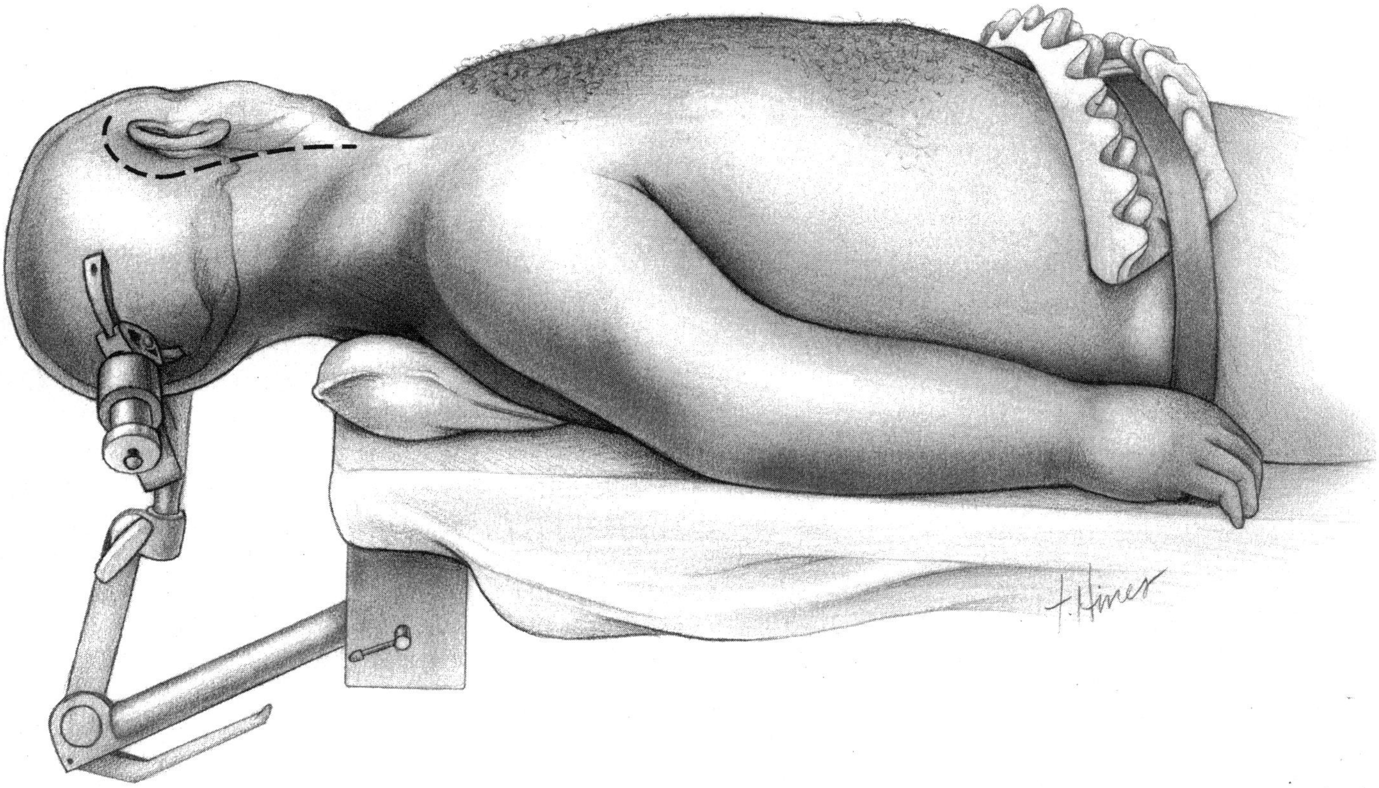

Figure 82–3 Positioning for the craniocervical approach. The patient is placed supine with the head in three-point fixation. The head is rotated to the contralateral side and a crescent-shaped skin incision is made from above the ear, passing 4 cm behind the mastoid tip, and down the anterior border of the sternocleidomastoid muscle to the cricoid cartilage. (Reprinted with permission from Tew JM, van Loveren HR, Keller JT: *Atlas of Operative Microneurosurgery*, Volume II. WB Saunders. In press.)

Initially the mastoid is decorticated from its tip inferiorly to the supramastoid crest (floor of the middle fossa) superiorly and from the posterior wall of the external auditory canal anteriorly to the sigmoid plate over the sigmoid sinus posteriorly. Resection of mastoid air cells exposes the cortical bony plates of the sigmoid sinus, temporal plate, canalicular plate, and sinodural angle. As the air cells are removed, the antrum is entered posterior and deep to the spine of Henle in Macewen's triangle. The lateral process of the incus and the lateral semicircular canal can be identified through the antrum. Exposure of the digastric ridge, the posteroinferior cortical indentation of the mastoid tip produced by the digastric muscle, serves as a landmark to the stylomastoid foramen and the distal end of the fallopian canal. The lateral, posterior, and superior semicircular canals are then further exposed. The remaining retrofacial air cells are removed to skeletonize the facial nerve in the fallopian canal from its external genu at the inferior edge of the lateral semicircular canal to the stylomastoid foramen. The chorda tympani is also identified at its origin from the vertical segment of the facial nerve. The sigmoid plate is further decorticated, and ultimately the thin shell of bone over the sigmoid sinus is removed. This dissection is carried inferiorly to expose the jugular bulb. Exposing the middle and posterior fossa dura and the intervening superior petrosal sinus reveals the superior semicircular canal (Fig. 82–4B). For patients with irreversible hearing loss a labyrinthectomy may be performed to expand the exposure.

Management of the facial nerve is an important component of surgical approaches to the jugular foramen.[78] Pensak and Jackler[79] suggested three options for facial nerve management, depending on the extent of tumor: (1) intact canal wall without facial nerve rerouting, (2) canal wall-down without facial nerve rerouting, (3) canal wall-down with anterior facial nerve rerouting. The first option maintains the physiologic structure of the ear canal and middle ear to preserve auditory functions, but is limited in its anterior exposure. The use of the canal wall-down approach without facial nerve rerouting is indicated when the ear canal or middle ear is extensively involved by tumor. Extended retrofacial exposure can be performed after transection of the chorda tympani with creation of a fallopian bridge (circumferential skeletonization of the fallopian canal) (Fig. 82–4C). With the fallopian bridge technique, tumors can be dissected posterior, lateral, and medial to the ICA after drilling of the carotid ridge. Preserving the normal anatomic position of the facial nerve

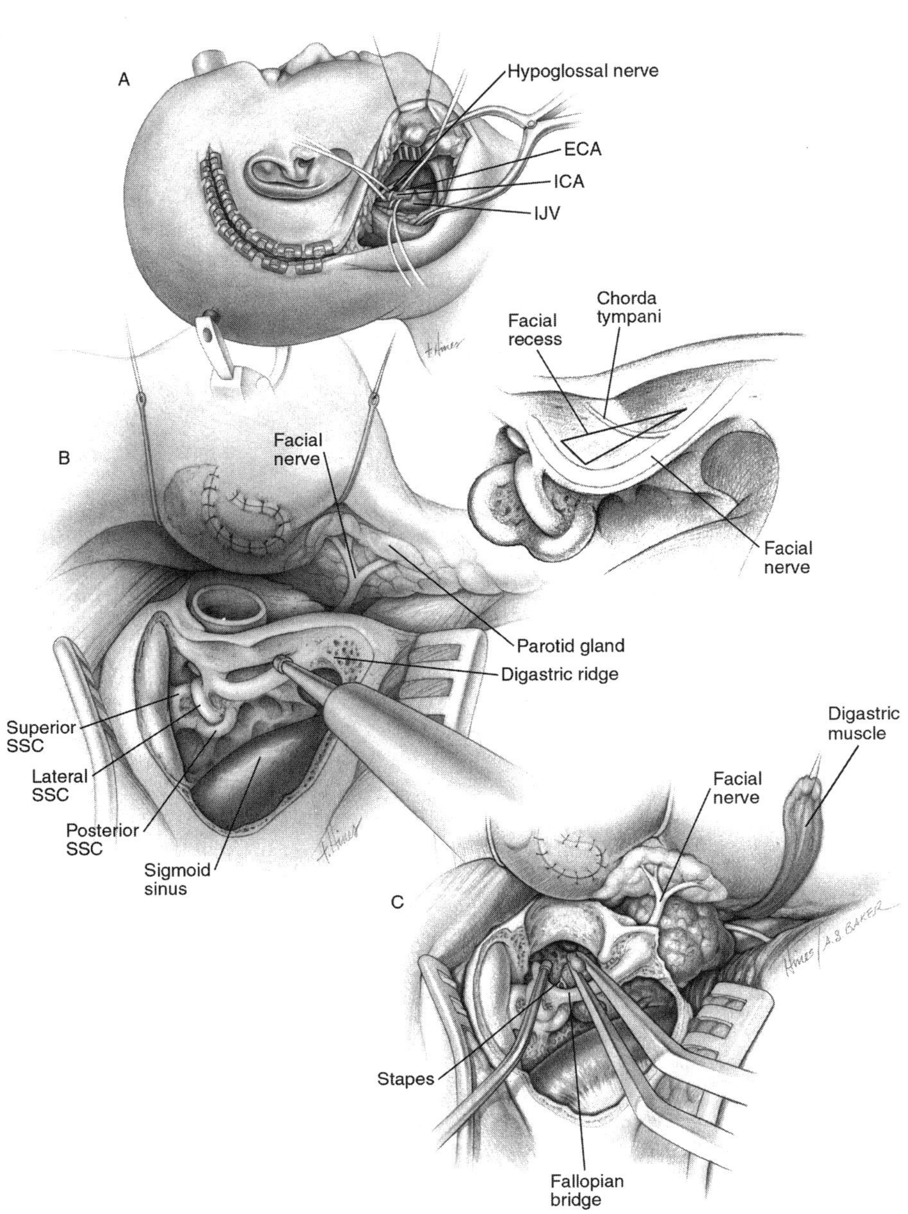

Figure 82–4 **(A)** The sternocleidomastoid muscle (SCM) is retracted laterally and dissection continues through the cervical fascia to the carotid sheath. The common facial vein is ligated and the hypoglossal nerve is identified as it crosses the carotid bifurcation. The ICA (internal carotid artery), ECA (external carotid artery), and IJV (internal jugular vein) are isolated with color-coded Silastic loops. **(B)** The skin and muscles over the mastoid area are reflected and the external ear canal is transected and closed in three layers and oversewn with a periosteal flap. The standard mastoidectomy is expanded by removing bone anterior to the facial nerve, called the facial recess (triangle), and sacrificing the chorda tympani nerve. **(C)** The posterior canal wall is thinned to eggshell thickness and removed (canal wall-down). The incus, malleus, and tympanic membrane are removed. Retrofacial air cells are removed with a high-speed drill, effectively creating a fallopian bridge containing the facial nerve. Bone of the mastoid tip is thinned and removed to the level of the digastric ridge. (Reprinted with permission from Tew et al.[84])

increases the likelihood of normal postoperative facial nerve function. The third option with facial nerve rerouting, originally described by Fisch,[77] is reserved for the infrequent tumor with extension anterior to the carotid genu. Mobilization of the mandible may also be necessary in this circumstance, if there is significant middle fossa and infratemporal extension.

TUMOR EXCISION—NEUROSURGEON

The third portion of the craniocervical approach to jugular foramen tumors is performed by the neurosurgeon of the skull base team. Any remaining bone over the posterior aspect of the jugular bulb is removed with a high-speed drill to better expose the jugular bulb/jugular vein junction (Fig. 82–5A). A small, low retrosigmoid suboccipital craniotomy extending to the foramen magnum can be performed to gain proximal isolation of the lower CNs. For tumors that occlude the inferior portion of the sigmoid sinus, the internal jugular vein is ligated and transected in the neck (Fig. 82–5B). In instances in which the tumor is on the dominant side of venous drainage an attempt should be made to preserve the sinus. The sigmoid sinus is ligated below the level of the superior petrosal sinus by opening the dura anterior (retrolabyrinthine) and posterior to the sinus, allowing the placement of hemoclips or sutures. All venous pathways, except the inferior petrosal sinus, are thus isolated so that the internal jugular vein and sigmoid sinus can be opened and tumor sharply dissected. The medial wall of the jugular bulb remains intact to preserve

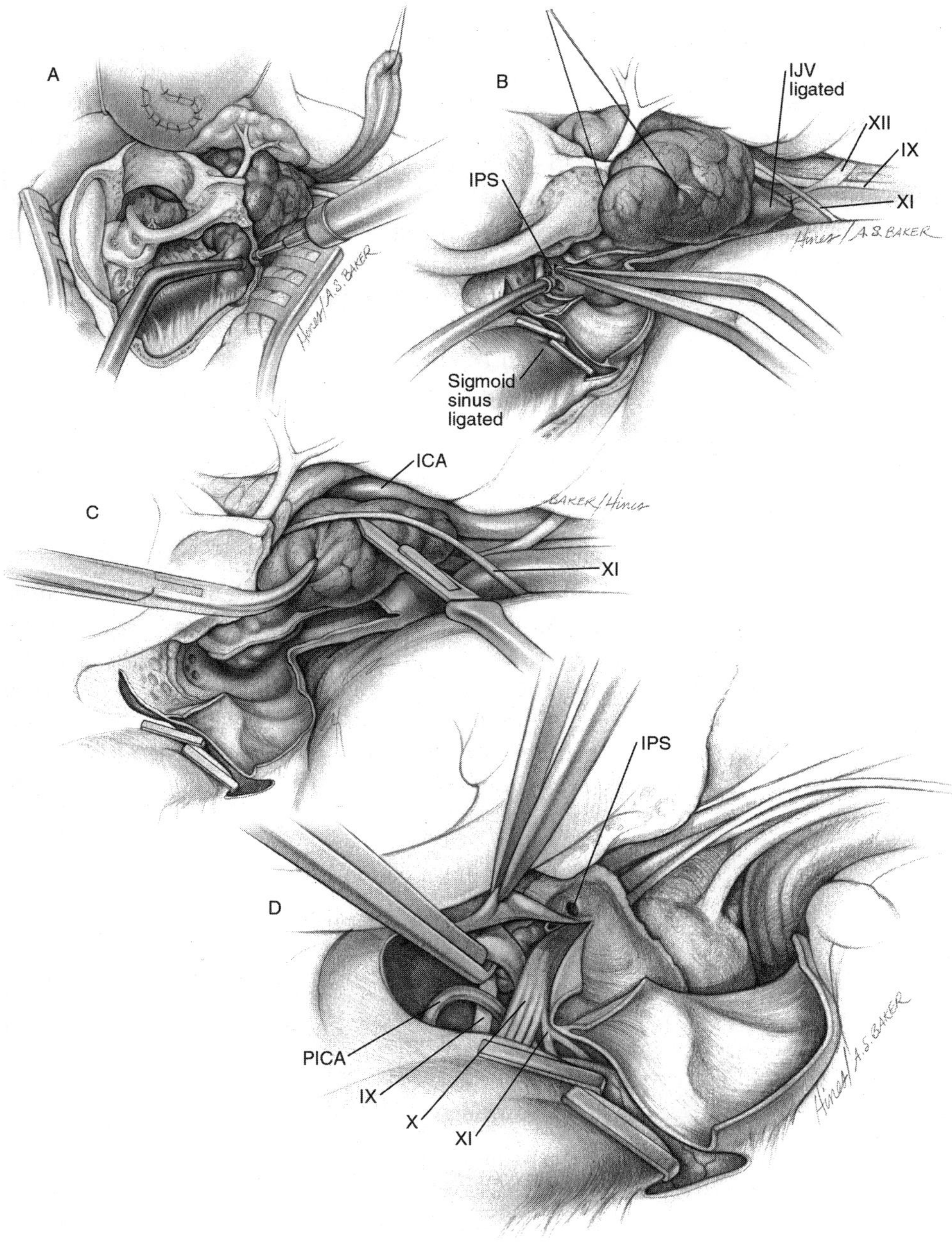

Figure 82–5 **(A)** After tumor is removed from the retrofacial air cells, any residual bone covering the jugular bulb is removed with a high-speed drill. This exposes the jugular bulb/jugular vein junction. **(B)** The sigmoid sinus is ligated below the petrosal sinus with hemoclips, and the internal jugular vein (IJV) is ligated below the pole of the tumor. The vein and sinus are opened along their length, and tumor is removed, revealing three to five inferior petrosal sinus (IPS) orifices. Bleeding from these orifices is controlled by packing with Oxycel and bone wax. The medial wall of the sinus is left intact with the posterior fossa dura. **(C)** The tumor is peeled from inferior to superior by dissecting from cranial nerves IX through XII and arterial feeders from the ascending pharyngeal artery. (ICA = internal carotid artery.) **(D)** The dura over the pars nervosa and IPS is incised with a No.15 blade to expose tumor intracranially in the jugular foramen along cranial nerve IX. A bone punch removes the occasional osseous bridge that divides the jugular foramen into pars nervosa and pars venosa compartments. (PICA = posterior inferior cerebellar artery.) (Reprinted with permission from Tew, et al.[84])

the orifices (usually 3 to 5) of the inferior petrosal sinus. Brisk venous bleeding encountered from the IPS is controlled with Oxycel cotton (Becton-Dickinson, Franklin Lakes, NJ). Care is taken to avoid overpacking the IPS that, thus, causes cranial nerve damage. Sharp dissection separates tumorous attachment to CNs IX through XII (Fig. 82–5C). Remaining tumor is dissected from the cranial nerves as they are traced intracranially from the jugular foramen to their extracranial course (Fig. 82–5D).

CLOSURE

Upon completion of the resection, the dura is reapproximated as well as possible and the remaining surgical defect obliterated with autologous tissue grafts, including adipose, fascia lata, and muscle as needed. A multilayer closure is then performed. Previously, all patients underwent intraoperative placement of a tracheostomy and feeding gastrostomy, but this is generally not necessary with current techniques and, therefore, is performed only as required.

Clinical Series—Outcomes, Complications

Clinical outcome for patients with tumors of the jugular foramen, including time to recurrence and neurologic morbidity, is, in part, related to the extent of tumor at the time of diagnosis. Smaller tumors are most amenable to complete resection with minimal risk of cranial nerve deficits. Patients with larger tumors are more likely to present with cranial nerve deficits and carry a higher risk of further cranial neuropathies postoperatively.[16,61,80] In their report on glomus jugulare tumors in 1962, Alford and

Guilford[36] reported a 6% postoperative recurrence rate for stage 0 tumors limited to the middle ear, and a 100% recurrence rate for the more extensive stage IV lesions eroding the petrous temporal bone and jugular foramen with intracranial extension. More contemporary series report gross total resections for jugular foramen tumors at 70 to 80%.[67,79] Facial nerve preservation (House–Brackman grade 1) is reported in more than 90% of these patients at 6 months of follow-up.[79]

RADIATION

Considerable debate remains in the literature as to whether radiation should be considered first-line therapy for glomus tumors and other tumors of the jugular foramen, rather than surgery.[16,60,63] In some large series of patients with glomus tumors, local control and survival have been achieved with radiotherapy in up to 90% of patients.[60,81,82] In his literature review of nearly 600 patients treated with either surgery or radiation as the primary modality for glomus tumors, Carrasco[81] found no significant differences in rates of tumor recurrence between these groups. In both groups high rates of salvage for recurrent tumors were demonstrated, whether with surgery, radiation, or a combination of both. Of these patients, even those with recurrence, fewer than 10% of patients died as a result of the glomus tumor. The incidence of posttreatment cranial neuropathies is low for radiotherapy.[47,83] The advent of stereotactic radiosurgery in recent decades provides a more precise technique for administering high-dose focal radiation, and preliminary reports indicate that this modality may have a role in the treatment of jugular foramen tumors.[82] One of the main differences between radiotherapy and surgery for glomus tumors is that radiotherapy is used as a means to control tumor growth, whereas surgery is used in an attempt to achieve a cure. Many patients irradiated for lesions of the jugular foramen require subsequent surgery for disease progression, and previously irradiated tissue presents many obvious difficulties for the surgeon.[16] In practicality, each of these modalities has clinical utility, and must be chosen separately or in combination as appropriate for individual patients.

Summary

In summary, pathological lesions of the jugular foramen remain a formidable challenge. Surgical resection requires intimate familiarity with the anatomic complexities of this region. Our general preference is for surgical resection of these lesions when possible. Embolization and radiation are also important adjuncts in the management of these diseases. Optimal patient outcomes are best achieved with a multidisciplinary approach to these complicated lesions.

REFERENCES

van Loveren et al.—CHAPTER 82

1. Stedman TL. *Stedman's Medical Dictionary*. 24th ed. Baltimore: Williams & Wilkins; 1982:548, 738
2. Katsuta T, Rhoton AL, Matsushima T. The jugular foramen: microsurgical anatomy and operative approaches. *Neurosurgery* 1997;41:149–202
3. Ayeni SA, Ohata K, Tanaka K, et al. The microsurgical anatomy of the jugular foramen. *J Neurosurg* 1995;83: 903–909
4. DiChiro G, Fisher RL, Nelson KB. The jugular foramen. *J Neurosurg* 1964;21:447–460
5. van Loveren HR, Liu SS, Pensak ML, et al. Anatomy of the jugular foramen: the neurosurgical perspective. *Opin Tech Otolaryngol Head Neck Surg* 1996;7:90–94
6. Bouthillier A, van Loveren HR, Keller JT. Segments of the internal carotid artery: a new classification. *Neurosurgery* 1996;38:425–433
7. Hovelacque A. Le crane dans son ensemble. In: *Osteologie*. Fascicule II. Paris: G. Doin & CE; 1934:155–161
8. Rhoton AL, Buza R. Microsurgical anatomy of the jugular foramen. *J Neurosurg* 1975;42:541–550
9. Shapiro R. Compartmentalization of the jugular foramen. *J Neurosurg* 1972;36:340–343
10. Miller CG, van Loveren HR, Keller JT, et al. Transpetrosal approach: surgical anatomy and technique. *Neurosurgery* 1993;33:461–469
11. Shao KN, Tatagiba M, Samii M. Surgical management of high jugular bulb in acoustic neurinoma via retrosigmoid approach. *Neurosurgery* 1993;32:32–36
12. Shiu PC, Hanafee WN, Wilson GH, et al. Cavernous sinus venography. *Am J Roentgenol Radium Ther Nucl Med* 1968; 104:57–62
13. Miller DL, Doppman JL, Chang R. Anatomy of the junction of the inferior petrosal sinus and the internal jugular vein. *AJNR* 1993;14:1075–1083
14. Lustig LR, Jackler RK. The variable relationship between the lower cranial nerves and jugular foramen tumors: implications for neural preservation. *Am J Otol* 1996;17:658–668
15. Saleh E, Najuib M, Aristegui M, et al. Lower skull base: anatomic study with surgical implications. *Ann Otol Rhinol Laryngol* 1995;104:57–61
16. Jackson CG, Cueva RA, Thedinger BA, et al. Cranial nerve preservation in lesions of the jugular fossa. *Otolaryngol Head Neck Surg* 1991;105:687–693

17. Kaufman BA, Francel PC, Roberts RL, et al. Chondroid chordoma of the lateral skull base. *Pediatr Neurosurg* 1995;2: 159–165
18. Rupa V, Rajsekhar V, Bhanu TS, et al. Primary chondroid chordoma of the base of the petrous temporal bone. *J Laryngol Otol* 1989;103:771–773
19. Harvey SA, Wiet RJ, Kazan R. Chondrosarcoma of the jugular foramen. *Am J Otol* 1994;15:257–263
20. Sabin HI, Bordi LT, Symon L. Epidermoid cysts and cholesterol granulomas centered on the posterior fossa: twenty years of diagnosis and management. *Neurosurgery* 1987;21: 798–805
21. Schweinfurth JM, Johnson JT, Weissman J. Jugular foramen syndrome as a complication of metastatic melanoma. *Am J Otolaryngol* 1993;14:168–174
22. Miyachi S, Negoro M, Saito K, et al. Myeloma manifesting as a large jugular tumor: case report. *Neurosurgery* 1990;27:971–977
23. Urbach H, Kristof R, Zentner J, et al. Sarcoidosis presenting as an intra- or extra-axial cranial mass: report of two cases. *Neuroradiology* 1997;39:516–519
24. Brown EW, Megerian CA, McKenna MJ, et al. Fibrous dysplasia of the temporal bone: imaging findings. *AJR* 1995; 164:679–682
25. Maruyama R, Nagaoka S, Todaka T, et al. Intracranial chondromyxoid fibroma extending into the jugular foramen. *Pathol Int* 1994;44:857–859
26. Han MH, Chang KH, Kim IO, et al. Non-Hodgkin lymphoma of the central skull base: MR manifestations. *J Comput Assist Tomogr* 1993;17:567–571
27. Matsumoto T. Amyloidomas in the cerebellopontine angle and jugular foramen. Case report. *J Neurosurg* 1985;62:592–596
28. Valentin G. Ueber eine gangliose Anschwellung in der Jacobsenschen Anastomose des Menschen. *Arch Anat Physiol Wissensch Med* 1840;89:287–290
29. Krause W. Die Glandula tympanica des Menschen. *Zentralbl Med Wiss* 1878;16:737–739
30. Guild SR. A hitherto unrecognized structure, the glomus jugularis, in man. *Anat Rec* 1941;79(suppl 2):28
31. Guild SR. The glomus jugulare, a nonchromaffin paraganglion, in man. *Ann Otol Rhinol Laryngol* 1953;62:1045–1071
32. Rosenwasser H. Carotid body tumor of the middle ear and mastoid. *Arch Otolaryngol* 1945;41:64–67
33. Winship T, Klopp CT, Jenkins WH. Glomus-jugularis tumors. *Cancer* 1948;1:441–448
34. Karas DE, Kwartler JA. Glomus tumors: a fifty-year historical perspective. *Am J Otol* 1993;14:495–500
35. Capps FCW. Glomus jugulare tumors of the middle ear. *J Laryngol Otol* 1952;66:302
36. Alford BR, Guilford FR. A comprehensive study of tumors of the glomus jugulare. *Laryngoscope* 1962;72:765–787
37. Oldring D, Fisch U. Glomus tumors of the temporal region: surgical therapy. *Am J Otolaryngol* 1979;1:7–18
38. Jenkins HA, Fisch U. Glomus tumors of the temporal bone, technique of surgical resection. *Arch Otolaryngol* 1981;107: 209–214
39. Glasscock ME, Jackson CG, Harris PF. Glomus tumors: diagnosis, classification and management of large lesions. *Arch Otolaryngol (Stockh)* 1982;108:401–406
40. Ebersold MF, Morita A, Olsen KD, et al. Glomus jugular tumors. In: Kaye AH, Laws ER, eds. *Brain Tumors.* New York: Churchill Livingstone; 1995:795–807
41. Rockley TJ, Hawke M. Glomus bodies in the temporal bone. *J Otolaryngol* 1990;19:51–56
42. Gulya AJ. The glomus tumor and its biology. *Laryngoscope* 1993;103(11 Pt 2; suppl 60):7–15
43. Robertson JH, Brodkey JA. Glomus jugulare tumors. In: Youmans JR, ed. *Neurological Surgery.* 4th ed. Philadelphia: WB Saunders; 1996:3084–3101
44. Watkins LD, Mendoza N, Cheesman AD, et al. Glomus jugulare tumours: a review of 61 cases. *Acta Neurochir (Wien)* 1994;130:66–70
45. Spector GJ, Druck NS, Gado MH. Neurological manifestations of glomus tumors in the head and neck. *Arch Neurol* 1976;33:270–274
46. Makek M, Franklin D, Zaho JC, et al. Neural infiltration of glomus temporale tumors. *Am J Otol* 1990;11:1–5
47. Robertson JH, Gardner G, Cocke EW. Glomus jugulare tumors. *Clin Neurosurg* 1993;41:39–61
48. Jackson CG, Harris PF, Glasscock ME, et al. Diagnosis and management of paragangliomas of the skull base. *Am J Surg* 1990;159:389–393
49. Kau R, Arnold W. Somatostatin receptor scintigraphy and therapy of neuroendocrine (APUD) tumors of the head and neck. *Acta Otolaryngol (Stockh)* 1996;116:345–349
50. Saito H, Saito S, Sano T, et al. Immunoreactive somatostatin in catecholamine producing extradural paraganglioma. *Cancer* 1982;50:560–565
51. Samii M, Babu RP, Tatagiba M, et al. Surgical treatment of jugular foramen schwannomas. *J Neurosurg* 1995;82:924–932
52. Samii M, Draf W. Surgery of tumors of the lateral posterior skull base and petrous bone. In: Samii M, Draf W, eds. *Surgery of the Skull Base: An Interdisciplinary Approach.* New York: Springer-Verlag; 1989:410–425
53. Last RJ. *Anatomy, Regional and Applied.* New York: Churchill Livingstone; 1984:584
54. Crumley RL, Wilson C. Schwannomas of the jugular foramen. *Laryngoscope* 1984;94:772–778
55. Symon L. Difficult to determine the origin of neuromas in jugular foramen (letter). *Surg Neurol* 1991;36:401
56. Taha J, Tew JM Jr, van Loveren HR, et al. Comparison of conventional and skull base approaches for the excision of trigeminal neurinomas. *J Neurosurg* 1995;82:719–725
57. Franklin DJ, Moore GF, Fisch U. Jugular foramen peripheral nerve sheath tumors. *Laryngoscope* 1989;99(10 pt 1): 1081–1087
58. Molony TB, Brackmann DE, Lo WW. Meningiomas of the jugular foramen. *Otolaryngol Head Neck Surg* 1992;106: 128–136
59. Brammer RE, Graham MD, Kemink JL. Glomus tumors of the temporal bone: contemporary evaluation and therapy. *Otolaryngol Clin North Am* 1984;17:499–512

60. Larner JM, Hahn SS, Spaulding CA, et al. Glomus jugulare tumors. Long-term control by radiation therapy. *Cancer* 1992; 69:1813–1817
61. Jackson CG. Diagnosis for treatment planning and treatment options. *Laryngoscope* 1993;103(11 Pt 2; suppl 60):17–22
62. Tali ET, Sener RN, Ibis E, et al. Familial bilateral glomus jugulare tumors. *Neuroradiology* 1991;3:171–172
63. van der Mey AG, Frijns JH, Cornelisse CJ, et al. Does intervention improve the natural course of glomus tumors? A series of 108 patients seen in a 32-year period. *Ann Otol Rhinol Laryngol* 1992;101:635–642
64. Parkin JL. Familial multiple glomus tumors and pheochromocytoma. *Ann Otol* 1981;90:6063
65. DeAngelis LM, Kelleher MB, Post KD, et al. Multiple paragangliomas in neurofibromatosis: a new neuroendocrine neoplasia. *Neurology* 1987;37:129–133
66. Tali ET, Yuh WT, Mayr NA, et al. Magnetic resonance imaging of bilateral familial paragangliomas. *Ann Otol Rhinol Laryngol* 1993;102:473–477
67. Patel SJ, Sekhar LN, Cass SP, et al. Combined approaches for resection of extensive glomus jugulare tumors. A review of 12 cases. *J Neurosurg* 1994;80:1026–1038
68. Carrier DA, Arriaga MA, Gorum MJ, et al. Preoperative embolization of anastomoses of the jugular bulb: an adjuvant in jugular foramen surgery. *AJNR* 1997;18:1252–1256
69. Murphy TP, Brackmann DE. Effects of preoperative embolization on glomus jugulare tumors. *Laryngoscope* 1989;99:1244–1247
70. Jackson CG. Basic surgical principles of neurotologic skull base surgery. *Laryngoscope* 1993;103(11 Pt 2; suppl 60):29–44
71. Fisch U, Fagan P, Valvanis A. The infratemporal fossa approach for the lateral skull base. *Otolaryngol Clin North Am* 1984;17:513–552
72. Glasscock ME. The history of glomus tumors: a personal perspective. *Laryngoscope* 1993;103(11 Pt 2; suppl 60):3–6
73. Green JD Jr, Brackmann DE, Nguyen CD, et al. Surgical management of previously untreated glomus jugulare tumors. *Laryngoscope* 1994;104(8 Pt 1):917–921
74. van Loveren HR, Aziz KM, Tauber M. Skull base exposures: posterior and lateral. In: McBlack P, Kaye A, eds. *Operative Neurosurgery*. London: Harcourt Brace; 2000: 1385–1398
75. Michelson RP, Connoly JE. Removal of glomus jugulare tumor utilizing complete occlusion of the cerebral circulation. *Laryngoscope* 1962;72:788–805
76. Jackson CG. Summary. *Laryngoscope* 1993;103(11 Pt 2; suppl 60):71–72
77. Fisch U. Infratemporal fossa approach to tumors of the temporal bone and base of the skull. *J Laryngol Otol* 1978;92: 949–967
78. Von Doersten PG, Jackler RK. Anterior facial nerve rerouting in cranial base surgery: a comparison of three techniques. *Otolaryngol Head Neck Surg* 1996;115:82–88
79. Pensak ML, Jackler RK. Removal of jugular foramen tumors: the fallopian bridge technique. *Otolaryngol Head Neck Surg* 1997;117:586–591
80. Kaye AH, Hahn JF, Kinney SE, et al. Jugular foramen schwannomas. *J Neurosurg* 1984;60:1045–1053
81. Carrasco V. Radiation therapy of glomus jugulare tumors. *Laryngoscope* 1993;103(11 Pt 2; suppl 60):23–27
82. Foote RL, Coffey RJ, Gorman DA, et al. Stereotactic radiosurgery for glomus jugulare tumors: a preliminary report. *Int J Radiat Oncol Biol Phys* 1997;38:491–495
83. Cole JM, Beiler D. Long-term results of treatment for glomus jugulare and glomus vagale tumors with radiotherapy. *Laryngoscope* 1994;104:1461–1465
84. Tew TM, van Loveren HR, Keller JT. *Atlas of Microneurosurgery*. Vol II. Philadelphia: WB Saunders; In press

Jugular Foramen Tumors

CHAPTER 83

Ugo Fisch, Thomas Linder, and Phillip Chang

The overwhelming majority of jugular foramen tumors are benign. Only 6% of the tumors are malignant. Paragangliomas, neurogenic tumors, and meningiomas account for more than 80% of lesions of the jugular foramen (Table 83–1). In spite of the benign histologic characteristics of these tumors, all are locally destructive. These tumors are clinically silent until they eventually cause embarrassment of the vital neurovascular structures that traverse, or are in close proximity to, the jugular foramen (Table 83–2). The lower cranial nerves, the facial nerve, and audiologic and vestibular function are all potentially compromised by the slow progression of jugular foramen tumors.

The clinician's ability to detect these lesions has been greatly enhanced with the advent and widespread availability of advanced imaging technology such as computed tomography (CT) and magnetic resonance imaging (MRI). Paragangliomas, schwannomas, and meningiomas are all known to be radioresistant. Surgery is the treatment of choice and provides the only chance of cure. With the current lateral otologic approaches of the skull base (Fig. 83–1), tumor control is excellent. Surgical morbidity is minimal but is still directly related to tumor size. For this reason, prompt diagnosis and treatment of jugular foramen tumors ensure an optimal outcome for the patient.

TABLE 83–1
Jugular Foramen Tumors; 1974–1994, at the University of Zurich ($n = 400$)

Tumor Type	*n*	%
Paragangliomas	*n* = 280	70
Temporal bone	240	
Glomus vagale	40	
Schwannomas	*n* = 41	10
IX, X	36	
XI	1	
XII	2	
Sympathetic trunk	2	
Others	*n* = 79	20
Chordoma	18	
Meningioma	10	
Infralabyrinthine cholesteatoma	10	
Papillary adenoma	8	
Various malignant tumors	24	
Various benign tumors	9	
Total	400	100

Anatomy of the Jugular Foramen

The normal jugular foramen averages 15 mm in length and 10 mm in width, and the smaller pars nervosa averages 5 mm in width.[1] There is a marked range in the dimensions and degree of asymmetry of the jugular foramen, due mainly to the pars vascularis. The right jugular vein and foramen are usually dominant.[1]

The glossopharyngeal, vagus, and cranial accessory nerves emerge in a line from along the medulla oblongata and then run laterally to the jugular foramen, where they leave the posterior cranial fossa through the jugular foramen. DiChiro *et al.*[1] describe the foramen as a canal coursing anteriorly, inferiorly, and laterally from an intracranial to an extracranial opening. A fibrous or bony septum separates the pars nervosa, containing the petrosal sinus and glossopharyngeal nerve, from the pars vascularis, containing the vagus and the accessory nerves along with the jugular vein.

The jugular foramen is anatomically significant, as it not only acts as a conduit for vital neurovascular structures, but is

TABLE 83–2
Signs and Symptoms of Jugular Foramen Tumors

Related to the mass effect
Aural (hearing loss, vertigo, tinnitus, otalgia, eustachian tube dysfunction)
Parapharyngeal (neck mass, parapharyngeal mass, dysphagia)
Neurologic
Lower cranial neuropathies (dysphagia, dysphonia, aspiration, shoulder weakness, dysarthria, hemiatrophy of the tongue
Facial nerve palsy
Vestibulocochlear nerve dysfunction
Trigeminal nerve dysfunction
Cerebellar dysfunction
Brain stem compression
Hydrocephalus
Paraneoplastic
Hyperdynamic state

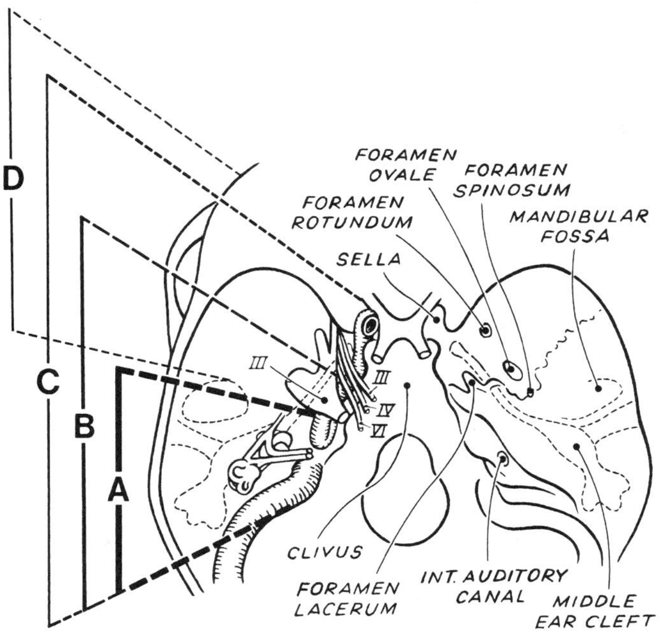

Figure 83–1 Schematic view of the lateral skull base approaches types A to D. The type A approach is the preferred access for jugular foramen tumors.

surrounded by vital neighboring structures. Both tumor progression and tumor resection may pose a potential threat to these structures.

Superior to the jugular foramen lies the cerebellopontine angle, the internal auditory canal, the inferobasal otic capsule, and the middle ear. Inferiorly, the jugular foramen leads to the carotid sheath and the cervical sympathetic chain. Medially lies a partition of bone separating the jugular foramen from the hypoglossal canal. Lateral is the stylomastoid foramen and the mastoid and proximal extratemporal portion of the facial nerve. The carotid crest separates jugular foramen from the carotid foramen and artery situated more anteriorly.

Typically, there are three glomus bodies or paraganglia in each temporal bone from which paragangliomas may arise.[2] The paraganglia are usually found accompanying Jacobson's (cranial nerve IX), Arnold's (cranial nerve X) nerve or in the adventitia of the dome of the jugular bulb. Temporal bone paragangliomas therefore more commonly originate from the jugular bulb and hypotympanum (glomus jugulare) than on the mucosa of the promontory (glomus tympanicum). Especially with large tumors, the site of origin of these tumors can often only be surmised.

Paraganglia are nonencapsulated and consist of lobules, intimately surrounded and interlaced with a rich network of capillaries. The lobules contain sustentacular cells (modified Schwann cells) and darker chief cells, arranged into groups known as *Zellballen* (cell balls). Derived from the neural crest, chief cells are members of the diffuse neuroendocrine system (DNES) and therefore have the capability of synthesizing catecholamines.

Schwannomas arising from the any of the lower cranial nerves will tend to expand the foramen[1,3-6] Like their vestibular counterpart, jugular foramen schwannoma arise at the transition zone between central and peripheral myelin.

With meningiomas, the jugular foramen may be the site of origin or, more frequently, may act as a conduit for the its extracranial extension. The jugular foramen and the foramen lacerum are the most common foramina, serving as pathways for the extracranial extension of a primary intracranial meningioma.

Temporal Bone Paragangliomas

Paragangliomas of the temporal bone (60%) and glomus vagale (10%) account for the vast majority of jugular foramen tumors (70%) (Table 83–1). Currently, the term *paraganglioma* is preferable, as it refers to the fact that these tumors arise from the paraganglia situated in perivascular locations, arising from neuroectodermal tissues. The term *glomus* is a misnomer and, although inaccurate, will no doubt persist.

In the head and neck, two anatomic groups of paragangliomas can be differentiated: temporal bone paragangliomas and cervical paragangliomas. Temporal bone paragangliomas can be classified as glomus tympanicum and glomus jugulare, in those cases in which the site of origin of the tumor can be determined. The term *cervical paragangliomas* describes glomus caroticum and glomus vagale. The jugular foramen can be affected by temporal bone paragangliomas and glomus vagale.

EPIDEMIOLOGY

Temporal bone paragangliomas are much more common than any other middle ear neoplasm. These tumors are second only to vestibular schwannoma as the most common tumor affecting the temporal bone.[7] Temporal bone paragangliomas account for 15% of all neoplasms at the skull base.[8] The incidence of this tumor is 1 : 1,300,000. The peak incidence is at 45 and 55 years of age, although this is highly variable. There is a predominant incidence in females[7,9] with a sex ratio of 4 : 1. There is no racial or ethnic predilection.

Although paragangliomas arise sporadically, a positive family history has been reported in 9.5 to 50% of patients.[10-12] The mode of inheritance in the familial form is currently attributed to the genetic imprinting mode of inheritance.[12]

The familial form is distinct from the nonfamilial form in that there is no female preponderance, and it is associated with a higher incidence (48%) of multicentric paragangliomas.[12] Multicentricity is found in about 5 to 15% of patients with the nonfamilial form. The most common second tumor is a carotid body tumor.

Pathology

Temporal bone paragangliomas are typically vascular reddish purple lobulated masses. Histologically, paragangliomas resemble paraganglia, displaying the same organoid pattern with *zellballen* composed of chief cell-like elements. Mitotic figures are rare. The histopathology is characterized by a rich vascularity.

Although usually histologically benign, paragangliomas of the temporal bone are characterized as locally destructive. Their growth is characteristically very slow, but rapid progression can occur and is unpredictable.[13,14] Spread occurs along the pathways of least resistance, often initially after the air cell tracts of cancellous and spongiotic temporal bone. Eventually, the tumor spreads outside the temporal bone via the jugular foramen and other neurovascular foramina.[15,16]

Paragangliomas overall have an incidence of malignancy of 2 to 4%, but this is far less common with temporal bone paragangliomas than with glomus vagale tumors. There is no histologic distinction between benign and malignant lesions. Malignancy is reserved for the presence of local, regional, and distal metastases. Distal metastases occur most commonly to the lungs.

Functional activity in skull base paragangliomas is 1 to 2%.[8,17-19] In these cases, the continuous or episodic secretion of catecholamines may produce clinical symptoms mimicking a pheochromocytoma. These features include persistent or paroxysmal hypertension, tachycardia, excessive perspiration, and anxiousness. When manipulated surgically, catecholamine-secreting paragangliomomas can potentially initiate a life-threatening hypertensive crisis, constituting an anesthetic emergency.

Paragangliomas of the temporal bone are associated with other neoplasms, both benign and malignant, in 7% of patients.[7] Tumors most commonly associated are pheochromocytomas, thyroid C-cell carcinoma, parathyroid adenomas, and visceral neoplasms of neural crest origin. There is also a reported association with the multiple endocrine neoplasm (MEN) syndromes.

TABLE 83–3
Fisch Staging of Temporal Paraganglioma

Class A: Tumor limited to the middle ear cleft

Class B: Tumor limited to the tympanomastoid area without destruction of bone in the infralabyrinthine compartment

Class C: Tumor extending into, and destroying, bone of the infralabyrinthine and apical compartments of the temporal bone

- C1: Tumor erodes the carotid foramen, but does not invade the carotid artery
- C2: Tumor destroys the vertical carotid canal between the carotid foramen and the carotid bend
- C3: Tumor extends along the horizontal portion of the carotid artery but does not reach the foramen lacerum
- C4: Tumor grows to the foramen lacerum along the carotid artery to the cavernous sinus

Class D: Tumor with intracranial extension

- De1: Tumor with intracranial extradural extension ≤2 cm in diameter
- De2: Tumor with intracranial extradural extension >2 cm in diameter
- Di1: Tumor with intracranial intradural extension ≤2 cm in diameter
- Di2: Tumor with intracranial intradural extension >2 cm in diameter
- D3: Tumor with inoperable intracranial extension

STAGING

Fisch staging of temporal bone paragangliomas classifies these paragangliomas according to the extent of the tumor on imaging. Each of the four categories of tumor requires a different therapeutic approach. Tympanic, tympanomastoid, infralabyrinthine and intracranial tumors are described as class A, B, C, and D, respectively[20-23] (Table 83–3).

CLINICAL PRESENTATION

The presentation of temporal bone paragangliomas is characterized by an insidious onset, and the slow progression of symptoms. Glomus jugulare tumors arising from the jugular foramen tend to be clinically silent until they eventually embarrass the function of the lower cranial nerves and encroach on the middle and inner ear.

At presentation, almost all patients have developed hearing loss (83%) and pulsatile tinnitus (83%).[16,24] The hearing loss is initially conductive in nature, with sensorineural hearing loss the hallmark of labyrinthine invasion. Patients may also complain of aural discharge, otalgia, and aural fullness.

Symptoms related to the lower cranial neuropathies, such as dysphonia (44%), dysphagia (36%), and shoulder weakness (33%), indicate significant jugular foramen involvement.[24] Because the onset of these lower cranial nerve palsies often occurs over years, excellent compensation is common at presentation.[24-26] Facial nerve weakness (33 to 36%) invariably indicates neural infiltration, usually in the mastoid portion.[24,27]

Physical examination consists of a complete otologic, head and neck, and cranial nerve examination. The hallmark of a temporal bone paraganglioma tumor is a red or reddish blue mass hypomesotympanic (70%) seen behind the tympanic membrane, referred to as the "sunset sign."[26] An aberrant carotid artery or a high jugular bulb may mimic this otoscopic appearance. In rare cases, a friable bleeding polyp in the external auditory canal may be the presenting sign of lateral growth of the tumor.[26] The neck is examined for bruits, concurrent tumors of the carotid body, vagus, thyroid, and parathyroid. Cervical lymphandenopathy may indicate malignant paraganglioma.

INVESTIGATION

The diagnosis of temporal bone paraganglioma is made on clinical evaluation, in collaboration with imaging. Biopsy of the tumor is unwarranted, with the undue risk of hemorrhage.

Audiologic function is documented with an audiogram. Screening for urine catecholamine metabolites (vanillylmandelic acid [VMA], normetanephrine, and metanephrine) is recommended only for those patients with hypertension and for those with pheochromocytoma-like symptoms.

When urinary catecholamine levels are elevated, a search should be undertaken for other functional tumors, including pheochromocytomas.[28] The search to localize other catecholamine-secreting paragangliomas may require comprehensive MRI, 131-metaiodobenzylguanidine nuclear scanning, and selective catheterization for venous samples for plasma norepinephrine determination.[29]

CT scan provides precise evaluation of bony destruction and erosion, which is a hallmark of temporal bone paragangliomas (Table 83–4). Destruction of the infralabyrinthine compartment and the anterolateral base of the skull determines the stage of temporal bone paraganglioma.[20,30] Temporal bone CT also provides useful preoperative information about the position of the jugular bulb, and the size and presence of the contralateral sigmoid sinus. Any evidence of erosion into the basal turn of the cochlea allows the surgeon to warn the patient of the attendant high risk of sensorineural hearing loss.

Complementing the CT evaluation of bone destruction, MRI with gadolinium-DPTA enhancement offers superior soft tissue resolution and differentiation. MRI confirms the diagnosis of paraganglioma with a typical salt-and-pepper appearance. MRI is also important in determining the intracranial extension of the tumor (intra- or extradural) and extension into the cavernous sinus.

Angiography confirms the diagnosis with its characteristic rapid vascular blush. It is also important in determining the blood supply and angioarchitecture of the tumor, as well as the integrity of the internal carotid artery and the collateral circulation.

For large temporal bone paragangliomas in which the preoperative imaging indicates encasement or invasion of the internal carotid artery, permanent preoperative balloon occlusion should be considered.[22,31,32] This is performed only if an awake temporary balloon occlusion of the internal carotid artery is tolerated by the patient.

Preoperative embolization considerably improves surgical conditions in skull base paraganglioma surgery.[22] This technique

TABLE 83–4

Radiologic Characteristics of Jugular Foramen Tumors

Technique	Paraganglioma	Schwannoma	Meningioma
High-resolution computer tomography	Irregular margin of tumor	Smooth margin of tumor	Smooth margin of tumor
	Irregular bony erosion of the jugular foramen	Smooth bony erosion of the jugular foramen, producing an ovoid defect	Smooth bony erosion of the jugular foramen
	No reactive sclerosis or hyperosteosis	Bony margin may show reactive sclerosis; no hyperosteosis	Bony margin may show reactive sclerosis and hyperosteosis
	No intralesional calcification	Intralesional calcification rare	Intralesional calcification common
	Marked contrast enhancement	Mild contrast enhancement	Moderate contrast enhancement
MRI with gadolinium	Isointense on T_1- and hyperintense on T_2-weighted images	Hypointense on T_1- and hyperintense on T_2-weighted images	Isointense on both T_1- and T_2-weighted images
	Salt-and-pepper appearance due the signal void of high-flow vascular channels	More homogeneous	More homogeneous
	Bright enhancement with gadolinium	Moderate enhancement with gadolinium	Moderate enhancement with gadolinium
Angiography	Highly vascular with a bright rapid-filling blush	Relatively avascular with a much slower, less vivid tumor blush	Relatively avascular with a much slower, less vivid tumor blush

decreases intraoperative hemorrhage and improves the demarcation of the tumor from the surrounding tissue, shortening the operating time.[33] Temporal bone paragangliomas derive their blood supply initially from the external carotid artery, predominantly the postauricular, ascending pharyngeal, and occipital arteries. As the tumor enlarges, it may also receive branches from the internal carotid artery (caroticotympanic) or the vertebrobasilar system.

MANAGEMENT

Surgery

Surgery has been established as the principal primary treatment of temporal bone paraganglioma.[21-23,34-36] Surgery offers the only chance of cure. With the modern microsurgical techniques and advances in anesthesia and interventional radiology, temporal bone paragangliomas are currently removed with minimal morbidity, excellent control rate, and good quality of life[23,24] In contrast, radiotherapy may, at best, arrest tumor growth with a significant side effect profile. For this reason radiotherapy is reserved when resection of the tumor is impossible or incomplete.[37-39]

In planning treatment, the objective—whether cure or palliation—is determined by a balance of patient, tumor, and treatment factors. Of these considerations, tumor stage is the most important in surgical planning. Tumor stage alone dictates the surgical approach. The infratemporal approach provides the necessary exposure to remove paragangliomas up to Fisch class C4De2Di1[23] (Fig. 83–2).

Surgery is contraindicated when the tumor is deemed unresectable or the risk of associated morbidity is unacceptably high. Surgery is contraindicated in Fisch class C and CD temporal bone paragangliomas when there is carotid involvement and the collateral cerebral circulation is poor. In patients who have a contralateral vagal palsy, surgery that compromises the only functional vagus is also contraindicated.

Class A Tumors Class A temporal bone paragangliomas are removed with a conventional transmastoid approach with hearing preservation. They tend to be more extensive than anticipated on preoperative imaging.

Class B Tumors As in Fisch class A, Fisch class B temporal bone paragangliomas may prove to be larger than indicated on preoperative imaging. In this case, both the surgeon and the patient must be prepared to progress from a conventional transmastoid approach to a subtotal petrosectomy, should there be extension into retrofacial air cells or deep infiltration of the spongiotic bone in the infralabyrinthine compartment of the temporal bone. If the tumor is found to invade the jugular bulb or the carotid foramen, an infratemporal type A approach is indicated.

Class C Tumors Fisch C class lesions are resectable via a infratemporal type A approach. The Fisch type A approach is a craniotemporocervical approach. It exposes the infralabyrinthine and apical compartments of the temporal bone, the mandibular fossa, and the posterior infratemporal fossa. It does so by subtotal petrosectomy and by anterior transposition of the facial nerve.[23] Dissection of the superior neck permits proximal and distal control

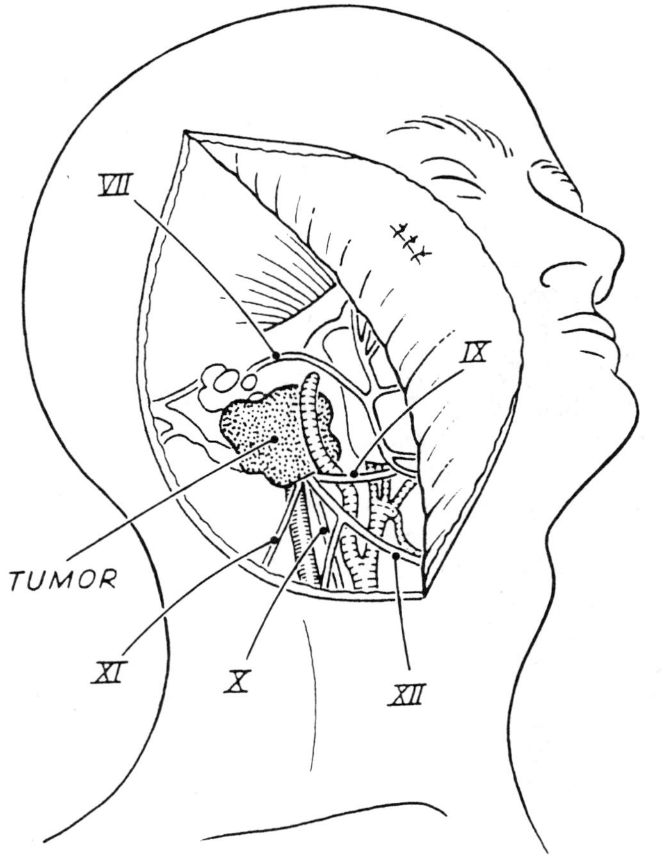

Figure 83–2 Schematic view of type A craniotemporocervical exposure for the removal of temporal paragangliomas class C.

of the jugular and carotid systems, essential for success in resection of these tumors.

More advanced temporal bone paragangliomas growing along the horizontal segment of the internal carotid artery to the foramen lacerum (Fisch class C3) require more extended infratemporal approaches. Removal of the most anterior portion of Fisch class C4 lesions within the foramen lacerum and cavernous sinus necessitates a combined Fisch type A and B approach. Extension into the cavernous sinus requires a switch from the Fisch type A to the Fisch type C approach.

Class D Tumors The intradural extension of a glomus tumor can only be removed at the same time as the main tumor mass, if the extension is < 2 cm (class Di1). Otherwise, a planned two-stage procedure is advisable, as intracranial intradural extension of > 2 cm may be strongly attached to the pons and medulla. Removal of tumor from this region often results in bleeding from the pontomedullary veins. Second-stage removal of large intracranial intradural tumors avoids serious complications, including sizable cerebrospinal fluid (CSF) leaks due to the persistent cough and aspiration that may arise when swallowing is affected at both a central and peripheral neurologic level.

After incomplete resection of a Di2 lesions, patients do not require an immediate two-stage procedure. These patients are first followedup with regular imaging every year, to monitor the progression of the residual tumor. Only 25% of residual intradural tumors require irradiation or neurosurgical intervention because of clinical or radiologic progression.

For class Di3 tumors, selected patients may benefit from removal of the extradural component of the tumor. This decompresses the posterior cranial fossa and devascularizes the rest of the tumor. Postoperative irradiation can be started 4 weeks after surgery.

Radiotherapy

Temporal bone paraganglioma has been proved to be radioincurable.[27,40] Rapid tumor progression after radiation has been well documented.[41-44] Failure rates vary from 15% to 30%.[41-44] At the Univerisity of Zurich, 30% of the patients operated on presented with tumor progression in spite of planned curative preoperative irradiation with 5000 to 7000 R.[22]

The biologic response of this benign tumor to radiotherapy differs from that of malignant neoplasms. The effectiveness of irradiation is limited by the low mitotic rate of chief cells. Chief cells have been shown to persist for years after therapeutic doses of irradiation.[7,38] Histologic analysis of surgical specimens of irradiated glomus tumors following surgical salvage has demonstrated formations of intact islands of vital chief cells.[27] For all these reasons, radiation is indicated for the progression of unresectable lesions or progressing residual tumor.

OUTCOME

Since 1974, 270 temporal bone paragangliomas have been resected at the University of Zurich. The percentage of tumors completely excised is 80% (Table 83–5). The operating time using the infratemporal approaches is acceptable[33] (Table 83–6). Within 2 years of surgery, 97% of the patients operated at the University of Zurich returned to their normal social life and previous occupation.[24]

TABLE 83–5

Results of Surgery for Temporal Paraganglioma: Total Excision of Tumor, 1974–1999 ($n = 270$)

Tumor Size	*n*	%
A	14/14	100
B	13/14	93
C1	29/30	97
C2	74/78	95
C3	80/110	73
C4	15/24	63
De1	25/26	96
De2	18/27	67
Di1	41/50	82
Di2	16/32	50
Total	325/405	80

TABLE 83–6

Operation Time for Fisch Type A, B, and C Surgical Approaches

Fisch Infratemporal	Operating Time	
Approach	Average	Range
Type A	6 h, 50 min	4:00–9:30
Type B	6 h, 35 min	5:00–7:00
Type C	5 h, 30 min	2:30–7:00

Neurogenic Tumors of the Jugular Foramen

Schwannomas and neurfibromas comprise the vast majority of nerve sheath tumors of the jugular foramen. The growth and presentation of these tumors are variable and may not necessarily be associated with lower cranial neuropathies.

EPIDEMIOLOGY

Although schwannomas are the second most common tumor of the jugular foramen, after paragangliomas, these tumors are relatively uncommmon. They account for only 10% of jugular foramen tumors and 3% of intracranial schwannomas[45,46] (Table 83–1).

PATHOLOGY

Schwannomas are usually isolated, well-encapsulated lesions that push axons aside. They are not associated with von Recklinghausen's disease. These tumors have the characteristic histologic patterns of Antoni type A and B type tissues. Neurofibromas, in contrast, are often multiple, nonencapsulated deeply infiltrating lesions that incorporate the axon within the substance of the tumor. These tumors are frequently seen in von Recklinghausen's disease.[47,48]

As with vestibular schwannomas, jugular foarmen schwannomas originate at the transition zone between central and peripheral myelin. Most jugular foramen schwannomas (88%) arise from the glossopharyngeal and vagus nerves.[47,49,50] Schwannomas originating from the accessory, hypoglossal, and sympathetic trunk are far less common.

There are three growth patterns of neurogenic tumors of the jugular foramen, depending on their point of origin along the nerve as they pass through the pars nervosa.[4,51] The tumors arising in the distal portion of the jugular foramen expand inferiorly out of the base of the skull, whereas those arising more proximally enlarge into the posterior cranial fossa. Tumors arising from the midregion of the foramen tend to expand primarily into the bone and become bilobed like a "saddlebag."[4]

STAGING

Neurogenic tumors of the jugular foramen originate from either the cranial nerves IX to XI, and XII, or the sympathetic ganglia. According to the tumor location they can be classified into separate groups[49,53] (Table 83–7).

CLINICAL PRESENTATION

Presentation is variable and may not necessarily be associated with neuropathies of the lower cranial nerves.[52] The site of origin of schwannomas along cranial nerves IX and X in the pars nervosa of the jugular foramen determines the pattern of growth and the clinical presentation.

The proximal lesions enlarge into the posterior cranial fossa and present with the signs of a cerebellopontine angle lesion. A tumor of this type may present without palsies of cranial nerves IX, X, and IX, even as the lesion reaches quite a large size. Sensorineural hearing loss, vertigo, and ataxia are more typical of these jugular foramen schwannomas with a predominant intracranial component.[52]

In contrast, the more distal jugular foramen schwannomas tend to enlarge inferiorly through the foramen of the skull base. Therefore, lower cranial nerve involvement is more common.[4,52] These patients present with elements of jugular foramen syndrome (Vernet or Jackson syndrome).[4,5] Symptoms tend to be of longer standing in those with tumors mainly involving the bone at the base of the skull, and shorter in those patients with entirely extracranial tumors.[4] As these more distal lesions enlarge, symptoms and signs referable to a mass effect within the parapharyngeal space may develop.

TABLE 83–7
Fisch Staging of Jugular Foramen Schwannomas

Type	Description	
A	Tumor confined to the soft tissue of the neck	
B	Primary involvement of the neck with extension up to the jugular foramen	
C	Tumor fills the jugular foramen with resultant bone expansion showing	
	Type C1	No involvement of the ICA above the carotid foramen
	Type C2	Involvement of the vertical segment of the ICA
	Type C3	Involvement of the horizontal segment of the ICA
	Type C4	Tumor extending into the foramen lacerum
D	Intracranial extension	
	Type De	Extradural
	Type Di	Intradural

ICA, interior carotid artery.

INVESTIGATION

As in paraganglioma, high-resolution computed tomography (HRCT) is superior in defining skull base bony erosion. Imaging should include the posterior cranial fossa, skull base, and the upper cervical region. On CT, schwannomas display ovoid enlargement of the jugular foramen, involving predominantly the pars nervosa, with smooth indistinct sclerotic margins.[1,4] In contrast, temporal bone paragangliomas causes irregular enlargement of the jugular foramen, with indistinct margins (Table 83–4). Lesions in the pars nervosa of the jugular foramen, may often be distinguished from hypoglossal schwannomas, which often present as dumbbell-shaped with intra- and extracranial extension.[54]

On MRI, their appearance is similar to that of a vestibular schwannoma. Carotid and vertebral angiography may help differentiate neural sheath tumors from a temporal bone paraganglioma, since the paraganglioma is highly vascular, while schwannoma has only slight, but variable, vascularity.[4,54]

MANAGEMENT

The surgical approach consists of a cervicoparotid approach, which can be combined with an infratemporal fossa approach type A. This approach permits removal of the tumor from the skull base with optimal vision of the skull base and of the vertical and horizontal portions of the internal carotid artery. The intracranial intradural extension can be removed in one stage even for D2 tumors because it is usually not attached to the surrounding structures and is lateralized by the CSF pressure as long as the arachnoid remains intact.

Meningiomas of the Jugular Foramen

Meningiomas are usually benign tumors that originate from the meningothelial arachnoid cells that tend to cluster around the tips of the arachnoid villi. Their preferential site corresponds closely with the location where arachnoid villi are most frequently encountered.[55-57] Therefore, the most common location for meningioma is the parasaggital area, the lateral cerebral convexities and the sphenoid ridge. The jugular foramen is an uncommon site for meningioma. Apart from the jugular foramen, other predilective sites of origin of meningiomas within the temporal bone are the internal auditory canal, the geniculate ganglion, and the sulci of the greater and lesser petrosal nerves.[58-60]

EPIDEMIOLOGY

Although meningiomas account for 13 to 18% of all intracranial tumors, meningiomas of the jugular foramen are relatively rare.[59] At the University of Zurich, meningiomas account for only 2.5% of jugular foramen tumors, with only 10 cases encountered over 20 years (Table 83–1).

Meningiomas more frequently affect females than males in the ratio of 2 : 1.[59] Intracranial meningiomas occur at any age. The peak incidence is at the age of 45. Temporal bone meningiomas have a clear predilection for the middle and later decades of life.[59]

PATHOLOGY

Grossly, meningiomas are firm well-circumscribed tumors, appearing smooth or lobulated, gray-white, tan, or pink. Microscopically, four histologic patterns are described: (1) syncitial which is most common; (2) fibroblastic; (3) transitional, and (4) angioblastic. The angioblastic pattern has the greatest predilection for locally aggressive behaviour, malignancy, and the worse prognosis.[59] Psammoma bodies and a whorled parenchymal pattern can be found in all types. Mitoses are usually rare or absent.[61-64]

Jugular foramen meningiomas may represent (1) the extracranial extension of a primary intracranial meningioma tumor; (2) a tumor arising in the jugular foramen; (3) a tumor arising from the arachnoidal cell clusters within the trunk or perineural sheath of one of the lower cranial nerves within or near the jugular foramen; or (4) a metastasis to cervical lymph nodes from a primary intracranial meningioma.[59,65]

Meningiomas spread along preformed bony channels. The most common pathway for extracranial meningioma to extend beyond the confines of the skull is through the jugular foramen into the parapharyngeal space.[59] The vascular spongiotic spaces may be diffusely infiltrated by tumor cells. Intracranial meningiomas that develop an extracranial extension via the jugular foramen assume an hourglass or dumbbell tumor configuration. The adjacent bone may show evidence of the classic reactive sclerosis and hyperostosis. In contrast, meningiomas originating from within the jugular foramen follow the direction of least resistance as they increase in size. They extend extracranially into the parapharyngeal space and neck, without entering the posterior cranial fossa.[59] Origin within the foramen of the skull base is evident by the extracranial paraphargeal location of these tumors, their firm attachment to the skull base at the jugular foramen, and the absence of any tumor tissue within the posterior cranial fossa.[59]

Meningiomas are usually solitary, slow-growing tumors that compress, rather than invade, the lower cranial nerves and the jugular vein within the jugular foramen. However, they may be multiple and, in rare cases, may invade vessels and nerves. Tumor extension along the lumen of the internal jugular vein has been reported, but is not characteristic.[66] In patients with extracranial meningiomas or multiple meningiomas or who are younger than 30 years of age, the central form of neurofibromatosis should be suspected.[67]

CLINICAL PRESENTATION

The clinical manifestations of jugular foramen meningioma may be due to compression of the cranial nerves within the foramen, or related to a superior intracranial or inferior cervical tumor component. Tumors superior to the jugular foramen within the posterior cranial fossa or within the middle ear manifest with deafness and tinnitus, headache, vertigo, and facial paresis. Raised intracranial pressure and cerebellar or brain stem compression are late, sinister signs. Tumor extension inferiorly into the cervical region may manifest as a parapharyngeal or neck mass.

INVESTIGATION

On CT, meningiomas of the jugular foramen typically show evidence of hyperostosis, calcification, bony erosion, and homogenous enhancement with contrast (Table 83–4). MRI usually shows isointensity on both T_1- and T_2-weighted images, while gadolinium-DTPA yields uniform enhancement. Angiography may, on occasion, be required to differentiate meningioma from temporal bone paraganglioma.

MANAGEMENT

The treatment of choice is surgical excision via the Fisch infratemporal approaches. Meningiomas do not respond favourably to irradiation and this modality is reserved for the inoperable lesions. Recurrence is particularly frequent in the angioblastic variant.[68] In the presence of diffuse infiltration of bone surrounding nerves, tumor removal may be associated with considerable functional losses. Therefore, in such a case, surgery is advisable in the presence of a symptomatic or clearly growing tumor.

Other Tumors of the Jugular Foramen

Apart from paragangliomas, schwannomas, neurofibromas, and meningiomas, other benign lesions affecting the jugular foramen include chordomas, lymphosarcomas, papillary adenomas of the middle ear, chondroblastomas, osteoblastomas, and haemangiomas (Table 83–1).

The most common malignant tumor of the jugular foramen is a secondary metastasis of the temporal bone. The most common site of the primary tumor in order of frequency is breast, kidney, lung, stomach, larynx, prostate, and thyroid gland.[69] Hematologic neoplasm of the temporal bone, including leukemia, lymphoma, and multiple myeloma, may all present with jugular foramen syndrome.

Summary

Jugular foramen tumors are uncommon lesions, dominated by benign tumors (paragangliomas, schwannomas, neurofibromas, and meningiomas). In spite of their benign histopathology, these lesions are chararcterized by locally destructive behaviour. Presentation is often insidious and the diagnosis delayed. Radiotherapy is inappropriate for the treatment of these radioresistant lesions in generally otherwise healthy patients. Surgical excision by the lateral otologic approaches in established skull base surgical units permits complete resection of these lesions with minimal morbidity and maximum tumor control.

REFERENCES

Fisch et al.—CHAPTER 83

1. DiChiro G, Fisher RL, Nelson KB. The jugular foramen. *J Neurosurg* 1964;21:447–460
2. Guild SR. Glomus jugulare, a nonchromaffin paraganglion in man. *Ann Otol Rhinol Laryngol* 1953;62:1015–1021
3. Arenberg IK, McCreary HS. Neurilemmomma of the jugular foramen. *Laryngoscope* 1971;81:544–557
4. Kaye AH, Hahn, JF, Kinney, SE, et al. Jugular foramen schwannomas. *J Neurosurg* 1984;60:1045–1053
5. Svien HJ, Baker HL, Rivers MH. Jugular foramen syndrome and allied syndromes. *Neurology* 1963;13:797–809
6. Pluchino G, Crivelli G, Vaghi MA. Intracranial neurinomas of the nerves of the jugular foramen. Report of 12 personal cases. *Acta Neurochir* 1975;31:201–221
7. Spector GJ, Maisel RH, Ogura JH. Glomus tumors in the middle ear. I. An analysis of 46 patients. *Laryngoscope* 1973;83:1652–1672
8. Kuhweide R, Lanser MJ, Fisch U. Catecholamine-secreting pargangliomas at the skull base. *Skull Base Surg* 1996;6:35–45
9. Alford BR, Guilford, FR. A comprehensive study of tumors of the glomus jugulare. *Laryngoscope* 1962;1:765–787
10. van Baars F, Cremers C, Van Den Broek P, et al. Genetic aspects of nonchromaffin paragangliomas. *Hum Genet* 1982; 60:305–309
11. Grufferman S, Gillman MW, Pasternak LR, et al. Familial carotid body tumors (case report and epidemiologic review). *Cancer* 1980;46:2116–2122
12. van der Mey AGL, Maaswinkel-Mooy PD, Cornelisse CJ, et al. Genomic imprinting in hereditary glomus tumors: evidence for new genetic theory. *Lancet* 1989;2:1291–1294
13. Bickerstaff ER, Howell JS. The neurological importance of tumors of the glomus jugulare. *Brain* 1953;76:576–593
14. Steinberg N, Holz WG. Glomus jugularis tumors. *Arch Otolaryngol* 1965;82:387–394
15. Gulya AJ. The glomus tumor and its biology. *Laryngoscope* 1993;103:7–15
16. House WF, Glasscock ME. Glomus tympanicum tumors. *Arch Otolaryngol* 1968;87:124–128
17. Glasscock ME, Jackson CG, Dickins JRE, Wiet RJ. Panel discussion: glomus jugulare tumors of the temporal bone. The surgical management of glomus tumors. *Laryngoscope* 1979; 89:1640–1654
18. Lack EE, Cubilla AL, Woodruff JM, Farr HW. Paragangliomas of the head and neck region. *Cancer* 1977;39:397–409
19. Glenner GG, Grimley PM. Tumors of the extra-adrenal paraganglion system (including chemoreceptors). In: Harlan I, Firminger MD, eds. *Atlas of Tumor Pathology.* Washington, DC: Armed Forces Institute of Pathology; 1973
20. Oldring D, Fisch U. Glomus tumors of the temporal region: surgical therapy. *Am J Otol* 1979;1:7–18
21. Fisch U. Infratemporal fossa approach for glomus tumors of the temporal bone. *Ann Otol Rhinol Laryngol* 1982;91:474–479
22. Fisch U, Fagan PA, Valavanis A. The infratemporal fossa approach for the lateral skull base. *Otolaryngol Clin North Am* 1984;17:513–552
23. Fisch U, Mattox D. *Microsurgery of the Skull Base.* NewYork: Georg Thieme Verlag; 1988:136–353
24. Briner HR, Linder TE, Pauw BP, Fisch U. Long-term results of surgery for temporal bone paraganglioma. *Laryngoscope* 1999;109:577–583
25. Lustig LR, Jackler RK. The variable relation between the lower cranial nerves and jugular foramen tumors: implications for neural preservation. *Am J Otol* 1996;17:658–668
26. Woods CI, Strasnick B, Jackson CG. Surgery for glomus tumors: the otology group experience. *Laryngoscope* 1993;103:65–70
27. Makek M, Franklin DJ, Zhao J, Fisch U. Neural infiltration of glomus temporale tumors. *Am J Otol* 1990;11:1–5
28. Nelson MD, Kendal BE. Intracranial catecholamine secreting paragangliomas. *Neuroradiology* 1987;29:277–282
29. Jackson CG. Neurotologic surgery for skull base tumors: diagnosis for treatment planning and treatment options. *Laryngoscope* 1993;103:17–27
30. Lo WWM, Solti-Bohman LG, Lambert PR. High-resolution CT in the evaluation of glomus tumors of the temporal bone. *Radiology* 1984;150:737–742
31. Andrews JC, Valavanis A, Fisch U. Management of the internal carotid artery. *Laryngoscope* 1989;99:1224–1229
32. Palaskas CW, Fisch U, Valavanis A, Pfaltz M. Permanent preoperative carotid artery occlusion and carotid body tumor surgery. *Skull Base Surg* 1993;3:22–31
33. Schmid S, Moe KS, Fisch U. The internal carotid artery in skull base surgery. In: Gates GA, ed. *Current Therapy in*

Otolaryngology, Head and Neck Surgery. St Louis; MO: Mosby; 1994:111–115
34. Fisch U. Infratemporal fossa approach for lesions in the temporal bone and base of the skull. *Adv Otorhinolaryngol* 1984;34:254–266
35. Gjuric M, Seidinger L, Wigand ME. Long-term results of surgery for temporal bone paraganglioma. *Skull Base Surg* 1996;6:147–152
36. Jackson CG, Haynes DS, Walker PA, et al. Hearing conservation surgery for glomus jugulare tumors. *Am J Otol* 1996;17:425–437
37. Boyle JO, Shimm DS, Coulthard SW. Radiotherapy for paragangliomas of the temporal bone. *Laryngoscope* 1990;100:896–901
38. Hawthorne MR, Makek MS, Harris JP, Fisch U. The histopathological and clinical features of irradiated and nonirradiated temporal paragangliomas. *Laryngoscope* 1988;98: 325–331
39. Lalwani AK, Jackler RK, Gutin PH. Lethal fibrosarcoma complicating radiation therapy for benign glomus jugulare tumor. *Am J Otol* 1993;14:398–402
40. Brackmann DE, House WF, Terry R, et al. Glomus jugulare tumors: effects of irradiation. *Trans Am Acad Ophthamol Otolaryngol* 1972;76:1423–1431
41. Spector GJ, Fierstein J, Ogura JH. A comparison of therapeutic modalities of glomus tumors in the temporal bone. *Laryngoscope* 1976;86:690–696
42. Sharma PD, Johnson AP, Whitton AC. Radiotherapy for jugulotympanic paragangliomas (glomus jugulare tumors). *J Laryngol Otol* 1984;98:621–629
43. Gibbin KP, Henk, JM. Glomus jugulare tumors in South Wales. A twenty year review. *Clin Radiol* 1978;29:607–609
44. Spector GJ, Compagno J, Perez CA, et al. Glomus jugulare tumors: effects of radiotherapy. *Cancer* 1975;35:1316–1321
45. Tan LC, Bordi L, Symons L, Cheesman AD. Jugular foramen neuromas. *Surg Neurol* 1990;34:205–211
46. Horn KL, Hankinson H. Tumors of the jugular foramen. In: Brcakmann DE, ed. *Neurotology.* St Louis, MO: CV Mosby; 1994:1059–1068
47. Roland P, Glasscock M.E III, Bojrab DI. Neuromas of the skull base. *Otolaryngol Head Neck Surg* 1986;94:539–547
48. Crumley RL, Wilson C. Schwannomas of the jugular foramen. *Laryngoscope* 1984;94:772–778
49. Franklin DJ, Moore GF, Fisch U. Jugular foramen peripheral nerve sheath tumors. *Laryngoscope* 1989;99:1081–1087
50. Gibson FB, Nichols, ML, Weiss RL, Calhoun KH. Pathologic quiz case 2. Plexiform neurofibroma. *Arch Otolaryngol Head Neck Surg* 1992;118:772–773, 775
51. Kinney SE, Dohn DF, Hahn JF, et al. Neuromas of the jugular foramen. In: Brackmann DE, ed. *Neurological Surgery of the Ear and Skull Base.* New York: Raven Press; 1982:361–367
52. Horn KL, House WF, Hitselberger WE. Schwannomas of the jugular foramen. *Laryngoscope* 1985;95:761–765
53. May JS, Fisch U. Neoplasms of the ear and lateral skull base. In: Bailey BJ, ed. *Head and Neck Surgery—Otolaryngology.* Philadelphia: JB Lippincott; 1993:1575–1576
54. Linder TE, Garvis WJ, Huwyler M, Fisch U. Pediatric–adolescent otologic skull base surgery. In: de Souza C, Stankiewicz JA, Pellitteri PK, eds. CA: *Textbook of Pediatric Otorhinolaryngology—Head and Neck Surgery.* San Diego, CA: Singular Publishing Group; 1998
55. Al-Mefty O. *Meningioma.* New York: Raven Press; 1991:37–57
56. Gagnon NB, Lavigne F, Mohr G, et al. Extracranial and intracranial meningiomas. *J Otolaryngol* 1986;15:380–384
57. Kepes JJ. *Biology, Pathology and Differential Diagnosis.* Philadelphia: Masson USA; 1982
58. Luetje CM, Syms CA, Luxford WE, et al. Meningiomas intrinsic to the geniculate ganglion. *Am J Otol* 1997;18:393–397
59. Nager GT, Heroy J, Hoeplinger M. Meningiomas invading the temporal bone with extension into the neck. *Am J Otolaryngol* 1983;4:297–324
60. Nager GT, Masica DN. Meningioma of the cerebellopontine angle and their relation to the temporal bone. *Laryngoscope* 1970;80:863–895
61. Austin MB, Mills SE. Neoplasms and neoplasm-like lesions involving the skull base. *Ear Nose Throat* 1986;65:57–73
62. Barnes L, Kapadia SB. The biology and pathology of selected skull base tumors. *J Neurooncol* 1994;20:213–240
63. Kennedy JD, Haines SJ. Review of skull base surgery approaches: with special reference to paediatric patients. *J Neurooncol* 1994;20:291–312
64. Shah MV, Haines, SJ. Paediatric skull, skull base, and meningeal tumors. *Neurosurg Clin North Am* 1992;3:893–924
65. Hoye JS, Hoar CS, Murray JE. Extrcranial meningioma presenting as a tumor of the neck. *Am J Surg* 1960;100:486–489
66. Schmidt D, Mackay B, Luna MA, Goepfert H. Aggressive meningioma with jugular vein extension. *Arch Otolaryngol* 1981;107:635–637
67. Friedman CD, Costantino PD, Teitelbaum B, et al. Primary extracranial meningioma of the head and neck. *Laryngoscope* 1990;100:41–48
68. Rubinstein LJ. *Tumors of the Central Nervous System.* Fascicle 6. Washington, DC: Armed Forces Institute of Pathology, 1972
69. Schucknedt HF. *Pathology of the Ear.* Phiadelphia: Lea & Febiger, 1993:488–489

Jugular Foramen Tumors

Peter G. Smith

CHAPTER 84

The best way to care for a patient who has a jugulotympanic paraganglioma continues to be debated by surgical and radiation oncologists. I believe that the fundamental reasons for the controversy include the overlapping information derived from currently available imaging studies, the protracted clinical course of these histologically benign tumors, the complications associated with a single therapeutic modality, and the clinical bias of the oncologist. In preparing this work, I struggled to resolve my own issues about the subject through a review of the literature. I was left, however, with more questions than answers. What follows, then, is a description of my current approach to helping patients with jugulotympanic paragangliomas. The algorithm reflects my own bias, and I expect it to change with an accumulation of more experience and knowledge derived from controversy.

Clinical Features

Traditionally called glomus tumors, jugulotympanic paragangliomas are second only to vestibular schwannomas as the most common neoplasms of the temporal bone. Replicating normal paraganglia, the tumors are characterized histologically by a rather vascular framework that surrounds nests of specialized cells.[1] Paragangliomas that arise in the jugular fossa are more common than those that originate within the middle ear. I have found the following clinical characteristics useful in making diagnostic or management decisions:

- Paragangliomas grow very slowly and usually have an extended clinical course.
- The most common presenting symptoms are a hearing loss and pulse-synchronous tinnitus in the affected ear.
- A middle ear mass with a vascular hue is almost always detected on a microscopic examination of the affected ear.
- Other symptoms and signs include progressive facial nerve paralysis and isolated or combined neuropathies of the basal cranial nerves.
- A person with a family history of paraganglioma is at a higher risk of having multicentric tumors.
- Less than 1% of jugular paragangliomas are functional or catecholamine-secreting.
- Few jugulotympanic paragangliomas are malignant.

Diagnosis

A jugulotympanic paraganglioma has such a characteristic otoscopic appearance that there is seldom an indication for a biopsy. A high jugular bulb might be mistaken for the superior pole of jugular paraganglioma; however, its smooth, pale blue margin helps distinguish it from a tumor. Although another middle ear neoplasm can mimic a paraganglioma, there is frequently something in the clinical history or examination that just does not fit that of the more common paraganglioma. Thus far, I have not had to biopsy a middle ear mass that I believed was a paraganglioma in order to formulate a treatment plan. Instead, I have frequently complemented the clinical findings with a radiologic evaluation that might include computed tomography (CT), magnetic resonance imaging (MRI), and angiography. However, not every patient suspected of having a jugulotympanic paraganglioma requires neuroradiologic evaluation. I believe, for example, that a patient with a small tympanic paraganglioma that can be seen in its entirety requires no additional evaluation. When the margins of a tumor are obscure, however, I do recommend a radiographic examination. The frequency with which improvements are made in imaging technology preclude insistence on one imaging technique over another. From my perspective, the choice of an initial imaging modality should be based on the information needed, the availability of imaging equipment, and the level of knowledge and experience of the consulting radiologist.

I still use high-resolution computed tomography (HRCT) of the cranial base with contrast enhancement as an initial imaging tool. Whether the lesion is a large tympanic paraganglioma or a sizable jugular variant is not therapeutically important to me. I have found that the study gives me a reliable assessment of the integrity of bone in the area of the jugular fossa, the carotid canal, and the facial canal, as well as an estimate of the extent of the neoplasm.

If the information derived from CT is equivocal or incomplete, I then use gadolinium-enhanced MRI for its superior soft tissue contrast resolution. MRI, for example, can distinguish between tumor and a serous or mucoid effusion, fat, muscle, and brain. I also use MRI to screen for synchronous tumors when clinically indicated. Finally, I use this imaging technique to screen for residual or recurrent disease, particularly if the patient has had prior treatment.

Early on, I had almost every patient with a large jugulotympanic tumor go through carotid and vertebral arteriography, regardless of what vascular structures were involved. I am still not sure of the origin of this philosophy. It may have evolved as a result of using the vertebral study to assess whether a tumor extended through the posterior cranial fossa and using the venous phase of the arteriogram to determine the status of the venous return. When there was radiologic evidence of encroachment of the carotid canal, I usually requested an assessment of the patient's tolerance to carotid artery sacrifice in the study. Over the course of 15 years, however, I have learned that (1) arteriography, especially carotid artery occlusion testing, has a known morbidity, regardless of how the patient is monitored; (2) I have yet to resect an internal carotid artery in a patient with a paraganglioma; (3) the one death I have witnessed was a young woman who passed carotid occlusion testing and died of postoperative stroke due to an embolus that developed behind a transiently constricted internal carotid artery[2]; (4) when coupled with CT and MRI findings, the information I obtained from angiography has not changed my treatment recommendations; and (5) the study is not cheap. Today, I use angiography in the context of adjuvant or therapeutic embolization to decrease the blood supply to a paraganglioma.

Management

I am not aware of a more controversial area regarding jugulotympanic paragangliomas than that of their treatment. Treatment alternatives include observation, surgery, radiation, a combination of surgery and radiation, or embolization. Regrettably, there are no clear-cut guidelines that can be followed to choose one treatment over another. Factors that affect my recommendation include the epicenter, size, and extent of the tumor, associated or combined neuropathies, and the person's age and medical condition. Each factor is intellectually weighted on the basis of my experience and integrated with the others to formulate a therapeutic recommendation. For example, I might suggest radiation therapy to a 45-year-old man with diabetes-related cardiovascular disease who has a combined vagal paralysis from a 3-cm jugular paraganglioma and surgery to a 70-year-old otherwise healthy woman who has a similar set of circumstances.

I used to believe that I just had to "do something" for someone who had a paraganglioma. Today, I am becoming more comfortable in offering observation as a valid option to some patients. The major question I usually have is who would best be served by this seldom-mentioned choice. I consider it in two different circumstances, both of which need the understanding consent of the patient. The first is when I believe that the patient will, in all likelihood, never require any intervention. Consider for example, the case of a 79-year-old woman in good health who has tolerable pulsatile tinnitus and a mild hearing loss from a tympanic paraganglioma. Although her tumor could be irradiated or removed, I would suggest that she be followed clinically through a semiannual otologic examination.

The second instance in which I am tempted to recommend observation constitutes a temporizing measure for someone whose tumor involves the jugular fossa, but has yet to induce a neuropathy of one of the basal cranial nerves. To the same extent that I am awed by the body's ability to adjust to slowly evolving neurologic deficits, I am dismayed by the potentially life-threatening problems that arise from acute, iatrogenic paralyses of the lower cranial nerves. With this in mind, I wonder whether it is in the patient's best interest to wait until the tumor has done slowly what I would most likely create abruptly in removing the tumor. This idea of "expectant waiting" was first proposed to me by a skilled head and neck surgeon whose task it has been to fix defects in pharyngolaryngeal function resulting from surgically induced neuropathies. Although some of us may call this option heretical, I think it makes a lot of sense. Since it was first suggested, I have not evaluated someone for whom it would apply. If the opportunity arises, however, I will offer it as an alternative, coupled with a semiannual MRI to screen for an unanticipated increase in the growth rate of the tumor.

I suggest surgery to a patient when the procedure would, in all likelihood, be curative. Although it is beyond the scope of this work to detail the approaches[3] used to remove these tumors, I have found the following guidelines helpful in planning and performing a resection:

- I screen a patient for a catecholamine-secreting tumor who has a history of high blood pressure, dysrrhythmia, or unexplained restiveness. If functional activity is found, antiadrenergic agents are used during the perioperative period.
- Angiographic embolization of a jugulotympanic paraganglioma that involves the jugular fossa is attempted the day preceding surgery.
- The surgical approach is tailored to include exposure of the tumor margins and adjacent neurovascular structures before the tumor is resected. In this way, the patient is, in a real sense, removed from the tumor, decreasing the potential for unexpected, and sometimes life-ending, complications. The exposure needed, for instance, can range from an extended elevation of the eardrum to avoid injury to the ossicular chain to combining an infratemporal fossa approach, a transcondylar approach, and a pterional approach to protect the integrity of the brain stem and the vertebral and internal carotid arteries. Irrespective of the approach, I try very hard to keep mobilization the facial nerve to a minimum. I have not enjoyed the success that others have had in maintaining the preoperative level of mimetic function when I have had to mobilize the nerve.
- The ablative defect is reconstituted or obliterated with reliable tissue. Simple extracranial soft tissue and bony defects can usually be repaired with free abdominal fat. Unfortunately, dural defects cannot be repaired primarily, and I have had limited success in using free fat grafts to partition the cerebrospinal fluid (CSF) space. Today, I prefer to use vascularized regional myogenous or free flaps to both obliterate the defect and seal the cerebrospinal fluid space.

- Correction of the sometimes frightening dysfunction resulting from acute-onset paralyses of the basal cranial nerves is not delayed; rather, it is begun during, or immediately after, the reconstructive phase of the operation.
- I usually have a sense of how long it will take to remove a given tumor. If the estimated anesthesia time for the ablative phase of the procedure is more than 10 h, I usually fill the wound with an antibiotic-impregnated packing, place an appropriate dressing, and arrange to have to have the patient slept overnight in an intensive care unit. The reconstructive and rehabilitative surgeons perform their procedures the next day. I have not witnessed an increase in the rate of wound infection with this policy.

I suggest radiation as a primary treatment to a patient with a jugulotympanic tumor who would, in all probability, require no further intervention during his or her lifetime. More frequently, I have used adjuvant therapy in patients who undergo surgery for a residual or recurrent tumor and still have physical or radiographic evidence of persistent disease. Removing a residual or recurrent paraganglioma is no different from removing similar disease elsewhere in the body. It is hard to differentiate between neoplastic and normal tissue, and the likelihood of leaving some disease is understandably greater. Since its availability in my geographic area, I have referred a few patients to a center that has a Gamma knife. My patients' experience with this and other forms of stereotactic radiosurgery is too limited to favor the modality over external-beam irradiation. Finally, I do recommend combined surgery and postoperative radiation to patients who have a tumor that has clinical or radiographic features suggestive of a rare malignant variant of a paraganglioma. I must emphasize, however, that the surgical objective and guidelines in this setting are not altered.

At the suggestion of an interventional radiologist, I recently had one woman undergo palliative embolization to relieve her of intractable pulsatile tinnitus from a paraganglioma that has persisted despite multiple, seemingly complete, resections and adjuvant radiation therapy. Her favorable response has prompted me to consider the modality in other patients with a similar history.

Summary

I have briefly described my current attitude toward helping people who have jugulotympanic paragangliomas. My suggestion to the reader is to take what he or she believes to be useful and incorporate it in an individual diagnostic and management strategy for patients who have these tumors.

REFERENCES

Smith—CHAPTER 84

1. Smith PG, Diemer DP, Schwaber MK, Levine RS. Clinical evaluation of glomus tumors of the ear and skull base. In: Thawley SE, Panje WR, Batsakis JG, Lindberg RD, eds. *Comprehensive Management of Head and-Neck Tumors.* 2nd ed. Philadelphia: WB Saunders; 1998:424–441
2. Smith PG, Killeen TE. Carotid artery vasospasm complicating extensive skull base surgery: cause, prevention and management. *Otolaryngol Head and Neck Surg* 1987:97:1–7
3. Jackson CG, Bohrer PS. Glomus tumors. In: Thawley SE, Panje WR, Batsakis JG, Lindberg RD, eds. *Comprehensive Management of Head and Neck Tumors.* 2nd ed. Philadelphia: WB Saunders; 1998:442–465

INDEX

Note: page numbers followed by f and t represent figures and tables respectively.